MW01277407

Management of Prostate Cancer

Michel Bolla • Hendrik van Poppel
Editors

Management of Prostate Cancer

A Multidisciplinary Approach

Second Edition

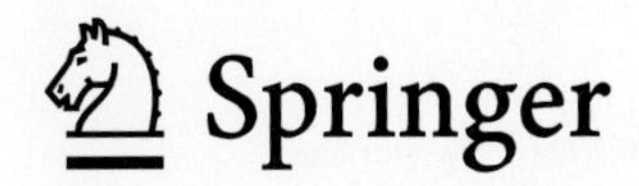

Editors
Michel Bolla
Department of Radiation Oncology
Hôpital Albert Michallon
Grenoble
France

Hendrik van Poppel
Department of Urology
University Hospitals Leuven
Leuven
Belgium

ISBN 978-3-319-42768-3 ISBN 978-3-319-42769-0 (eBook)
DOI 10.1007/978-3-319-42769-0

Library of Congress Control Number: 2016963566

Printed on acid-free paper

This Springer imprint is published by Springer Nature
The registered company is Springer International Publishing AG
The registered company address is: Gewerbestrasse 11, 6330 Cham, Switzerland

Preface

Prostate cancer is the first ranked cancer in men in Europe. Despite the 10-year overall survival improvement provided by the ERSPC, there is no European mass screening as for breast or colon and rectum cancers, but early diagnosis is possible among men aged 50–75 years managed by general practitioners and/or urologists provided an informed consent is obtained, taking into account age, family history of cancer, co-morbidity, baseline PSA, prostate volume, PSA density and velocity, as well as information about biopsy modalities and potential side effects. Random biopsies become more precise thanks to the matching of magnetic resonance imaging and ultrasound acquisitions to guide them on the index lesion. Once clinical workup is done, TNM and d'Amico classifications are established, the medical charts of the patients are discussed in tumour board and individualized treatments are proposed according to national and/or EAU guidelines to be explained later on to the patients. Phase III randomized trials have contributed to set up a multidisciplinary approach between pathologists, urologists, radiation oncologists and medical oncologists. The pathologist has a key role in helping to define risk factors on the surgical specimen – tumour volume, tumour stage and Gleason grade and particularly margin status – to decide about the indication for immediate post-operative or deferred salvage radiotherapy. Urologists are the first experts to announce the diagnosis and discuss the therapeutic options: the patients with a poor IPSS and/or uroflowmetry data are candidates to surgery as well as those who prefer to quickly eradicate the cancer or who need to know the precise analysis of the extension. The patients who cannot be operated on for technical or medical reasons or who are worried about the potential risk of incontinence or impotence can prefer radiotherapy and will discuss with the radiation oncologist the action of radiotherapy, its modalities – brachytherapy, high dose high precision external irradiation – the potential acute and late toxicity, the modalities of surveillance and the possibilities of treatment after relapse. The more we know the less aggressive we are, and patients with very low risk will be allowed to choose active surveillance to be treated later on at pre-defined triggers. Others can be oriented towards deferred treatment in case of less aggressive tumours, due to limited life expectancy or older age. In daily practice, open or laparoscopic (robot-assisted) radical prostatectomy and intensity-modulated radiotherapy remain the gold standard knowing that surgical and/or radiation innovations need feasibility, quality assurance, human resources and evaluation of local control and health-related quality of life. The indication and the duration of androgen deprivation therapy combined with radiotherapy are based on clinical stage, prognostic factors, WHO performance status, co-morbidity and sexual health: to mitigate side effects, modalities and chronology of the follow-up must be organized and shared harmoniously between specialists, and practitioners, cardiologists and endocrinologists concerned with the patients. The risk of relapse after local treatment must be explained as well as the available salvage modalities. PSA thresholds are well defined to declare biochemical relapse after surgery or radiotherapy and multi-parametric MRI and PET choline are very useful to authenticate the site of the relapse. Indeed salvage radiotherapy is possible in case of biochemical relapse after surgery, while salvage radical prostatectomy, high intensity focused ultrasound, brachytherapy or cryosurgery can be done after radiotherapy, radical prostatectomy remaining the reference. When a distant relapse arises, LHRH agonists or antagonists are the standard of care, given continuously or intermittently in case of metastatic disease. Maximal androgen blockade will benefit to a selected group of advanced prostate cancer patients. Since the publication of recent works, chemotherapy with docetaxel added to the primary hormonal manipulation benefits significantly to the survival in newly diagnosed metastatic prostate cancer patients, and this benefit is more pronounced in patients with a high metastatic burden. The landscape of patients resistant to chemical castration has changed and medical oncologists have an enriched pharmacopoeia with docetaxel and cabazitaxel in symptomatic patients, and CYP 17 inhibitors like abiraterone acetate or more potent antiandrogens like enzalutamide for others, while vaccines may be reserved to some kind of biochemical relapse. This new edition benefits from the more recent breakthroughs and offers an updated overview from epidemiology to therapeutic algorithms with new insights concerning genomics, radiologic investigations, nuclear medicine and medical treatments. Physicians must keep in mind that more science requires more consciousness and ethics to maintain a good relation with the patients to give them more therapeutic education to anticipate the near future. While the cure rate is increasing the patients have an important role to play, to participate in clinical research, a kind of joint venture which may be beneficial for them today or for others tomorrow. Patients who are not cured may have an extended survival, new therapeutic approaches giving the illness the appearance of a chronic disease, and the challenge is therefore to give duration and quality to the prolonged life.

Grenoble, France Michel Bolla
Leuven, Belgium Hendrik Van Poppel

Contents

Epidemiology of Prostate Cancer in Europe: Patterns, Trends and Determinants

Freddie Bray and Lambertus A. Kiemeney

1 Introduction

Malignant neoplasms of the prostate, hereafter referred to as prostate cancer (ICD-10 C61), usually originate in the glandular tissue. While these cancers, mainly adenocarcinomas, are often indolent, there is a subset of men who are diagnosed with highly malignant prostate cancers associated with poor prognosis. The disease poses a substantial public health burden worldwide and in Europe: it is the second most frequently diagnosed cancer and the fifth leading cause of cancer death among men globally, with an estimated 1.1 million new cases diagnosed and 307,000 deaths from the disease in 2012 [16]. Among European men, it is the most common neoplasm and third-ranked cause of cancer death, with almost 400,000 cases and over 92,000 deaths

Incidence rates of prostate cancer are heavily influenced by the diagnosis of latent cancers by serum prostate-specific antigen (PSA) testing of asymptomatic individuals, and by the detection of latent cancer in tissue removed during prostatectomy operations, or at autopsy. When PSA became commercially available in the mid-1980s in the USA and the late 1980s in Europe, the intensive use of the test by general practitioners and urologists as an early detection and diagnostic tool led to inflated incidence rates first in the USA [21] and within a few years in Greater Europe, notably in several Nordic countries [26].

During the early to mid-1990s, the detection of a substantial number of early-stage prostate cancers brought about rapid increases in population-level incidence rates across the higher-income countries of Northern, Western and Southern Europe. The extent to which prostate cancer incidence is now (as estimated in 2012) the leading form of cancer occurrence in men in these regions can be visibly grasped in Fig. 1. An East–west divide can be seen in Europe that combines differences in diagnostic intensity and the prominent cause of cancer in the region: in Central and Eastern Europe, PSA testing has been historically lower but male tobacco consumption higher and declining later, relative to elsewhere in Europe. Indeed, lung cancer remains the leading cancer in the eastern areas of Europe, prostate cancer in the west. In contrast, only in Sweden is prostate cancer the leading cause of cancer death, a country in which the male population did not take up the smoking habit like neighbouring countries; lung cancer ranks as the most important form of cancer death in men in all of the 39 remaining countries in Europe.

F. Bray (✉)
Section of Cancer Surveillance, International Agency for Research on Cancer, 150, Cours Albert Thomas, F-69372 Lyon Cedex, Lyon, France
e-mail: brayf@iarc.fr

L.A. Kiemeney
Radboud University Medical Center, Radboud Institute for Health Sciences, Department for Health Evidence & Department of Urology, Nijmegen, The Netherlands

M. Bolla, H. van Poppel (eds.), *Management of Prostate Cancer*,
DOI 10.1007/978-3-319-42769-0_1

Prostate (24)
Lung (15)
Colorectum (1)
No data
The boundaries and names shown and the designations used on this map do not imply the expression of any opinion whatsoever on the part of the World Health Organization concerning the legal status of any country, territory, city or area or of its authorities, or concerning the delimitation of its frontiers or boundaries. Dotted and dashed lines on maps represent approximate border lines for which there may not yet be full agreement.
Data source: GLOBOCAN 2012
Map production: IARC
World Health Organization
World Health Organization
© WHO 2015. All rights reserved

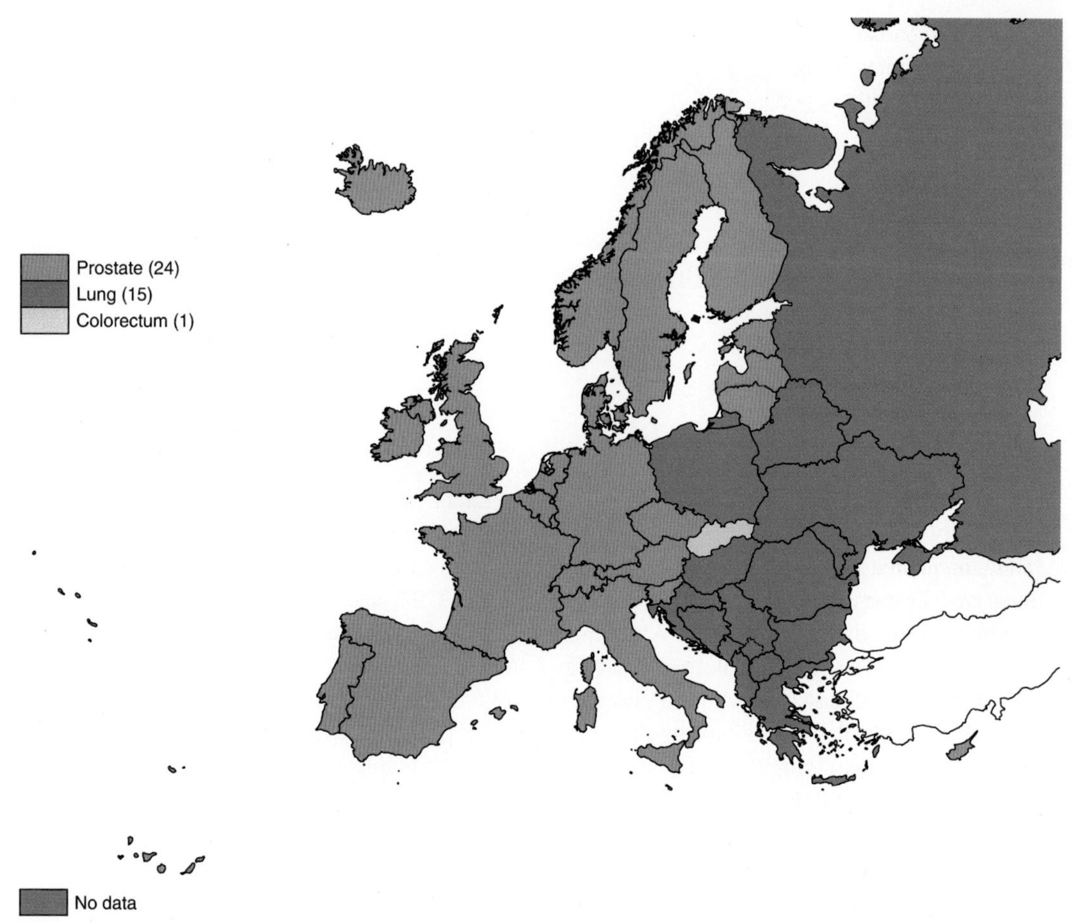

Fig. 1 Most common type of cancer in 40 European countries, based on the frequency of new cases as estimated in 2012 (Source: GLOBOCAN (http://globocan.iarc.fr))

Trends in incidence and mortality are not static, however, and prostate cancer incidence rates are to a great extent dependent on GP and urologist practices with respect to PSA testing. Conversely, prostate cancer mortality rates tend to be a better marker of extended disease and case fatality than of early diagnosis of asymptomatic cancers. Moderate declines in mortality rates have provided critical evidence of the favourable effect of increased curative treatment, particularly of early-diagnosed prostate cancer, within the last two decades.

1.1 Aims of Chapter

The aims of this chapter are threefold: (i) to describe the current profile of prostate cancer in Europe, (ii) to compare and contrast how recent trends in incidence and mortality are changing and (iii) to assess the factors that contribute to this evolving landscape, with a focus on the epidemiology of prostate cancer, the underlying risk factors and prospects of prevention. This chapter begins with a brief exploration of the global statistics of prostate cancer, followed by a more thorough comparison of the incidence and mortality burden and rates across European countries by region, and within these populations over time.

1.2 Data Sources and Methods

In presenting recent geographic variations, national incidence and mortality estimates of prostate cancer were available by country, sex and age and extracted from GLOBOCAN database for the year 2012 (http://globocan.iarc.fr). Temporal comparisons make use of recorded incidence of the disease in 1975–2014 from national and regional population-based cancer registries of high quality complied in successive volumes of *Cancer Incidence in Five Continents* (http://ci5.iarc.fr) and in corresponding recorded mortality available nationally from the WHO mortality databank (http://www-dep.iarc.fr/WHOdb/WHOdb.htm); we obtained more recent data from published or online sources for a number of European populations, including the Nordic countries (http://ancr.nu) and the Netherlands (http://www.cijfersoverkanker.nl/). To enable comparison adjusted for the effects of differing age composition and population ageing over time, all incidence and mortality rates presented in this chapter are age-standardised to the world standard population [14], and are denoted *ASR*. In deciphering incidence and mortality trends over time, joinpoint regression models [25] were fitted to identify sudden linear changes in annual rates and to estimate the direction and magnitude of the slope within these distinct periods of time.

2 Prostate Cancer Incidence and Mortality

2.1 Global Patterns and Trends

By 2012, prostate cancer became the fourth most common cancer in the world, ranking third in importance in men, and the most frequent male cancer in 91 countries worldwide. While the estimated total annual number of 1.1 million cases represents about 15 % of all male cancers, it is a less prominent cause of cancer mortality, with just over 300,000 deaths estimated annually, or almost 7 % of male cancer deaths. The relatively low case fatality signifies many men are alive years after their initial diagnosis of prostate cancer – an estimated 3.9 million at 5 years in 2012 – making this by far the most prevalent form of cancer in men. Prostate cancer is also a cancer of the elderly, with three-quarters of a million cases diagnosed (68 %) in men aged 65 years or more.

Worldwide, recorded incidence is very high where health-seeking behaviour and health-care systems are advanced, and estimates of national incidence rates vary at least 25-fold (Fig. 2a). As a result of a substantial diagnosis of latent cancers through PSA testing of asymptomatic individuals, rates are often elevated in the high-income countries within Oceania, Northern America, and Western and Northern Europe, and low in many Asian populations, particularly in Southern Asia. Incidence rates are intermediate to high in many regions and countries in economic transition, where PSA testing is not likely to be highly prevalent, including the Caribbean, South America and Sub-Saharan Africa. A combination of genetic (ethnic) risk differences and environmental, dietary and lifestyle factors are at play, although the specific risk components are largely unknown. Clearly, rates are higher in populations where men of African-Caribbean origin is a key risk factor; in the USA, rates among blacks remain 35 % higher than those in whites.

With almost 60,000 new cases estimated in 2012, cancer of the prostate is the most frequently diagnosed cancer in Sub-Saharan African men, with the risk of developing prostate cancer before age 75 of 3.4 % (i.e. affecting almost 1 in 30 men) equivalent to the lifetime risks of breast (3.5 %) and cervical cancer (3.8 %) among women in the region [31]. While the disease is the most frequent neoplasm among men, there is a tenfold variation in prostate cancer incidence rates in Sub-Saharan countries with a cumulative risk ranging from 0.8 % in Ethiopia to greater than 8 % in the Republic of South Africa in 2012. Even in the latter country, rates are modest compared with those in men of African descent in the USA and Caribbean [16] [], although the

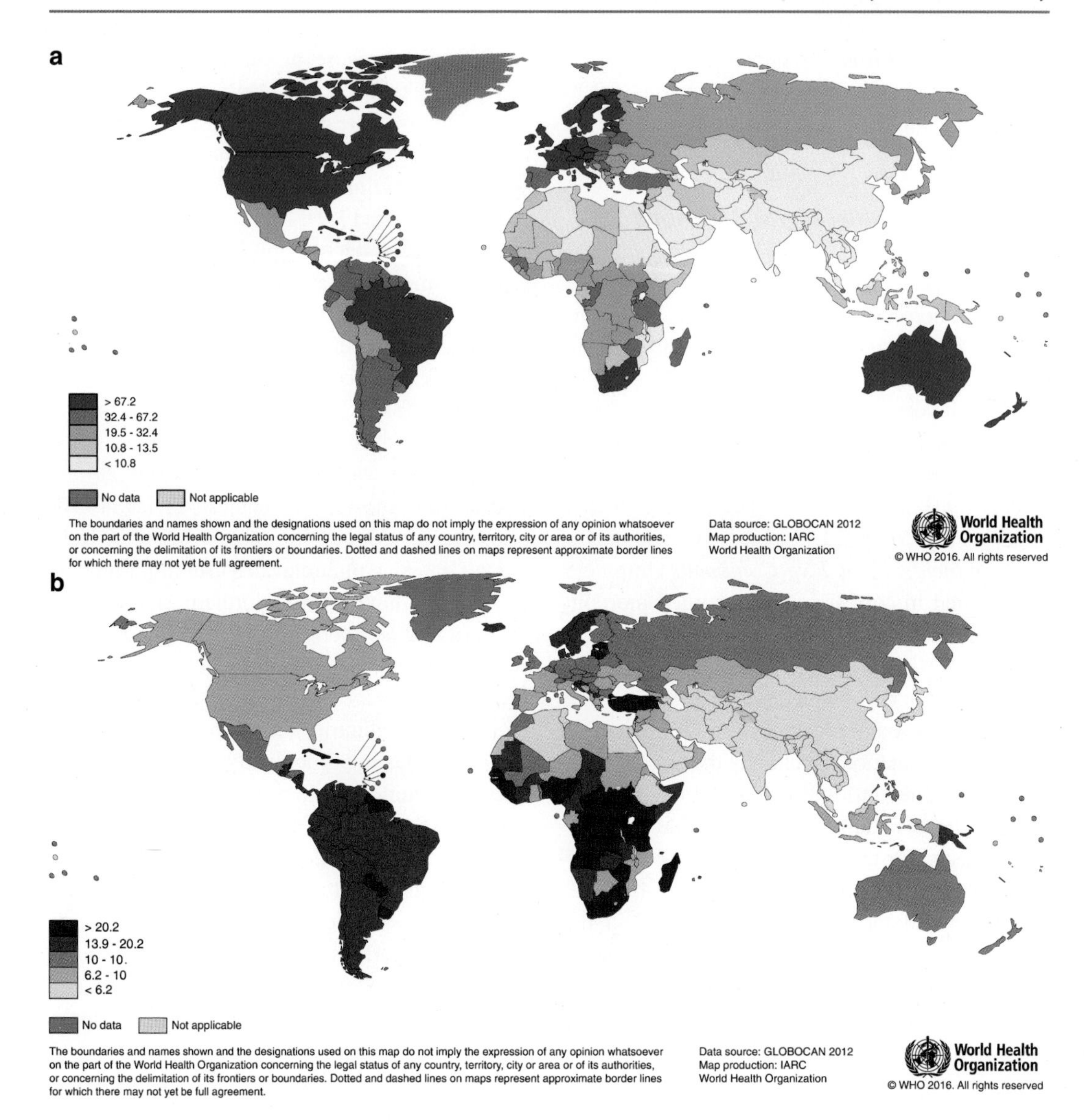

Fig. 2 (**a**) Global map of prostate cancer incidence in 184 countries, based on age-standardised rates (World). Source: GLOBOCAN (http://globocan.iarc.fr). (**b**) Global map of prostate cancer mortality in 184 countries, based on age-standardised rates (World) (Source: GLOBOCAN (http://globocan.iarc.fr))

incidence is markedly increasing in a number of African populations, for example, in Kampala [35] and in the black population of Harare [10].

Mortality rates are less affected by early diagnosis of asymptomatic disease, and although a better marker of underlying risk of extended prostate cancer, they are also heavily dependent on the treatment options available in a given country (Fig. 2b). Mortality rates are high in North America, Northern and Western Europe, Australia/New Zealand, but also in parts of Latin America (Brazil) and the Caribbean, and in much of Sub-Saharan Africa. Indeed of the 42 countries where prostate cancer is the leading cause of cancer death among men, 19 are in Sub-Saharan Africa, 13 in Central and South America and 9 are in the Caribbean. Mortality rates are low in most Asian populations and in North Africa.

Using data from population-based cancer registries, five distinct time trend patterns have been demonstrated in prostate cancer incidence globally according to age [38]. Notably, incidence rates have been observed to peak among men aged over 75 years in most high-income populations, reflecting declining PSA screening at older ages and diagnosis at younger ages. In contrast, rates for men aged 45–54 years have not clearly stabilised or declined in most populations, and PSA testing is not likely to fully explain the rapidly rising rates of early-onset prostate cancer. In fact, decreasing overall prostate cancer mortality rates during the last decade has been reported mainly for North America, Oceania, Western Europe and parts of Northern Europe, where PSA testing has been more intensively implemented. This contrasts with the rising prostate cancer mortality rates observed in Central and Eastern Europe, and in parts of Asia and Africa [9]. The declining mortality rates may suggest that treatment and possibly earlier diagnosis have had an impact, whereas the rising rates could reflect an increasing diagnosis of prostate cancer; in both instances, the contribution of a changing prevalence and distribution of the underlying risk factors cannot be discounted.

2.2 Current Patterns in Europe

As with a global exposition of prostate cancer, the interpretation of observed variations in incidence in Europe – including any elucidation of potential risk determinants – is hampered by likely differences in the prevalence of PSA testing. Understanding the equivalent rates of mortality is also difficult given multiple contributory factors: the advent of curative treatment at about the same time as the increasing utilisation of the PSA test, and underlying this, the changing prevalence of one more (largely unknown) determinants of the disease. Each of these may have contributed to the levels of prostate cancer mortality in a given European population.

Geographic Variations in Incidence and Mortality

With over 400,000 new cases of prostate cancer, the disease is the leading cause of cancer in men, ahead of lung and colorectal cancer in second and third place, respectively. The disease is responsible for 22 % of the 1.8 million cancer cases among European men in 2012 and ranks fourth most frequent cancer in both sexes. Figure 3a, b, respectively, map the prostate cancer incidence and mortality rates in 2012 in 40 European countries, while Fig. 4 compares the ranking of mortality versus incidence. Rates of incidence vary tenfold in Europe, with the highest rates (125–160 per 100,000) in Lithuania, France, each of the Nordic countries as well as Switzerland and Ireland. Rates are intermediate (100–125) in Austria, Germany, Italy and England and Wales, and low (<50) in the Eastern European countries of Poland, Belarus, the Russian Federation and Bulgaria.

Approximately 92,000 deaths from prostate cancer were estimated to have occurred in 2012 in Europe, and thus the third-ranked cause of cancer death among men, after lung and colorectal cancer. In contrast to incidence, mortality rates vary only by a factor of 3, with some geographic differences observed. As with incidence, the highest mortality rates are seen in Lithuania, with their Baltic neighbours, Latvia and Estonia, ranked in second and third position. Rates are also relatively high (>25 per 100,000) in several Nordic countries (Denmark, Norway and Sweden), and in several Southern European countries (Slovenia, Croatia and Portugal) but moderate in several others (Spain, Italy and Greece); as with incidence, many of the lowest rates are seen in Central and Eastern European countries. The lowest rate is in Belarus, among the countries compared.

Clearly, there is little correlation in the present rates of prostate cancer incidence and mortality in Europe (Fig. 5). There is considerably more variability in incidence, and while the lowest and highest rates of both measures are, respectively, seen in Lithuania and Belarus, there are instances where incidence in a given country is relatively low and mortality relatively high (Latvia, Croatia), and vice versa (France). Figure 5 portrays the incidence rates in 3–5 year-periods (1983–87, 1993–97 and

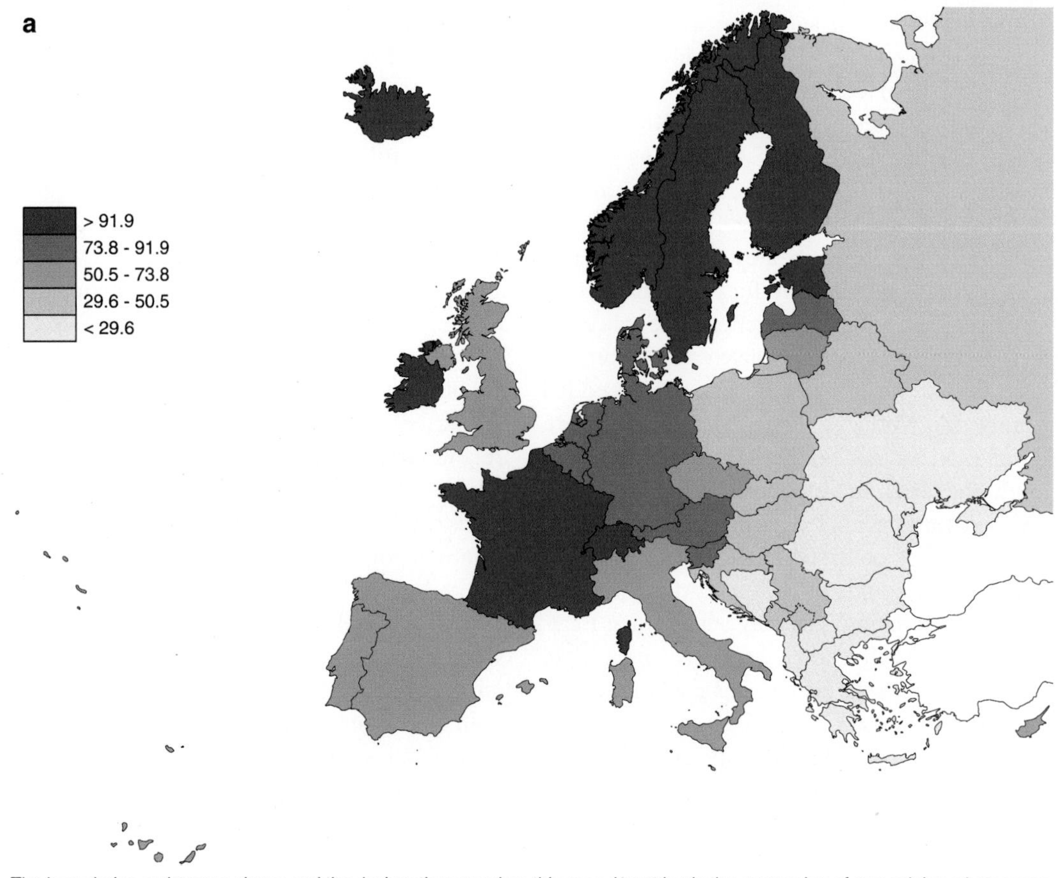

The boundaries and names shown and the designations used on this map do not imply the expression of any opinion whatsoever on the part of the World Health Organization concerning the legal status of any country, territory, city or area or of its authorities, or concerning the delimitation of its frontiers or boundaries. Dotted and dashed lines on maps represent approximate border lines for which there may not yet be full agreement.

Data source: GLOBOCAN 2012
Map production: IARC
World Health Organization

World Health Organization

Fig. 3 (**a**) European map of prostate cancer incidence in 40 countries, based on age-standardised rates (World) (Source: GLOBOCAN (http://globocan.iarc.fr)). (**b**) European map of prostate cancer mortality in 40 countries, based on age-standardised rates (World) (Source: GLOBOCAN (http://globocan.iarc.fr))

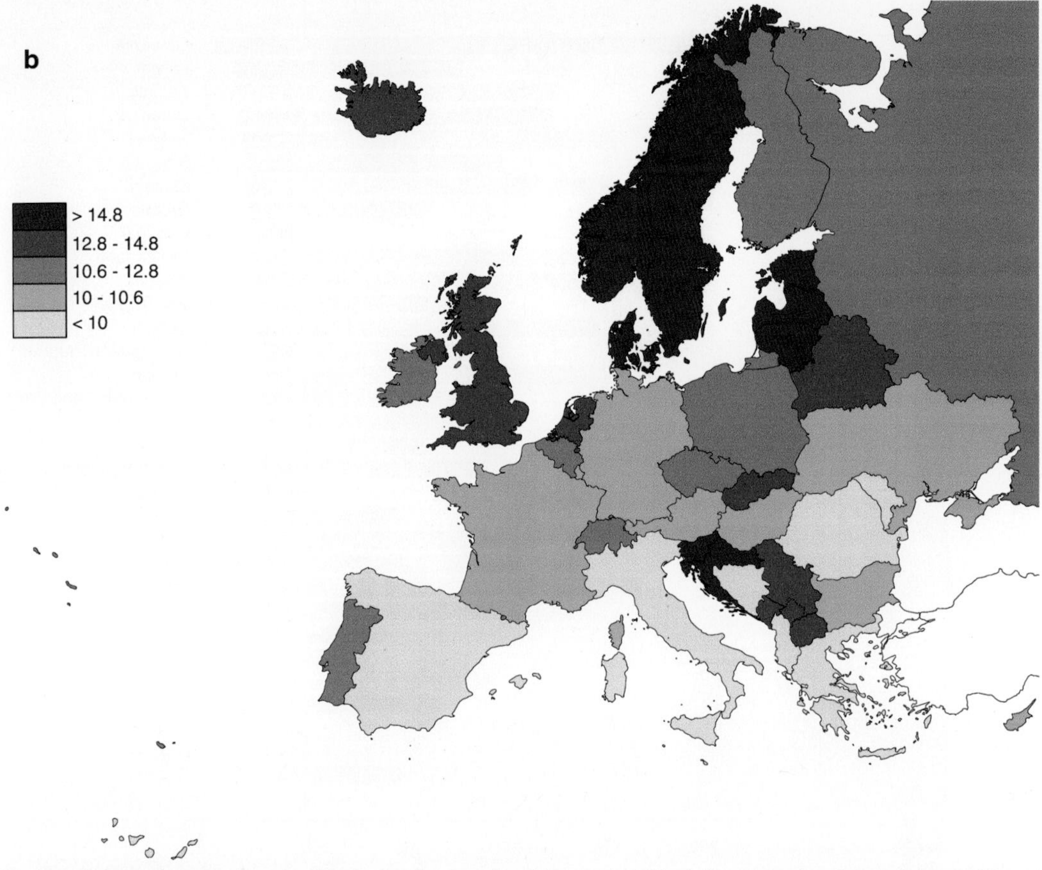

The boundaries and names shown and the designations used on this map do not imply the expression of any opinion whatsoever on the part of the World Health Organization concerning the legal status of any country, territory, city or area or of its authorities, or concerning the delimitation of its frontiers or boundaries. Dotted and dashed lines on maps represent approximate border lines for which there may not yet be full agreement.

Data source: GLOBOCAN 2012
Map production: IARC
World Health Organization

World Health Organization

Fig. 3 (continued)

2000–04) against mortality rates 5–10 years later (circa 1993, 2003, 2010). The correlation is reasonably strong between the two measures in the 1980s diagnostic era, with the mortality rates directly related to the prior level of incidence in a given population. That correlation appears to weaken over time, however, as one enters the era of PSA availability and its expanded use as a test in Europe, during the 1990s and early 2000s.

2.3 Comparative Trends by European Region

The incidence has increased rapidly over the past two decades, and rates are influenced by early diagnosis among asymptomatic individuals, and prior to the PSA testing era, detection of latent cancer in tissue removed during prostate surgery. Examining trends in prostate cancer incidence and mortality in 32 countries, the

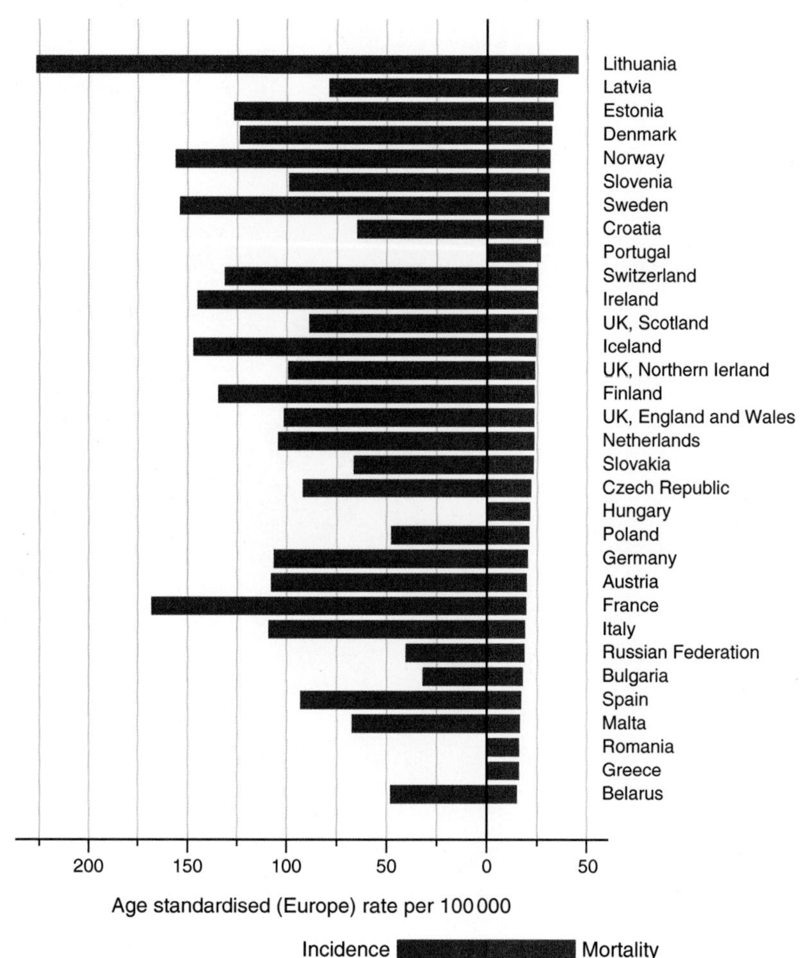

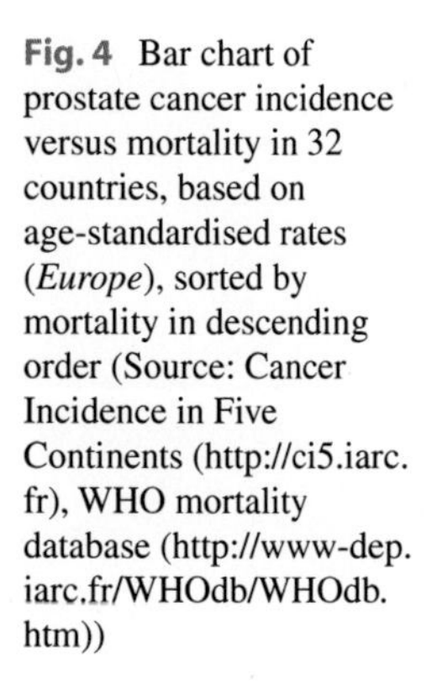

Fig. 4 Bar chart of prostate cancer incidence versus mortality in 32 countries, based on age-standardised rates (*Europe*), sorted by mortality in descending order (Source: Cancer Incidence in Five Continents (http://ci5.iarc.fr), WHO mortality database (http://www-dep.iarc.fr/WHOdb/WHOdb.htm))

trends are presented for various years spanning 1975–2014 for 17 Northern and Western countries (Fig. 6a) and 15 Southern and European countries (Fig. 6b); the estimated annual percentage change is given.

Increasing trends in the incidence of prostate cancer have been observed in all countries from the mid-1970s through to the early 2000s, and for the period 1990–2004, the rate of increase ranged from 6 to 10 % on average per annum in France, Spain, Ireland, Italy, Slovenia, the Russian Federation and the Baltic countries (Estonia, Latvia, Lithuania) to 3–5 % in the remaining countries shown in Fig. 7. Notable are the uniform declines in prostate cancer incidence seen from the mid-2000s in almost all Northern and Western European countries, with the possible exception of countries in the Baltic region and the UK (Fig. 6a and Table 1). These recent decreases are not seen in any country within Southern or Eastern Europe, except in Italy (Fig. 6b, Table 1).

There appears to be little relation between the extent of the increases in prostate cancer incidence (as estimated from 1990) and the subsequent mortality declines (as estimated from 1996, Tables 1 and 2). National mortality declines in prostate cancer mortality were observed from 1996 in 19 of the 27 countries where both incidence and mortality measures are available (Fig. 7); these ranged from 2 to 3 % declines in Austria, France, Switzerland, Germany, the Netherlands, Finland, Spain and Norway to less than 1 % declines in Denmark and Slovakia. In contrast, increases in mortality of 0.5 % (Poland)

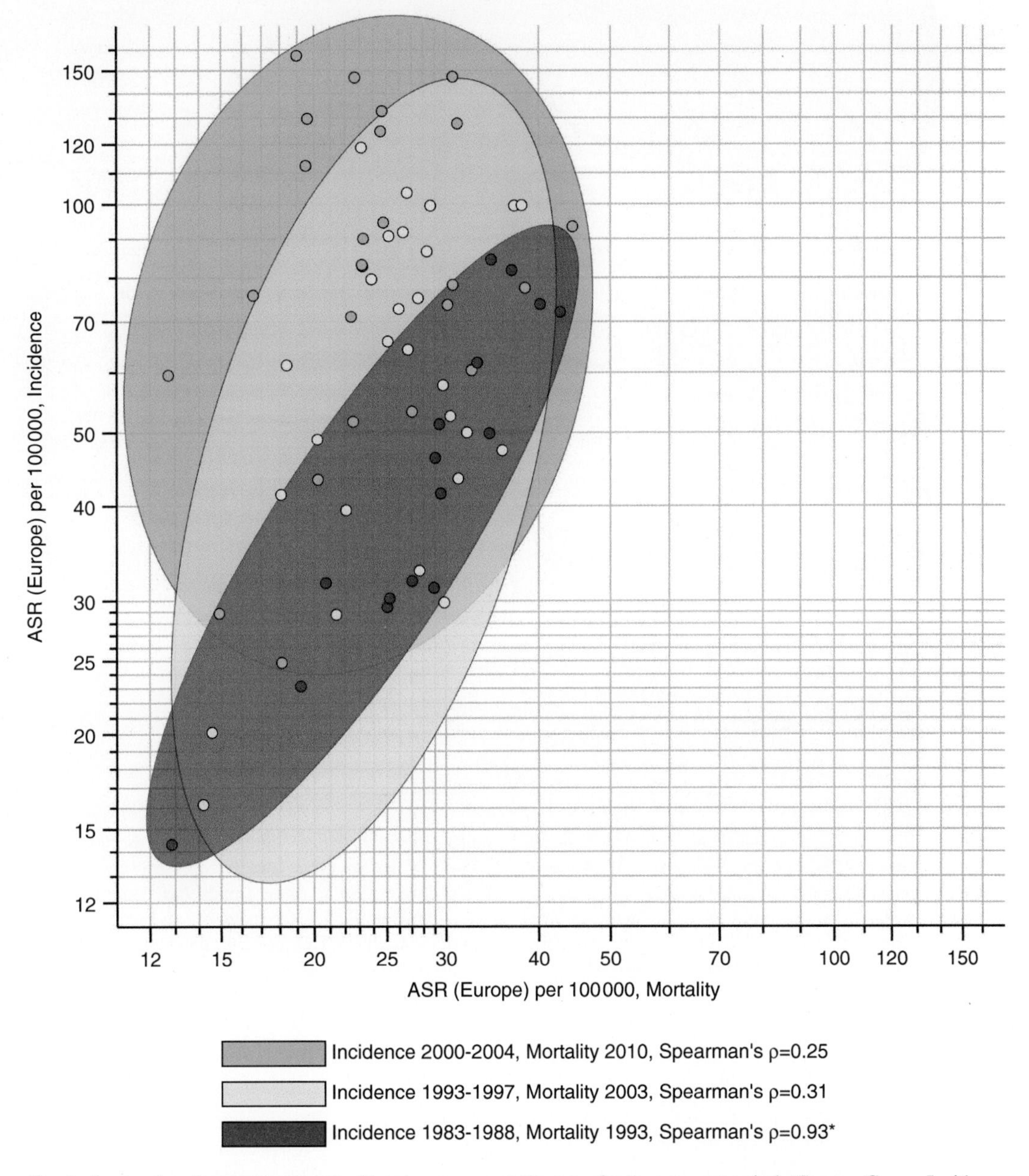

Fig. 5 Scatterplot of prostate cancer incidence versus mortality rates for three recent periods (Source: Cancer Incidence in Five Continents (http://ci5.iarc.fr), WHO mortality database (http://www-dep.iarc.fr/WHOdb/WHOdb.htm))

through to 4 % (Lithuania) are seen in the remaining eight countries in the Baltic region, Southern or Eastern Europe. Below is a more detailed exposition of the trends by region.

Northern Europe

In the five Nordic countries, rates have been uniformly increasing during the 1990s (Fig. 6a and Table 1). Notable are the very recent declines in rates seen during period 2004–8, although incidence rates in Finland subsequently increased in 2008 following a short-term decline from 2005. Significant mortality declines of 2–3 % per annum are observed in all Nordic countries (Table 2), with the declines beginning in 1992 in Iceland, through to 1998 in Sweden (Table 3).

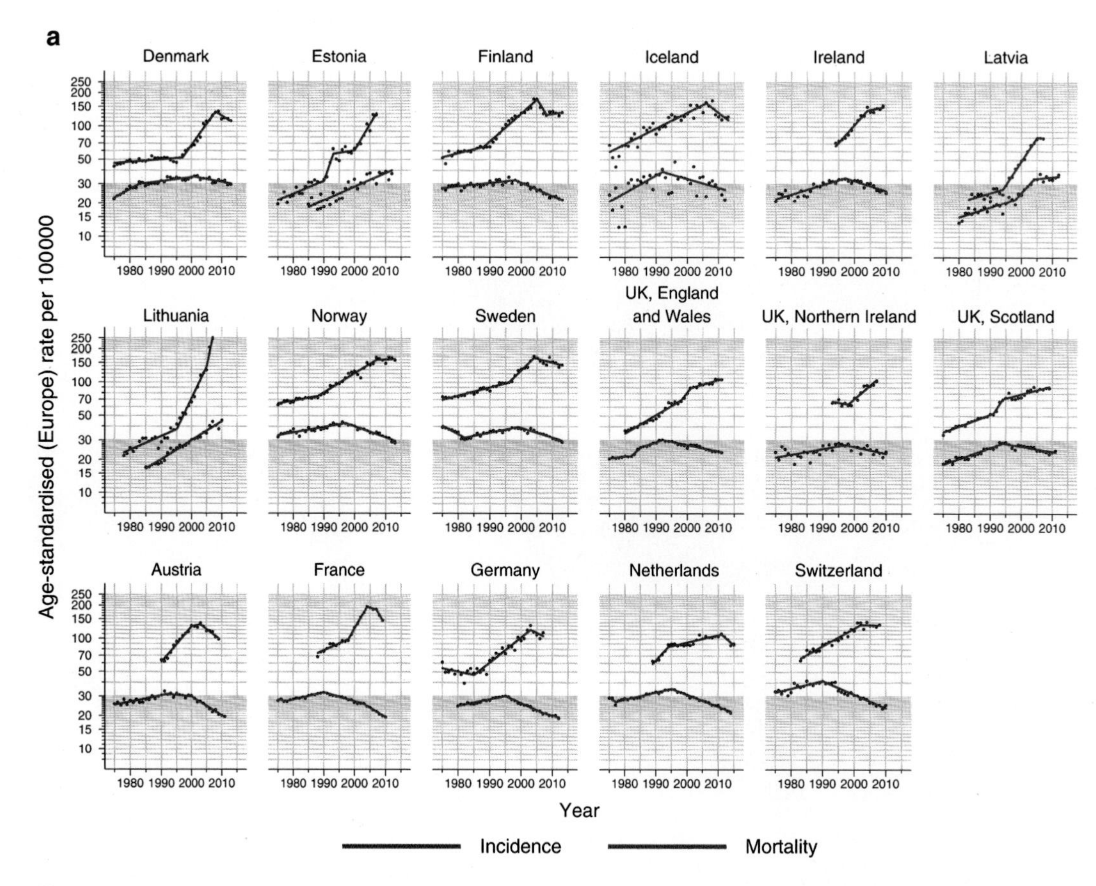

Fig. 6 (**a**) Line graphs of prostate cancer incidence versus mortality rates 1975–2014 in Northern and Western Europe. *Circles*: observed rates; Solid lines: trends based on Joinpoint regression (Source: Cancer Incidence in Five Continents (http://ci5.iarc.fr), WHO mortality database (http://www-dep.iarc.fr/WHOdb/WHOdb.htm)). (**b**) Line graphs of prostate cancer incidence versus mortality rates 1975–2014 in Southern and Eastern Europe. *Circles*: observed rates; *Solid lines*: trends based on Joinpoint regression (Source: Cancer Incidence in Five Continents (http://ci5.iarc.fr), WHO mortality database (http://www-dep.iarc.fr/WHOdb/WHOdb.htm))

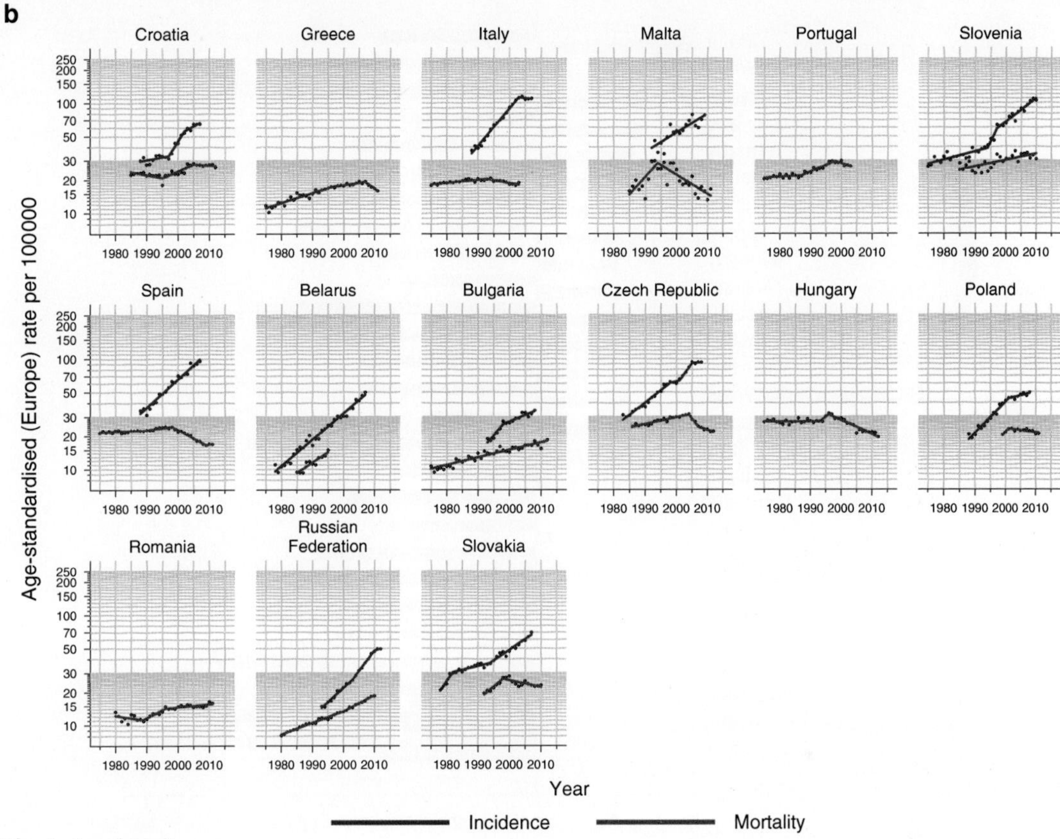

Fig. 6 (continued)

The incidence has also been increasing in the UK and Ireland but unlike their Nordic counterparts, no recent incidence declines are seen. Significant annual declines in mortality of slightly over 1 % were observed in the constituent countries of the UK. – as early as 1992 in England and Wales (Table 3) – with mean declines of 2.1 % observed in Ireland (since 1997). The Baltic countries have a very different prostate cancer profile, with significantly increasing rates of both incidence and mortality observed in the last decades; these correspond to 3 % in Estonia and 4 % in Lithuania (Fig. 6b and Table 2). A suggestion of a stabilisation of mortality rates can be observed in Latvia from 2004.

Western Europe

Increasing incidence rates are observed in all five countries since the mid-1980s, ranging from around 3 % per annum for the period 1990–2004 (Switzerland, the Netherlands) to almost 7 % (France). As seen in the Nordic countries, incidence rates have uniformly declined in Western Europe, with the decrease beginning during the period 2002–4 (Fig. 6a and Table 1). Some of the largest decreases in prostate cancer mortality in European men are seen in the region (Fig. 7), notably the close to 4 % rate declines in Austria and France, beginning in 2000 and 2003, respectively (Fig. 6b and Table 2).

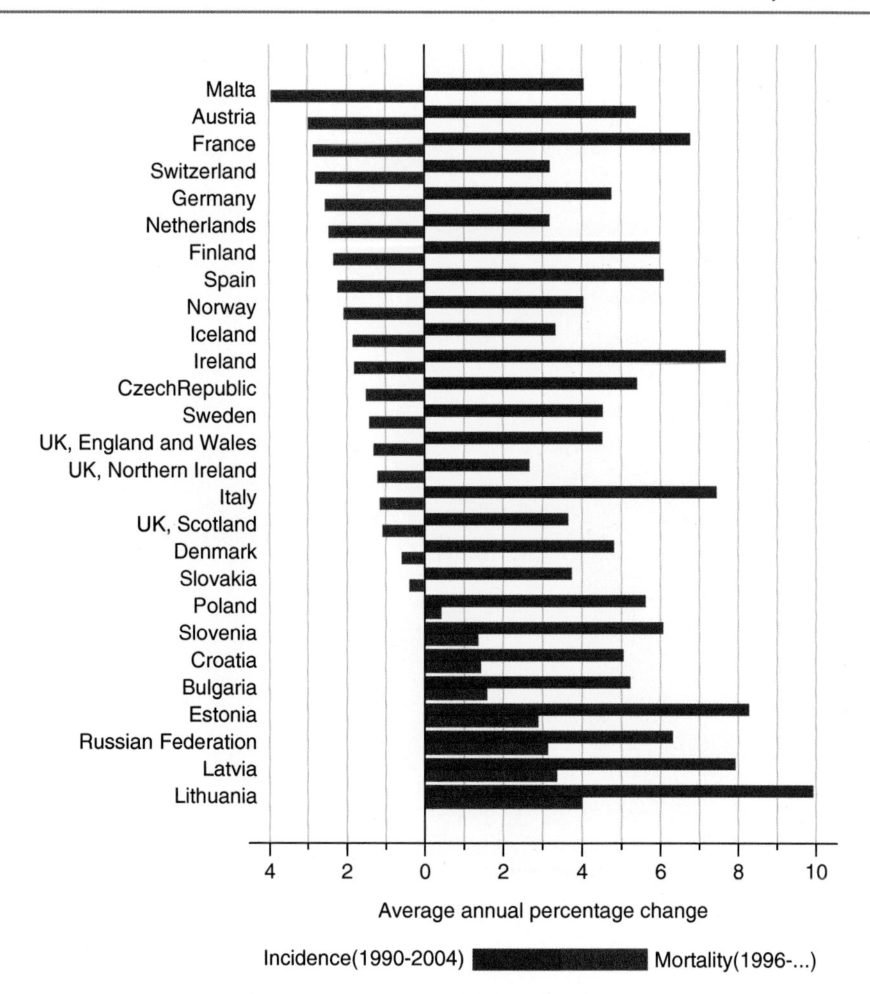

Fig. 7 Average annual percentage changes in prostate cancer incidence (1990–2004) and mortality trends (1996-) based on the joinpoint regression, sorted in ascending order of mortality trends (Source: Cancer Incidence in Five Continents (http://ci5.iarc.fr), WHO mortality database (http://www-dep.iarc.fr/WHOdb/WHOdb.htm))

Southern Europe
Incidence trends in the four Southern European countries are increasing rapidly, particularly in Italy, Slovenia and Spain where the mean annual increases are 6–7 % per annum from 1990 to 2004 (Fig. 6b and Table 1). The mortality trends showed more variability across the six countries examined, although decreasing rates are seen in all countries except Slovenia. Among the most impressive declines are the 3.4 % and 3.9 % per annum reductions in Spain 1998–2009 and Malta 1994–2011, respectively (Fig. 6b and Table 2).

Eastern Europe
Some of the largest rate increases in prostate cancer incidence are observed in the five Eastern European countries, including the Czech Republic and Russia, where the rates rose 9–10 % per year during the 2000s, although the increases have attenuated subsequently in very recent years (Fig. 6b and Table 1). In terms of mortality, there is greater variability; the long-term increases in the Russian Federation and Bulgaria of 2–3 % per annum contrast with the rapid declines of the same order of magnitude in Hungary (since 1996) and more recently in the Czech Republic and Slovakia (Fig. 6b and Table 2).

Table 1 Prostate cancer incidence: new cases, person and age-standardised (Europe) rates circa 2006–2010, data span available and joinpoint regression analysis by country within European region

Country	Mean incidence cases per year 2006–2010	Person-years 2006–2010	ASR (Europe) 2006–2010	Observed period	JP linear segment	EAPC CI (95 %)
Europe	129 210	153 918116				
Northern Europe	65 260	46 532 428				
Denmark	4 256	2 719 803	123.8	1975–2013	1975–1997 1997–2008 2008–2013	0.5[a] (0.0; 1.0) 9.1[a] (7.9; 10.3) −4.0[a] (−6.3; −1.6)
Estonia	691	620 195	106.3	1975–2007	1975–1990 1990–1993 1993–2000 2000–2007	2.7[a] (0.8; 4.7) 20.6 (−14.3; 69.6) 1.1 (−3.8; 6.1) 11.7[a] (8.6; 14.8)
Finland	4 479	2 604 531	134.6	1975–2013	1975–1988 1988–2005 2005–2008 2008–2013	1.7[a] (0.4; 3.0) 6.0[a] (5.4; 6.6) −10.2 (−19.5; 0.2) 1.0 (−1.3; 3.4)
Iceland	225	159 570	147.1	1975–2013	1975–2006 2006–2013	3.3[a] (2.8; 3.9) −4.9[a] (−7.9; −1.8)
Ireland	2 741	2 154 884	143.3	1994–2009	1994–2004 2004–2009	7.7[a] (6.5; 8.8) 1.3 (−1.0; 3.6)
Latvia	824	1059 911	75.1	1983–2007	1983–1994 1994–2005 2005–2007	1.9[a] (0.5; 3.4) 10.3[a] (9.0; 11.6) −0.8 (−11.0; 10.6)
Lithuania	2 555	1592 521	163.3	1978–2007	1978–1995 1995–2005 2005–2007	2.9[a] (1.7; 4.1) 13.8[a] (11.9; 15.8) 36.7[a] (23.4; 51.5)
Norway	4 264	2 377 718	156.2	1975–2013	1975–1988 1988–2007 2007–2013	1.2[a] (0.1; 2.2) 4.0[a] (3.5; 4.5) 0.2 (−1.7; 2.2)
Sweden	9 510	4 585 718	154.0	1975–2013	1975–1996 1996–2004 2004–2013	1.7[a] (1.3; 2.1) 6.6[a] (4.8; 8.4) −1.7[a] (−2.7; −0.7)
UK, England and Wales	32121	25 326 450	101.4	1980–2011	1980–1998 1998–2001 2001–2011	3.9[a] (3.4; 4.4) 8.7 (−2.7; 21.5) 1.9[a] (1.2; 2.7)

(continued)

Table 1 (continued)

Country	Mean incidence cases per year 2006–2010	Person-years 2006–2010	ASR (Europe) 2006–2010	Observed period	JP linear segment	EAPC CI (95 %)
UK, Northern Ireland	841	845 796	96.1	1993–2007	1993–1998 1998–2007	−1.1 (−6.1; 4.2) 5.8[a] (4.0; 7.7)
UK, Scotland	2 753	2 485 331	88.0	1975–2009	1975–1991 1991–1994 1994–2009	2.5[a] (1.8; 3.2) 10.5 (−3.7; 26.7) 1.7[a] (1.2; 2.2)
Western Europe	22 847	16148 556				
Austria	5 224	4 038 612	109.4	1990–2009	1990–2000 2000–2003 2003–2009	7.6[a] (6.5; 8.8) 1.3 (−9.1; 12.8) −4.7[a] (−6.5; −2.9)
France	5 992	2 984 699	172.2	1988–2009	1988–1998 1998–2004 2004–2007 2007–2009	2.9[a] (1.9; 3.9) 11.9[a] (9.8; 14.1) −1.9 (−8.6; 5.3) −11.1[a] (−17.6; −4.0)
Germany	837	511456	113.2	1975–2007	1975–1985 1985–2003 2003–2007	−1.4 (−3.9; 1.2) 5.4[a] (4.5; 6.3) −3.2 (−8.4; 2.3)
Netherlands	10 075	8 144 299	104.3	1989–2015	1989–1994 1994–2011 2011–2015	7.3[a] (3.1; 11.5) 1.5[a] (1.0; 2.1) −5.5[a] (−8.9; −2.0)
Switzerland	719	469 490	133.4	1983–2008	1983–2002 2002–2008	3.7[a] (3.2; 4.3) −0.1 (−2.5; 2.2)
Southern Europe	8 001	7172 636				
Croatia	1517	2138 032	62.2	1988–2007	1988–1997 1997–2002 2002–2007	1.2 (−0.7; 3.2) 11.1[a] (5.3; 17.2) 3.5[a] (0.5; 6.6)
Italy	3447	2 080 603	109.9	1988–2007	1988–2003 2003–2007	8.1[a] (7.6; 8.6) −0.9 (−3.3; 1.6)
Malta	156	203 268	69.2	1992–2009	1992–2009	4.1[a] (2.6; 5.5)
Slovenia	1146	997 043	99.0	1975–2010	1975–1994 1994–1997 1997–2010	1.8[a] (0.9; 2.6) 14.4 (−7.3; 41.3) 4.9[a] (4.2; 5.7)
Spain	1735	1753 690	87.9	1988–2007	1988–2007	6.1[a] (5.5; 6.6)
Eastern Europe	33102	84 064496				

Belarus	1750	4 572 634	43.3	1978–2007	1978–2007	5.7[a] (5.4; 6.0)
Bulgaria	1590	3 733 526	32.2	1993–2008	1993–1998	8.2[a] (4.2; 12.3)
					1998–2008	2.8[a] (1.7; 3.9)
Czech Republic	4 949	5 027 528	90.5	1983–2008	1983–1998	5.2[a] (4.7; 5.8)
					1998–2001	1.6 (−8.1; 12.3)
					2001–2005	9.6[a] (5.0; 14.5)
					2005–2008	0.3 (−3.4; 4.2)
Poland	1096	2 365 394	47.0	1988–2008	1988–2001	6.7[a] (5.9; 7.6)
					2001–2008	1.6[a] (0.1; 3.0)
Russian Federation	22 385	65 749 763	40.4	1993–2012	1993–2003	6.1[a] (5.3; 6.8)
					2003–2010	9.0[a] (7.9; 10.1)
					2010–2012	2.2 (−2.8; 7.4)
Slovakia	1 332	2615651	60.7	1978–2007	1978–1982	10.0[a] (3.7; 16.8)
					1982–1994	1.6[a] (0.6; 2.7)
					1994–2007	4.6[a] (4.0; 5.2)

CI confidence interval
[a]Statistically significant

Table 2 Prostate cancer mortality: new deaths, person and age-standardised (Europe) rates circa 2006–2010, data span available and joinpoint regression analysis by country within European region

Country	Mean incidence cases per year 2006–2010	Person-years 2006–2010	ASR (Europe) 2006–2010	Observed Period	JP linear segment	EAPC CI (95 %)
Europe	79 487	314 570 696				
Northern Europe	17 497	47 822 287				
Denmark	1 136	2 724 046	31.6	1975–2013	1975–1983	3.6[a] (2.1; 5.2)
					1983–2001	0.8[a] (0.4; 1.2)
					2001–2013	−1.2[a] (−1.7; −0.6)
Estonia	230	605 582	35.7	1985–2012	1985–2012	2.9[a] (2.3; 3.4)
Finland	807	2 606 774	24.2	1975–2013	1975–1998	0.7[a] (0.4; 1.0)
					1998–2013	−2.7[a] (−3.2; −2.3)
Iceland	49	159 355	28.4	1975–2012	1975–1992	3.7[a] (1.2; 6.3)
					1992–2012	−1.8[a] (−3.3; −0.3)
Ireland	525	2 162 832	26.6	1975–2010	1975–1997	2.0[a] (1.6; 2.5)
					1997–2010	−2.1[a] (−2.9; −1.3)
Latvia	365	979 270	34.4	1980–2012	1980–1998	2.1[a] (1.3; 2.9)
					1998–2004	7.4[a] (3.0; 12.0)
					2004–2012	0.6 (−1.1; 2.4)
Lithuania	547	1 456 969	41.6	1985–2010	1985–2010	4.0[a] (3.7; 4.3)
Norway	1 064	2 380 853	33.7	1975–2013	1975–1997	1.1[a] (0.9; 1.4)
					1997–2013	−2.3[a] (−2.6; −1.9)
Sweden	2 450	4 590 870	33.2	1975–2013	1975–1982	−3.5[a] (−4.8; −2.2)
					1982–1999	1.3[a] (1.0; 1.7)
					1999–2013	−2.0[a] (−2.4; −1.6)
UK, England and Wales	9 297	26 785 718	24.3	1975–2011	1975–1982	0.6 (−0.5; 1.7)
					1982–1985	6.2 (−1.2; 14.1)
					1985–1992	2.3[a] (1.2; 3.4)
					1992–2011	−1.3[a] (−1.5; −1.1)
UK, Northern Ireland	226	869 855	23.0	1975–2010	1975–1997	1.2[a] (0.6; 1.8)
					1997–2010	−1.4[a] (−2.5; −0.3)
UK, Scotland	801	2 500 163	23.7	1975–2011	1975–1994	2.3[a] (1.9; 2.7)
					1994–2011	−1.1[a] (−1.4; −0.7)
Western Europe	25 518	86 364 688				

Austria	1 117	4 059 464	21.5	1975–2011	1975–1992	1.3[a] (0.9; 1.7)
					1992–2000	−0.6 (−2.0; 0.7)
					2000–2011	−3.8[a] (−4.5; −3.2)
France	8 986	30 225 670	20.8	1975–2010	1975–1978	−0.7 (−3.1; 1.7)
					1978–1990	1.5[a] (1.2; 1.8)
					1990–2003	−1.8[a] (−2.1; −1.6)
					2003–2010	−3.9[a] (−4.3; −3.4)
Germany	12 010	40 815 102	20.7	1980–2012	1980–1995	1.4[a] (1.1; 1.6)
					1995–2007	−2.9[a] (−3.2; −2.6)
					2007–2012	−1.8[a] (−2.8; −0.7)
Netherlands	2 095	7 504 334	29.7	1975–2014	1975–1977	−5.0 (−10.5; 0.8)
					1977–1995	1.5[a] (1.3; 1.7)
					1995–2014	−2.4[a] (−2.6; −2.3)
Switzerland	1 310	3 760 118	25.0	1975–2010	1975–1990	1.6[a] (0.9; 2.3)
					1990–2010	−2.8[a] (−3.2; −2.4)
Southern Europe	17 095	63 803 923				
Croatia	660	2 101 797	27.4	1985–2012	1985–1995	−1.3[a] (−2.3; −0.2)
					1995–2005	2.9[a] (1.8; 4.0)
					2005–2012	−0.4 (−1.8; 0.9)
Greece	1 574	5 464 094	18.0	1975–2011	1975–1996	2.1[a] (1.8; 2.4)
					1996–2007	1.0[a] (0.2; 1.7)
					2007–2011	−4.6[a] (−7.2; −2.0)
Italy	7 197	27 744 064	18.4	1975–2003	1975–1993	0.6[a] (0.4; 0.8)
					1993–2003	−1.1[a] (−1.6; −0.7)
Malta	31	209 869	14.9	1985–2011	1985–1994	7.5[a] (2.4; 12.9)
					1994–2011	−3.9[a] (−5.5; −2.3)
Portugal	1 712	4 997 329	27.7	1975–2003	1975–1987	0.4 (−0.4; 1.3)
					1987–1998	2.8[a] (2.0; 3.6)
					1998–2003	−2.2[a] (−4.1; −0.2)
Slovenia	350	1 002 387	32.9	1985–2010	1985–2010	1.3[a] (0.8; 1.9)

(continued)

Table 2 (continued)

Country	Mean incidence cases per year 2006–2010	Person-years 2006–2010	ASR (Europe) 2006–2010	Observed Period	JP linear segment	EAPC CI (95 %)
Spain	5 571	22 284 383	17.3	1975–2011	1975–1989	0.3 (–0.1; 0.6)
					1989–1998	0.9[a] (0.3; 1.5)
					1998–2009	–3.4[a] (–3.8; –3.0)
					2009–2011	1.2 (–3.6; 6.2)
Eastern Europe	19 377	116 579 798				
Belarus	441	4 797 846	12.9	1985–1995	1985–1995	4.5[a] (3.1; 5.9)
Bulgaria	820	3 654 124	16.5	1975–2012	1975–2012	1.6[a] (1.4; 1.8)
Czech Republic	1 317	5 097 845	24.0	1986–2012	1986–2004	1.4[a] (1.2; 1.6)
					2004–2007	–8.0[a] (–14.0; –1.7)
					2007–2012	–2.3[a] (–3.7; –0.8)
Hungary	1 186	4 769 849	21.9	1975–2012	1975–1993	–0.0 (–0.4; 0.4)
					1993–1996	5.2 (–6.3; 18.0)
					1996–2012	–2.9[a] (–3.3; –2.5)
Poland	3 897	18 456 675	21.9	1999–2011	1999–2001	6.7 (–2.7; 17.0)
					2001–2011	–0.8[a] (–1.5; –0.2)
Romania	1 789	10 709 460	15.2	1980–2011	1980–1989	–1.0 (–2.4; 0.5)
					1989–1996	3.5[a] (1.0; 6.0)
					1996–2011	0.7[a] (0.2; 1.2)
Russian Federation	9 419	66 463 516	17.5	1980–2010	1980–2000	2.4[a] (2.3; 2.6)
					2000–2010	3.4[a] (3.0; 3.8)
Slovakia	508	2 630 483	23.0	1992–2010	1992–1998	5.6[a] (3.0; 8.3)
					1998–2010	–1.4[a] (–2.1; –0.6)

CI confidence interval
[a]Statistically significant

Table 3 Summary of recent declines in national prostate mortality in Europe: year which the downturn was first observed and the estimated annual per cent change (EAPC)

Country	Year decline identified	EAPC CI (95 %)
Northern Europe		
Denmark	2001	−1.2[a] (−1.7; −0.6)
Finland	1998	−2.7[a](−3.2; −2.3)
Iceland	1992	−1.8[a] (−3.3; 0.3)
Ireland	1997	−2.1[a] (−2.9; −1.3)
Norway	1997	−2.3[a] (−2.6; −1.9)
Sweden	1999	−2.0[a] (−2.4; −1.6)
UK, England and Wales	1992	−1.3[a] (−1.5; −1.1)
UK, Northern Ireland	1997	−1.4[a] (−2.5; −0.3)
UK, Scotland	1994	−1.1[a] (−1.4; −0.7)
Western Europe		
Austria	1992	−0.6 (−2.0; 0.7)
France	1990	−1.8[a] (−2.1; −1.6)
Germany	1995	−2.9[a] (−3.2; −2.6)
Netherlands	1995	−2.4[a] (−2.6; −2.3)
Switzerland	1990	−2.8[a] (−3.2; −2.4)
Southern Europe		
Croatia	2005	−0.4 (−1.8; 0.9)
Greece	2007	−4.6[a] (−7.2; −2.0)
Italy	1993	−1.1[a] (−1.6; −0.7)
Malta	1994	−3.9[a] (−5.5; −2.3)
Portugal	1998	−2.2[a] (−4.1; −0.2)
Spain	1998	−3.4[a] (−3.8; −3.0)
Eastern Europe		
Czech Republic	2004	−8.0[a] (−14.0; −1.7)
Hungary	1996	−2.9[a] (−3.3; −2.5)
Poland	2001	−0.8[a] (−1.5; −0.2)
Slovakia	1998	−1.4[a] (−2.1; −0.6)

CI confidence interval
[a]Statistically significant

Lastly, Table 3 indicates the 24 countries where prostate cancer mortality rates have declined, the year the downturn began and the extent of the decrease per annum. The first declines in prostate cancer mortality rates were seen in France and Switzerland in 1990, while the latest are observed in Greece in 2007, but in most countries rates began to fall during the mid- to late-1990s. There was considerable variability in the timing and order of magnitude of the year-on-year decreases, varying from approximately 0.6 % in Austria (from 1992) to 4–8 % for the quite recent declines observed in the Czech Republic and Greece.

2.4 Key Determinants of the Cancer Burden

Towards one-quarter (22 %) of all cancers diagnosed in men in Europe today are cancers of the prostate, compared with 11 % estimated in 1995 [5]. While the true impact of prostate cancer screening can be only evaluated indirectly, incidence rates are clearly heavily influenced by the radical changes in diagnostic capabilities and practice over the last decades. The increasing rates in European men can be partly attributed to TURP in the 1970s and 1980s, while the more marked upsurge in incidence over the last 15–20 years (as identified in many countries via the joinpoint analyses) can be largely attributed to the greater use of PSA testing and subsequent biopsy. The initial rise in PSA testing in the late 1980s, closely followed by increasing prostate cancer incidence rates, has been clearly demonstrated in the Nordic countries [24]; given the consistent observation of increases in incidence in European countries – ranging from 3 to 10 % per annum from the early to mid-1900s – it is likely that such practices have prevailed in all regions of Europe. Of note are the recent accelerations in the historically lower rates observed in Southern and Eastern Europe, including Croatia, Slovenia, the Czech Republic and Slovakia.

There is little correlation between incidence and mortality rates in different European populations, nor in the evolution in trends in the last 15 years. Where observable, the slow and steady increases in prostate cancer mortality in the 1970s and 1980s have been replaced uniformly by declining mortality rates that are now apparent in 24 countries in Europe, with only the Baltic countries, where mortality rates are stable or rising, the clear exception. The underlying reasons for the fall in mortality across Europe are likely to imitate those conjectured in the USA, at least in part; Brawley [5] has noted possible explanations for the rate declines since 1991 in the USA that include an effect of screening and treatment, changes in the attribution of cause of death, or improved treatment resulting in a genuine postponement of death for some men with metastatic disease. Ecologic studies have revealed that declines in prostate cancer mortality rates are seen too early to be solely attributed to PSA testing; some have postulated they may be the result of improving treatment of both localised and high-risk disease [18]. The extent to which underlying changes in the prevalence and distribution of risk factors contribute to these trends remains largely unexplored and unknown.

Still, incidence varies tenfold and detectable falls in incidence have occurred recently in many higher-income countries, particularly in Northern and Western Europe. The changing but persistent influence of PSA on incidence relates to the perceptions and practices of health-care professionals regarding its utility as a prognostic test as well as public awareness of the controversy surrounding prostate cancer screening; in France, public perceptions of screening have been observed to vary by age and socioeconomic status [20]. The evidence of the benefits and harms of screening have become increasingly evident, as has the question of whether PSA can reduce prostate cancer mortality via the European Randomised Study of Screening for Prostate Cancer (ERSPC) trial. Schroder et al. [32] have reported a 22 and 21 % risk reduction from PSA screening at 11 or 13 years of follow-up, respectively, although in absolute terms, one death from prostate cancer was prevented for every 781 men invited for screening at 13 years follow-up. With three-fifths of screen-detected cancers in the ERSPC trial classified as low risk, experts have stressed that decision-making must be informed by tools that are able to stratify risk of low or high grade cancers on biopsy; the extent to which the trial findings will influence PSA testing practices and PSA screening awareness in Europe will reveal itself in the temporal patterns of prostate cancer incidence in due course.

2.5 Caveats in Interpretation

There are several points of caution we should note in the above analysis linked to the availability and quality of the data sources and the methods applied. GLOBOCAN was utilised to present cancer incidence and mortality maps for 2012 worldwide and for Europe. These are estimates that rely upon the best available data on cancer incidence and mortality in a given country. In Europe, the methods used to estimate national rates involve projections of recent trends, where annual data are available prior to 2012 [17]. Incidence data derive from population-based cancer registries which may cover national populations or subnational areas; estimates in France, Spain and Italy are all based on national estimates based on regional rather than national coverage, for example. An aggregation of regional registry datasets was required, assuming that the pertaining cancer registries collectively represented national patterns and trends. Where no recorded incidence data were available or when they were considered to be lacking sufficient quality, as was the case in nine countries in Europe including Greece, Hungary and Romania, modelled estimates were derived by applying available national mortality to regional data from other countries. In Europe, almost all countries have national mortality data through death registration systems compiled in the WHO mortality database, the exceptions being Bosnia Herzegovina and Montenegro.

To further compare patterns and trends in prostate cancer in Europe, we focussed on 32 countries, predominantly with high quality incidence and mortality, the former measure based mainly on registries included in the recent volumes of the *Cancer Incidence in Five Continents* (CI5) series. Those compiled in these volumes have been assessed as having high quality incidence data following a peer-reviewed assessment of their comparability, completeness and accuracy; yet for a number of countries – including Germany, Italy and Spain – regional registries are used to convey national profiles. These regional proxies may be more or less representative in certain countries than others. Given the difficulties in interpreting contemporary rates of prostate cancer incidence and mortality in Europe, comparative data on PSA use, treatment modalities and stage information may have provided insight, but were not available.

One methodological shortcoming is the use of joinpoint regression [23]. Quantification of the trends within linear segments can be unduly influenced by the last data points, while joinpoints and arbitrary slopes are sometimes identified by the regression where the underlying data are subject to substantial random variation. The technique is, however, particularly suitable for prostate cancer, permitting, in this chapter, quantification of the rather abrupt linear trends in incidence and mortality in Europe over time.

3 Epidemiology and the Prospects for Prevention

This chapter closes with a review of the epidemiology of prostate cancer and by extension, the potential to reduce the burden via removal or reduction of the causes of the disease through primary prevention strategies. The first thing to note is that, for a disease as prevalent and incident as prostate cancer, relatively little is known about its exact aetiology. Convincing evidence has been produced for only a few risk factors: ageing, genetic predisposition, ethnicity and body fatness. Numerous scientific papers have suggested a long list of other risk factors, of which those most intensely investigated will be reported in this section. Results of these studies are quite inconsistent which makes any definitive conclusions difficult. Apart from the general problems in observational studies on risk factors for disease, in prostate cancer the definition of the disease is arbitrary. Because of the large impact of PSA testing on prostate cancer incidence and the differences between indolent and potentially lethal prostate cancers, epidemiological studies should preferably study the latter subgroup of tumours in order to validly identify risk factors for the disease [21].

Ageing

The most well-known risk factor for prostate cancer is ageing, as evidenced by the age-specific incidence rates in the previous paragraphs. Prostate cancer is rarely diagnosed before the age of 45. In most western communities the peak in the incidence rates lies between 65 and 75 years of age. In a recent review of postmortem studies, the estimated mean cancer prevalence in men who died from other causes increased in a nonlinear fashion from 5 % (95 % CI: 3–8 %) at age <30 years to 59 % (95 % CI: 48–71 %) by age >79 years [3]. This underlines one of the greatest dilemmas in prostate cancer diagnostics nowadays: most men who have prostate cancer will die with the disease, not from the disease. The pivotal issue of research in prostate cancer is the identification of discriminative tests that can accurately predict invalidating and lethal prostate cancer.

Family History and Genetics

Besides age, a positive family history of prostate cancer is the most well-established risk factor for prostate cancer. First-degree relatives of affected men carry a two- to threefold increased risk of being diagnosed with the disease themselves. It is estimated that 5–10 % of prostate cancers have a true genetic cause. But the identification of the genes underlying these Mendelian forms of prostate cancer has appeared to be much more problematic than in, for example, breast cancer. Apparently, familial prostate cancer is a far more heterogeneous disease with contributions from many more genetic loci than familial breast cancer [28]. Mutations in the few high-penetrance genes are so rare that testing in families with hereditary prostate cancer, that is, families with three or more first-degree relatives (or 2 first-degree relatives of young age) with prostate cancer [8] is not useful, possibly with the exception of two genes: *BRCA2* and *HOXB13*. Male carriers of a *BRCA2* mutation have a two- to sixfold increased risk of prostate cancer, occurring earlier in life and with a more aggressive phenotype. The G84E (rs138213197) mutation in *HOXB13* is something like a middle-penetrance mutation with a quite high population frequency of about 0.1–1.3 % and a fairly high risk ratio of 3.5–7 for prostate cancer [21, 25]. More and more clinical genetics centres around the world are starting to test for these genes in men at increased prostate cancer risk.

In addition to the handful of high-penetrance genes, since 2007, genome-wide association studies have identified approximately 100 low-penetrance genetic polymorphisms (single nucleotide polymorphisms – SNPs) that are associated with an increased risk of prostate cancer [28]. Some of these SNPs are in or near genes, for example, the *HNF1B* gene, the *KLK3* gene (PSA) and the *MSMB* gene, but many if not most are in intergenic regions with unknown functions. The 8q24 region is a good example of the latter type, containing multiple SNPs that are significantly associated with prostate cancer and other cancer types. Because of the design of the GWAS studies, the prevalence of these SNPs in the population is high. The direct consequence, however, is that their effect is weak: typically, odds ratios of 1.1–1.3 are found. Using combinations of SNPs, polygenic risk scores are being developed to aid in predicting the individual risk of prostate cancer. With such scores, it is possible to discriminate men with a very high or a very low risk Table 4 [1]. The problem, however, is that the proportion of men with a clinically relevant increased risk is still quite small while all men have to be genotyped to identify this small group. The challenge is how to counsel the men who are not in the highest risk category. Nevertheless, at some point in the near future, such polygenic risk scores will probably be used to individualise population screening programmes for prostate cancer.

Recently, it has been shown that the prevalence of low-penetrance SNPs is about the same, or a little bit higher, in patients from hereditary prostate cancer families as in patients from the general population [13]. This may be interpreted as evidence that the clustering of such SNPs rather than high-penetrance genes may cause a clustering of patients in families. The alternative explanation is, however, that so-called hereditary prostate cancer families are not strongly genetically determined but merely the result of increased awareness and PSA testing of men in such families. The finding that prostate cancer patients in these families have a better prognosis than patients from the general population supports this alternative explanation [12]. This emphasises the importance of considering the aggressiveness and method of diagnosis of prostate cancers in families before deciding that unaffected men in these families should be tested in order to avoid overdiagnosis.

Ethnicity

As shown in the previous section on incidence, enormous differences in prostate cancer incidence exist between ethnic populations. The lowest incidence is found in men of Asian descent, whereas men who live in North America and Northern

Table 4 Estimation of a Polygenic Risk Score (PRS) using 100 prostate cancer risk variants and comparison of risk by PRS percentiles (iCOGS data)

Percentiles (%)	OR (using PRS)	OR (using iCOGS)
<1	1 (baseline)	0.19 (0.13–0.27)
1–10	1.68 (1.13–2.50)	0.31 (0.28–0.35)
10–25	2.78 (1.88–4.10)	0.52 (0.48–0.55)
25–75	5.39 (3.67–7.92)	1 (baseline)
75–90	9.57 (6.50–14.09)	1.78 (1.68–1.88)
90–99	15.78 (10.71–23.26)	2.93 (2.75–3.12)
≥99	30.47 (20.14–46.09)	5.65 (4.83–6.62)

Europe have a very high prostate cancer risk. Particularly men of African-American heritage have a very high risk of prostate cancer. Ethnic differences are most probably caused by a combination of genetic factors, exposure to environmental risk factors and factors related to health-seeking behaviour. This is illustrated most clearly by the results of migration studies, which looked at prostate cancer incidence trends in Asian men (low incidence) who migrated to the USA (high incidence); prostate cancer incidence in these men increased markedly and significantly, but to a level that was intermediate between the incidence in the Japanese and the original American population [11]. A similar phenomenon was found for Japanese men who emigrated to Brazil [20].

Diet

It has long been thought that diet is an important factor in the development and progression of prostate cancer. And it probably is, considering the observation that second and following generation migrants adopt the risks of their new countries, combined with the fact that there are no other lifestyle factors that can easily explain this observation. The paradox here is that the strongest evidence for the role of diet comes from the weakest study designs, such as migrant studies. Designs that are supposedly stronger such as prospective cohort studies and randomised trials have yielded inconsistent results. A clear example of this is the SELECT trial (Selenium and Vitamin E Cancer Prevention Trial) [25]. This large prospective trial, in which 31,000 men were included, studied the effect of vitamin E, selenium, and the combination of both vs. placebo. No effect on prostate cancer incidence was found for administering selenium, either alone or in combination. This refuted the result found in the Nutrition Prevention of Cancer (NPS) trial [15], which observed a 50 % reduction in prostate cancer incidence in men randomised to selenium supplements. The Continuous Update Program of the World Cancer Research Fund brings expert nutritional epidemiologists together from around the globe and continuously reviews the literature on diet and cancer in a meticulous way. It concluded in 2014 that there is no diet or nutritional factor that is convincingly or probably associated with prostate cancer [36] (http://www.wcrf.org/int/research-we-fund/continuous-update-project-findings-reports/prostate-cancer). On the contrary, the CUP project concludes that there is strong evidence that beta-carotene, either through food or supplements, is unlikely to have a substantial risk on the risk of prostate cancer. So, the numerous studies on dietary fats, red and processed meat, vitamin E, selenium, lycopene, cruciferous vegetables, green tea, tomato products and many other nutritional factors have not resulted in any clarity about the role of diet in prostate cancer. The recent report [36] specifically concludes that:

- The evidence that a higher consumption of dairy products increases the risk of prostate cancer is limited.
- The evidence that diets high in calcium increase the risk of prostate cancer is limited.
- The evidence that low plasma alpha-tocopherol concentration (vitamin E) increases the risk of prostate cancer is limited.
- The evidence that low plasma (blood) selenium concentrations increases risk of prostate cancer is limited.

One has to question, however, whether the best designs to study aetiology are really the best designs in the field of nutritional epidemiology. For example, most randomised trials on supplements and cohort studies on nutritional factors start with study populations over 50 years of age. If diet has its most important effect in puberty or even earlier in childhood or pre-conception, these designs will not be able to validly assess any effect. Other problems have to do with misclassification of food intake over the years, variable within-person eating habits, arbitrary dosages of interventions in trials and so forth. Possibly, the weakest study designs (ecological migrant studies) are the best when it comes to nutritional epidemiology. Unfortunately, these designs cannot come up with any specific conclusion beyond typical diets in certain parts of the world.

Body Fatness

In its 2014 report on prostate cancer, the World Cancer Research Fund concludes that greater body fatness (marked by BMI, waist circumference and waist-hip ratio) is probably a cause of advanced prostate cancer. In a meta-analysis of 23 studies ($N=11,149$) on advanced prostate cancer, a statistically significant 8 % increased risk was found per 5 kg/m2 increase in body mass index (BMI) [36]. A meta-analysis of four studies on waist circumference ($N=1,781$) showed a statistically significant 12 % increased risk per 10 cm and a meta-analysis of 4 studies on waist-hip ratio resulted in a significant 15 % higher risk per 0.1 unit increase. It is not entirely clear what the mechanism is behind this association. Obesity influences the levels of quite a few hormones and growth factors such as insulin and leptin, which can promote the growth of cancer cells. In men, obesity is associated with lower testosterone levels, although the importance of this is not really clear. Serum testosterone levels do not seem to have a strong effect on prostate cancer risk but because it is essential for differentiation of prostate epithelium, decreased levels may facilitate the growth of a less differentiated, aggressive prostate cancer phenotype. Obesity is also associated with a low-grade chronic inflammatory state which can promote cancer development. Obese adipose tissue is characterised by macrophage infiltration, an important source of inflammation. Fat cells produce pro-inflammatory factors, leading to elevated concentrations of circulating TNF-alpha, IL-6 and CRP.

Adult Attained Height

In a meta-analysis of 34 studies ($N=79,387$), the WCRF report found a statistically significant 4 % increased risk per 5 cm taller height: RR 1.04 (95 % CI 1.03–1.05). Adult height is related to the rate of growth during foetal life and childhood. Health and nutrition status in the neonatal period and childhood may impact on the age of sexual maturity. Resulting effects on circulating levels of growth factors, insulin, and other endocrine or tissue specific mediators may influence cancer risk.

Diabetes

Most data on the association between diabetes and prostate cancer come from studies on diabetes type 2. The results from epidemiological studies are somewhat inconsistent but, overall, there seems to be a reduced risk [30]. This contradicts the finding that body fatness is a risk factor for prostate cancer. Because the link between diabetes type 2 and prostate cancer is mainly observed in studies from the PSA era, diabetes is known to decrease the serum PSA value, and the association is stronger for low-grade than for high-grade prostate cancer; it is possible that the association is caused by detection bias. In addition, it is extremely difficult to disentangle the effects of diabetes and its treatment.

In a recent cohort study using five nationwide registers of persons with type 1 diabetes (Australia, Denmark, Finland, Scotland and Sweden), 553 prostate cancers were diagnosed among 2 million male person-years of follow-up. A reduced risk of prostate cancer was found ($HR=0.56$; 95 % CI 0.51–0.61) [7].

Androgens

Because the function of the prostate is so dependent on androgens and because hormonal treatment is used in metastasised prostate cancer, it has long been believed that having higher levels of testosterone in the blood may increase the risk of prostate cancer. And indeed, clinical trials with 5-alpha reductase inhibitors (5-ARIs), the Prostate Cancer Prevention Trial (PCPT), in which men were treated with finasteride 5 mg daily or placebo for 7 years, and the REduction by DUtasteride of prostate Cancer Events (REDUCE) trial, in which patients were treated with dutasteride 0.5 mg daily or placebo for 4 years [2, 34] suggested a decrease in risk (see Chapter 2 by Bertrand Tombal). However, the results of these trials may have been influenced by several factors such as end-of-study biopsies. In the non-trial situation, a link between androgens and prostate cancer development is not clear [31]. Recently, a large prospective study from Finland, Sweden and Norway confirmed the absence of an association between prediagnostic serum testosterone levels and prostate cancer development [27]. More research is needed to clarify the link between diabetes and prostate cancer.

Vasectomy
Several recent meta-analyses of the association between vasectomy and prostate cancer have concluded that there is no link between the two (e.g. [37]). US-based studies found a positive association (RR = 1.54) but non-USA studies did not (RR = 0.74). Probably, some studies that did find a positive association have suffered from bias due to differences in health-seeking behaviour by vasectomised and non-vasectomised men.

Aspirin
There is some evidence in the literature that aspirin and other NSAIDS slightly reduce the risk of prostate cancer. However, a recent analysis of the Health Professionals Follow-up Study among 48,000 men did not find any effect of regular aspirin use on prostate cancer risk [6].

Physical Activity
It is not clear whether being more physically active reduces the risk of prostate cancer. A review and meta-analysis of 43 studies did report a decreased risk (pooled RR = 0.90; 95 % CI 0.84–0.95) but because many low-quality studies were included, a definitive conclusion is impossible [26].

Prostatitis
Despite the fact that a definitive causative infectious agent or agents has yet to be identified, accumulating evidence both in human studies and in animal models indicate that infections may contribute to potentially tumour-promoting chronic prostatic inflammation [33].

In conclusion, because ageing, genetic predisposition and ethnicity are not modifiable, until harder evidence becomes available on other suspected risk factors, maintaining a healthy weight is the only lifestyle factor that can lower the risk of prostate cancer.

Acknowledgements We thank Mathieu Laversanne for development of the tables and figures included in this chapter.

References

1. Al Olama AA. A meta-analysis of 87,040 individuals identifies 23 new susceptibility loci for prostate cancer. Nat Genet. 2014;46(10):1103–9.
2. Andriole GL, Bostwick DG, Brawley OW, et al. Effect of dutasteride on the risk of prostate cancer. N Engl J Med. 2010;362(13):1192–202.
3. Bell KJ, Del Mar C, Wright G, Dickinson J, Glasziou P. Prevalence of incidental prostate cancer: a systematic review of autopsy studies. Int J Cancer. 2015;137:1749–57.
4. Bray F, Ferlay J, Laversanne M, Brewster DH, Gombe Mbalawa C, Kohler B, Piñeros M, Steliarova-Foucher E, Swaminathan R, Antoni S, Soerjomataram I, Forman D. Cancer incidence in five continents: inclusion criteria, highlights from volume X and the global status of cancer registration. Int J Cancer. 2015;137(9):2060–71.
5. Brawley OW. Trends in prostate cancer in the United States. J Natl Cancer Inst Monogr. 2012;2012(45):152–6.
6. Cao Y, Nishihara R, Wu K, Wang M, Ogino S, Willett WC, Spiegelman D, Fuchs CS, Giovannucci EL, Chan AT. Population-wide impact of long-term use of aspirin and the risk for cancer. JAMA Oncol. 2016;2:762–9. doi:10.1001/jamaoncol.2015.6396.
7. Carstensen B, Read SH, Friis S, Sund R, Keskimäki I, Svensson AM, Ljung R, Wild SH, Kerssens JJ, Harding JL, Magliano DJ, Gudbjörnsdottir S, Diabetes and Cancer Research Consortium. Cancer incidence in persons with type 1 diabetes: a five-country study of 9,000 cancers in type 1 diabetic individuals. Diabetologia. 2016;59(5):980–8. [Epub ahead of print].
8. Carter BS, Bova GS, Beaty TH, et al. Hereditary prostate cancer: epidemiologic and clinical features. J Urol. 1993;150(3):797–802.
9. Center MM, Jemal A, Lortet-Tieulent J, Ward E, Ferlay J, Brawley O, Bray F. International variation in prostate cancer incidence and mortality rates. Eur Urol. 2012;61(6):1079–92.

10. Chokunonga E, Borok MZ, Chirenje ZM, Nyakabau AM, Parkin DM. Trends in the incidence of cancer in the black population of Harare, Zimbabwe 1991–2010. Int J Cancer. 2013;133(3):721–9.
11. Cook LS, Goldoft M, Schwartz SM, et al. Incidence of adenocarcinoma of the prostate in Asian immigrants to the United States and their descendants. J Urol. 1999;161(1):152–5.
12. Cremers RG, Aben KK, Van Oort IM, Sedelaar JP, Vasen HF, Vermeulen SH, Kiemeney LA. The clinical phenotype of hereditary versus sporadic prostate cancer: HPC definition revisited. Prostate. 2016;76(10):897–904. doi:10.1002/pros.23179. [Epub ahead of print].
13. Cremers RG, Galesloot TE, Aben KK, van Oort IM, Vasen HF, Vermeulen SH, Kiemeney LA. Known susceptibility SNPs for sporadic prostate cancer show a similar association with "hereditary" prostate cancer. Prostate. 2015;75(5):474–83.
14. Doll R, Payne P, Waterhouse J. Cancer incidence in five continents: a technical report. New York: UICC/ Springer; 1966.
15. Duffield-Lillico AJ, Dalkin BL, Reid ME, et al. Selenium supplementation, baseline plasma selenium status and incidence of prostate cancer: an analysis of the complete treatment period of the Nutritional Prevention of Cancer Trial. BJU Int. 2003;91(7):608–12.
16. Ferlay J, Soerjomataram I, Dikshit R, Eser S, Mathers C, Rebelo M, Parkin DM, Forman D, Bray F. Cancer incidence and mortality worldwide: sources, methods and major patterns in GLOBOCAN 2012. Int J Cancer. 2015;136(5):E359–86.
17. Feletto E, Bang A, Cole-Clark D, Chalasani V, Rasiah K, Smith DP. An examination of prostate cancer trends in Australia, England, Canada and USA: Is the Australian death rate too high? World J Urol. 2015 Nov;33(11):1677-87. doi:10.1007/s00345-015-1514-7. PubMed PMID: 25698456; PubMed Central PMCID:PMC4617845.
18. Ferlay J, Steliarova-Foucher E, Lortet-Tieulent J, Rosso S, Coebergh JW, Comber H, Forman D, Bray F. Cancer incidence and mortality patterns in Europe: estimates for 40 countries in 2012. Eur J Cancer. 2013;49(6):1374–403.
19. Eisinger F, Morère JF, Touboul C, Pivot X, Coscas Y, Blay JY, Lhomel C, Viguier J. Prostate cancer screening: contrasting trends. Cancer Causes Control. 2015 Jun;26(6):949-52. doi: 10.1007/s10552-015-0573-9. PubMed PMID: 25822574.
20. Gudmundsson J, Sulem P, Gudbjartsson DF, Masson G, Agnarsson BA, Benediktsdottir KR, Sigurdsson A, Magnusson OT, Gudjonsson SA, Magnusdottir DN, Johannsdottir H, Helgadottir HT, Stacey SN, Jonasdottir A, Olafsdottir SB, Thorleifsson G, Jonasson JG, Tryggvadottir L, Navarrete S, Fuertes F, Helfand BT, Hu Q, Csiki IE, Mates IN, Jinga V, Aben KK, van Oort IM, Vermeulen SH, Donovan JL, Hamdy FC, Ng CF, Chiu PK, Lau KM, Ng MC, Gulcher JR, Kong A, Catalona WJ, Mayordomo JI, Einarsson GV, Barkardottir RB, Jonsson E, Mates D, Neal DE, Kiemeney LA, Thorsteinsdottir U, Rafnar T, Stefansson K. A study based on whole-genome sequencing yields a rare variant at 8q24 associated with prostate cancer. Nat Genet. 2012;44(12):1326–9. doi:10.1038/ng.2437. Epub 2012 Oct 28.
21. Hankey BF, Feuer EJ, Clegg LX, Hayes RB, Legler JM, Prorok PC, et al. Cancer surveillance series: interpreting trends in prostate cancer--part I: evidence of the effects of screening in recent prostate cancer incidence. J Natl Cancer Inst. 1999;91(12):1017–24.
22. Iwasaki M, Mameri CP, Hamada GS, et al. Secular trends in cancer mortality among Japanese immigrants in the state of Sao Paulo, Brazil, 1979–2001. Eur J Cancer Prev. 2008;17(1):1–8.
23. Jahn JL, Giovannucci EL, Stampfer MJ. The high prevalence of undiagnosed prostate cancer at autopsy: implications for epidemiology and treatment of prostate cancer in the Prostate-specific Antigen-era. Int J Cancer. 2015;137(12):2795–802. doi:10.1002/ijc.29408. Epub 2015 Jan 8. Review.
24. Karlsson R, Aly M, Clements M, Zheng L, Adolfsson J, Xu J, Grönberg H, Wiklund F. A population-based assessment of germline HOXB13 G84E mutation and prostate cancer risk. Eur Urol. 2014;65:169–76.
25. Kim HJ, Fay MP, Feuer EJ, Midthune DN. Permutation tests for joinpoint regression with applications to cancer rates. Stat Med. 2000;19(3):335–51.
26. Kvåle R, Auvinen A, Adami HO, Klint A, Hernes E, Møller B, Pukkala E, Storm HH, Tryggvadottir L, Tretli S, Wahlqvist R, Weiderpass E, Bray F. Interpreting trends in prostate cancer incidence and mortality in the five Nordic countries. J Natl Cancer Inst. 2007;99(24):1881–7.
27. Lippman SM, Klein EA, Goodman PJ, et al. Effect of selenium and vitamin E on risk of prostate cancer and other cancers: the Selenium and Vitamin E Cancer Prevention Trial (SELECT). JAMA. 2009;301(1):39–51.
28. Liu Y, Hu F, Li D, Wang F, Zhu L, Chen W, Ge J, An R, Zhao Y. Does physical activity reduce the risk of prostate cancer? A systematic review and meta-analysis. Eur Urol. 2011;60:1029–44.
29. Lumme S, Tenkanen L, Langseth H, Gislefoss R, Hakama M, Stattin P, Hallmans G, Adlercreutz H, Saikku P, Stenman UH, Tuohimaa P, Luostarinen T, Dillner J. Longitudinal biobanks-based study on the joint effects of infections, nutrition and hormones on risk of prostate cancer. Acta Oncol. 2016;15:1–7. [Epub ahead of print].
30. Lynch HT, Kosoko-Lasaki O, Leslie SW, Rendell M, Shaw T, Snyder C, D'Amico AV, Buxbaum S, Isaacs WB, Loeb S, Moul JW, Powell I. Screening for familial and hereditary prostate cancer. Int J Cancer. 2016;138:2579–91.
31. Parkin DM, Bray F, Ferlay J, Jemal A. Cancer in Africa 2012. Cancer Epidemiol Biomarkers Prev. 2014;23(6):953–66. doi:10.1158/1055-9965.EPI-14-0281.
32. Pierce BL. Why are diabetics at reduced risk for prostate cancer? A review of the epidemiologic evidence. Urol Oncol. 2012;30:735–43.

33. Roddam AW, Allen NE, Appleby P, Key TJ, Endogenous Hormones and Prostate Cancer Collaborative Group. Endogenous sex hormones and prostate cancer: a collaborative analysis of 18 prospective studies. J Natl Cancer Inst. 2008;100:170–83.
34. Schröder FH, Hugosson J, Roobol MJ, Tammela TL, Zappa M, Nelen V, Kwiatkowski M, Lujan M, Määttänen L, Lilja H, Denis LJ, Recker F, Paez A, Bangma CH, Carlsson S, Puliti D, Villers A, Rebillard X, Hakama M, Stenman UH, Kujala P, Taari K, Aus G, Huber A, Van der Kwast TH, Van Schaik RH, de Koning HJ, Moss SM, Auvinen A, ERSPC Investigators. Screening and prostate cancer mortality: results of the European Randomised Study of Screening for Prostate Cancer (ERSPC) at 13 years of follow-up. Lancet. 2014;384(9959):2027–35.
35. Sfanos KS, Isaacs WB, De Marzo AM. Infections and inflammation in prostate cancer. Am J Clin Exp Urol. 2013;1(1):3–11.
36. Thompson IM, Goodman PJ, Tangen CM, et al. The influence of finasteride on the development of prostate cancer. N Engl J Med. 2003;349(3):215–24.
37. Wabinga HR, Nambooze S, Amulen PM, Okello C, Mbus L, Parkin DM. Trends in the incidence of cancer in Kampala, Uganda 1991–2010. Int J Cancer. 2014;135(2):432–9. doi:10.1002/ijc.28661. Epub 2014 Feb 27.
38. WCRF. http://www.wcrf.org/sites/default/files/Prostate-Cancer-2014-Report.pdf. 2014.
39. Zhang XL, Yan JJ, Pan SH, Pan JG, Ying XR, Zhang GF. Vasectomy and the risk of prostate cancer: a meta-analysis of cohort studies. Int J Clin Exp Med. 2015;8(10):17977–85. eCollection 2015.
40. Zhou CK, Check DP, Lortet-Tieulent J, Laversanne M, Jemal A, Ferlay J, Bray F, Cook MB, Devesa SS. Prostate cancer incidence in 43 populations worldwide: an analysis of time trends overall and by age group. Int J Cancer. 2016;138(6):1388–400.

Chemoprevention

Antonino Battaglia, Thomas Van de Broeck, Lisa Moris, Lorenzo Tosco, Wouter Everaerts, Maarten Albersen, Frank Claessens, Gert De Meerleer, Hendrik Van Poppel, Paolo Gontero, Daimantas Milonas, and Steven Joniau

1 Introduction

There is strong interest in prostate cancer (PCa) in the field of cancer chemoprevention because of its slow development which can be used to stratify the disease at different steps of carcinogenesis, offering different targets for chemoprevention. Although the clinical presentation of PCa is heterogeneous, a considerable number of tumors remain indolent [1]. Even clinically significant prostate tumors progress slowly compared to other types of cancer (such as pancreatic cancer or small-cell lung carcinoma) [3]. Thus, the EAU Prostate Cancer Guidelines recommend that curative therapy should only be offered when a patient is expected to live more than 10 years [2]. The ideal preventive therapy would prevent cancer development or slow progression in such a way that active therapy would no longer be necessary. There are geographical differences in PCa

A. Battaglia
Department of University Urology, Città della Salute e della Scienza – Molinette, Turin, Italy

Department of Development and Regeneration, University Hospitals Leuven, Urology, Leuven, Belgium

T. Van de Broeck • L. Moris
Department of Development and Regeneration, University Hospitals Leuven, Urology, Leuven, Belgium

KU Leuven, Laboratory of Molecular Endocrinology, Leuven, Belgium

L. Tosco
Department of Development and Regeneration, University Hospitals Leuven, Urology, Leuven, Belgium

KU Leuven, Nuclear Medicine and Molecular Imaging, Leuven, Belgium

W. Everaerts • M. Albersen • H. Van Poppel
Department of Development and Regeneration, University Hospitals Leuven, Urology, Leuven, Belgium

F. Claessens
KU Leuven, Laboratory of Molecular Endocrinology, Leuven, Belgium

G. De Meerleer
Department of Oncology, University Hospitals Leuven, Radiation Oncology, Leuven, Belgium

P. Gontero
Department of University Urology, Città della Salute e della Scienza – Molinette, Turin, Italy

D. Milonas
Department of Urology, Lithuanian Health Science University, Eiveniu 2, 50009 Kaunas, Lithuania

Department of Urology, Hospital of Lithuanian University of Health Sciences Kauno Klinikos, Kaunas, Lithuania

S. Joniau (✉)
Department of Development and Regeneration, University Hospitals Leuven, Urology, Leuven, Belgium
e-mail: steven.joniau@uzleuven.be

M. Bolla, H. van Poppel (eds.), *Management of Prostate Cancer*,
DOI 10.1007/978-3-319-42769-0_2

incidence and mortality, with a higher risk in Western countries (e.g., North America) when compared to Eastern countries (e.g., Japan). However, when a Japanese man moves to the USA and adopts a Western lifestyle, his PCa phenotype reflects that of an American man. This has led to the hypothesis that not only genetic background but also environment can influence prostate carcinogenesis. The air that we breathe, the work that we do, and the food that we choose to eat everyday could all potentially play roles in prostate carcinogenesis. Although no definitive proof is currently available regarding the protective effect of any specific dietary factors, investigating the use of dietary supplements remains an attractive option. Currently no dietary or lifestyle elements are known to influence the risk of developing PCa. Another strategy in preventive medicine is to target the prostate on a molecular level. Prostate development and carcinogenesis are both driven by androgens activating the androgen receptor, causing it to be the most studied target for prevention. Chronic inflammation, which is an immune response to perturbed tissue homeostasis, seems to also play an important role in general carcinogenesis. Thus, aspirin and other anti-oxidizing agents have been investigated as promising candidates for chemoprevention. In this chapter we will discuss the development and preventive effects of natural elements, drugs, and dietary lifestyle. Unfortunately, data are often inconclusive or conflicting. Nevertheless, evidence shows that chemoprevention is a possible concept.

2 What We Learned from the SELECT (Table 1)

Selenium is a nutritionally essential mineral that enters the food from the soil. Therefore, selenium concentrations can vary based on the selenium content of the soil. The richest sources are nuts, eggs, fish, cereals, and cruciferous vegetables. The recommended dietary allowance (RDA) for selenium is 55 μg/day [4].

Vitamin E is a group of elements that includes tocopherols, with α-tocopherol being the most biologically active form in this group. The recommended daily intake is 15 mg/day for adults. Vitamin E is found in different types of oils (sunflower, almond, wheat germ, palm, and olive), vegetables (spinach, beet greens, avocados, broccoli), and butter.

The Selenium and Vitamin E Cancer Prevention Trial (SELECT) represents one of the largest cancer chemoprevention trials conducted to date [5]. The SELECT was based on the results of two previous trials (Nutritional Prevention of Cancer (NPC) [6] and Alpha-Tocopherol, Beta-Carotene Cancer Prevention (ATBC) [7]) reporting a reduction in PCa with the use of vitamin E (α-tocopherol) and selenium.

The SELECT was a phase 3, four-arm, randomized, placebo-controlled trial comparing selenium (200 μg/day), vitamin E (400 IU/day), selenium + vitamin E, and placebo to determinate whether one or both of these substances can help prevent PCa when taken as dietary supplements. Patient inclusion started in July 2001, enrolling 35,533 men from 427 different centers, with a follow-up until October 2008, which was later extended to 2011. The inclusion criteria were ≥50 years of age for African Americans and >55 years of age for all other men, no previous diagnosis of PCa, prostate-specific antigen (PSA) baseline ≤4 ng/mL, and a normal digital rectal examination (DRE). The trial had a first median overall follow-up of 5.46 years and 5.1 % loss to follow-up. The primary end point was the incidence of PCa. The trial found no evidence of a benefit of using selenium or vitamin E at the testes with doses and formulations among the four groups with a significant rate. The hazard ratio was 1.13 (99 % confident interval (CI), 0.95–1.35) in the vitamin E group, 1.04 (99 % CI, 0.87–1.24) in the selenium group, and 1.05 (99 % CI, 0.88–1.25) in the selenium + vitamin E group, compared to placebo. These results seemed to be in conflict with the results of the ATBC, a trial of the effect of vitamin E and beta-carotene in lung cancer prevention, in which one of the secondary findings was a reduction in the incidence of PCa. The main difference between the SELECT and ATBC trial is that the ATBC trial was not designed to determinate PCa incidence, so this finding could have been introduced by selection bias. Furthermore, the vitamin E dose used in the SELECT was much

Table 1 Role of Selenium and Vitamin E

	Principal sources	Daily recommended intake	Conclusion
Selenium	Nuts, eggs, fish, cereals	55 μg/day	No evidence suggests a chemoprevention role
Vitamin E (α-tocopherol)	Sunflowers, almond, spinach	15 mg/day	Probable role in reducing aggressiveness of PCa Selective role in chemoprevention in smokers (see below)

PCa prostate cancer

higher (400 IU/day) than the dose used in the ATBC trial (50 IU/day). This could be explained by a possible U-shaped response curve with moderate vitamin E levels being protective, but doses at both ends of the spectrum (very high/very low) being deleterious. An update in 2011 [8] extended the analysis of the long-term effect of vitamin E and selenium concluding that the risk of PCa at 7 years is 17% at a dose of 400 IU/day vitamin E, warning against unregulated consumption of easily available products containing a high concentration of multivitamins and supplements in the absence of strong evidence of a demonstrated clinical benefit. After the results of the SELECT became available, several studies were designed to try to explain the failure of the preventive role of selenium and vitamin E in PCa prevention. One such study conducted in 2015 in North Carolina and Louisiana (North Carolina-Louisiana Prostate Cancer Project (PCaP) [9]) tried to show the action of vitamin E at different doses in people diagnosed with PCa, taking into account the ethnic differences between African Americans and European American. Dietary vitamin E was estimated from a food frequency questionnaire, supplement use from questionnaire/inventory, and the concentration of vitamin E from abdominal adipose samples. The chosen doses of vitamin E were 30, 100, 200, 400, 600, or 800 IU/day. The results of this study showed that the intake of vitamin E is inversely associated with PCa aggressiveness in European American men, but this was not significant in African American men too. A Cochrane review published in 2014 [10], including 55 prospective observational studies (including approximately one million participants) and eight randomized controlled trials (RCTs) with a total of 44,000 participants, concluded that there was no evidence suggesting that selenium supplements prevent cancer in humans, although an inverse association was found in some observational studies. The optimal dose for both supplements has not yet been defined, necessitating better clarification of the pathogenic mechanism of selenium and α-tocopherol in prostate cells. Furthermore, which subpopulation may actually benefit from this preventive therapy should be determined.

3 The Role of Vitamin D and IGF-1

In 1990, Schwartz and Hulka [11] described an association between PCa risk and vitamin D deficiency that correlates with age, race, and latitudes. In vitro analyses have shown that vitamin D metabolites 25(OH)D and 1,25(OH)2D may have a chemopreventive effect. Serum vitamin D was examined from the PCPT (Prostate Cancer Prevention Trial) and SELECT. The SELECT [12], a randomized placebo-controlled trial of selenium and vitamin E on PCa risk, showed a linear decrease in the risk of high-grade PCa in African Americans and U-shaped curves in other men. In contrast, PCPT, a double-blind placebo-controlled trial of finasteride for the primary prevention of PCa, showed a linear decrease in the risk of detecting high-grade PCa. Different studies have been conducted, none with a clear scientific relevance on the others. What ultimately emerges is that supplementation with vitamin D must be assessed only if the patient exhibits a deficiency and must be dispensed with attention.

The insulin-like growth factor (IGF) pathway has been shown to play an important role in PCa growth [13]. Increased serum IGF-1 levels are positively associated with an increased risk of PCa. The activation of IGF-1 receptor (IGF-1R) is mandatory for prostate cell proliferation; and inhibitors of this receptor may have therapeutic value with regard to chemoprevention. Metformin (1,1-dimethylbiguanide hydrochloride) is a biguanide drug widely used for the treatment of type 2 diabetes and represents one of the most commonly prescribed oral hypoglycemic agents worldwide [14, 15]. The antitumor mechanism of metformin includes activation of the AMPK/mTOR pathway and direct inhibition of IGF. Because of these possible antitumoral effects, different studies have proposed a role for metformin in the chemoprevention of PCa. One of the first studies to try to establish a role of metformin in the prevention of PCa was the Reduction by Dutasteride of Prostate Cancer Events (REDUCE) study, designed as a randomized clinical trial to compare the effect of dutasteride on PCa diagnosis among men with a negative biopsy. Diabetic patients that did not receive treatment were compared to diabetic patients treated with metformin or another antidiabetic drug. However, no significant association was found between the use of metformin or non-metformin antidiabetic medication and PCa risk [16]. In a meta-analysis conducted by Wu et al. in August 2015 [17] that included six cohort studies and four case-controls studies involving a total of 863,769 patients showed a significant reduction in PCa risk in the cohort studies, but no association in the case-control studies. In population-based studies, metformin seems to be associated with a dose-dependent reduction in PCa risk [18]. More high-quality studies are needed to confirm the role of metformin in PCa chemoprevention.

4 The Unusual Role of the Smoking

Smoking cigarettes is a well-established risk factor for several cancers, even urological cancers such as bladder cancer; but the correlation with PCa is still unclear. The European Prospective Investigation into Cancer and Nutrition (EPIC) study is a large prospective cohort study of 145,112 European men included during 1992–2000 and analyzed during 2004–2008 with a median follow-up of 11.9 years [19]. At the inclusion visit data on smoking status (current, past, or never smoker), a number of cigarettes and average were gathered, as well as information on other diet and lifestyle factors. The results of this study showed that active smokers have a significantly lower risk of PCa than men who have never smoked with a relative risk of 0.90 (95 % CI, 0.83–0.97). This association was shown for localized and low-grade PCa, but not for advanced and high-grade disease. Former smokers (with an exposure of more than 40 years) have an increased risk of advanced PCa compared to men who have never smoked. Furthermore, active smokers have a nonsignificant increased risk of PCa mortality compared to men who have never smoked. Heavy smokers (defined as more than 25 cigarettes/day) have an increased risk of lethal PCa and higher risk of dying from the disease. A potential correlation between supplement use by smokers and the probability of PCa has also been investigated [20]. The Third National Health and Nutrition Examination Survey (NHANES III) was a cross-sectional study performed from 1988 to 1994 that enrolled 33,944 men representing the US population. From this cohort, 1457 men were selected to measure serum levels of sex steroid hormones and α-tocopherol. The authors found an inverse correlation between serum α-tocopherol and circulating sexual hormones such as testosterone, estradiol, and sex hormone-binding globulin (SHBG) in men exposed to cigarettes. Thus, vitamin E may influence sexual hormone production which can provide support for the hypothesis that vitamin E can be a selectively chemopreventive agent for the incidence of PCa in smokers.

5 Natural Compounds: Lycopene, Polyphenols, Sulforaphane, and (Iso) Flavonoids (Table 2)

Prostate cancer presents high rates of morbidity and mortality especially in Western countries. A lower incidence is observed Eastern countries, such as China and Japan. Migrants from the East have a risk of developing cancer equal to those of Western countries. Thus environmental influences, including diet, may play a role in prostate

Table 2 Role of Flavonoids, Polyphenols, Lycopene and Sulforaphane

	Food	Conclusion
Flavonoids	Olives, onion, romaine lettuce	Attention to infant exposure Dose-dependent role in localized PCa
Polyphenols	Green tea, red wine, chocolate, coffee	Chemoprotective role, not clear on localized or advanced PCa
Lycopene	Tomatoes, carrots	Contrasting evidence if protective on advanced or localized PCa
Sulforaphane	Broccoli, brussels sprouts, and cauliflowers	Promising results in vitro

PCa prostate cancer

carcinogenesis. Therefore, many scientists are trying to identify dietary components that could exert an anticarcinogenic effect in PCa.

The flavonoids [21] are one of the most representative elements of polyphenolic compounds. The name is derived from Latin *flavus*, meaning yellow. According to the International Union of Pure and Applied Chemistry (IUPAC) nomenclature, they can be classified into flavonols, isoflavonoids, and neoflavonoids. Of particular interest for chemoprevention are the subcategories of flavonols (quercetin, kaempferol, myricetin, and fisentin) and isoflavonoids (genistein and daidzein). The flavonols can be found in olives, onions, romaine lettuce, and cranberries. Their ability to act on PCa by inhibiting tumor growth, invasion, and metastatic potential has been demonstrated both in vitro and in vivo [22]. The chemical structures are reminiscent of estrogens, leading to the hypothesis that flavonoids could exert their effect by interacting with the androgen receptor (AR). How they might affect AR activity is still unclear, though it has been hypothesized that it might be by acting on 5- α-dihydrotestosterone. The efficacy of flavonols has already been shown in many other types of cancers such as colon and lung cancer, but this effect is not dependent on AR activity. This class of flavonoids may also act as epigenetic modulators. Several observational studies correlating isoflavonoid intake with PCa risk have been performed in the Far East because of the high consumption of isoflavonoids. The first large study to investigate the correlation between isoflavones and PCa was performed by the Japan Public Health Center (JPHC) and showed that high plasma genistein levels are associated with a dose-dependent decrease in localized PCa incidence [23]. There was no significant correlation with the risk of advanced PCa. Kurahashi et al. performed a prospective study including 307 men with newly diagnosed PCa to investigate the correlation between isoflavone intake and risk of PCa. Men with high isoflavone intake exhibited a dose-dependent decrease in the risk of localized PCa [24]. Notably, infant exposure to isoflavones may lead to carcinogenesis and several anomalies of the reproductive system because of its estrogenic activity disrupting the endocrine system [25]. Therefore, careful precautions must be considered when isoflavones are used as chemoprevention for PCa.

Polyphenols owe their name to the presence of multiple phenol structural units. Polyphenols can be found in many kinds of fruits and vegetables, green and black tea, red wine, chocolate, and coffee. The mode of action of polyphenols has not yet been fully determined [26]. In 2006 a randomized, double-blind, placebo-controlled study reported a 90 % reduction in progression from high-grade prostatic intraepithelial neoplasia (HG-PIN) to PCa [27, 28]. The possible protective effect was also investigated in another study of 272 patients with HG-PIN in which polyphenol intake significantly reduce serum PSA levels [29]. Although the results seem to be encouraging, larger clinical trials of the protective effect in men at risk of PCa or with low-grade disease are needed. One of the most studied sources of polyphenols is green tea. Green tea has been suggested to act on different pathways related to carcinogenesis: anti-oxidative actions, inhibition of inflammation, and inhibition of topoisomerase. The Japan Public Health Center completed a study of 49,920 men that included 404 cases of newly diagnosed of PCa. The consumption of green tea was dose-dependent associated with the rate of PCa risk, with high levels of consumption being associated with a decrease in the risk of advanced PCa. In conclusion, green tea consumption seems to reduce the risk of PCa diagnoses, but not the risk of advanced PCa [30].

Lycopene is a carotene and carotenoid pigment responsible for the bright red color of fruits and vegetables such as tomatoes, carrots, and watermelons. Like all carotenoids, lycopene is a polyunsaturated hydrocarbon. Although not an essential nutrient for humans, it is commonly found in most diets. Due to its color, it is often used as a food additive (E160d). Due to its strong antioxidant properties, it is postulated as a candidate chemopreventive agent. A Cochrane review performed in 2011 [31] showed an inverse correlation between lycopene intake and PCa. Three RCTs were included with a total of 154 participants. However, there is still insufficient evidence to support or refute the use of lycopene for the prevention of PCa. Analysis by experts of the World Cancer Research Fund concluded that there is sufficient evidence for the protective effect of lycopene on PCa. However, some studies do not support this conclusion, maybe because its chemopreventive effect is more evident in the early stages of PCa. Whether lycopene may or may not protect against PCa is still open for debate. Notably, two important studies published both in 2015 came to different conclusions. Chen et al. [32] performed a systematic review and the first dose-response meta-analysis describing a significant reduction of PCa incidence with a linear correlation between lycopene intake and PCa reduction, with doses ranging between 9 and 21 mg/day. For plasma concentrations of lycopene ranging between 2.17 and 85 μg/dL, there was a nonlinear dose-response correlation with PCa reduction and no association for plasma values >85 μg/dL. In contrast, Key et al. [33] conducted a pooled analysis determining at possible association of carotenoids, retinol, and vitamin E with the risk of PCa. Their analysis included 11,239 cases and 18,541 controls from 15 different studies. In this study, neither lycopene nor any of the carotenoids was associated with a reduction in PCa risk. Stratifying for clinical disease, lycopene varies significantly by stage and aggressiveness and is associated with a reduction in the overall risk of PCa, but only before 1990 (before the PSA era). Retinols do not change for stage and aggressiveness of PCa and are positively associated in men >70 years of age but not those who are younger. Vitamin E is associated with a decrease risk of advanced and aggressive PCa, but not localized or advanced. An inverse correlation of PCa risk has been found in current and past smokers, but not in never smokers, and it is not statistically relevant. Therefore, this pooled study showed an association between lycopene intake and a reduction of developing advanced PCa, but not overall PCa risk. In regard to vitamin E, there is no association with the overall risk of PCa. However, retinols are significantly associated with PCa, with a 13 % higher risk in men with high retinol concentrations. In summary lycopene and vitamin E are inversely associated with the risk of aggressive PCa; retinol is positively associated with overall PCa risk.

Sulforaphane [34] is an organosulfur compound obtained from cruciferous vegetables such as broccoli, brussels sprouts, and cauliflowers. Different anticarcinogenic effects are attributed to sulforaphane, including enhance protection against oxidative stress, apoptosis induction, suppressed progression, and inhibited angiogenesis. In vitro and animal experiments have shown that sulforaphane has an excellent protective effect, but this has not yet been confirmed in humans. Cohort studies have concluded there is little or no association with the risk of developing PCa. However, in the last few decades, some studies have found that people who eat a large quantity of cruciferous vegetables have a lower risk of PCa.

6 Medical Drugs: 5-α-RIs and NSAIDs (Table 3)

Drugs like finasteride and dutasteride alter androgen level by inhibiting 5-α-reductase, which converts testosterone into 5- α-dihydrotestosterone,

Table 3 Clinical trials on 5 Alpha-reductase inhibitors

	Primary end point	Study population	Study design	Follow-up	Conclusion
REDUCE (Reduction by Dutasteride of Prostate Cancer Events)	Dutasteride and PCa (detected on biopsy at 2 and 4 years)	6729 participants 50–75 years PSA: 2.5–10 ng/mL Biopsy negative within 6 months	Multicentric Randomized Double-blind Placebo-controlled parallel group	4 years	Dutasteride reduces incidence of PCa detected on biopsy (mainly GS 5–6), between 3rd and 4th year; upgrading in PCa in dutasteride group (GS 8–10) may be due to reduction in prostate volume
PCPT (Prostate Cancer Prevention Trial)	Finastride and PCa	18,882 participants >55 years DRE not suspected PSA <3 ng/mL	NA	7 years	Finasteride prevents or delays PCa Increased risk of high-grade PCa Sexual side effects
CombAT (The Combination of Avodart and Tamsulosin)	Combination therapy with dutasteride and tamsulosin in BPH	4844 participants ≥50 years PSA: 1.5–10 ng/mL	Multicentric Randomized Double-blind Parallel group	4 years	Dutasteride alone or with tamsulosin reduces the risk of PCa in men with BPH undergoing annual DRE and PSA
PLESS (Proscar Long-Term Efficacy and Safety Study)	Finasteride, PCa and PSA	3040 participants 45–78 years PSA <10 ng/mL Pre-randomization biopsy	Double-blind Placebo controlled	4 years	Multiplying PSA by 2 and using normal ranges, the PSA for PCa screening is preserved

PCa prostate cancer, *DRE* digital rectal examination, *NA* not available, *GS* Gleason score, *BPH* benign prostatic hyperplasia

the strongest endogenous ligand of AR. Therefore, these compounds influence prostatic proliferation and could potentially control tumor growth. Different studies have looked for a correlation between 5-α-reductase inhibitors (5-α-RIs) and PCa, some as the primary end point (Prostate Cancer Prevention Trial, PCPT [35], and REDUCE [36]) and others for effects on benign prostatic hyperplasia (BPH) (Combination of Avodart and Tamsulosin (CombAT) [37, 38]). Yet others studies have explained the reading of PSA in 5-α-RIs treatments (Proscar Long-Term Efficacy and Safety Study (PLESS) [39]). The two main questions these trials have tried to answer are whether 5-α-RIs can reduce the incidence of PCa or high-grade PCa. In the REDUCE study, a reduction in the overall incidence of PCa was observed in the group treated with dutasteride compared to placebo. Increased diagnosis of high-grade PCa with Gleason score ≥8 was significant in the dutasteride group after the 3rd and the 4th year of treatment. This finding was attributed to the reduction in prostate volume, resulting in a greater chance of finding biopsy cores positive for high-grade PCa. After adjusting for possible confounding variables, no significant increase in dutasteride was observed over the 4 years of treatment. The PCPT showed a difference in the rate of high-grade disease already in the first year of the study. Histologic changes are induced by finasteride, but it is possible that it also results in a relatively higher incidence of high-grade tumors by selectively inhibiting low-grade tumors. Notably, biopsy at inclusion was not mandatory in the PCPT, and the real cancer status was not clear before the study. Despite this limitation, in both studies a higher incidence of poorly differentiated PCa was observed in the treatment group compared to the placebo group, but these findings were not confirmed in latter studies [40, 41].

The various studies were analyzed in a Cochrane review [42] in order to assess in absolute terms the correlation between 5-α-RIs and PCa. The results and clinical interpretations demonstrate some limitations. First, the above studies include patients who undergo regular screening with PSA and DRE lacking the impact on the population that is not actively screened. No data are available regarding at what age and for how long chemoprevention is needed. In conclusion 5-α-RIs can reduce PCa in men who receive regular screening with PSA and DRE (eventually biopsies) but not in absolute terms depending on different factors such as race, family history, age, and baseline PSA.

Aspirin and other NSAIDs act on cyclooxygenase-2 (COX-2), an inducible enzyme overexpressed in PCa tissues. These drugs may also inhibit angiogenesis, promote invasion, and induce apoptosis. Because of these potential antitumoral mechanisms, several studies have assessed their effect on PCa prevention. Mahmud et al. [43] conducted a systematic review and meta-analysis to assess the strength and consistency of the relationship between NSAIDs and cancer incidence. One major limitation is that the optimal dose, time, and duration of these compounds in the preventive setting have not been analyzed. With a reduced risk of PCa (OR 0.85 for prospective studies 95 % CI 0.77–0.94 and OR 1.01 for retrospective studies 95 % CI 0.86–1.18), the authors concluded that aspirin does reduce the risk of developing PCa, and the protective effects seem to be stronger with advanced stages than for total incidence. In the Finnish Prostate Cancer Screening Trial (FinPCST) [44] (median follow-up of 7.5 years), 6535 patients with newly diagnosed PCa between 1996 and 2009 received a prescription for NSAIDs (aspirin, coxibs, acetaminophen) and the amount and dose recorded. Post-diagnostic NSAID use was associated with worse PCa-specific survival. However, when analyzing the use at the last 3 years before the end of follow-up, NSAID groups had a lower risk of PCa death. Aspirin was also not significantly associated with PCa survival, except in the last 3 years. Pre-diagnostic use of NSAIDs is associated with worse survival in high-grade PCa, but this was not confirmed in men with low-grade PCa. Therefore, a decrease in specific PCa survival is concluded in men receiving NSAIDs, which is controversial but can explained by the different indication of the use of NSAIDs with respect to other studies. In this study the prescription is for the relief of symptoms in advanced PCa, such as bone pain and secondary metastatic disease. The protective effect of aspirin is detected with its use in the years preceding diagnosis. Data from the REDUCE study [45] correlate NSAID use and PCa incidence. Remembering the inclusion criteria of a baseline biopsy and PSA 2.5–10 ng/mL, the use of NSAIDs was recorded without information on dose and frequency. The authors found a reduction in total and high-grade PCa in NSAID users. Liu et al. [46] performed a meta-analysis in 2014 that included 39 observational studies showing a 14 % decrease in PCa-specific mortality in aspirin users. Unfortunately, most studies do not provide the dose, frequency, and duration of aspirin use. RCTs could give us conclusive data on the actual protective effect of aspirin, including the required dose and frequency.

7 Can Diet Prevent Prostate Cancer? (Table 4)

Although different studies have investigated the correlation between diet and PCa incidence, a common consensus is lacking. The consumption of meat, particularly well-cooked and processed red meat, has been investigated as a potential risk factor [47]. The generation of heterocyclic amines is thought to be the cause of carcinogenesis [48, 49]. The European Prospective Investigation into Cancer and Nutrition (EPIC), including a total of 11,928 men demonstrated no association between heterocyclic amines and

Table 4 Role of meat, milk and fish

Meat	Processed meat	Weak significant risk of total prostate cancer
Milk	Cow's milk	Strong evidence of a risk of prostate cancer
Fish	Fish and fish oil	Nonstatistical influence on the risk of prostate cancer

PCa. Bylsma and Alexander [50] conducted the most recent review and meta-analysis in terms of the association between meat and PCa. More than 700,000 male participants were included from 26 prospective studies, with an average of follow-up of 6–22 years. For fresh red meat, including fresh or unprocessed beef, lamb, and pork, no significant associations were observed for White, Black, or Asian men, even after stratifying for dose. For processed meat such as ham, hot dogs, sausage, and bacon, the results showed a minor but significantly elevated risk of PCa for the whole population, but lost its significance when stratified for race.

Even milk and dairy products are being investigated for any possible effects on PCa risk [51]. An effect may be due to a combination of fat intake and subsequent suppression of circulating vitamin D. Some studies have found almond milk to have a suppressive effect on cancer cell growth. Song et al. [52] confirmed the effect of milk in a prospective cohort study. Higher intake of skim and low-fat milk is associated with increased PCa risk. The Health Professionals Study demonstrated a strong association between calcium intake and PCa risk. Dairy proteins are a significant dietary source of calcium. A 35 g/day increase in the consumption of diary protein was demonstrated to be associated with a 32 % increased risk of developing PCa. Importantly, only calcium from diary proteins is positively associated with PCa risk. Is there a molecular answer? The mammalian target of rapamycin complex (mTORC) signaling pathway is being studied to answer this question. mTORC links amino acid, growth factor, and energy availability to prostate epithelial cell growth and carcinogenesis. There are two types of mTORC, but only type 1 acts as a special protagonist in cellular nutrition and energy. mTORC1 is an energy-dependent regulator of AMPK, an energy sensor target of metformin. One of the most important amino acids that acts on mTORC1 is leucine, and insulin is not able to activate mTORC1 if cells are deprived of amino acids. Evidence suggests that only milk proteins have the unique ability to increase both insulin/IGF-1 and leucine signaling. mTORC1 is upregulated in nearly 100 % of advanced PCa. Metformin inhibits insulin, which on its own, acts on mTORC1 pathways, together with leucine signaling. In conclusion, cow's milk signals via insulin/IGF-1 and leucine inducing early promotion of mTORC1. We should not forget the demonstrated role of cruciferous vegetables in decreased PCa. Broccoli, brussels sprouts, and cauliflowers inhibit mTORC1 attenuating its activation due to the high consumption of leucine. In vitro studies suggest that green tea affects mTORC1. Thus, if there is a correlation between food and prostate carcinogenesis, it can be explained by the role of mTORC1 in prostate cells. More in vitro and in vivo studies are needed to better specify the pathways induced by food, particularly the damage of milk proteins and the protective role of metformin and vegetables such as cruciferous and green tea.

In the past fish and fish oil have been demonstrated to be protective for chronic inflammatory diseases [53]. As chronic inflammation is one of the mechanisms underlying carcinogenesis, fish and fish oil have been proposed as possible chemopreventive agents. In light of this, Lovegrove et al. performed a systematic review in 2015 investigating the association of fish and fish oil with PCa risk. Thirty-seven articles were included with a total of 495,321 participants. No significant protective effect of a fish-rich diet on PCa risk of PCa aggressiveness was found.

8 Chemoprevention in Precancerous Prostatic Lesion

Clinical trials enriched for patients at the highest risk of developing PCa provide a way to rapidly evaluate the possible chemopreventive effect of a drug, and men with HG-PIN represent such a population. Patients at high risk of developing PCa, such as patients with HG-PIN, are an attractive target that could benefit from chemoprevention. Several chemoprevention trials of nutritional supplements and other compounds have been conducted in men with HG-PIN.

The first single-arm study investigating this population was conducted in 2007 by Joniau et al. [54], enrolling 100 men with isolated HG-PIN in at least one biopsy core. This subgroup received Prevalon® (selenium 100 μg + vitamin E 30 mg + isoflavonoids 50 mg) twice a day. In a large number of patients, the level of PSA remained stable or decreased from baseline, and in this subgroup the overall risk of PCa development was lower than in patients with rising PSA levels. As discussed above, high doses of supplements are correlated with an increased risk of PCa. The results of later randomized placebo-controlled studies with various agents in the HG-PIN population were mostly negative. Taneja et al. [55] included 1590 men with HG-PIN to investigate a possible effect of 20 mg toremifene on PCa prevention. Estrogen receptor-α acts as a mediator of growth-stimulating signal transduction through the initiation of a stromal paracrine effect on PCa epithelium, and low concentrations of toremifene inhibit the α-receptor. Despite promising results in a phase II study, after 3 years using annual re-biopsies, no difference in the PCa detection rate was found for toremifene vs. placebo (32.3 % vs. 34.7 %, respectively) [56]. The SWOG S9917 study reported no PCa-preventive effect of selenium in patients with HG-PIN over a 3-year period [57]. Fleshner et al. [58] from the Canadian Clinical Trials Group presented similar data for the preventive effects of vitamin E, selenium, and soy protein on the progression of HG-PIN to PCa. In 2014 Gontero et al. [59] conducted a double-blind RCT in men diagnosed with atypical small acinar proliferation (ASAP) or multifocal high-grade prostatic intraepithelial neoplasia (mHG-PIN). The subjects received high nontoxic doses of lycopene (35 mg), selenium (55 μg), and green tea catechins (600 mg). After 37 months of follow-up, the high doses of supplementation resulted in a threefold increase in PCa risk. Thus, this study confirms the need for well-designed dose-response trials, which seem to be crucial for any dietary supplements before proceeding to trails investigating chemoprevention.

Conclusion

Different inconsistencies have been shown, and no one can conclude definitively a predominant role among chemopreventive agents due to differences in study design, sample size, administered dose, and plasma concentrations. As shown in this chapter, several agents are being investigated. There are no conclusive studies or trials that may or may not confirm the effectiveness of a substance in reducing PCa. Conclusions often conflict or overlap even with the same agents. Reviews and meta-analysis have been conducted but are not conclusive. Certainly some points remain. First, in nature there are available elements that can play a chemopreventive role in PCa which can lead to thinking that, with an adjusted diet, we can prevent or at least reduce the incidence and eventual aggressiveness of PCa. "We are what we eat," meaning we can control the incidence and aggressiveness of PCa through the food that we choose to eat each day, as it becomes part of our cellular and molecular mechanisms. Supplements like vitamins or concentrated natural extracts can help in this way, but an excessive amount may lead to the opposite desired effect. Do not forget the role of some widely used medications such as metformin for diabetes or aspirin. Using these drugs to care for other pathologies, we can determinate a role in the chemoprevention of PCa. The enthusiastic beginning of 5-α RI was dampened by conflicting conclusions, and the Food and Drug Administration (FDA) does not recommend using it for chemoprevention. The role of mTORC1 in prostate cells seems to be promising. A unique molecular pathway may be found for mTORC1 in which different environmental and diet factors overlap: metformin, cruciferous vegetables, and green tea inhibit its activation leading a protective role in the chemoprevention of PCa, compared to a diet rich of leucine like cow's milk and cheese which can promote PCa risk. Much remains to be done in this sense, especially by applying studies, ecological or prospective, confirming the role of mTORC1 in the pathogenesis of PCa. At the present time, there are no substances, drugs, or food that can reassure the chemoprevention of prostate cancer. What emerges is that much is being done in this field using known data from literature and designing new in vitro and in vivo studies that can help increase understanding. Much has been done in the past and there is still much to do. Chemoprevention remains a topic of great interest, especially because of the hope of preventing rather than curing cancer with the support of molecular data and laboratory tests. In particular, due to the slow molecular carcinogenesis and development of PCa, we could modulate its aggressiveness through the application of supplements, natural substances, and dietary factors. The road is still long, but much of it has already been traveled.

References

1. Breslow N, et al. Latent carcinoma of prostate at autopsy in seven areas, The International Agency for Research on Cancer, Lyons, France. Int J Cancer. 1977;20:680.
2. Mottet N. et al. EAU-ESTRO-SIOG guidelines on prostate cancer. Eur Urol. 2016. http://dx.doi.org/10.1016/j.euro.2016.08.003 (Epub ahead of print).
3. Kristal AR, et al. Baseline selenium status and effects of selenium and vitamin E supplementation on prostate cancer risk. J Natl Cancer Inst. 2014;106(3):djt456.
4. Nicastro HL, Dunn BK. Selenium and prostate cancer prevention: insights from the Selenium and Vitamin E Cancer Prevention Trial (SELECT). Nutrients. 2013;5:1122–48.
5. Lippman SM, et al. Effect of selenium and vitamin E on risk of prostate cancer and other cancers. The selenium and vitamin E cancer prevention trial (SELECT). JAMA. 2009;301(1):39–51.
6. Clark LC, et al. Nutritional Prevention of Cancer Study Group. Effects of selenium supplementation for cancer prevention in patients with carcinoma of the skin: a randomized controlled trial. JAMA. 1996;276(24):1957–63.
7. The Alpha-Tocopherol, Beta Carotene Cancer Prevention Study Group. The effect of vitamin E and beta carotene on the incidence of lung cancer and other cancers in male smokers. N Engl J Med. 1994;330(15):1029–35.
8. Klein EA, et al. Vitamin E and the risk of prostate cancer. The Selenium and Vitamin E Cancer Prevention trial (SELECT). JAMA. 2011;306(14):1549–56.
9. Antwi SO, et al. Dietary, supplement, and adipose tissue tocopherol levels in relation to prostate cancer aggressiveness among African and European Americans: the North Carolina-Louisiana Prostate Cancer Project (PCaP). Prostate. 2015;75:1419–35.
10. Vinceti M, et al.. Selenium for preventing cancer. Cochrane Database Syst Rev. 2014;(3):CD005195.
11. Schwarts GG, Hulka BS. Is vitamin D deficiency a risk factor for prostate cancer? (Hypothesis). Anticancer Res. 1990;10(5A):1307–11.
12. Schwarts GG. Vitamin D in blood and risk of prostate cancer: lessons from the Selenium and Vitamin E Cancer Prevention Trial and the Prostate Cancer Prevention Trial. Cancer Epidemiol Biomarkers Prev. 2014;23(8):1447–9.
13. Pollack M, et al. Insulin-like growth factors and prostate cancer. Cancer Metastasis Rev. 1998;17:383–90.
14. Margel D, et al. Association between metformin use and risk of prostate cancer and its grade. J Natl Cancer Inst. 2013;105:1123–31.
15. Kato H, et al. Metformin inhibits the proliferation of human prostate cancer PC-3 cells via the downregulation of insulin-lie growth factor 1 receptor. Biochem Biophys Res Commun. 2015;461:115–21.
16. Feng T, et al. Metformin use and risk of prostate cancer: results from the REDUCE study. Cancer Prev Res (Phila). 2015;8(11):1055–60.
17. Wu GF, et al. Metformin therapy and prostate cancer risk: a meta-analysis of observational studies. Int J Clin Ext Med. 2015;8(8):13089–98.
18. Zhang ZJ, et al. The prognostic value of metformin for cancer patients with concurrent diabetes: a systematic review and meta-analysis. Diabetes Obes Metab. 2014;16:707–10.
19. Rohrmann S, et al. Smoking and the risk of prostate cancer in the European Prospective Investigation into Cancer and Nutrition. Br J Cancer. 2013;108:708–14.
20. Mondul AM, et al. Association of serum α-tocopherol with sex steroid hormones and interactions with smoking: implications for prostate cancer risk. Cancer Causes Control. 2011;22:827–36.
21. Dixon RA, Pasinetti GM. Flavonoids and isoflavonoids: from plant biology to agriculture and neuroscience. Plant Physiol. 2010;154:453–7.
22. Boam T. Anti-androgenic effects of flavonols in prostate cancer. Ecancermedicalscience. 2015;9:585.
23. Kurahashi N, et al. Plasma isoflavones and subsequent risk of prostate cancer in a nested case-control study: the Japan Public Health Center. J Clin Oncol. 2008;26(36):5923–9.

24. Kurahashi N, et al. Soy product and isoflavone consumption in relation to prostate cancer in Japanese men. Cancer Epidemiol Biomarkers Prev. 2007;16(3): 538–45.
25. Zhang HY, et al. Isoflavones and prostate cancer: a review of some critical issues. Chin Med J. 2016;129: 341–7.
26. Van Poppel H, Tombal B. Chemoprevention of prostate cancer with nutrients and supplements. Cancer Manag Res. 2011;3:91–100.
27. Bettuzzi S, et al. Chemoprevention of human prostate cancer by oral administration of green tea catechins in volunteers with high-grade prostate intraepithelial neoplasia: a preliminary report from a one-year proof-of-principle study. Cancer Res. 2006;66(2):1234–40.
28. Brausi S, et al. Chemoprevention of human prostate cancer by green tea catechins: two years later. A follow-up update. Eur Urol. 2008;54(2):472–3.
29. McLarty J, et al. Tea polyphenols decrease serum levels of prostate-specific antigen, hepatocyte growth factor, and vascular endothelial growth factor in prostate cancer patients and inhibit production of hepatocyte growth factor and vascular endothelial growth factor vitro. Cancer Prev Res (Phila). 2009;2(7): 673–82.
30. Kurahashi N, et al. Green tea consumption and prostate cancer risk in Japanese men: a prospective study. Am J Epidemiol. 2008;167:71–7.
31. Ilic D, et al. Lycopene for the prevention of prostate cancer. Cochrane Database Syst Rev. 2011;(11): CD008007.
32. Chen P, et al. Lycopene and risk of prostate cancer. Medicine. 2015;94(33):1–14.
33. Key TJ, et al. Carotenoids, retinol, tocopherols, and prostate cancer risk: pooled analysis of 15 studies. Am J Clin Nutr. 2015;102:1142–57.
34. Watson GW, et al. Phytochemicals from cruciferous vegetables epigenetics, and prostate cancer prevention. AAPS J. 2013;15(4):951–61.
35. Thompson IM, et al. The influence of finasteride on the development of prostate cancer. N Engl J Med. 2003;349:3. p 215–24.
36. Andriole GL, et al. Effect of dutasteride on the risk of prostate cancer. N Engl J Med. 2010;362:13. p 1192–202.
37. Roehrborn CG, et al. The effects of combination therapy with dutasteride and tamsulosin on clinical outcomes in men with symptomatic benign prostatic hyperplasia: 4-year results from CombAT study. Eur Urol. 2010;57:123–31.
38. Roehrborn CG, et al. Effect of dutasteride on prostate biopsy rates and the diagnosis of prostate cancer in Men with lower urinary tract symptoms and enlarged prostates in the Combination of Avodart and Tamsulosin trial. Eur Urol. 2011;59:244–9.
39. Andriole GL, et al. Treatment with finasteride preserves usefulness of prostate-specific antigen in the detection of prostate cancer: results of a randomized, double-blind, placebo-controlled clinical trial. Urology. 1998;52:195–202.
40. Fleshner NE, et al. Dutasteride in localised prostate cancer management: the REDEEM randomised, double-blind, placebo-controlled trial. Lancet. 2012;379:24–30.
41. Ross AE, et al. Effect of treatment with 5-α reductase inhibitors on progression in monitored men with favourable-risk prostate cancer. BJU Int. 2012;110: 651–7.
42. Wilt TJ, et al. 5-α-Reductase inhibitors for prostate cancer chemoprevention: an updated Cochrane systematic review. BJU Int. 2010;106:1444–51.
43. Mahmud S, et al. Prostate cancer and use of nonsteroidal anti-inflammatory drugs: systematic review and meta-analysis. Database of Abstracts of Reviews of Effects 2015 Issue 2. Original article: Br J Cancer. 2004;90(1):93–99.
44. Veitonmäki T, et al. Use of non-steroidal anti-inflammatory drugs and prostate cancer survival in the Finnish prostate cancer screening trial. Prostate. 2015; 75:1394–402.
45. Vidal AC, et al. Aspirin, NSAIDs, and risk of prostate cancer: results from the REDUCE study. Clin Cancer Res. 2015;21(4):756–62.
46. Liu Y, et al. Effect of aspirin and other non-steroidal anti-inflammatory drugs on prostate cancer incidence and mortality: a systematic review and meta-analysis. BMC Med. 2014;12:55.
47. Zhijun W, et al. Nutraceuticals for prostate cancer chemoprevention: from molecular mechanism to clinical application. Expert Opin Investig Drugs. 2013; 22(12):1613–36.
48. Mandair D, et al. Prostate cancer and the influence of dietary factors and supplements: a systematic review. Nutr Metab. 2014;11:30.
49. Wu K, et al. Associations between unprocessed red and processed meat, poultry, seafood and egg intake and the risk of prostate cancer: a pooled analysis of 15 prospective cohort studies. Int J Cancer. "Accepted article". doi:10.1002/ijc.29973.
50. Bylsma LC, Alexander DD. A review and meta-analysis of prospective studies of red and processed meat, meat cooking methods, heme iron, heterocyclic amines and prostate cancer. Nutr J. 2015;14:125.
51. Melnik BC, et al. The impact of cow's milk-mediated mTORC1-signaling in the initiation and progression of prostate cancer. Nutr Metab. 2012;9:74.
52. Song Y, et al. Whole milk intake is associated with prostate cancer-specific mortality among U.S. male physicians. J Nutr. 2013;143(2):189–96.
53. Lovegrove C, et al. Systematic review of prostate cancer risk and association with consumption of fish and fish-oils: analysis of 495,321 participants. Int J Clin Pract. 2015;69(1):87–105.
54. Joniau S, et al. Effect of nutritional supplement challenge in patients with isolated high-grade prostatic intraepithelial neoplasia. Urology. 2007;69:1101–6.

55. Taneja SS, et al. Prostate cancer diagnosis among men with isolated high-grade intraepithelial neoplasia enrolled onto a 3-year prospective phase III clinical trial of oral toremifene. J Clin Oncol. 2013;31:523–9.
56. Price D, et al. Toremifene for the prevention of prostate cancer in men with high grade prostatic intraepithelial neoplasia: results of a double-blind, placebo controlled, phase IIB clinical trial. J Urol. 2006;176:965–70.
57. Marshall JR, et al. Phase III trial of selenium to prevent prostate cancer in men with high-grade prostatic intraepithelial neoplasia: SWOG S9917. Cancer Prev Res. 2011;4:1761–9.
58. Fleshner NE, et al. Progression from high-grade prostatic intraepithelial neoplasia to cancer: a randomized trial of combination Vitamin-E, soy, and selenium. J Clin Oncol. 2011;29:2386–90.
59. Gontero P, et al. A randomized double-blind placebo controlled phase I-II study on clinical and molecular effects of dietary supplements in men with precancerous prostatic lesions. Chemoprevention or "chemopromotion"? Prostate. 2015;75:1177–86.

Individual and Population-Based Screening

Kai Zhang, Chris H. Bangma,
Lionne D.F. Venderbos, and Monique J. Roobol

1 Introduction

Prostate cancer (PCa) is the second most frequently diagnosed cancer and fifth common cause of cancer death among men in the world [1]. In Europe, there were 416,732 new PCa patients diagnosed, and 92,247 men died from their disease in 2012 [2]. In the United States, the lifetime risk of being diagnosed with PCa is approximately 1 in 7, which is the highest among all male cancers [3]. Even in Asian countries where the incidence and mortality of PCa are the lowest, a rapid increase in the incidence and mortality rates has been noted over the past two decades (Table 1), mainly due to the introduction of prostate-specific antigen (PSA) testing [4, 5]. Although high-quality, population-based PCa data are limited, current studies point toward a significant increasing trend of PCa incidence in several African countries, such as Uganda, Zimbabwe, and Mali [6, 7]. These figures indicate that PCa is an important public health issue worldwide.

The PSA test is a simple and effective tool, which is widely used for the early diagnosis of PCa with the rationale that early detection might avoid suffering from metastases and lower disease-specific mortality. Several PSA-based screening trials with the aim to evaluate the effect of PSA-based population screening have been completed or are ongoing. The two largest randomized trials are the prostate arm of the Prostate, Lung, Colorectal, and Ovarian Cancer Screening Trial (PLCO) and the ongoing European Randomized Study of Screening for Prostate Cancer (ERSPC) study (Table 2). After 13 years of follow-up, the PLCO trial reported no difference in PCa mortality between the screening and control arm [9], while the ERSPC study reported a significant PCa mortality reduction (21 %) in favor of the screening arm [8].

Although the results on mortality are contradictory, both trials have one thing in common: PSA-based screening leads to large numbers of unnecessary biopsies and detection of potentially indolent PCa. This so-called overdiagnosis often coincides with overtreatment [10]. As many as 75 % of men with a raised PSA (≥3 ng/ml) have a benign biopsy result [11], and the rate of overdiagnosis within the ERSPC trial is estimated to be approximately 50 % [12], which leads many patients to needless curative treatment with the consequences of high costs and side effects.

In this chapter, first PSA and other conventional screening instruments like digital rectal examination (DRE) and transrectal ultrasound (TRUS) will be discussed. Then some new emerging tools, like proPSA, Prostate Health

K. Zhang, MD • C.H. Bangma, MD, PhD
L.D.F. Venderbos, PhD • M.J. Roobol, PhD (✉)
Department of Urology, Erasmus University Medical Center, Rotterdam, The Netherlands
e-mail: m.roobol@erasmusmc.nl

M. Bolla, H. van Poppel (eds.), *Management of Prostate Cancer*,
DOI 10.1007/978-3-319-42769-0_3

Table 1 Trends in prostate cancer incidence in Asian countries and regions

Country	Period	Average annual percent change
China (2 registries)	1993–2002	12.1
Japan (4 registries)	1993–2002	7.2
Philippines (2 registries)	1993–2002	3.1
Republic of Korea	1999–2007	13.8
Singapore	1993–2002	4.6
Thailand (2 registries)	1993–2002	3.1
India, Chennai	1996–2005	−0.5

Adapted from Center et al. [4]

Table 2 Comparison of the ERSPC and the PLCO study

Feature	ERSPC [8]	PLCO [9]
Country	8 European countries	The United States
Period	1993-	1993-2001, screening completed in 2006
Centers involved	9	10
No. participants	162,338	76,693
Age group (years)	55–69	55–74
Randomized	Yes	Yes
PCa mortality reduction	21 %	No

Index (PHI), multiparametric MRI (mpMRI), and multivariate risk prediction tools, will be discussed – all having the potential to reduce unnecessary biopsies and potential overdiagnosis. Finally, conclusions will be drawn and future directions sketched.

2 Conventional Screening Instruments

2.1 PSA

PSA is a kallikrein-like serine protease. This enzyme is almost exclusively produced by the epithelial cells of the prostate, making it an organ-specific marker. In 1987, PSA was introduced in the USA to evaluate treatment response after intended curative therapy. Soon after, PSA was widely used for opportunistic screening. PSA, however, is not cancer-specific. Prostatitis, benign prostatic hyperplasia (BPH), and urethral or prostatic trauma can also increase the serum PSA. Furthermore, (clinically significant) PCa can be present in men without elevated PSA levels [13].

Besides PSA not being PCa-specific, serum levels are subject to variability as well. First of all, the serum PSA test is available through several companies with different test properties leading to different test results if compared directly [14]. To overcome this issue, the World Health Organization (WHO) developed the standard assay of PSA in 1999 which has been introduced by most clinics nowadays [15]. Second, PSA levels vary from day to day. To assess variability of PSA levels, a total of 1686 men with serum PSA levels between 3 and 10 ng/ml in the STHLM3 trial underwent a second PSA test within eight weeks of the first PSA test and before biopsy. Results showed that PSA levels decreased with more than 20 % among 19 % of men and increased more than 20 % among 15 % of men. Up to 17 % of men had repeated PSA levels ≤3 ng/ml, which meant those men might not have an indication for biopsy. This study suggested that a repeated PSA value could serve as a decision aid for the decision to undergo a biopsy [16].

The continuum of PCa risk for different PSA ranges is presented on the basis of data coming from the Prostate Cancer Prevention Trial (PCPT) and the ERSPC study [17, 18]. These studies showed that the sensitivity decreased with increasing PSA levels, while the specificity increased with increasing PSA levels. Lowering PSA cutoff levels consequently led to a higher PCa detection rate, but also resulted in an increase of unnecessary biopsies and of the overdiagnosis of potentially indolent cancers [19]. In the case that a physician would like to have 80 % confidence not missing a PCa, he/she should apply a PSA cutoff value of 1.1 ng/ml as indication for biopsy. This would however result in 60 % of the biopsy being negative [20].

The assessment of PSA kinetics, PSAV (PSA velocity, the increase of the absolute level of PSA during one year) and PSADT (PSA doubling time), has been used to assess both overall PCa risk and risk of aggressive PCa. PSAV is primarily used at the time of diagnosis, whereas PSADT is primarily used in the posttreatment setting as a surrogate marker of disease progression [21]. The ERSPC and PCPT study, taking into account only men actually biopsied, demonstrated that PSAV added very little predictive value to the decision whether or not to take a prostate biopsy, i.e. PSAV was of no added value in a PCa screening setting [22, 23]. However, for men with a sudden unexpected rise in their PSA level, when evidence of prostatitis is absent, a prostate biopsy might be indicated [24].

Increasing age is associated with an increase of the serum PSA level. As a reference, age-specific median PSA values are 0.7, 0.9, 1.2, and 1.5 ng/ml for men in their 40s, 50s, 60s, and 70s, respectively [25]. However, applying these cutoffs for further assessment (biopsy) may increase the risk of a delayed diagnosis of high-grade PCa despite the benefit of fewer biopsies [26].

PSA is also strongly related to total prostate or transition zone volume, as more PSA leaks into the serum possibly due to the fact that in large glands the prostate capsule is more disrupted. PSAD (PSA density, PSA/gland volume) improves PSA sensitivity and specificity, and knowing the size of the prostate is often the basis for the number of biopsies [27].

On the basis of the data above, we have to conclude that there is no optimal absolute PSA cutoff value to recommend prostate biopsy. Hence, the decision to perform biopsy should not only be based on PSA but should also take into account other relevant factors, such as age, DRE result, family history, prostate volume, having had a previous negative biopsy, and additional predictive markers that maintain sensitivity but increase specificity.

2.2 DRE

DRE is an integral component of the assessment of the prostate gland and is the classical method for the detection of PCa. A recently published study in Ireland shows that DRE alone had a sensitivity and specificity of 81 % and 40 %, respectively, in diagnosing PCa, with a positive predictive value of 42 % [28]. However, in men with low PSA levels, DRE has a low sensitivity and predictive value and tends to diagnose the tumors when they are already pathologically advanced and potentially beyond cure [29–31]. Therefore, DRE is not an optimal tool for the early detection of PCa. A DRE can, however, provide information on the size of the prostate. This information can be used to correct for the rise in PSA level caused by the presence of BPH [32], i.e., PSAD. It is important to note that DRE holds a more subjective character than PSA and that DRE results differ among physicians. The inter-observer variation, for estimating prostate size, noted as the Kappa score, has shown to be 0.532 between urologists and general practitioners [33].

2.3 TRUS

The transrectal ultrasound (TRUS) is used since the early 1980s and is the standard tool for guiding systematic diagnostic prostate biopsy. Lesions suspicious for the presence of PCa on TRUS usually appear as a hypoechoic focal lesion in the peripheral zone. However, these lesions have a variable appearance which considerably overlaps with benign lesions. Therefore, the sensitivity and specificity of grayscale TRUS in the detection of PCa is low. Inspection of the gland should focus on identifying asymmetry, areas of increased vascularity, hypoechogenicity, and the presence of focal bulges, irregularity, or breaches of the capsule. These features are associated with the presence of cancer and should be documented, but are not sufficiently reliable to make a diagnosis without obtaining a biopsy [34].

TRUS, like DRE, is also a highly subjective examination. When five well-trained physicians were given 18 records of TRUS videotape to decide whether or not to perform prostate biopsy, a Kappa value of 0.2 was found, indicating that the agreement between physicians is very poor [35]. TRUS does, however, has the advantage of facilitating a more precise measurement of prostate size as compared to DRE [34].

2.4 TRUS-Guided Biopsy

TRUS-guided biopsy plays a crucial role in the diagnosis of PCa, but more as a guidance tool for systematic prostate biopsy [36]. The random TRUS-guided biopsy technique has its flaws and over the past decade there has been a trend to sample more biopsy cores to increase the sensitivity [34]. The current standard, as recommended by the European Association of Urology, is a 10–12 core biopsy scheme because it has been shown that taking more than 12 cores is not significantly more conclusive [37].

Recently, new emerging technologies in TRUS-guided biopsy have been introduced and showed potential in the diagnosis of PCa. Ultrasound contrast agent studies provide information regarding vascularity of the lesion. Molecular imaging for targeting specific biomarkers could be applied for detecting PCa angiogenesis and surface biomarkers [36]. Elastography is an ultrasound technique that provides information regarding tissue elasticity and stiffness [36]. A prospective study of 353 patients has shown that elastography-guided biopsy can improve PCa detection compared to grayscale ultrasound guidance (51.1 % vs. 39.4 %), but cannot replace the systematic biopsy due to the low sensitivity (60.8 %) [38]. Up to now, there are no large, multicenter studies with standardization of technique nor high-quality prospective trials to clarify the role of these techniques. A crucial disadvantage of the ultrasound-based techniques is that the sampling approach of biopsy is essentially "blind" to any local tissue characteristics. The advent of MRI-guided prostate biopsy has solved this problem with direct visualization of suspicious lesions and is being increasingly used worldwide [39]. It is therefore questionable whether these ultrasound techniques will become widely used while it must be noted that TRUS-guided biopsy has the advantage of being simple and inexpensive.

Whatever guidance is used, a prostate biopsy is not without risks. Common side effects include hematospermia, hematuria, pain, infection, and urine retention [40] (Table 3). A recently published Cochrane review of randomized trials on antibiotic prophylaxis for TRUS-guided biopsy shows that antibiotic prophylaxis is effective in preventing infectious complications following prostate biopsy. The study showed that long-term (3 days) antibiotic treatment is not superior to short-term (1 day), and multiple-dose therapy is not better than single-dose [41].

Table 3 The rates of main complications after 5676 prostate biopsy procedures, Rotterdam section of the ERSPC study

Complication	Rate, %
Minor complications[a]	
Hematospermia	50.4
Hematuria >3 days	22.6
Rectal bleeding	1.3
Voiding problems	0.8
Major complications[b]	
Pain after biopsy	7.5
Fever	3.5
Use of antibiotics	3.3
Hospitalization	0.5
Urinary retention	0.4
Nausea/sickness	0.3
Use of analgesics	0.3
Allergic reaction to antibiotic prophylaxis	0.1

Adapted from Penzkofer et al. [39]

[a]Minor complications: expected side effects causing minimal or no discomfort, and requiring no additional treatment

[b]Major complications: adverse effects causing significant discomfort, disability, or requiring additional treatment

In this context, it is important to realize the increase of antibiotic resistance. In a 10-year population-based cohort study, a rapid increase was seen in ciprofloxacin-resistant bacterial blood stream infection after prostate biopsy, from 0 % in 2003 to 19 % in 2012. The same pattern has been observed for some other antibiotics, i.e., extended spectrum b-lactamase (ESBL), trimethoprim–sulfametoxazole, and cefotaxime [42]. This situation prompts urologists to find more optimal tools and strategies to reduce unnecessary prostate biopsies.

3 New Predictive Makers and mpMRI

3.1 PSA Subforms

PSA is present in the serum in two forms, the complex and the free form (free PSA, fPSA). The fPSA molecular subform proPSA contains a seven amino acid proleader peptide. Different truncated forms of proPSA have been identified and all of them are enzymatically inactive. Three forms of proPSA in serum ([−2], [−4], and [−5/−7] proPSA) are known where [2] proPSA (p2PSA) is the most stable form [43, 44].

PHI was developed by Beckman Coulter, Inc. in partnership with the NCI Early Detection Research Network and was approved by the FDA in 2012. This new blood test is actually a mathematical formula of three PSA-based biomarkers – (p2PSA/fPSA)×PSA½ [45] and has the advantage that the outcome is, just like the PSA test, one number which can be used as a cutoff for further assessment.

A European two-center study included 756 patients to investigate the performance of p2PSA and PHI in PCa detection [46]. It showed that between men with and without PCa, the p2PSA and PHI levels were significantly different [46]. PHI achieved the highest PCa predictive value in both centers with areas under the curve (AUC) of 0.750 and 0.709, compared to tPSA (AUC: 0.585 and 0.534) and %fPSA (fPSA/tPSA, AUC: 0.675 and 0.576). Also, %p2PSA (p2PSA/fPSA) showed significantly higher AUCs compared to tPSA and %fPSA (AUC: 0.716 and 0.695, respectively).

In another observational prospective study, 646 patients from five European urologic centers with a tPSA range of 2–10 ng/ml underwent initial prostate biopsy [47]. It was shown that p2PSA, %p2PSA, and PHI significantly improved the predictive accuracy of PCa with a Gleason score ≥7 by 6.4 %, 5.6 %, and 6.4 %, respectively (all $p<0.001$). If a PHI cutoff of 27.6 was applied, 15.5 % of biopsies could have been avoided [47]. An American study also concluded that compared to tPSA, PHI had significantly higher predictive value for detection of Gleason 7 or greater PCa (AUC: 0.707 vs. 0.551 for tPSA) and clinically significant PCa (Gleason 7 or greater, 3 or more positive cores, and more than 50 % involvement of any core, AUC 0.698 vs. 0.549 for tPSA) [48]. Moreover, at a 90 % sensitivity cutoff point for PHI, 30.1 % of patients could have been prevented from unnecessary biopsies. Similar results were found in some Asian trials [49–51], which further confirms the clinical validity and utility of p2PSA and PHI.

Also based on PSA isoforms, the so-called four-kallikrein panel (4 K panel) has shown to be of added value in predicting the presence of a biopsy-detectable (significant) PCa. The commercially available 4 K score test, based on tPSA, free PSA, intact PSA, and kallikrein-related peptidase 2 (hK2), gives a probability that a man will have a significant PCa detected at prostate biopsy [52]. A recent study compared the 4 K panel with PHI for the predictive value for PCa in a group of 531 men. It was shown that the 4 K panel and PHI had similar performance in predicting PCa (AUC: 0.690 vs. 0.704) and high-grade PCa (AUC: 0.718 vs. 0.711) [53].

To date, p2PSA and PHI are not widely available, most likely due to financial reasons. Especially in some developing countries where population-based PSA screening is not common practice yet, these new markers could be of benefit despite the higher costs. It is in these countries where the consequences of PSA-based testing, unnecessary testing and overdiagnosis could still be avoided and as such make the new test although more expensive, cost-effective. An American study hypothesized a health plan with 100,000 male members aged 50–75 years old, tested with PSA and applying a PSA 4 ng/ml as cutoff for prostate biopsy, would be cost-effective even with adding p2PSA to PSA and %fPSA. The costs would increase with $13,611 (1-year costs). These additional costs would be neutralized by the savings on the costs of potentially unnecessary biopsies (−$98,650), office visits (−$8664), and laboratory tests (−$516) [54].

To summarize, compared to the currently used tPSA and fPSA levels, p2PSA and PHI test results are more accurate, most likely cost-effective, and as such improve the process of early detection of PCa.

3.2 Genetic Markers

Progress in gene research made it possible to develop genetic marker tests such as the prostate cancer gene 3 (PCA3) and the transmembrane protease, serine 2 (TMPRSS2): v-ets erythroblastosis virus E26 oncogene homolog (ERG) tests. Both of them can be tested in human urine, which is noninvasive, simple, and convenient for patients [55].

PCA3 is a noncoding RNA and is only expressed in human prostate tissue [55]. In 1999, PCA3 was found highly overexpressed in PCa tissue compared to normal prostate tissue [56], which would make it an appropriate indicator for the presence of PCa. PCA3 has been approved by the US Food and Drug Administration (FDA) for estimating PCa risk following a negative biopsy in 2012.

In a study of 809 men at initial or repeat prostate biopsy in Europe and North America, PCA3 showed higher predictive value than PSA for PCa detection (AUC: 0.679 vs. 0.527) [57]. However, in another study of 721 prescreened men within the Dutch part of the ERSPC study, ROC analyses showed an AUC of 0.635, a limited improvement as compared to the AUC of tPSA (AUC: 0.581, $p=0.143$) [58].

TMPRSS2: ERG is a fusion gene and can be found in approximately 50 % of PCa patients [54]. In a study including 78 men with PCa-positive biopsies and 30 men with PCa-negative biopsies, the TMPRSS2: ERG showed a rather low sensitivity of 37 %, however, a high specificity of 93 %, and a positive predictive value of 94 % [59]. However, in the largest study of 1180 PCa patients with a median follow-up of 12.6 years after radical prostatectomy, it was shown that TMPRSS2: ERG overexpression was only associated with tumor stage, but not with Gleason score, metastases, biochemical recurrence, and cancer-related and overall mortality, suggesting that TMPRSS2: ERG might not be a strong predictive marker in PCa patients [60].

The combination of several markers is likely to improve test performance. In a recent large-sample study, urine samples were collected from 1244 men [61]. It demonstrated that for predicting PCa, the AUCs of PSA, PSA plus TMPRSS2: ERG, and PSA plus PCA3 were 0.585, 0.693, and 0.726, respectively; for predicting high-grade PCa (Gleason score >6), the AUCs of PSA, PSA plus TMPRSS2: ERG, PSA plus PCA3, and PSA plus T2: ERG plus PCA3 were 0.651, 0.729, 0.747, and 0.772, respectively. These data show that if more relevant information is added to multivariate prediction models, their predictive capability increases. However, clinical usefulness and cost-effectiveness should never be overlooked.

In terms of genetic risk factors, genome-wide association studies (GWAS) have identified over 1000 single nucleotide polymorphisms (SNPs) associated with PCa risk [62]. In a recent study, a prediction model for PCa was built with 65 established risk SNPs and 68 novel SNPs [63], showing that the 65 established SNPs provided AUC between 0.64 and 0.69 for different populations. When adding an additional 68 novel SNPs, the AUC increased from 0.67 to 0.68 ($p=0.0012$) [63]. In the recent STHLM study, however, the added value of SNPS in a multivariate model with clinical parameters and serum-based biomarkers (subforms of PSA) seemed rather low [64]. Although many new markers have proven better predictive ability than tPSA, the latter is still the most widely and frequently used marker worldwide, most likely since we lack long-term data of the effect on disease-specific mortality when some clinically significant PCa cases are being missed when avoiding diagnoses at the cost of saving unnecessary biopsies and potential overdiagnosis. It is exactly here where informed- and shared decision making come in and every man must balance his potential benefit and harm.

3.3 MRI-Guided Biopsy

Magnetic resonance imaging (MRI) has been used in prostate imaging since the 1980s. Initially, only T1-weighted (T1W) and T2-weighted

(T2W) pulse sequences were used for morphologic assessment on prostate MRI which had limited capability to distinguish benign node and clinically insignificant PCa from significant cancer [65]. mpMRI is a new technology were anatomic T@W imaging is combined with diffusion-weigthed imaging (DWI), apparent-diffusion coefficient (ADC) maps and dynamic contrast-enhanced (DCE) MRI [65].

Apart from the tumor microenvironment information, mpMRI can also offer anatomic insight and possibly qualitative, semi-quantitative, and fully quantitative imaging biomarkers, which might reflect the underlying tumor histopathology and biological behavior, making that mpMRI has better performance on PCa detection [66]. There are several different scoring systems classifying suspicious lesions on prostate mpMRI, such as a three-point scale (low, moderate, high suspicion), or a five-point scale ranging from 1 (no suspicion) to 5 (high suspicion), which is known as The Prostate Imaging-Reporting and Data System (PI-RADS) [67, 68]. After the process of fusion with real-time ultrasonographic maps, mpMRI can be used as guidance at prostate biopsy [67].

A recent US-based prospective study reported the results of 1003 men undergoing both mpMRI-guided and standard TRUS-guided random biopsy from 2007 to 2014. The study showed that mpMRI-guided biopsy improved the detection rate of high-risk PCa by 30 % and reduced the detection of low-risk PCa by 17 % compared to standard biopsy (both $P<.001$) [69]. Moreover, in the subgroup including 170 patients with pathological results after radical prostatectomy, mpMRI-guided biopsy had a greater predictive value for distinguishing low-risk PCa from moderate- and high-risk PCa than standard biopsy or combined biopsy.

In a systematic review, a total of 1926 patients from 16 studies with a positive MRI were evaluated [70]. The PCa prevalence in the whole group was 59 %. It demonstrated that MRI-guided biopsy did not outperform TRUS-guided biopsy in overall PCa detection. MRI-guided biopsy did show a greater detection rate for significant PCa compared to TRUS-guided biopsy (individual sensitivity of 0.91 vs. 0.76), as well as a lower detection rate for insignificant PCa (individual sensitivity of 0.44 vs. 0.83). In the subgroup analysis for men with an initial biopsy, MRI- and TRUS-guided biopsy showed similar results for overall PCa detection, and a small difference in significant PCa detection, but for men with a previous negative biopsy, MRI-guided biopsy had remarkable better performance on overall PCa detection (relative sensitivity 1.62) [70].

An important concern regarding the use of mpMRI in the detection of PCa is the learning curve. A current study showed that the mpMRI-PCa detection rate by two radiologists nearly doubled (42–81 %) in 2-year study period [71], suggesting that some PCa, even clinically significant PCa, might be missed in the early stage of the application of mpMRI. Therefore, it is recommended that mpMRI imaging for PCa detection should be analyzed by radiologists with sufficient expertise.

It is clear that mpMRI significantly improves the diagnostic accuracy for significant PCa. According to the currently available evidence, there is still place for the standard systematic TRUS-guided biopsy but in men with a previous negative random biopsy, mpMRI-guided biopsy has proven to be of clear added value.

4 Individual Screening

4.1 PCa Risk Calculators

As already pointed out earlier on in this chapter, PCa screening is associated with a reduction of metastatic disease and disease-specific mortality but also with unnecessary biopsies, overdiagnosis, and overtreatment. The balance between benefits and harms is still not well established. Hence, we urgently need an approach to detect potential aggressive PCa early enough to prevent those progressing to an advanced stage beyond cure. It is therefore recommended switching from screening every man within a certain age range to screening a certain population at a relative higher risk of PCa. With this in mind, PCa risk calculators are being developed using relevant prebiopsy information to identify those men who are at risk of a potential aggressive PCa and as such may actually benefit from early detection.

The two most frequently used PCa risk calculators are the PCPT and ERSPC risk calculators [72, 73]. The PCPT risk calculator is designed using data from 5519 men of the placebo group of the PCPT who underwent prostate biopsy [73]. This risk calculator is based on PSA value, family history, outcome of DRE, and prior biopsy. The PCPT risk calculator development study showed a predictive value (expressed as AUC) of 0.702, which was only slightly higher than the AUC of PSA alone (0.678) in this dataset. Most likely, the absence of prostate volume may explain this. The PCPT risk calculator has been externally validated in American and European populations, with AUC's ranging from 0.57 to 0.74 [74]. When applying the PCPT risk calculator to an Asian population, an AUC of 0.783 was found [75]. The PCPT risk calculator is available on the Internet (http://deb.uthscsa.edu/URORiskCalc/Pages/uroriskcalc.jsp).

The ERSPC risk calculator is developed in a European (Dutch) population and includes six steps based on different predictive models, including age, PSA value, DRE result, outcome of TRUS, family history, prostate volume, and previous biopsy status [76]. This calculator is easily accessible through the Internet (www.prostatecancer-riskcalculator.com) for both physician and patient or through a smartphone-app for the physician (App: Rotterdam Prostate Cancer Risk Calculator). The development study indicated that the AUC for the ERSPC risk calculator step 3 model (for men screened for the first time, including information on TRUS and prostate volume) reached 0 .77 compared to an AUC of 0.64 by PSA alone [73]. External validation studies conducted in Northern American and European populations reported AUCs between 0.71 and 0.80 [77–79], and calibration slopes between 0.61 and 0.83 [77, 78]. Similar results were found when ERSPC risk calculators (model 3 and 4 for patients undergoing initial biopsies and repeat biopsies) were validated in an Asian population, showing AUCs between 0.77 and 0.88 [75, 79, 80] and a calibration slope of 0.873 [75]. While discrimination of the ERSPC risk calculators in Asian populations is acceptable, calibration is not optimal. Most likely differences in prevalence and the percentage of significant PCa cases detected at prostate biopsy are the main reasons [79, 80]. The fact that the relationship between PSA levels and risk of a positive prostate biopsy varies is confirmed by an analysis of the so-called Prostate biopsy collaborative group. These differences are challenging when developing PSA-driven algorithms to determine whether biopsy is indicated [81].

Both risk calculators have been compared directly [82]. The results of a study comprising 525 European men showed that the AUC of the ERSPC calculator was significantly higher than the AUC of the PCPT calculator and PSA alone (0.801, 0.744, and 0.643, respectively). Furthermore, the ERSPC calculator showed better calibration than the PCPT calculator. As a result, higher net benefit was shown for the ERSPC calculator by decision curve analysis, suggesting that 9 % and 23 % of unnecessary biopsies could have been avoided if a risk threshold of 20 % and 30 % was applied, respectively. In contrast, the PCPT model showed limited net benefit. In other head-to-head comparisons, the ERSPC risk calculator showed superiority over the PCPT model [75, 77, 80, 83].

In addition to the classical risk factors, some of the new markers such as PHI have the potential to improve the predictive capability of a risk calculator. When a total of 2001 patients from 6 Irish centers were analyzed using the PCPT and ERSPC risk calculator formulae, it was found that PHI can increase the AUC of the ERSPC model (model 3 + DRE for patients at initial biopsy and model 4 + DRE for patients at repeat biopsy) from 0.72 to 0.76 for PCa prediction in a subgroup of 222 patients for whom the PHI score was available. The recently developed ERSPC-PHI risk calculator showed better calibration and higher net benefit than the ERSPC model [83]. In another study, PCA3 was proven to add some predictive value to the so-called DRE-based ERSPC risk calculator (including a DRE-based estimate of prostate volume) which was reflected by an increase from AUC of 0.70 to 0.73 for detecting PCa in prescreened men [84].

In summary, risk calculators combining multiple risk factors show a higher predictive ability than PSA alone in PCa detection. The ERSPC risk calculator seems to outperform the PCPT risk calculator, but head-to-head comparisons, including more available risk calculators, are recommended where besides discrimination calibration should also be assessed. Hopefully, these types of analyses and subsequent local adaptations will encourage physicians to use these tools more often in their daily clinical practice.

4.2 Risk-Based Strategy

This brings us to the concept of risk stratification which implies using a certain PCa risk as a threshold for biopsy, with the aim to improve the efficiency of early PCa detection and to reduce its harms.

At the first screening round of the Dutch part of ERSPC, it has retrospectively been shown that with applying an additional risk threshold of 12.5 % in addition to the used PSA cutoff value of 3.0 g/ml to trigger biopsy could have avoided 33 % of biopsies [76]. With this approach, although 14 % of PCa cases would have been missed, up to 70 % of them could be considered as potentially indolent, and 17 of the 18 up to then deadly PCa cases would have been detected. Moreover, at repeat screening 4 years later, a similar strategy would result in 37 % fewer biopsies. Although 16 % of PCa would be missed, 81 % could be classified as likely indolent. By contrast, when PSA ≥ 4.0 ng/ml cutoff value would have been applied, similar numbers of unnecessary biopsies could have been saved, but the number of (significant) PC cases missed would be considerably higher (25 % at initial screening, 43 % at repeat screening).

Whether or not to perform a prostate biopsy is often a difficult decision in clinical practice. Both physician and patient need to balance the benefit of avoiding unnecessary biopsies against the harm of missing life-threatening PCa. With a risk-based strategy, used in addition to their clinical expertise physicians can more accurately distinguish between a possible diagnosis of low-risk (potentially indolent) or high-risk (potentially significant) PCa and, after discussion with the (potential) patient act accordingly.

A still unresolved issue is the age to start screening and start risk calculation, i.e., should men start PSA testing at a younger age like in their early 40s? In a Swedish study, PSA values were tested in archived blood plasma from 1312 participants later diagnosed with PCa and from 3728 matched controls. Blood samples were collected from 1974 to 1986 when men were aged 33–50 years. After a median follow-up of 23 years, the analyses showed that the PSA value at or before 50 was highly associated with subsequent diagnosis of PCa and advanced PCa (AUC: 0.719 and 0.751, respectively) [85]. This would imply that early risk stratification would allow large numbers of men to be screened less frequently and further testing will be focused on those men with a potential high risk of dying from PCa. However, it must be noted that when looking at these data more carefully, in men above the proposed cutoff of ≥1.6 ng/ml (only 10 % of the study population), only 44 % of all PCa deaths occurred. One can expect that such a strategy where further testing is to be delayed with at least 10 years in 90 % of the population but where 56 % of PCa deaths occurred will not be followed. What will be the result of starting testing at early age remains to be seen but it is likely that it will result in again unnecessary biopsies and treatment harm, exactly that what we want to avoid. In Germany, the so-called PROBASE study has been initiated that compares the effect of screening starting at age 45 or 50. Hopefully, this trial will provide more insight into this dilemma [86].

5 Conclusions and Way to Go

Obviously, PSA-based population screening for PCa should at the moment and it its current form not be recommended due to the high proportion of unnecessary biopsies, overdiagnosis, and overtreatment. However, it is still essential to detect those life-threatening PCa at a time when treatment is still possible. Therefore, we need an approach with which we can distinguish low-risk from high-risk disease and with which we can selectively identify men that can actually benefit from PCa screening.

PCa risk calculators, which are developed and derived from population-based studies, have proven to be of aid in considering further assessment. Their implementation into patient counseling and clinical decision making can help to avoid unnecessary biopsies. Whether or not to start screening or to perform a biopsy should be decided based on an individual multivariate risk assessment in combination with balanced information and shared decision making.

Once the decision to biopsy is made, the next question will be how to detect significant PCa more accurately. MpMRI-guided biopsy has the potential to replace conventional systematic TRUS-guided biopsy owing to its higher diagnostic accuracy for significant PCa, especially for men with a previous negative biopsy.

Finally, an interesting and controversial topic is whether population-based PCa screening programs are still needed. Currently, the use of the PSA test and subsequent biopsy is an integrated part of daily clinical practice. However, it has been shown that despite having guidelines on the early detection of PCa there are numerous examples of misuse of the PSA test in daily clinical practice [87–90]. Men are being tested who are very unlikely to benefit (i.e., men with very limited life expectancy) while others that should be referred for further testing are not. It is therefore time that we either adapt clinical practice, start following guidelines, and start implementing new techniques, or stop PSA screening in the clinical setting and introduce specialized screening units where, only after a diagnosis has been made, patients enter clinical practice.

References

1. Soerjomataram I, Lortet-Tieulent J, Parkin DM, et al. Global burden of cancer in 2008: a systematic analysis of disability-adjusted life-years in 12 world regions. Lancet. 2012;380(9856):1840–50.
2. Ferlay J, Steliarova-Foucher E, Lortet-Tieulent J, et al. Cancer incidence and mortality patterns in Europe: estimates for 40 countries in 2012. Eur J Cancer. 2013;49:1374–403.
3. Siegel RL, Miller KD, Jemal A. Cancer statistics, 2016. CA Cancer J Clin. 2016;66(1):7–30.
4. Center MM, Jemal A, Lortet-Tieulent J, et al. International variation in prostate cancer incidence and mortality rates. Eur Urol. 2012;61(6):1079–92.
5. Torre LA. Global cancer incidence and mortality rates and trends-an update. Cancer Epidemiol Biomarkers Prev. 2015;25(1):16–27.
6. Chu LW, Rithey J, Devesa SS, et al. Prostate cancer incidence rates in Africa. Prostate Cancer. 2011;2011:947870.
7. Wabinga HR, Nambooze S, Amulen PM, et al. Trends in the incidence of cancer in Kampala, Uganda 1991–2010. Int J Cancer. 2014;135(2):432–9.
8. Schroder FH, Hugosson J, Roobol MJ, et al. Screening and prostate cancer mortality: results of the European Randomised Study of Screening for Prostate Cancer (ERSPC) at 13 years of follow-up. Lancet. 2014;384(9959):2027–35.
9. Andriole GL, Crawford ED, Grubb 3rd RL, et al. Prostate cancer screening in the randomized Prostate, Lung, Colorectal, and Ovarian Cancer Screening Trial: mortality results after 13 years of follow-up. J Natl Cancer Inst. 2012;104(2):125–32.
10. Loeb S, Bjurlin MA, Nicholson J, et al. Overdiagnosis and overtreatment of prostate cancer. Eur Urol. 2014;65(6):1046–55.
11. Schroder FH, Hugosson J, Roobol MJ. Screening and prostate-cancer mortality in a randomized European study. N Engl J Med. 2009;360(13):1320–8.
12. Draisma G, Boer R, Otto SJ, et al. Lead times and overdetection due to prostate-specific antigen screening: estimates from the European Randomized Study of Screening for Prostate Cancer. J Natl Cancer Inst. 2003;95(12):868–78.
13. Ankerst DP, Thompson IM. Sensitivity and specificity of prostate-specific antigen for prostate cancer detection with high rates of biopsy verification. Arch Ital Urol Androl. 2006;78:125–9.
14. Blijenberg BG, Yurdakul G, Van Zelst BD, et al. Discordant performance of assays for free and total prostate-specific antigen in relation to the early detection of prostate cancer. BJU Int. 2001;88(6):545–50.
15. Foj L, Filella X, Alcover J, et al. Variability of assay methods for total and free PSA after WHO standardization. Tumour Biol. 2014;35(3):1867–73.
16. Nordstrom T, Adolfsson J, Gronberg H, et al. PSA test before biopsy decisions: STHLM3 results. 2016 Annual Congress of EAU, Abstract 97.

17. Thompson IM, Pauler DK, et al. Prevalence of prostate cancer among men with a prostate-specific antigen level<or =4.0 ng per milliliter. N Engl J Med. 2004;350(22):2239–46.
18. Schroder FH, Carter HB, Wolters T, et al. Early detection of prostate cancer in 2007. Part 1: PSA and PSA kinetics. Eur Urol. 2008;53(3):468–77.
19. Postma R, Schroder FH, van Leenders GJ, et al. Cancer detection and cancer characteristics in the European Randomized Study of Screening for Prostate Cancer (ERSPC)--Section Rotterdam. A comparison of two rounds of screening. Eur Urol. 2007;52(1):89–97.
20. Thompson IM, Ankerst DP. Prostate-specific antigen in the early detection of prostate cancer. CMAJ. 2007;176(13):1853–8.
21. Greene KL, Albertsen PC, Babaian RJ, et al. Prostate specific antigen best practice statement: 2009 update. J Urol. 2013;189(1 Suppl):S2–11.
22. Roobol MJ, Kranse R, de Koning HJ, et al. Prostate-specific antigen velocity at low prostate-specific antigen levels as screening tool for prostate cancer: results of second screening round of ERSPC (ROTTERDAM). Urology. 2004;63(2):309–13; discussion 313–5.
23. Loughlin KR. PSA velocity: a systematic review of clinical applications. Urol Oncol. 2014;32(8):1116–25.
24. Vickers AJ, Wolters T, Savage CJ, et al. Prostate-specific antigen velocity for early detection of prostate cancer: result from a large, representative, population-based cohort. Eur Urol. 2009;56(5):753–60.
25. Loeb S, Roehl KA, Catalona WJ, et al. Is the utility of prostate-specific antigen velocity for prostate cancer detection affected by age? BJU Int. 2008;101(7):817–21.
26. Reed A, Ankerst DP, Pollock BH, et al. Current age and race adjusted prostate specific antigen threshold values delay diagnosis of high grade prostate cancer. J Urol. 2007;178(5):1929–32.
27. Djavan B, Remzi M, Zlotta AR, et al. Complexed prostate-specific antigen, complexed prostate-specific antigen density of total and transition zone, complexed/total prostate-specific antigen ratio, free-to-total prostate-specific antigen ratio, density of total and transition zone prostate-specific antigen: results of the prospective multicenter European trial. Urology. 2002;60(4 Suppl 1):4–9.
28. Walsh AL, Considine SW, Thomas AZ, et al. Digital rectal examination in primary care is important for early detection of prostate cancer: a retrospective cohort analysis study. Br J Gen Pract. 2014;64(629):e783–7.
29. Thompson IM, Rounder JB, Teague JL, et al. Impact of routine screening for adenocarcinoma of the prostate on stage distribution. J Urol. 1987;137(3):424–6.
30. Schroder FH, van der Maas P, Beemsterboer P, et al. Evaluation of the digital rectal examination as ascreening test for prostate cancer. Rotterdam section of the European Randomized Study of Screening for Prostate Cancer. J Natl Cancer Inst. 1998;90(23):1817–23.
31. Bozeman CB, Carver BS, Caldito G, et al. Prostate cancer in patients with an abnormal digital rectal examination and serum prostate-specific antigen less than 4.0 ng/mL. Urology. 2005;66(4):803–7.
32. Roobol MJ. Digital rectal examination can detect early prostate cancer. Evid Based Med. 2015;20(3):119.
33. Varenhorst E, Berglund K, Lofman O, et al. Inter-observer variation in assessment of the prostate by digital rectal examination. Br J Urol. 1993;72(2):173–6.
34. Harvey CJ, Pilcher J, Richenberg J, et al. Applications of transrectal ultrasound in prostate cancer. Br J Radiol. 2012;85(1):S3–S17.
35. Mottet N, Lehmann M, Cicorelli S, et al. Transrectal ultrasonography in prostatic cancer: interexaminer variability of interpretation. Eur Urol. 1997;32(2):150–4.
36. Hwang SI, Lee HJ. The future perspectives in transrectal prostate ultrasound guided biopsy. Prostate Int. 2014;2(4):153–60.
37. Heidenreich A, Bastian PJ, Bellmunt J, et al. EAU guidelines on prostate cancer. part 1: screening, diagnosis, and local treatment with curative intentupdate 2013. Eur Urol. 2014;65:124–37.
38. Brock M, von Bodman C, Palisaar RJ, et al. The impact of real-time elastography guiding a systematic prostate biopsy to improve cancer detection rate: a prospective study of 353 patients. J Urol. 2012;187(6):2039–43.
39. Penzkofer T, Tempany-Afdhal CM. Prostate cancer detection and diagnosis: the role of MR and its comparison to other diagnostic modalities – a radiologist's perspective. NMR Biomed. 2014;27(1):10.
40. Raaijmakers R, Kirkels WJ, Roobol MJ, et al. Complication rates and risk factors of 5802 transrectal ultrasound-guided sextant biopsies of the prostate within a population-based screening program. Urology. 2002;60(5):826–30.
41. Zani EL, Clark OA, Rodrigues Netto Jr N. Antibiotic prophylaxis for transrectal prostate biopsy. Cochrane Database Syst Rev. 2011;5:CD006576.
42. Aly M, Dyrdak R, Nordstrom T, et al. Rapid increase in multidrug-resistant enteric bacilli blood stream infection after prostate biopsy – A 10-year population-based cohort study. Prostate. 2015;75(9):947–56.
43. Mikolajczyk SD, Grauer LS, Millar LS, et al. A precursor form of PSA (pPSA) is a component of the free PSA in prostate cancer serum. Urology. 1997;50:710–4.
44. Mikolajczyk SD, Millar LS, Wang TJ, et al. A precursor form of prostate-specific antigen is more highly elevated in prostate cancer compared with benign transition zone prostate tissue. Cancer Res. 2000;60:756–9.

45. Sartori DA, Chan DW. Biomarkers in prostate cancer: what's new? Curr Opin Oncol. 2014;26(3):259–64.
46. Jansen FH, van Schaik RH, Kurstjens J. Prostate-specific antigen (PSA) isoform p2PSA in combination with total PSA and free PSA improves diagnostic accuracy in prostate cancer detection. Eur Urol. 2010;57(6):921–7.
47. Lazzeri M, Haese A, de la Taille A, et al. Serum isoform [-2]proPSA derivatives significantly improve prediction of prostate cancer at initial biopsy in a total PSA range of 2-10 ng/ml: a multicentric European study. Eur Urol. 2013;63(6):986–94.
48. Loeb S, Sanda MG, Broyles DL, et al. The prostate health index selectively identifies clinically significant prostate cancer. J Urol. 2015;193(4):1163–9.
49. Ito K, Miyakubo M, Sekine Y, et al. Diagnostic significance of [-2]pro-PSA and prostate dimension-adjusted PSA-related indices in men with total PSA in the 20-100 ng/mL range. World J Urol. 2013;31:305–11.
50. Ng CF, Chiu PK, Lam NY, et al. The Prostate Health Index in predicting initial prostate biopsy outcomes in Asian men with prostate-specific antigen levels of 4-10 ng/mL. Int Urol Nephrol. 2014;46:711–7.
51. Na R, Ye D, Liu F, et al. Performance of serum prostate-specific antigen isoform [-2]proPSA (p2PSA) and the prostate health index (PHI) in a Chinese hospital-based biopsy population. Prostate. 2014;74(15):1569–75.
52. Vickers AJ, Cronin AM, Aus G, et al. A panel of kallikrein markers can reduce unnecessary biopsy for prostate cancer: data from the European Randomized Study of Prostate Cancer Screening in Göteborg. Sweden BMC Med. 2008;6:19.
53. Nordström T, Vickers A, Assel M, et al. Comparison between the four-kallikrein panel and prostate health index for predicting prostate cancer. Eur Urol. 2015;68(1):139–46.
54. Nichol MB, Wu J, An JJ, Huang J, Denham D, Frencher S, et al. Budget impact analysis of a new prostate cancer risk index for prostate cancer detection. Prostate Cancer Prostatic Dis. 2011;14:253–61.
55. Sanguedolce F, Cormio A, Brunelli M, et al. Urine TMPRSS2: ERG fusion transcript as a biomarker for prostate cancer: literature review. Clin Genitourin Cancer. 2015;17:117–21.
56. Bussemakers MJ, van Bokhoven A, Verhaegh GW, et al. DD3: a new prostate-specific gene, highly overexpressed in prostate cancer. Cancer Res. 1999;59:5975–9.
57. Chun FK, de la Taille A, van Poppel H, et al. Prostate cancer gene 3 (PCA3): development and internal validation of a novel biopsy nomogram. Eur Urol. 2009;56(4):659–67.
58. Roobol MJ, Schroder FH, van Leeuwen P, et al. Performance of the prostate cancer antigen 3 (PCA3) gene and prostate-specific antigen in prescreened men: exploring the value of PCA3 for a first-line diagnostic test. Eur Urol. 2010;58(4):475–81.
59. Hessels D, Smit FP, Verhaegh GW, et al. Detection of TMPRSS2-ERG fusion transcripts and prostate cancer antigen 3 in urinary sediments may improve diagnosis of prostate cancer. Clin Cancer Res. 2007;13(17):5103–8.
60. Pettersson A, Graff RE, Bauer SR, et al. The TMPRSS2:ERG rearrangement, ERG expression, and prostate cancer outcomes: a cohort study and meta-analysis. Cancer Epidemiol Biomarkers Prev. 2012;21(9):1497–509.
61. Tomlins SA, Day JR, Lonigro RJ, et al. Urine TMPRSS2:ERG plus PCA3 for individualized prostate cancer risk assessment. Eur Urol. 2015;15:45.
62. Al Olama AA, Kote-Jarai Z, Berndt SI, et al. A meta-analysis of 87,040 individuals identifies 23 new susceptibility loci for prostate cancer. Nat Genet. 2014;46(10):1103–9.
63. Szulkin R, Whitington T, Eklund M, et al. Prediction of individual genetic risk to prostate cancer using a polygenic score. Prostate. 2015;75(13):1467–74.
64. Grönberg H, Adolfsson J, Aly M, et al. Prostate cancer screening in men aged 50-69 years (STHLM3): a prospective population-based diagnostic study. Lancet Oncol. 2015;16(16):1667–76.
65. Weinreb JC, Barentsz JO, Choyke PL, et al. PI-RADS Prostate Imaging – Reporting and Data System: 2015, Version 2. Eur Urol. 2016;69(1):16–40.
66. Diaz de Leon A, Costa D, Pedrosa I. Role of multiparametric MR imaging in malignancies of the urogenital tract. Magn Reson Imaging Clin N Am. 2016;24(1):187–204.
67. Pinto PA, Chung PH, Rastinehad AR, et al. Magnetic resonance imaging/ultrasound fusion guided prostate biopsy improves cancer detection following transrectal ultrasound biopsy and correlates with multiparametric magnetic resonance imaging. J Urol. 2011;186:1281–5.
68. Barentsz JO, Richenberg J, Clements R, et al. ESUR prostate MR guidelines 2012. Eur Radiol. 2012;22(4):746–57.
69. Siddiqui MM, Rais-Bahrami S, Turkbey B, et al. Comparison of MR/ultrasound fusion-guided biopsy with ultrasound-guided biopsy for the diagnosis of prostate cancer. JAMA. 2015;313(4):390–7.
70. Schoots IG, Roobol MJ, Nieboer D, et al. Magnetic resonance imaging-targeted biopsy may enhance the diagnostic accuracy of significant prostate cancer detection compared to standard transrectal ultrasound-guided biopsy: a systematic review and meta-analysis. Eur Urol. 2015;68(3):438–50.
71. Gaziev G, Wadhwa K, Barrett T, et al. Defining the learning curve for multiparametric magnetic resonance imaging (MRI) of the prostate using MRI-transrectal ultrasonography (TRUS) fusion-guided transperineal prostate biopsies as a validation tool. BJU Int. 2016;117(1):80–6.
72. Kranse R, Roobol M, Schroder FH. A graphical device to represent the outcomes of a logistic regression analysis. Prostate. 2008;68:1674–80.

73. Thompson IM, Ankerst DP, Chi C, et al. Assessing prostate cancer risk: results from the prostate cancer prevention trial. J Natl Cancer Inst. 2006;98(8):529–34.
74. Zhu X, Albertsen PC, Andriole GL, et al. Risk-based prostate cancer screening. Eur Urol. 2012;61(4):652–61.
75. Zhu Y, Wang JY, Shen YJ. External validation of the Prostate Cancer Prevention Trial and the European Randomized Study of Screening for Prostate Cancer risk calculators in a Chinese cohort. Asian J Androl. 2012;14(5):738–44.
76. Roobol MJ, Steyerberg EW, Kranse R, et al. A risk-based strategy improves prostate – specific antigen – driven detection of prostate cancer. Eur Urol. 2010;57:79–85.
77. Trottier G, Roobol MJ, Lawrentschuk N, et al. Comparison of risk calculators from the Prostate Cancer Prevention Trial and the European Randomized Study of Screening for Prostate Cancer in a contemporary Canadian cohort. BJU Int. 2011;108(8 Pt 2):E237–44.
78. van Vugt HA, Roobol MJ, Kranse R, et al. Prediction of prostate cancer in unscreened men: external validation of a risk calculator. Eur J Cancer. 2011;47(6):903–9.
79. Yoon DK, Park JY, Yoon S, et al. Can the prostate risk calculator based on Western population be applied to Asian population? Prostate. 2012;72(7):721–9.
80. Lee DH, Jung HB, Park JW, et al. Can Western based online prostate cancer risk calculators be used to predict prostate cancer after prostate biopsy for the Korean population? Yonsei Med J. 2013;54(3):665–71.
81. Vickers AJ, Cronin AM, Roobol MJ, Hugosson J, Jones JS, Kattan MW, Klein E, Hamdy F, Neal D, Donovan J, Parekh DJ, Ankerst D, Bartsch G, Klocker H, Horninger W, Benchikh A, Salama G, Villers A, Freedland SJ, Moreira DM, Schröder FH, Lilja H. The relationship between prostate-specific antigen and prostate cancer risk: the Prostate Biopsy Collaborative Group. Clin Cancer Res. 2010;16(17):4374–81.
82. Cavadas V, Osório L, Sabell F, et al. Prostate cancer prevention trial and European randomized study of screening for prostate cancer risk calculators: a performance comparison in a contemporary screened cohort. Eur Urol. 2010;58(4):551–8.
83. Oliveira M, Marques V, Carvalho AP, et al. Head-to-head comparison of two online nomograms for prostate biopsy outcome prediction. BJU Int. 2011;107(11):1780–3.
84. Foley RW, Maweni RM, Gorman L, et al. The ERSPC risk calculators significantly outperform the PCPT 2.0 in the prediction of prostate cancer; a multi-institutional study. BJU Int. 2016.
85. Lilja H, Cronin AM, Dahlin A, et al. Prediction of significant prostate cancer diagnosed 20 to 30 years later with a single measure of prostate-specific antigen at or before age 50. Cancer. 2011;117(6):1210–9.
86. Arsov C, Becker N, Hadaschik BA, et al. Prospective randomized evaluation of risk-adapted prostate-specific antigen screening in young men: the PROBASE trial. Eur Urol. 2013;64(6):873–5.
87. Loeb S. Guideline of guidelines: prostate cancer screening. BJU Int. 2014;114(3):323–5.
88. Nordström T, Aly M, Clements MS, Weibull CE, Adolfsson J, Grönberg H. Prostate-specific antigen (PSA) testing is prevalent and increasing in Stockholm County, Sweden, Despite no recommendations for PSA screening: results from a population-based study, 2003–2011. Eur Urol. 2013;63(3):419–25.
89. Moss S, Melia J, Sutton J, Mathews C, Kirby M. Prostate-specific antigen testing rates and referral patterns from general practice data in England. Int J Clin Pract. 2016;14:312.
90. Van der Meer S, Löwik SA, Hirdes WH, Nijman RM, Van der Meer K, Hoekstra-Weebers JE, Blanker MH. Prostate specific antigen testing policy worldwide varies greatly and seems not to be in accordance with guidelines: a systematic review. BMC Fam Pract. 2012;13:100.

Anatomo-pathology

S. Prendeville and T.H. Van der Kwast

1 Gross Anatomy of the Prostate: Clinical Importance

Accurate localization of prostate cancer(s) within the gland may have implications for both diagnosis and treatment, including the potential for focal therapies which have been developed in recent years. Detailed anatomic knowledge forms the basis of different approaches to surgical dissection (interfascial, intrafascial, extrafascial). In addition, knowledge of the boundaries of the prostate and the fascial anatomy is also essential for accurate pathological staging of prostatectomy specimens. The official anatomic terminology of the prostate and its contiguous structures has been revised several times in the past and current recommendations try to accommodate clinical concepts within an updated terminology [52] as highlighted in an authoritative and well-illustrated review of the topic [79], which was recently updated [80]. It is worth noting, however, that certain aspects of the anatomy of the prostate remain controversial with variable terminology used in the published literature.

S. Prendeville • T.H. Van der Kwast (✉)
Department of Pathology, University Health Network and University of Toronto, Toronto, ON, Canada
e-mail: theodorus.vanderkwast@uhn.ca

1.1 The Boundaries of the Prostate

The prostate gland lies posterior to the pubic symphysis and anterior to the rectum and it merges proximally with the bladder neck and distally (at its apex) with the external urethral sphincter. The prostate gland is not surrounded by a true capsule but rather a "pseudocapsule" comprising a condensation of fibromuscular stroma at the outer edge of the prostate which has a variable appearance [80]. Surrounding this are the periprostatic fascial layers and the neurovascular bundles. Anteriorly, the prostate is also covered by smooth muscle bundles arising from the outer longitudinal detrusor muscle of the bladder (detrusor apron) and by the dorsal vascular complex (Figs. 1 and 2).

1.1.1 Periprostatic Fascia

The anterior surface of the prostate, detrusor apron, and dorsal vascular complex are covered by a layer of visceral endopelvic fascia, which is fused in the midline with the anterior fibromuscular stroma of the prostate. Laterally, the prostate is covered by a layer of fascia termed the prostatic fascia and, external to this, the levator ani fascia.

The posterior surface of the prostate and seminal vesicles are closely covered by Denonvilliers' fascia, or the posterior prostatic and seminal vesicle fascia [79]. Denonvilliers' fascia consists of a

M. Bolla, H. van Poppel (eds.), *Management of Prostate Cancer*,
DOI 10.1007/978-3-319-42769-0_4

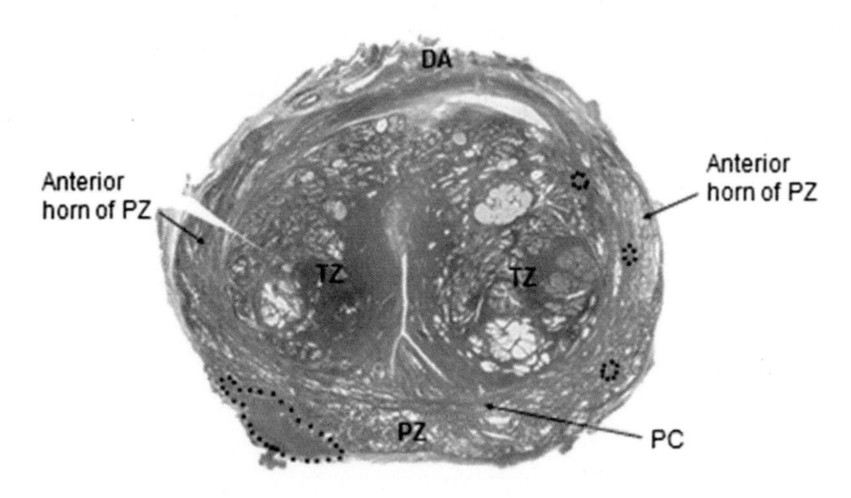

Fig. 1 Wholemount section of radical prostatectomy specimen, with multifocal prostate cancer (marked by *dotted line*). *DA* detrusor apron, *PC* posterior commissure, *PZ* peripheral zone, *TZ* transition zone, *U* urethra. The index tumor is located in the posterior peripheral zone, and one small cancer is located in the transition zone of the anterior prostate

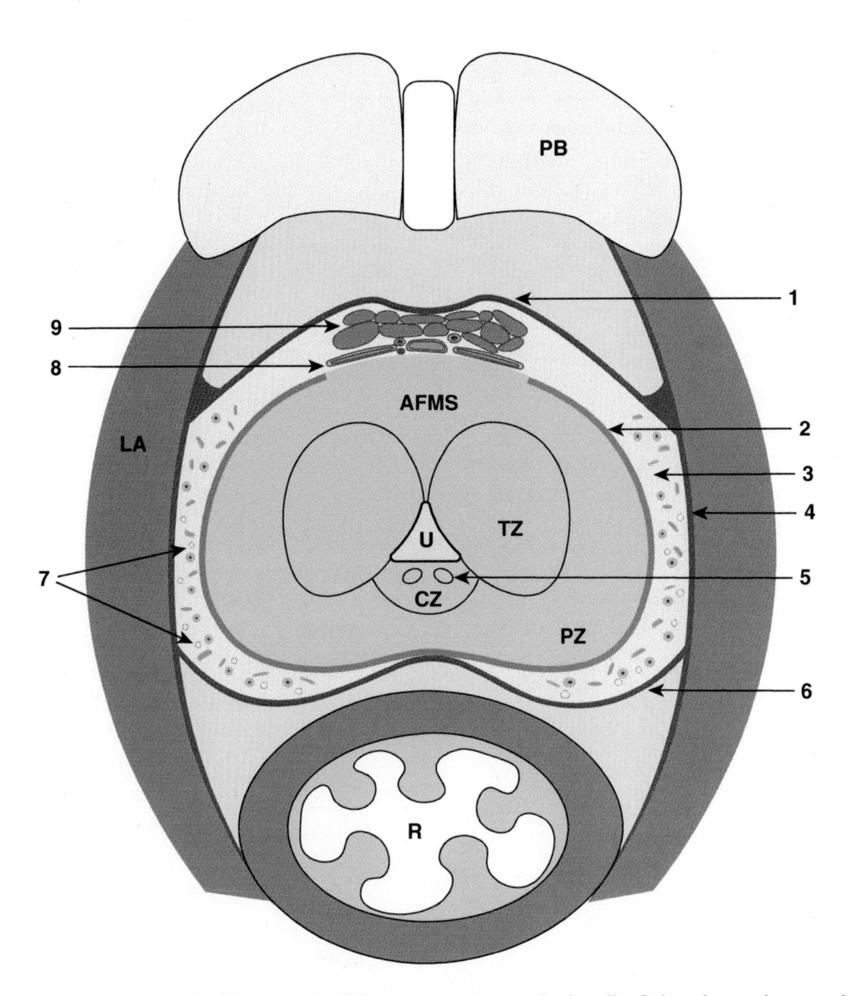

Fig. 2 Schematic illustration of midprostate (axial section) and surrounding structures. *1* visceral endopelvic fascia, 2 prostatic pseudocapsule, 3 prostate fascia, 4 levator ani fascia, 5 ejaculatory duct, 6 Denonvilliers' fascia, 7 neurovascular bundle, 8 dorsal vascular complex, 9 detrusor apron, *AFMS* anterior fibromuscular stroma, *CZ* central zone, *LA* levator ani muscle, *PB* pubic bone, *PZ* peripheral zone, *R* rectum, *TZ* transition zone, *U* urethra

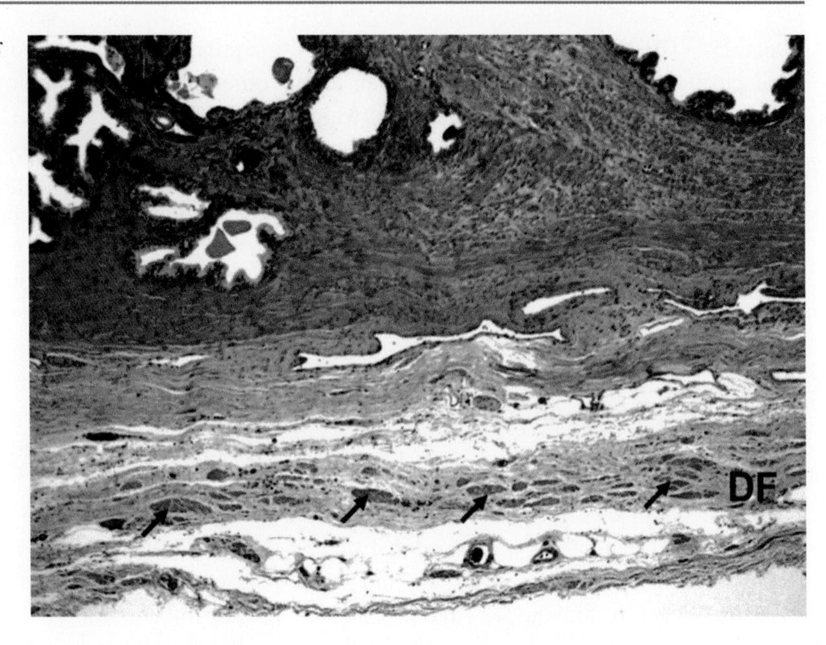

Fig. 3 Section of posterior margin of the prostate, displaying Denonvilliers' fascia (*DF*) with small bundles of smooth muscle (*arrows*) embedded in fibrous tissue of low cellularity. Here Denonvilliers' fascia is separated from the outer prostate by a thin layer of loose connective tissue

single layer of loose connective tissue and interlacing leaves of elastic tissue or smooth muscle and is adherent to the prostate at the base near the seminal vesicles [51] (Fig. 3). The neurovascular bundles are generally located posterolaterally in the region medial to the levator ani fascia and anterior to Denonvilliers' fascia. However, this is subject to interindividual variation and remains controversial, with recent evidence for a more complex nerve distribution [57]. At prostatectomy, increasing amounts of periprostatic tissue will be resected with intra-, inter-, and extrafascial approaches, respectively. Extrafascial dissection is carried out lateral to the levator ani fascia and posterior to Denonvilliers' fascia. While this is the most oncologically safe dissection, it includes complete resection of the neurovascular bundle [80]. Conversely, an intrafascial approach allows preservation of the neurovascular bundle but carries an increased risk of prostatic incision [79].

1.1.2 The Superior and Inferior Boundaries of the Prostate

At the superior boundary of the prostate, the bladder neck is formed from prostatic tissue, the vesical sphincter, and detrusor muscle of urinary bladder origin [80]. The prostate apex (inferior boundary) represents the site where the intermediate or membranous part of the urethra exits the prostate. This part of the urethra is surrounded by the external urethral sphincter, which is a distinct muscular structure, separated from the pelvic floor musculature by a thin fibrous layer [67]. The sphincter is composed of two layers: an outer horseshoe-shaped layer of striated muscle and an inner circumferential smooth muscle layer [80].

1.1.3 Anatomical Implications for Tumor Staging at Prostatectomy

The anatomy of the prostate can pose challenges for accurate pathological staging in relation to extraprostatic extension [26]. This is particularly true at the anterior border, apex and bladder neck, where prostatic stroma may blend with smooth muscle of the detrusor apron, skeletal muscle of the urinary sphincter and smooth muscle of the urinary bladder detrusor muscle, respectively (see Sect. 4.4).

1.2 Prostate Lobes

Clinically, during digital rectal examination, a lobulation of the prostate may be noted, which can be due to the indentation of the rectal surface or a preferential growth of the transition zone in elder men, commonly referred to as benign prostatic hyperplasia (BPH) [52]. In the midposterior urethral position, BPH may result in median lobe hyperplasia, also known as Home's lobe, which protrudes as a ball valve into the bladder lumen just inferior to the trigone. Although the vast majority of contemporary carcinomas do not present as a nodule, prostate cancers identified by positive digital rectal examination are pathologically advanced in over 50 % of men [27].

1.3 McNeal's Four Prostate Regions

In 1988, McNeal proposed a model of zonal anatomy of the prostate gland, abolishing the previous concept of a lobular organization of the gland structure [43]. In his model, the prostate is divided into four regions: (1) the anterior fibromuscular stroma, (2) the central zone, (3) the transition zone, and (4) the peripheral zone (Figs. 1 and 2). These four regions can be identified by T2-weighted magnetic resonance imaging (MRI).

1.3.1 The Anterior Fibromuscular Stroma

The anterior fibromuscular stroma extends along the anteromedial aspect of the prostate and merges with the striated muscle of the external sphincter at the apex and the vesical sphincter of the bladder neck. The distal (apical) portion of the anterior fibromuscular stroma is rich in striated muscle and is important in voluntary sphincter function, whereas at its proximal end smooth muscle becomes a dominant feature with an important role in involuntary sphincter function [30]. The anterior fibromuscular stroma contains few if any prostatic glands.

1.3.2 The Central Zone

The central zone is a cone-shaped area between the ejaculatory ducts and the bladder neck, situated posterior to the ascending prostatic urethra, and occupies about 30 % of the prostatic glandular mass. Histologically, the prostatic glands in the central zone have a distinct and more complex architecture often with cribriform and papillary features as compared to those in the other zones. For pathologists, it is important to recognize central zone glands, because their nuclear features may resemble high-grade prostatic intraepithelial neoplasia (H-PIN), a precursor lesion of prostate cancer [7] (see Sect. 3).

1.3.3 The Transition Zone and Peripheral Zone

The transition zone is mainly located lateral and anterior to the urethra (Figs. 1 and 2) and may be separated from the peripheral zone by a band of denser fibromuscular stroma that is the posterior commissure [52]. The transition zone normally comprises only about 5 % of prostatic glandular tissue. The peripheral zone comprises about 65 % of the prostatic glandular tissue with the majority occupying the inferior (apical) and posterior part of the prostate, although it also extends anteriorly as the lateral horn of the peripheral zone. Thus, the anterior prostate comprises both peripheral zone (lateral) and transition zone (mediolateral) components as well as the midline anterior fibromuscular stroma [25].

1.4 Prostate Zones and Cancer

About 70 % of prostate cancers originate in the peripheral zone, most of them at a posterior or posterolateral localization [43]. This coincides with the frequent occurrence of the cancer precursor high-grade prostatic intraepithelial neoplasia (H-PIN) in the peripheral zone and its much rarer occurrence in the transition zone [7]. In several patient series, it was shown that in spite of significantly higher PSA levels as well as greater tumor volume when compared with those of peripheral zone cancers, tumors from the transition zone showed similar biochemical cure rates following radical prostatectomy [76]. This would suggest a less aggressive phenotype for transition zone cancers when compared to tumors from the peripheral zone. However, contradictory findings have also been reported, e.g., Augustin et al. [4] found that the zonal location was not an independent prognostic factor on multivariate analysis.

The determination of the zonal origin of prostate carcinoma by the pathologist is more challenging on standard quadrant sections of prostatectomy specimens when compared to wholemount sections [25]. Often a prostate cancer involves both the peripheral and transition zone and anterior transition zone carcinomas may extend into the midline anterior fibromuscular stroma.

2 Microscopic Anatomy of the Prostate

Histologically, the prostate is composed of acini and ducts, both of which are lined by a dual cell population that is an inner layer of luminal or secretory cells and an outer rim of basal cells. Each of the three anatomically distinct zones of the prostate has its own set of periurethral main prostatic ducts. The lining of the latter structures often displays a hyperplasia of basal cells and here the luminal cells may have a columnar (ductal) appearance [58]. The periurethral ducts give off branches, with tributaries adopting the more rounded architecture with cuboidal luminal cell morphology of prostatic acini as they progress upstream from the urethra, until eventually ducts and acini are no longer distinguishable. Interspersed within the glandular lining of the ducts and acini are the neuroendocrine cells which secrete regulatory neuropeptides. Only the luminal cells express prostate-specific antigen, which is under androgen regulation. Androgen receptors can be found in the nuclei of luminal cells and most of the fibromuscular stromal cells (Fig. 4), whereas the neuroendocrine cells and most of the basal cells lack androgen receptors [37].

2.1 Age-Related Microscopic Changes

In aging men, hyperplasia of both the glandular and/or fibromuscular components (BPH) occurs almost uniquely in the transition zone. By contrast, the peripheral zone is more often subject to glandular atrophy. Histologically, usual type atrophy is characterized by a flattening of the luminal cells resting on a single conspicuous layer of cuboidal basal cells, while the glands lose their infoldings to a straighter outline. However, various different morphological forms of atrophy exist (and often coexist), including partial atrophy, cystic atrophy (Fig. 5), sclerotic atrophy, and

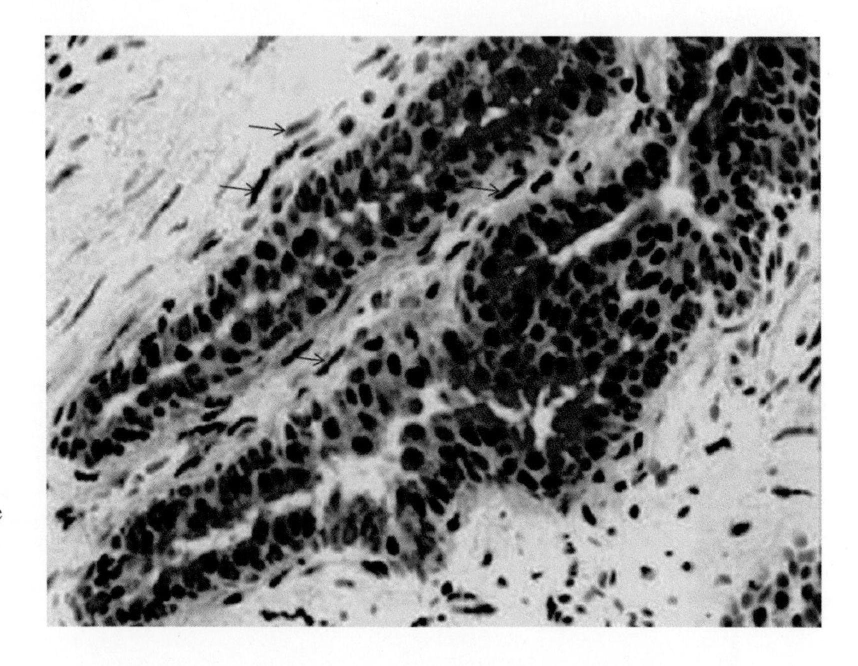

Fig. 4 Microscopic image of prostate tissue immunostained for PSA (*red*) and androgen receptor (*brown*). Blue nuclei are unstained. Both stromal cells (*arrows*) and PSA-positive luminal cells are positive for androgen receptor, while basal cells are negative for androgen receptor

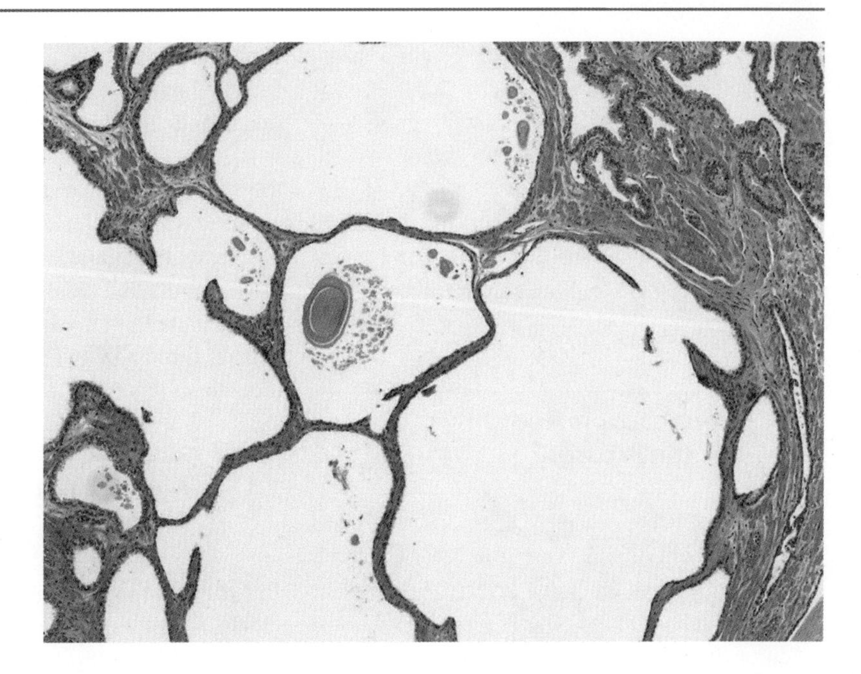

Fig. 5 Microscopic image of prostate glands showing cystic atrophy, adjacent to normal prostate glands at the right

hyperplastic atrophy/postatrophic hyperplasia. Recent studies suggested that the presence of atrophy [48] and a greater extent of acute and chronic inflammation [49] in a negative prostate biopsy is associated with a lower risk of subsequent carcinoma. Thus, although it is not current standard practice to specifically report on these parameters in negative biopsies, they may potentially provide useful information in the future.

2.2 Androgen Deprivation-Induced Changes

It is well established that long-term use of aromatase inhibitors, such as Dutasteride leads to an average reduction in prostate gland volume by 17.5 % after 2 years, mainly attributed to its effect on BPH [3]. Microscopic changes of the normal tissues during long-term administration of aromatase inhibitors have not been described. This is in contrast to the pronounced effects of antiandrogens and lutein hormone releasing hormone agonists. After androgen deprivation to castration levels, the entire prostate will shrink to about 80 % of its original size within 3 months of treatment. This reduction in volume is associated with a profound remodeling of the prostate tissue [73], which is different for the peripheral and transition zone of the normal prostate. In the peripheral zone, a general atrophy of prostatic glands is noted while the transition zone glands display more prominent basal cell hyperplasia and the glands become smaller and more rounded.

3 Precursor Lesions of Prostate Cancer (H-PIN)

High-grade prostatic intraepithelial neoplasia (H-PIN) is widely accepted as the main precursor lesion for prostate cancer. However, there is also recent evidence that some cases of H-PIN may actually represent intra-acinar spread of invasive carcinoma rather than a true precursor, and this is an area of ongoing research [15]. In addition, other glandular proliferations have been proposed as potential precursor lesions, e.g., adenosis (atypical adenomatous hyperplasia) has been put forward as a potential precursor to carcinomas arising in the transition zone ([15]). Intraductal carcinoma (IDC-P) is discussed in Sect. 4.3.

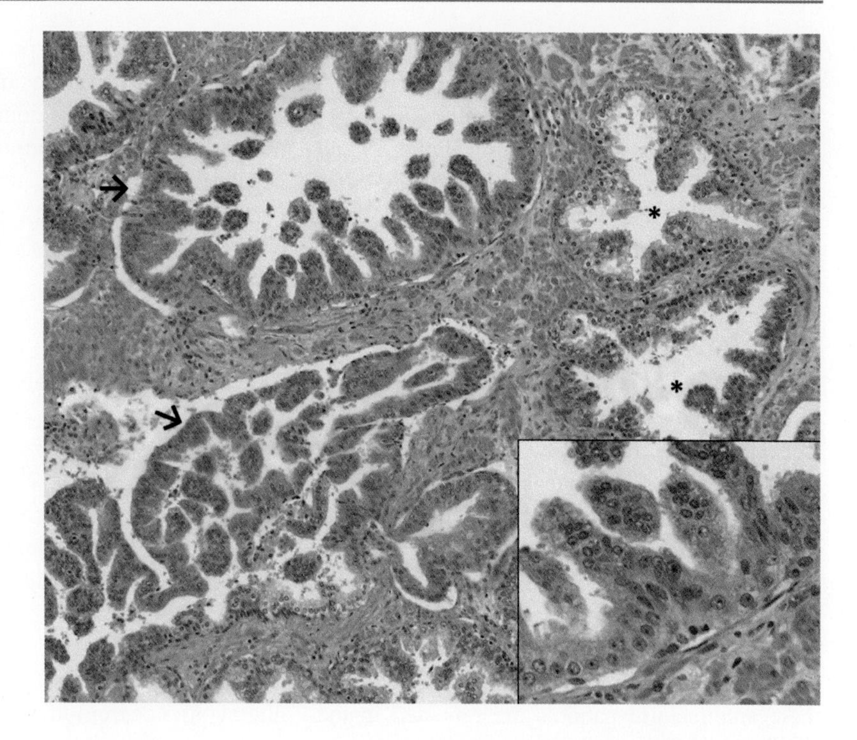

Fig. 6 Micrograph showing H-PIN (*arrows*) with admixed benign glands (*). *Inset*: high power view demonstrating prominent nucleoli which are the hallmark of H-PIN

3.1 High-Grade Prostatic Intraepithelial Neoplasia (H-PIN)

H-PIN is characterized by the presence of dysplastic features in the luminal cells lining prostatic glands or ducts, while retaining the antecedent architecture of benign glands (Fig. 6). The morphologic hallmark of H-PIN is the presence of prominent nucleoli in cells lining prostatic glands or ducts with a luminal (but not basal) cell morphology and location [7]. Montironi et al. [47] reported that H-PIN was found in association with invasive carcinoma in 70 % of cystoprostatectomy specimens with an incidental prostate cancer and in 50 % of specimens without prostate cancer. Because of this association of H-PIN with carcinoma, their similarity in cytonuclear features, their close spatial association in the prostate, and shared specific genetic changes, H-PIN is considered a precursor for prostate cancer [18]. It remains unclear, however, which proportion of H-PIN actually progresses over time to invasive prostate cancer. Accordingly, most guidelines do not recommend repeat biopsy for isolated H-PIN; however, multifocal H-PIN (>1 core involved) has been shown to be associated with a higher risk of subsequent carcinoma [45].

4 Prostate Cancer

Prostate cancer is a very common finding in elder men, and its clinical course is highly variable. The histopathological features of prostate cancer and its spatial extension have been shown to be the strongest predictors of their behavior.

4.1 Types and Variants of Adenocarcinoma

Conventional acinar adenocarcinoma accounts for the vast majority of cases; however, other types of prostate cancer may also be encountered. Some of the latter constitute histological variants of acinar adenocarcinoma, while others represent distinct tumor entities, as outlined out in the World Health Organization (WHO) classification of tumors of the urinary system and male genital tract [46]. Some of these variants and tumor types may have prognostic implications, or they may occur in certain clinical situations, e.g., following prior non-surgical treatment including radiation and hormonal manipulation. Examples of the latter include small and large cell neuroendocrine carcinoma and the very rare adenosquamous carcinoma.

4.1.1 Conventional Acinar Adenocarcinomas and Its Variants

Conventional acinar adenocarcinoma is the most common type of prostate cancer, representing over 95 % of cases. This type of adenocarcinoma displays a remarkable morphologic heterogeneity, which may coexist within the same tumor focus. Most common is the formation of small- to medium-sized glands, but these glands may fuse, or form cribriform or ragged sheets of cells and these architectural patterns are reflected in the histopathological grading of adenocarcinoma (see Sect. 4.2.2). A number of histopathological variants exist, some of which are of significance as they may cause diagnostic difficulty for pathologists, including the pseudohyperplastic, foamy gland, atrophic, and microcystic variants. Other variants confer a worse prognosis compared with conventional acinar adenocarcinoma [32], including the signet ring cell like, pleomorphic giant cell, and sarcomatoid variants. Mucinous (colloid) carcinoma is diagnosed at prostatectomy when >25 % of the tumor contains extracellular mucin pools. This very rare variant comprises 0.2 % of prostate cancers [28] and was initially thought to be more aggressive than conventional acinar adenocarcinoma, although more recent studies have suggested that it may in fact have a better prognosis [56].

4.1.2 Ductal Adenocarcinoma

Although in the current WHO classification of prostate cancer [46] ductal adenocarcinoma is coined as a distinct type of prostate adenocarcinoma, some would consider it a variant of conventional adenocarcinoma. Ductal adenocarcinoma as a dominant pattern accounts for a mere 0.2–0.8 % of all prostate cancers (IARC 2016), but it is more frequently seen as a smaller component of conventional acinar adenocarcinoma. These tumors involve the large periurethral ducts and may become clinically manifest as an exophytic papillary mass in the prostatic urethra. Consistent with the features of large periurethral duct epithelium (see Sect. 2), the columnar neoplastic cells form a pseudostratified layer, often lining papillary structures with true fibrovascular cores, and their nuclei are mostly elongated or oval often with a single macronucleolus. Recognizing ductal adenocarcinoma is important, as it is more aggressive than conventional acinar adenocarcinoma [63]. In terms of grading, ductal adenocarcinoma is assigned Gleason pattern 4, or Gleason pattern 5 if comedo necrosis is present (IARC 2016). An uncommon variant termed prostatic intraepithelial neoplasia-like ductal adenocarcinoma exists which behaves similar to Gleason score 6 adenocarcinoma [72] and is therefore important to recognize and grade accordingly.

4.1.3 Neuroendocrine Carcinoma

The presence of scattered neuroendocrine cells, as identified by immunohistochemical staining, is a relatively common finding in otherwise conventional acinar adenocarcinoma. The clinical significance of this type of neuroendocrine differentiation is controversial; however, it is generally regarded as not being prognostically significant [19, 34]. Poorly differentiated neuroendocrine carcinomas of the prostate include small cell carcinoma and large cell neuroendocrine carcinoma. Small cell carcinoma appears morphologically similar to its counterpart at other sites, being composed of sheets of cells with a high nuclear:cytoplasmic ratio, nuclear molding and frequent mitoses, apoptosis, and necrosis. There is a history of conventional acinar adenocarcinoma in 40–50 % of cases [19], and in many cases, small cell carcinoma emerges following androgen deprivation treatment [53]. Immunohistochemistry is helpful to demonstrate neuroendocrine differentiation, using antibodies against synaptophysin, chromogranin A, and CD56, while the tumors generally lack expression of androgen receptors and PSA. When the tumor occurs in its pure form, a metastasis from another primary site should be excluded clinically. This distinction cannot be readily made on the basis of morphological or immunohistochemical features and it is worth noting that the lung/thyroid cancer marker TTF-1 is commonly positive in small cell carcinomas of primary prostatic origin. Fluorescence in situ hybridization (FISH) or reverse transcriptase polymerase chain reaction (RT-PCR) to detect TM-PRSS2-ERG gene fusion may be helpful to confirm a primary prostatic origin [62], while it is worth noting that ERG immunohistochemistry is not reliable in this setting [19, 62]. Large cell neuroendocrine carcinomas of the prostate are exceptionally rare, especially in their pure form, with limited published data available [24]. They are composed of large nests of cells with peripheral palisading, necrosis, and immunohistochemical evidence of neuroendocrine differentiation. These tumors show cytological features that are distinct from those of small cell carcinoma, including prominent nucleoli, clumped chromatin and abundant cytoplasm [19]. Both small and large cell neuoroendocrine carcinomas show an aggressive behavior similar to poorly differentiated neuroendocrine carcinoma at other body sites. Finally, adenocarcinoma with Paneth cell-like neuroendocrine differentiation is important for pathologists to recognize as Paneth cell-like areas may show high-grade architectural features (Gleason pattern 5), even though these tumors generally have a favorable prognosis [70]. As a result, grading may not be applicable in these areas [19, 70].

4.1.4 Other Rare Prostate Cancer Types

Other types of prostate cancer that may rarely be encountered include basal cell carcinoma, squamous cell carcinoma, and adenosquamous carcinoma. The latter two entities may develop in the setting of androgen deprivation therapy and/or radiotherapy for prostate cancer.

4.2 Grading of Prostate Cancer

The Gleason grading system was first developed in the 1960s with modifications in 2005 and 2014. This system originally accounted for the heterogeneity of prostate cancer by identifying 5 grades on the basis of tumor architecture, ranging from 1 (most differentiated) to 5 (least differentiated). By adding the primary and secondary architectural growth patterns, a nine-tiered total score of ascending aggressiveness from 2 to 10 is obtained. In biopsy specimens, this score is calculated by adding the most dominant pattern and the worst/highest of the remaining patterns, while in prostatectomy specimens, the score is based on the most dominant and second most dominant patterns. In contemporary practice, Gleason scores 1 and 2 are virtually never reported such that prostate specimens are generally assigned a Gleason score ranging from 6 to 10. In prostatectomy cases with more than two architectural patterns, a tertiary grade may be reported. When a small volume of a high grade pattern (4 or 5) is present, it is usually assigned as a minor or tertiary pattern if it comprises <5 % of the tumor volume. A meta-analysis by [31] has shown convincingly that the presence of a tertiary grade 5 component has an unfavorable prognostic impact. On the other hand, most studies have shown that a < 5 % grade 4 component in an otherwise Gleason score 6 (3 + 3) carcinoma hardly affects the prognosis.

4.2.1 ISUP 2014 Grade Groups

Recently, a new grading system comprising 5 "Grade Groups," which are based on the modified Gleason grading patterns, was adopted by the International Society of Urological Pathology (ISUP) [21] and incorporated into the current WHO classification [46]. This five-tiered system (see Table 1) provides a simpler grading model for patients and clinicians [23] and also allows more accurate tumor stratification, particularly with regard to Gleason score 3 + 4 vs. 4 + 3 cancers, which have significantly different prognoses [12, 85]. In addition, given that Gleason score 6 cancers have an insignificant

Table 1 Grade groups and corresponding Gleason score

Grade Group	Gleason score
1	3+3=6 or less
2	3+4=7
3	4+3+7
4	4+4=8; 3+5+8; 5+3=8
5	4+5=9; 5+4=9, 5+5=10

risk of metastasis [60], labeling these tumors as grade 1, the lowest possible grade in the new system, provides a more logical terminology to help patients better understand the favorable prognosis of their disease and avoid overtreatment in these cases. In current practice, the convention is to report both the Gleason score and the corresponding ISUP 2014 Grade Group in parallel [50].

4.2.2 Quantification of High-Grade Carcinoma

One of the limitations of grading is interobserver variability, in particular with regard to the diagnosis of "poorly formed glands" as Gleason pattern 4, where the differential diagnosis includes tangentially sectioned pattern 3 glands [86]. Quantification of the percentage of high-grade cancer (pattern 4 or 5) on biopsy and prostatectomy specimens has been proposed to help further refine grading and provide additional prognostic information to aid decision making. A recent study, which included a large number of cases, has shown a continuous increase in the risk of PSA recurrence with increasing percentage of Gleason pattern 4 identified [61], while previous studies also found the amount of high-grade cancer to be an independent prognostic factor [78]. These findings suggest that additional clinically relevant information can be derived from morphologic grading as a continuum as compared with categorical grading. This is of particular relevance in the scenario of active surveillance of patients with low risk cancer. In many centers, active surveillance is only considered for cases with Gleason 3 + 3 disease; however, cases with a low volume (e.g., <5 %) of Gleason pattern 4 may also be deemed suitable. These issues are the subject of many ongoing studies which seek to further refine and standardize the clinically relevant information that prostate cancer grading provides.

4.2.3 Gleason Grade 4 Subpatterns

Of the Gleason architectural patterns, Gleason 4 is the most heterogeneous as it can comprise a variety of different patterns including cribriform structures, glomeruloid structures, fused glands, and poorly formed glands (Fig. 8). This heterogeneity translates into clinical behavior, in particular with regard to cribriform growth which has been shown to be a strong independent predictor for distant metastasis and disease-specific death in Gleason score 7 cancer at prostatectomy [39]. Invasive cribriform carcinoma often shows morphologic overlap with intraductal carcinoma (IDC-P) and immunohistochemical staining for basal cells may be required to differentiate the two entities. This distinction is necessary when there is potentially isolated IDC-P on a prostate core biopsy or when any associated carcinoma is low grade (e.g., Gleason 3 + 3, Grade Group 1), as IDC-P is not included when grading invasive carcinoma [19]. Given that any amount of IDC-P or cribriform carcinoma has an important prognostic implication ([38, 74] no longer in press), it is now recommended that their presence should be routinely reported in all diagnostic specimens [50].

4.3 Intraductal Carcinoma

Intraductal carcinoma of the prostate (IDC-P) is characterized histologically by an expansile, lumen-spanning proliferation of malignant epithelial cells within large ducts which retain an intact basal cell layer (Fig. 7). IDC-P is distinguished from H-PIN on the basis of a greater degree of architectural and/or cytological atypia [29]. This distinction is critical as IDC-P is often associated with high-grade invasive carcinoma [59] and is an adverse prognostic marker in biopsy and prostatectomy specimens [54, 75, 80, 86]. It is postulated that IDC-P represents intraductal propagation of an aggressive carcinoma

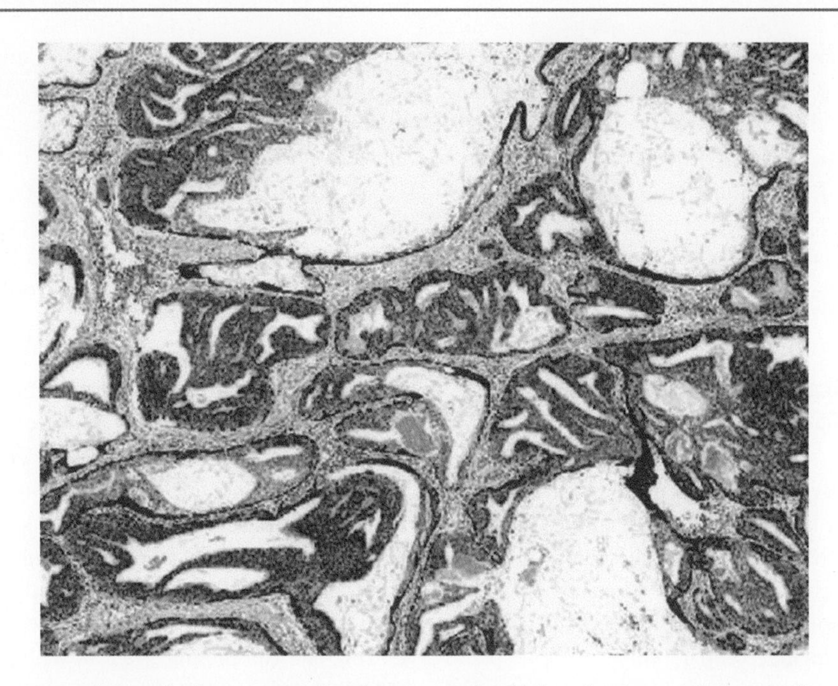

Fig. 7 Low power micrograph of an extensive intraductal carcinoma of the prostate immunostained for alpha-methyl coenzyme A (*red*) racemase and the basal cell marker high molecular weight keratin (*brown*). Glands and ducts are distended by a large mass of neoplastic cells (*red*), but remain lined by basal cells (brown)

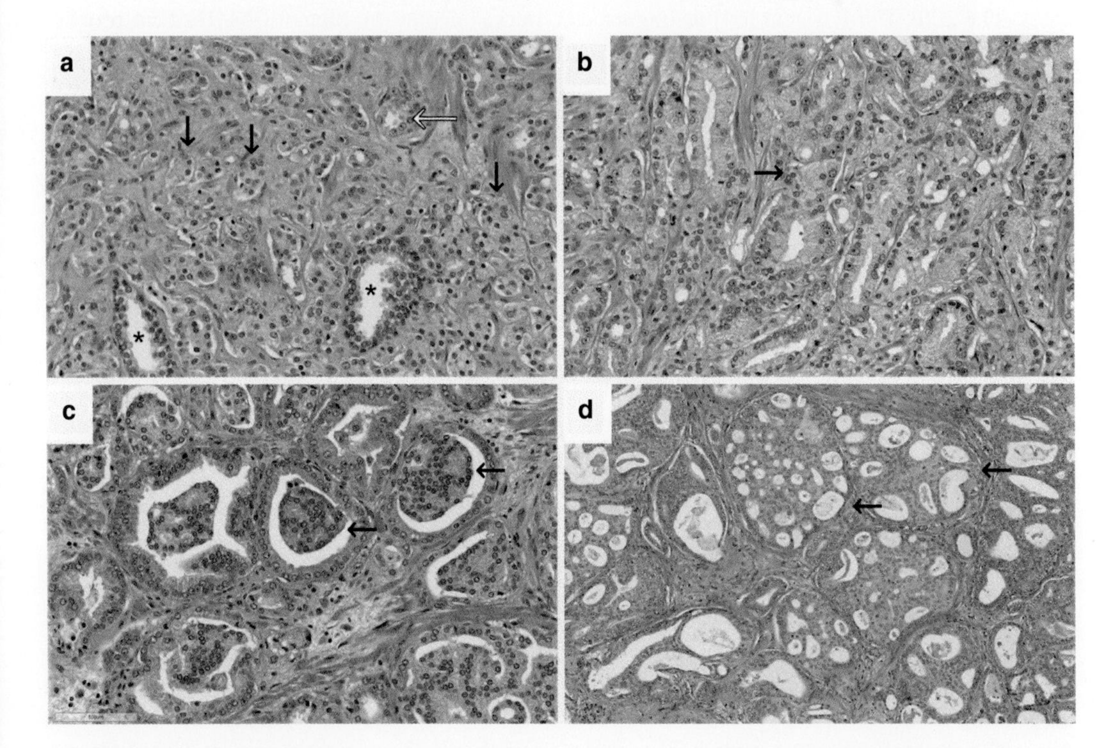

Fig. 8 The heterogeneity of Gleason grade 4 prostate cancer is displayed in these four micrographs. (**a**) Ill-formed malignant glands without lumina (*black arrow*). Some well-formed malignant glands with lumina (*white arrow*) and benign glands (*) are also present. (**b**) Fused glands. (**c**) Glomeruloid structures. (**d**) Cribriform architecture

[36, 44]; however, it may also represent a precursor lesion distinct from H-PIN. The latter theory is supported by the occasional finding of IDC-P without an associated invasive carcinoma at prostatectomy [59]. A finding of isolated IDC-P on biopsy, without an associated invasive carcinoma, should prompt either immediate rebiopsy or definitive treatment.

4.4 Staging of Prostatectomy Specimens

The objective of staging is to (1) group malignancies which have an apparently similar prognosis so as to inform a uniform therapeutic approach, (2) assist clinical trials and research studies by defining homogeneous patient populations, and (3) promote the comparability of clinicopathologic data from multiple hospitals and research groups. In general, pathologic substaging of tumors should maintain symmetry with clinical substaging, thus allowing direct comparison of cases. The 2009 TNM system [64] distinguishes organ confined (pT2) and nonorgan confined prostate cancers (pT3a,b/pT4) to describe the extent of cancer in a radical prostatectomy specimen.

4.4.1 Stage pT2 Prostate Cancer

Organ confined or localized prostate cancers are stage pT2, which means they are within the confines of the prostate, including its outer fibromuscular border. Pathological substaging of T2 cancers is optional, given its lack of clinical and academic value [76]. Although clinical substaging of T2 prostate cancer is of value, the clinical substages do not correspond with the pathological substages.

4.4.2 Stage pT3a Prostate Cancer

Extraprostatic extension (EPE) is defined as tumor extension beyond the confines of the prostate. Although the definition is simple, diagnosing EPE is not always straightforward due to the absence of a true histological capsule [5]. Unequivocal EPE can be diagnosed when tumor is identified in contact with adipose tissue (Fig. 10), as intraprostatic fat is rarely if ever encountered [68]. In the posterolateral aspects of the gland, EPE can also be diagnosed when tumor is identified within loose connective tissue or perineural spaces of the neurovascular bundles, or as a distinct tumor nodule within desmoplastic stroma which bulges beyond the normal contour of the gland [42]. At the anterior fibromuscular stroma, diagnosing EPE may be more difficult as the prostate stroma may blend imperceptibly with extraprostatic muscle. At this site, clear tumor extension beyond the prostate contour or into the adipose tissue at the sides [9] should help determine the presence of EPE (Fig. 9). In the apex, benign glands are frequently admixed with striated muscle, and as a consequence, the finding of malignant glands within striated muscle does not represent extraprostatic extension [42]. Bladder neck invasion is diagnosed when malignant glands are identified within smooth muscle bundles of the bladder neck, beyond the plane of any benign prostate glands.

Since in contemporary series at least 50 % of patients with extraprostatic extension at radical prostatectomy do not show tumor progression over a 10-year follow-up period, methods to improve the prognostication of EPE have been examined [42]. In general, EPE is subclassified as focal/minimal or nonfocal/established and different methods exist to make this distinction based on the number of glands [20], the number of high power fields [81] or radial extent of EPE [69]. While there is no clear consensus on which method to use, each categorization system has been shown to have prognostic significance.

4.4.3 Stage pT3b Prostate Cancer

Seminal vesicle invasion as defined by the invasion of the muscular wall of the extraprostatic seminal vesicles (stage pT3b) conveys a highly unfavorable prognosis. The carcinoma can invade the seminal vesicles by (1) spreading along the ejaculatory duct and/or (2) by

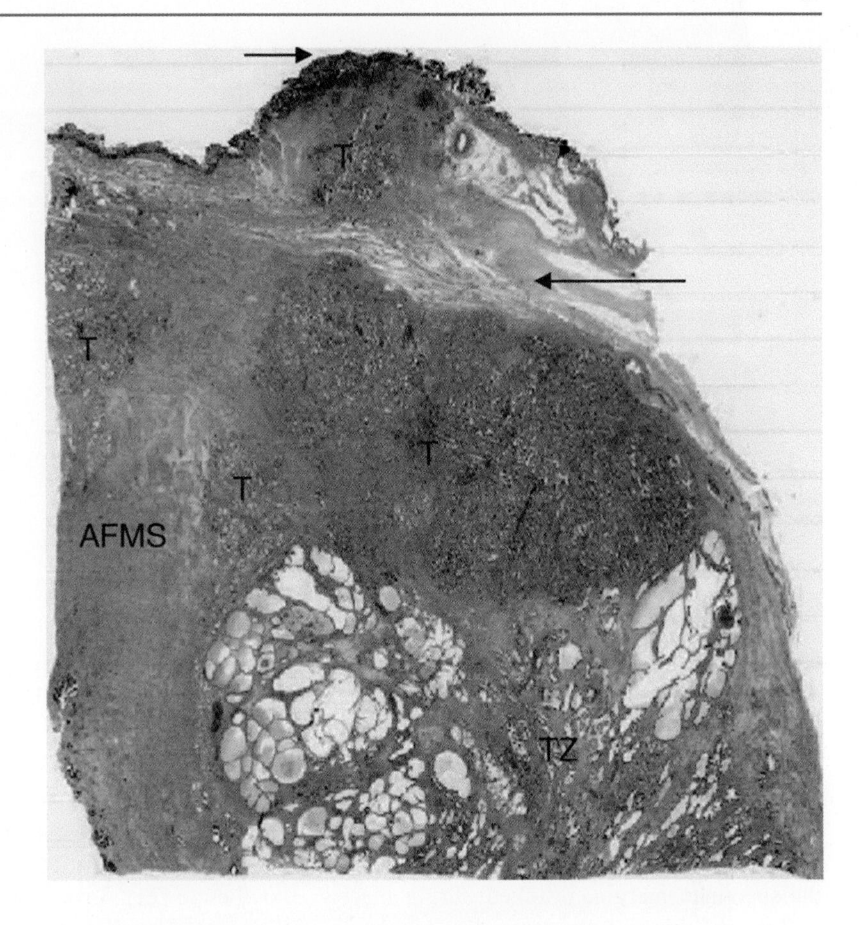

Fig. 9 Upper right quadrant section of prostatectomy specimen with a larger anterior cancer (T) of the transition zone (*TZ*), penetrating the anterior surgical margin (*short arrow*). The long arrow indicates the plane separating the prostate from the anterior extraprostatic tissue. The tumor is adjacent to and infiltrates the anterior fibromuscular stroma (*AFMS*)

direct invasion at the base of the prostate and/or (3) by extending first into periseminal vesicle soft tissue and then subsequently into the wall of the seminal vesicle. Rarely, discontinuous metastases in blood vessels in the seminal vesicle are present as an isolated finding [6]. As for the latter, there is no consensus whether this should be considered stage pT3b or not. Irrespective of staging, the presence of any lymphovascular space invasion should be routinely reported [42].

4.4.4 Stage pT4 Prostate Cancer

The designation of stage pT4 in a prostatectomy is highly restricted now: pT4 urinary bladder neck involvement by prostatic carcinoma includes only prostate cancer with gross or radiographic extension into the bladder neck. It is allowable to assign a pT4 stage associated with radical prostatectomy if an associated biopsy of urinary bladder, rectum, or pelvic side wall is positive for prostatic carcinoma that is directly invading these structures, as assessed clinically or radiologically [42]. A positive surgical margin at the bladder neck does not constitute stage pT4 cancer but is reported as pT3a margin positive cancer [10].

4.5 Surgical Margins

Approximately 10–35 % of radical prostatectomy specimens are reported to have positive surgical margins on pathologic evaluation. Biochemical progression-free survival for men with surgical margin positivity on radical prostatectomy is about 60 % as compared to 80 % in patients with negative surgical margins [13,

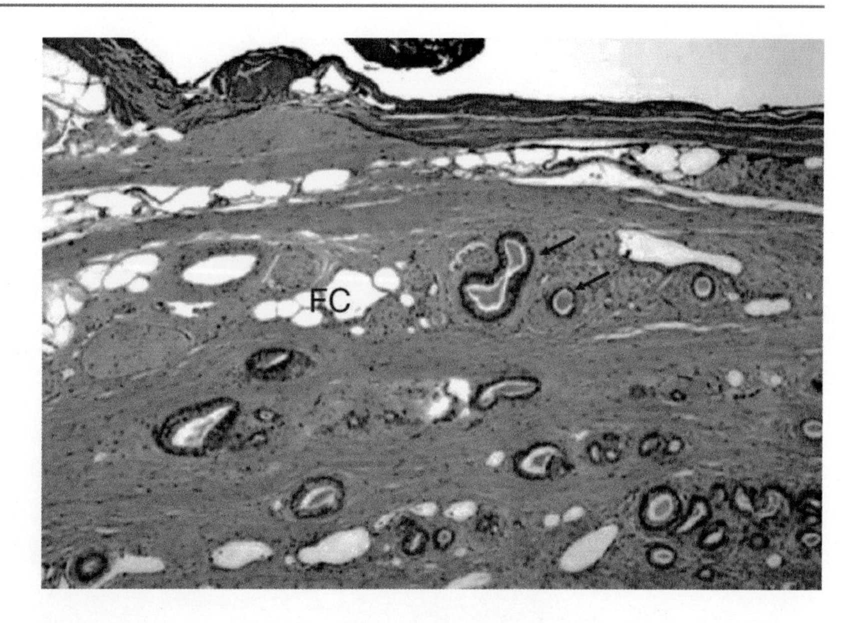

Fig. 10 A few tumor glands (*arrows*) are found at the level of fat cells (*FC*), indicating focal extraprostatic extension

55]. Most but not all investigators have been able to confirm the independent prognostic impact of this parameter in multivariable analyses [71].

4.5.1 Definition of Positive Margins

The outer surface of the prostate, representing the specimen margin, is inked during macroscopic evaluation of prostatectomy specimens. The margin is considered positive when tumor cells are microscopically identified directly in contact with this inked surface. Lacerations in the outer margin may cause tracking of ink and this can be a cause of a false-positive margin [14] (Fig. 11). In addition, the presence of tumor cells at the outer surface of a section which is *not* covered by ink should be regarded as a negative margin. In the case of a negative surgical margin, there is conflicting evidence as to whether the tumor distance to the margin has prognostic significance. Initial studies found no association between margin distance and disease recurrence rate [16, 17, 22]. As a result, the margin is interpreted as negative even when tumor is microscopically very close, e.g., <0.1 mm, and a measurement of tumor distance to the margin is not routinely reported [71]. However, recent large studies which have reported a significant association between close margins (<0.1 mm) and biochemical recurrence suggest that a close margin may be prognostically significant [33, 41].

4.5.2 Location, Extent, and Grade of Positive Surgical Margin

Published reports on the impact of the location of positive surgical margins on outcome have been conflicting [71]. Several studies have shown that the extent of tumor at the surgical margin correlates with postoperative disease recurrence, but a large study by [66] demonstrated that neither location nor extent of positive margin improved the predictive accuracy of a nomogram compared to one in which surgical margin status was modeled as positive vs. negative. Recent studies have also suggested that the Gleason grade of the tumor at the positive margin has prognostic significance [11, 35, 77] as a lower grade tumor at the margin is associated with more favorable pathologic features and a decreased risk of early biochemical recurrence [35].

4.6 Anterior Prostate Cancers

Transition zone cancers, particularly when in an anterior location, tend to be detected late, since they are generally not targeted by the standard biopsy scheme which focuses mainly on cancers in the posterior location [8]. Often they have reached

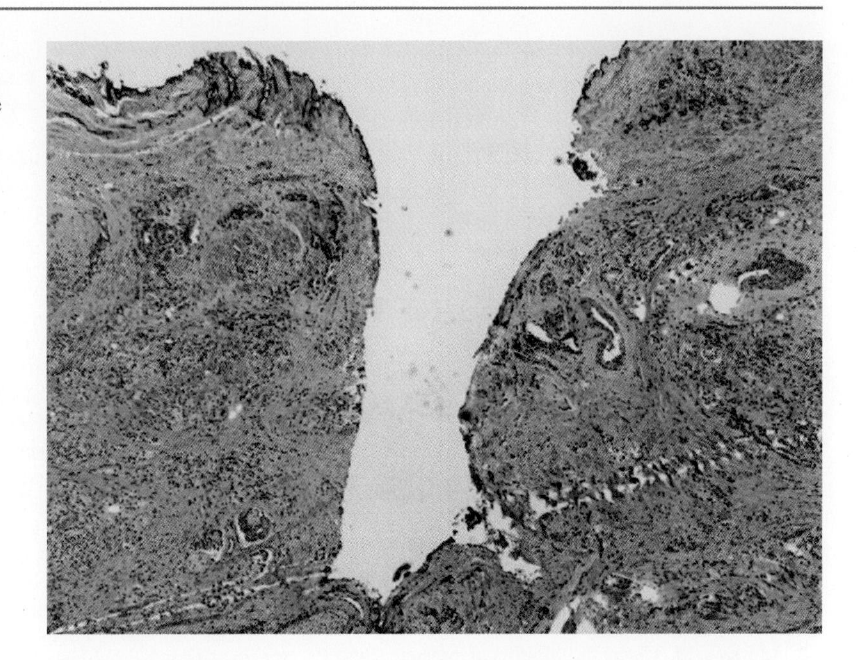

Fig. 11 A laceration into the prostatic tissue. Although tumor cells are here in contact with the ink, this should not be considered as a true positive margin

a large size and/or transformed into an aggressive higher grade cancer before their detection, and under these circumstances there is a greater risk of a positive margin and biochemical failure when prostatectomy is performed (Fig. 9). Anterior prostate cancers are not uncommon, with about 35 % of the anterior prostate cancers originating from the anterior horn of the peripheral zone, thus representing peripheral zone carcinomas [1].

The acronym PEATS (i.e., prostatic evasive anterior tumor syndrome) alludes to the phenomenon of anterior cancers detected at a stage too advanced to be cured [40]. It is obvious that in patients enrolled in an active surveillance program it remains a challenge to identify the presence of these hidden aggressive anterior tumors. Magnetic resonance imaging-guided biopsies targeting anterior zone abnormalities play an increasing role in this clinical setting.

4.7 Multifocality and Index Tumor

Multifocality of prostate cancer (Fig. 1) is very common, with 2–5 tumors of variable size found in 80 % of prostatectomy specimens [82]. The concept of an index or dominant tumor was derived from the Stanford group who measured the volume of the largest tumor nodule in wholemount sections and demonstrated its independent clinical significance [65]. The advancement of focal therapy for the treatment of prostate cancer has made this concept more relevant, but it has been challenged in the past on two grounds. Firstly, several subsequent studies have failed to demonstrate the independent prognostic significance of tumor volume [83], and secondly, the dominant nodule does not always represent the component of tumor having the highest Gleason score or the most advanced pathological stage [2]. In particular, pT stage and Gleason grade/score may need to be included in the defining characteristics such that, in the case of a multifocal cancer, the index tumor would represent the tumor with the worst prognostic features.

5 Concluding Remarks

As reflected in this chapter, the approach to the diagnosis and management of prostate cancer is underpinned by an understanding of the anatomic and histopathological features of the disease. New insights into diagnostic and prognostic histopathological parameters, including a new approach to cancer grading, help to risk stratify tumors and guide therapeutic decision making. With advances in technology, there is an expanding role for imaging studies in the diagnosis and management of prostate cancer, in particular with regard to the diagnosis of anteriorly located tumors and the use of focal therapies. Ultimately, an awareness of the potential for overtreatment of indolent prostate cancers continues to drive the search for improved pathological, molecular-genetic, and imaging parameters that can accurately predict behavior and prognosis.

References

1. Al-Ahmadie HA, Tickoo SK, Olgac S, et al. Anterior-predominant prostatic tumors: zone of origin and pathologic outcomes at radical prostatectomy. Am J Surg Pathol. 2008;32:229–35.
2. Andreoiu M, Cheng L. Multifocal prostate cancer: biologic, prognostic, and therapeutic implications. Hum Pathol. 2010;41:781–93.
3. Andriole GL, Bostwick DG, Brawley OW, et al. REDUCE Study Group. Effect of dutasteride on the risk of prostate cancer. N Engl J Med. 2010;362: 1192–202.
4. Augustin H, Hammerer PG, Blonski J, et al. Zonal location of prostate cancer: significance for disease-free survival after radical prostatectomy? Urology. 2003;62: 79–85.
5. Ayala AG, Ro JY, Babaian R, Troncoso P, Grignon DJ. The prostatic capsule: does it exist? Its importance in the staging and treatment of prostatic carcinoma. Am J Surg Pathol. 1989;13(1):21–7.
6. Berney DM, Wheeler TM, Grignon DJ, ISUP Prostate Cancer Group, et al. International Society of Urological Pathology (ISUP) Consensus Conference on Handling and Staging of Radical Prostatectomy Specimens. Working group 4: seminal vesicles and lymph nodes. Mod Pathol. 2011;24:39–47.
7. Bostwick DG, Liu L, Brawer MK, et al. High-grade prostatic intraepithelial neoplasia. Rev Urol. 2004;6:171–9.
8. Bott SR, Young MP, Kellett MJ, et al. Contributors to the UCL Hospitals' Trust Radical Prostatectomy Database. Anterior prostate cancer: is it more difficult to diagnose? BJU Int. 2002;89:886–9.
9. Bouyé S, Potiron E, Puech P, et al. Transition zone and anterior stromal prostate cancers: zone of origin and intraprostatic patterns of spread at histopathology. Prostate. 2009;69:105–13.
10. Buschemeyer 3rd WC, Hamilton RJ, Aronson WJ, et al. Is a positive bladder neck margin truly a T4 lesion in the prostate specific antigen era? Results from the SEARCH Database. J Urol. 2008;179:124–9.
11. Cao D, Kibel AS, Gao F, et al. The Gleason score of tumor at the margin in radical prostatectomy is predictive of biochemical recurrence. Am J Surg Pathol. 2010;34:994.
12. Chan TW, Partin AW, Walsh PC, Epstein JI. Prognostic significance of Gleason score 3+4 versus Gleason score 4+3 tumor at radical prostatectomy. Urology. 2000;56(5):823–7.
13. Cheng L, Darson MF, Bergstralh EJ, et al. Correlation of margin status and extraprostatic extension with progression of prostate carcinoma. Cancer. 1999;86:1775–82.
14. Chuang AY, Epstein JI. Positive surgical margins in areas of capsular incision in otherwise organ-confined disease at radical prostatectomy: histologic features and pitfalls. Am J Surg Pathol. 2008;32:1201–6.
15. De Marzo AM, Haffner MC, Lotan TL, Yegnasubramanian S, Nelson WG. Premalignancy in Prostate Cancer: Rethinking What we Know. Cancer Prev Res (Phila). 2016;9(8):648–56.
16. Emerson RE, Koch MO, Daggy JK, et al. Closest distance between tumor and resection margin in radical prostatectomy specimens. Lack of prognostic significance. Am J Surg Pathol. 2005;29:225–9.
17. Epstein JI. Evaluation of radical prostatectomy capsular margins of resection: the significance of margins designated as negative, closely approaching, and positive. Am J Surg Pathol. 1990;14:626–32.
18. Epstein JI. Precursor lesions to prostatic adenocarcinoma. Virchows Arch. 2009;454:1–16.
19. Epstein JI, Amin MB, Beltran H, et al. Proposed morphologic classification of prostate cancer with neuroendocrine differentiation. Am J Surg Pathol. 2014;38(6): 756–67.
20. Epstein JI, Carmichael MJ, Pizov G, et al. Influence of capsular penetration on progression following radical prostatectomy: a study of 196 cases with long-term follow-up. J Urol. 1993;150:135–41.
21. Epstein JI, Egevad L, Amin MB, et al. The 2014 International Society of Urological Pathology (ISUP) Consensus Conference on Gleason Grading of Prostatic Carcinoma: Definition of Grading Patterns and Proposal for a New Grading System. Am J Surg Pathol. 2016;40(2):244–52.
22. Epstein JI, Sauvageot J. Do close but negative margins in radical prostatectomy specimens increase the risk of postoperative progression? J Urol. 1997;157(1): 241–3.
23. Epstein JI, Zelefsky MJ, Sjoberg DD, et al. A contemporary prostate cancer grading system: a validated alternative to the Gleason Score. Eur Urol. 2016;69(3): 428–35.
24. Evans AJ, Humphrey PA, Belani J, et al. Large cell neuroendocrine carcinoma of prostate: a clinicopathologic summary of 7 cases of a rare manifestation of advanced prostate cancer. Am J Surg Pathol. 2006;30:684–93.
25. Fine SW, Al-Ahmadie HA, Gopalan A, et al. Anatomy of the anterior prostate and extraprostatic space: a contemporary surgical pathology analysis. Adv Anat Pathol. 2007;14:401–7.

26. Fine SW, Reuter VE. Anatomy of the prostate revisited: implications for prostate biopsy and zonal origins of prostate cancer. Histopathology. 2012;60(1): 142–52.
27. Gosselaar C, Roobol MJ, Roemeling S, et al. The role of the digital rectal examination in subsequent screening visits in the European randomized study of screening for prostate cancer (ERSPC), Rotterdam. Eur Urol. 2008;54:581–8.
28. Grignon DJ. Unusual subtypes of prostate cancer. Mod Pathol. 2004;17(3):316–27.
29. Guo CC, Epstein JI. Intraductal carcinoma of the prostate on needle biopsy: histologic features and clinical significance. Mod Pathol. 2006;19:1528–35.
30. Hammerich KH, Ayala GE, Wheeler TM (2009) Anatomy of the prostate gland and surgical pathology of prostate cancer. Cambridge University 1–10
31. Harnden P, Shelley MD, Coles B, et al. Should the Gleason grading system for prostate cancer be modified to account for high-grade tertiary components? A systematic review and meta-analysis. Lancet Oncol. 2007;8:411–9.
32. Humphrey PA. Histological variants of prostatic carcinoma and their significance. Histopathology. 2012;60(1): 59–74.
33. Izard JP, True LD, May P, et al. Prostate cancer that is within 0.1 mm of the surgical margin of a radical prostatectomy predicts greater likelihood of recurrence. Am J Surg Pathol. 2014;38(3):333–8.
34. Jeetle SS, Fisher G, Yang ZH, et al. Neuroendocrine differentiation does not have independent prognostic value in conservatively treated prostate cancer. Virchows Arch. 2012;461(2):103–7.
35. Kates M, Sopko NA, Han M, Partin AW, Epstein JI. Importance of reporting the Gleason Score at the positive surgical margin site: analysis of 4,082 consecutive radical prostatectomy cases. J Urol. 2016;195(2):337–42.
36. Kovi J, Jackson MA, Heshmat MY. Ductal spread in prostatic carcinoma. Cancer. 1985;56:1566–73.
37. Krijnen JL, Janssen PJ, Ruizeveld de Winter JA, et al. Do neuroendocrine cells in human prostate cancer express androgen receptor? Histochemistry. 1993;100:393–8.
38. Kweldam CF, Kümmerlin IP, Nieboer D et al. Disease-specific survival of patients with invasive cribriform and intraductal prostate cancer at diagnostic biopsy. Mod Pathol. 2016;29(6):630–6
39. Kweldam CF, Wildhagen MF, Steyerberg EW, et al. Cribriform growth is highly predictive for postoperative metastasis and disease-specific death in Gleason score 7 prostate cancer. Mod Pathol. 2015;28(3): 457–64.
40. Lawrentschuk N, Haider MA, Daljeet N, et al. 'Prostatic evasive anterior tumours': the role of magnetic resonance imaging. BJU Int. 2010;105:1231–6.
41. Lu J, Wirth GJ, Wu S, et al. A close surgical margin after radical prostatectomy is an independent predictor of recurrence. J Urol. 2012;188(1):91–7.
42. Magi-Galluzzi C, Evans AJ, Delahunt B, ISUP Prostate Cancer Group, et al. International Society of Urological Pathology (ISUP) Consensus Conference on Handling and Staging of Radical Prostatectomy Specimens. Working group 3: extraprostatic extension, lymphovascular invasion and locally advanced disease. Mod Pathol. 2011;24(1): 26–38.
43. McNeal JE. Normal histology of the prostate. Am J Surg Pathol. 1988;12:619–33.
44. McNeal JE, Yemoto CE. Spread of adenocarcinoma within prostatic ducts and acini: morphologic and clinical correlations. Am J Surg Pathol. 1996;20: 802–14.
45. Merrimen JL, Jones G, Srigley JR. Is high grade prostatic intraepithelial neoplasia still a risk factor for adenocarcinoma in the era of extended biopsy sampling? Pathology. 2010;42(4):325–9.
46. Moch H, Humphrey PA., Ulbright TM, Reuter, VE (2016) WHO Classification of Tumours of the Urinary System and Male Genital Organs. International Agency for Research on Cancer
47. Montironi R, Mazzucchelli R, Santinelli A, et al. Incidentally detected prostate cancer in cystoprostatectomies: pathological and morphometric comparison with clinically detected cancer in totally embedded specimens. Hum Pathol. 2005;36(6):646–54.
48. Moreira DM, Bostwick DG, Andriole GL, et al. Baseline prostate atrophy is associated with reduced risk of prostate cancer in men undergoing repeat prostate biopsy. J Urol. 2015;194(5):1241–6.
49. Moreira DM, Nickel JC, Andriole GL, Castro-Santamaria R, Freedland SJ. Greater extent of prostate inflammation in negative biopsies is associated with lower risk of prostate cancer on repeat biopsy: results from the REDUCE study. Prostate Cancer Prostatic Dis. 2016;19(2):180–4.
50. Mottet N, Bellmunt J, Bourke L et al (2016). Members of the EAU Guidelines Panel on Prostate Cancer. EAU-ESTRO-SIOG Pocket Guidelines on Prostate Cancer. Edn. presented at the EAU Annual Congress Munich 2016. ISBN 978-90-79754-86-1.
51. Muraoka K, Hinata N, Morizane S, et al. Site-dependent and interindividual variations in Denonvilliers' fascia: a histological study using donated elderly male cadavers. BMC Uro. 2015; 15:42.
52. Myers RP, Cheville JC, Pawlina W. Making anatomic terminology of the prostate and contiguous structures clinically useful: historical review and suggestions for revision in the 21st century. Clin Anat. 2010;23: 18–29.
53. Nadal R, Schweizer M, Kryvenko ON, Epstein JI, Eisenberger MA. Small cell carcinoma of the prostate. Nat Rev Urol. 2014;11(4):213–9.
54. O'Brien BA, Cohen RJ, Wheeler TM, et al. A post-radical-prostatectomy nomogram incorporating new pathological variables and interaction terms for improved prognosis. BJU Int. 2011;107:389–95.

55. Ohori M, Wheeler TM, Kattan MW, et al. Prognostic significance of positive surgical margins in radical prostatectomy specimens. J Urol. 1995;154:1818–24.
56. Osunkoya AO, Nielsen ME, Epstein JI. Prognosis of mucinous adenocarcinoma of the prostate treated by radical prostatectomy: a study of 47 cases. Am J Surg Pathol. 2008;32(3):468–72.
57. Park YH, Jeong CW, Lee SE. A comprehensive review of neuroanatomy of the prostate. Prostate Int. 2013;1(4):139–45.
58. Pickup M, Van der Kwast TH. My approach to intraductal lesions of the prostate gland. J Clin Pathol. 2010;60:856–65.
59. Robinson BD, Epstein JI. Intraductal carcinoma of the prostate without invasive carcinoma on needle biopsy: emphasis on radical prostatectomy findings. J Urol. 2010;184:1328–33.
60. Ross HM, Kryvenko ON, Cowan JE, et al. Do adenocarcinomas of the prostate with Gleason score (GS) ≤6 have the potential to metastasize to lymph nodes? Am J Surg Pathol. 2012;36(9):1346–52.
61. Sauter G, Steurer S, Clauditz TS, et al. Clinical utility of quantitative Gleason grading in prostate biopsies and prostatectomy specimens. Eur Urol. 2016;69(4): 592–8.
62. Schelling LA, Williamson SR, Zhang S, et al. Frequent TMPRSS2-ERG rearrangement in prostatic small cell carcinoma detected by fluorescence in situ hybridization: the superiority of fluorescence in situ hybridization over ERG immunohistochemistry. Hum Pathol. 2013;44(10):2227–33.
63. Seipel AH, Wiklund F, Wiklund NP, Egevad L. Histopathological features of ductal adenocarcinoma of the prostate in 1,051 radical prostatectomy specimens. Virchows Arch. 2013;462(4):429–36.
64. Sobin LH, Gospodariwicz M, Wittekind C (2009) TNM Classification of Malignant Tumors 7th edn. Wiley-Blackwell: Oxford, UK International Union Against Cancer (UICC) 243–248
65. Stamey TA, McNeal JE, Yemoto CM, et al. Biological determinants of cancer progression in men with prostate cancer. JAMA. 1999;281:1395–400.
66. Stephenson AJ, Wood DP, Kattan MW, et al. Location, extent and number of positive surgical margins do not improve accuracy of predicting prostate cancer recurrence after radical prostatectomy. J Urol. 2009;182:357–63.
67. Stolzenburg JU, Schwalenberg T, Horn LC, et al. Anatomical landmarks of radical prostatectomy. Eur Urol. 2007;51(3):629–39.
68. Sung MT, Eble JN, Cheng L. Invasion of fat justifies assignment of stage pT3a in prostatic adenocarcinoma. Pathology. 2006;38(4):309–11.
69. Sung MT, Lin H, Koch MO, et al. Radial distance of extraprostatic extension measured by ocular micrometer is an independent predictor of prostate-specific antigen recurrence: a new proposal for the substaging of pT3a prostate cancer. Am J Surg Pathol. 2007;31: 311–8.
70. Tamas EF, Epstein JI. Prognostic significance of paneth cell-like neuroendocrine differentiation in adenocarcinoma of the prostate. Am J Surg Pathol. 2006;30(8):980–5.
71. Tan PH, Cheng L, Srigley JR, et al. International Society of Urological Pathology (ISUP) Consensus Conference on Handling and Staging of Radical Prostatectomy Specimens. Working group 5: surgical margins. Mod Pathol. 2011;24(1):48–57.
72. Tavora F, Epstein JI. High-grade prostatic intraepithelial neoplasia like ductal adenocarcinoma of the prostate: a clinicopathologic study of 28 cases. Am J Surg Pathol. 2008;32(7):1060–7.
73. Têtu B, Srigley JR, Boivin JC, Dupont A, et al. Effect of combination endocrine therapy (LHRH agonist and flutamide) on normal prostate and prostatic adenocarcinoma. A histopathologic and immunohistochemical study. Am J Surg Pathol. 1991;15:111–20.
74. Trudel D, Downes MR, Sykes J, et al. Prognostic impact of intraductal carcinoma and large cribriform carcinoma architecture after prostatectomy in a contemporary cohort. Eur J Cancer. 2014;50(9):1610–6.
75. Van der Kwast T, Al Daoud N, Collette L, et al. Biopsy diagnosis of intraductal carcinoma is prognostic in intermediate and high risk prostate cancer patients treated by radiotherapy. Eur J Cancer. 2012;48:1318–25.
76. Van der Kwast TH, Amin MB, Billis A, ISUP Prostate Cancer Group, et al. International Society of Urological Pathology (ISUP) Consensus Conference on Handling and Staging of Radical Prostatectomy Specimens. Working group 2: T2 substaging and prostate cancer volume. Mod Pathol. 2011;24: 16–25.
77. Viers BR, Sukov WR, Gettman MT, et al. Primary Gleason grade 4 at the positive margin is associated with metastasis and death among patients with Gleason 7 prostate cancer undergoing radical prostatectomy. Eur Urol. 2014;66:1116.
78. Vis AN, Roemeling S, Kranse R, et al. Should we replace the Gleason score with the amount of high-grade prostate cancer? Eur Urol. 2007;51:931–9.
79. Walz J, Burnett AL, Costello AJ et al. A critical analysis of the current knowledge of surgical anatomy related to optimization of cancer control and preservation of continence and erection in candidates for radical prostatectomy. Eur Urol 2010; 57(2):179–192
80. Walz J, Epstein JI, Ganzer R et al. A Critical Analysis of the Current Knowledge of Surgical Anatomy of the Prostate Related to Optimisation of Cancer Control and Preservation of Continence and Erection in Candidates for Radical Prostatectomy: An Update. Eur Urol. 2016;70(2):301–11.
81. Watts K, Li J, Magi-Galluzzi C, Zhou M. Incidence and clinicopathological characteristics of intraductal carcinoma detected in prostate biopsies: a prospective cohort study. Histopathology. 2013;63(4):574–9.
82. Wheeler TM, Dillioglugil O, Kattan MW, et al. Clinical and pathological significance of the level and

extent of capsular invasion in clinical stage T1-2 prostate cancer. Hum Pathol. 1998;29:856–62.
83. Wise AM, Stamey TA, McNeal JE, et al. Morphologic and clinical significance of multifocal prostate cancers in radical prostatectomy specimens. Urology. 2002;60:264–9.
84. Wolters T, Roobol MJ, van Leeuwen PJ, et al. Should pathologists routinely report prostate tumor volume? The prognostic value of tumor volume in prostate cancer. Eur Urol. 2010;57:821–9.
85. Wright JL, Salinas CA, Lin DW. Prostate cancer specific mortality and Gleason 7 disease differences in prostate cancer outcomes between cases with Gleason 4+3 and Gleason 3+4 tumors in a population based cohort. J Urol. 2009;182(6):2702–7.
86. Zhao T, Liao B, Yao J, et al. Is there any prognostic impact of intraductal carcinoma of prostate in initial diagnosed aggressively metastatic prostate cancer? Prostate. 2015;75:225–32.

Biomarkers for Prostate Cancer

S. Dijkstra, R.J. Hendriks, G.H.J.M. Leyten,
P.F.A. Mulders, and J.A. Schalken

1 Introduction

Traditionally, clinical diagnosis and management of the individual patient are based on clinical cohort-based studies. The heterogeneity within 'risk cohorts' can still be considerable which impairs decision-making for an individual patient. Therefore, we urgently need improved methods to accurately predict the biological behaviour, and therapy response for well-stratified/homogeneous groups of patients. In the last decade, revolutionary advancements in molecular profiling technologies have been made resulting in new diagnostic algorithms. It is noteworthy that it is just 60 years ago that the double-helix model for the structure of DNA was first described. Molecular biology developed quickly and with nucleic acid amplification technologies whole genome gene and expression profiling became feasible. The field expanded beyond the traditional/core genes that follow Francis Crick's dogma (gene<−>RNA>protein) by the discovery of non coding RNAs, including microRNAs (miRNAs). This enables us to identify the individual in a different way from the way we did before. These advances have marked the beginning of a new era for modern medicine: individualized medicine. This is an approach that strives for a 'customized' healthcare; a patient-specific strategie instead of the standard 'one-size-fits-all' approach.

Biomarkers are important tools in individualized medicine. A biomarker can be defined as a characteristic that is objectively measured and evaluated as an indicator of normal biological processes, pathogenic processes or pharmacologic responses to a therapeutic intervention [18]. This includes physiological measurements and clinical imaging, but also specific cells, molecules, genes, gene products, enzymes or hormones.

Biomarkers in cancer (can) have several valuable applications:

- Improve diagnosis
- Improve staging
- Indicate disease prognosis (e.g., indolent vs. clinical significant prostate cancer)
- Monitor response to treatment
- Select patients for different treatment options
- Surrogate endpoint in trials
- Therapeutic target

In prostate cancer, prostatic acid phosphatase (PAP) is considered the first known biomarker. This enzyme was discovered to be increased in men with metastasized prostate cancer in 1938 [71]. The use of PAP was not useful for diagnosis, and was only used to monitor prostate cancer

S. Dijkstra (✉) • R.J. Hendriks • G.H.J.M. Leyten
P.F.A. Mulders • J.A. Schalken
Radboud University Medical Center, Department of Urology, Nijmegen, The Netherlands
e-mail: siebren.dijkstra@radboudumc.nl

M. Bolla, H. van Poppel (eds.), *Management of Prostate Cancer*,
DOI 10.1007/978-3-319-42769-0_5

patients after diagnosis. In the 1980s, prostate-specific antigen (PSA) was introduced into clinical practice. This is to date the only widely used biomarker in prostate cancer. The introduction of PSA has resulted in earlier detection of the disease, although it also has important limitations. Its use in screening and prognosis remains controversial due to the fact that it is an organ-specific marker and not a cancer-specific marker. Novel, prostate cancer–specific biomarkers are needed to differentiate indolent from aggressive disease to minimize overtreatment of clinically insignificant prostate cancer.

The ideal characteristics of a biomarker for prostate cancer are as follows:

- Only produced by tumour tissue
- Non-invasive test, easy to manage
- As inexpensive as possible
- Ability to detect prostate cancer at an early stage
- Differentiate between indolent and clinically significant tumours
- High sensitivity and specificity

Prostate cancers are usually heterogeneous, and recognition and identification of the most significant focus are important to predict disease progression. Combination of biomarkers with clinical risk factors will be also important to optimize predictive value. Prostate cancer biomarkers can be detected in different diagnostic substrates, each aiding different clinical decisions (Table 1).

Novel biomarkers can be identified through genetic epidemiological studies (evaluating inherited genetic predispositions in large cohorts, genome-wide association studies, GWAS) or molecular profiling studies, evaluating the molecular profile of the tumour. Around 20 GWAS studies have revealed a total of 77 single nucleotide polymorphisms (SNPs) that are associated with an increased chance to develop prostate cancer [56]. The observed relative risks are insufficient to individualize diagnosis [82], yet may be of use for pre-selection. This chapter will focus on established biomarkers and promising novel biomarkers identified by molecular profiling studies, arranged by tissue markers, blood markers and urine markers.

Table 1 Different diagnostic substrates for prostate cancer biomarkers

Diagnostic substrates	Invasive	Clinical decision
Urine	–	Biopsy
Blood	–	Biopsy, treatment
Biopsy specimen	+	Treatment
Prostatectomy specimen (Gleason score + pTNM)	++	Adjuvant treatment

2 Tissue Markers

Once tissue is available, important decisions have already been made, either a biopsy has been taken or the prostatic gland was surgically removed. Thus, the main clinical need is to accurately predict the biological behaviour of the malignant process. In case the pathologist is not sure about the diagnosis of invasive prostate cancer, immunohistochemistry using antibodies against the basal cell–specific high molecular weight keratins (34β E12) and AMACR has proven to be helpful [88]. In recent years, various genetic tests have become commercially available that use gene expression panels to predict tumour characteristics and the need of adjuvant treatment. Since better treatment modalities become available, adjuvant strategies are likely to be considered again and biomarkers indicative for biological behaviour can be helpful. In this part, we will focus on high potential biomarkers for which standardized methods are or can be developed and we will describe the current already commercially available tissue-based genetic tests.

2.1 Gene Fusions: TMPRSS2-ERG

The classic example of a gene fusion implicated in cancer development is the BCR:ABL fusion in patients with chronic myelogenous leukaemia. This fusion results from a reciprocal translocation

T(9;22), first recognized as the Philadelphia chromosome. This discovery has been revolutionary as it has led to the development of imatinib which is an inhibitor of the BCR:ABL gene fusion product which transformed the previously fatal leukaemia into a manageable chronic disease for many patients [51].

In prostate cancer, recurrent gene rearrangements were discovered in 2005: a fusion of the 5' untranslated region of TMPRSS2 (androgen-regulated trans-membrane protease, serine 2) to Ets family genes (oncogenic transcription factors) [148]. Oncogene ERG (v-ets erythroblastosis virus E26 oncogene homologue (avian)) is the most commonly involved Ets family member in gene fusions. TMPRSS2-ERG has been detected in approximately 50 % of Caucasian prostate cancer patients. This gene fusion is less frequently seen in men from other ethnic background. Magi-Gazulli et al. reported fusion-positive prostate cancers in 31 % of African-American men and only in 16 % of Japanese men [104]. Rearrangements with other Ets transcription factors have been identified in approximately 5–10 % of PSA-screened prostate cancers: ETV1 (ETS variant 1 gene), ETV4 and ETV5 [8, 74, 147]. In addition to TMPRSS2, other fusion partners involved in ETS fusions have been identified. Their possible clinical relevance is not clear.

As a result of the gene fusion with TMPRSS2, the expression of ERG becomes androgen regulated and thus overexpressed. ERG expression can be detected in prostate cancer patients by immunohistochemistry with a high specificity of >95 % and is not seen in benign prostate epithelium [113, 122]. This suggests that ERG immunostaining could be a solid diagnostic biomarker, albeit in approximately half of the prostate cancer patients. The clinical implications for patients with an Ets gene fusion-positive tumour are currently still under investigation. Results on a potential prognostic value are conflicting.

A recent study described that ERG overexpression was associated with Gleason score (≥8) and stage (T3-T4 tumours) [62]. This worse prognosis of fusion-positive cancers has been reported earlier by several other studies [52, 117, 162]. On the contrary, various studies found that TMPRSS2-ERG fusion did not predict reduced prostate cancer survival nor was it associated with biochemical recurrence, metastasis or overall survival [61, 67].

The largest study so far assessed the predictive value of ERG overexpression in a cohort including1180 men treated with radical prostatectomy. Overexpression was found in 49 % of the cases and correlated with a higher tumour stage. No association was found with Gleason score, metastases to distant organs and bones, biochemical recurrence after radical prostatectomy and prostate cancer–related death or all-cause mortality [124]. In a meta-analysis by the same authors, including 48 studies, TMPRSS2-ERG fusion was associated with advanced stage tumours at diagnosis, but not with biochemical recurrence or lethal disease. These results suggest that TMPRSS2-ERG is not a very strong prognostic marker for men treated with radical prostatectomy, although fusion presence might be associated with tumour stage [124].

2.2 Ki-67/MIB1-Labelling Index

Expression of the Ki-67 protein is strictly associated with cell proliferation. Ki-67 has therefore been extensively studied for its potential use as a proliferation marker in different types of cancer, including prostate cancer. Its name is derived from the city of origin (Kiel) and the number of the original clone in the 96-well plate [134]. Ki-67 can be determined by immunohistochemistry using the monoclonal antibody MIB-1 [36]. The proportion of tumour cells staining positive for Ki-67 is known as the Ki-67 labelling index. This proved to be an independent and significant prognostic biomarker for prostate cancer–specific survival [1, 22]. Furthermore, the Ki-67 labelling index has repeatedly shown to be a predictive marker for disease recurrence and progression after radical prostatectomy and radiotherapy [17, 28, 132]. Although its usefulness has been well established, the Ki-67 labelling index is currently not used in daily practice.

2.3 PTEN

PTEN (Phosphatase and TENsin homologue) is a tumour-suppressor gene, located on chromosome 10q23 [92]. This gene plays a key role in carcinogenesis. PTEN antagonizes the PI-3 K/Akt pathway and thereby modulating cell growth/survival and cell migration/adhesion [153]. In prostate cancer, PTEN loss has been associated with proliferation and survival of cancer cells, resistance to castration [137], chemotherapy [80, 126] and radiotherapy [3], bone metastasis [166] and recurrence after radical prostatectomy [15]. Ferraldeschi et al. studied the predictive value of PTEN expression in a post-docetaxel abiraterone treatment setting and demonstrated that loss of PTEN expression was associated with worse survival and shorter time on abiraterone treatment [60]. Thus, PTEN is assumed to be a potent prognostic and predictive marker and a clear target for novel (gene) therapies. However, this requires further research.

2.4 E-Cadherin

Cadherins are a family of epithelial cell-cell adhesion molecules that play a key role in preserving epithelial integrity [141]. Their function is dependent on calcium, hence their name ('calcium-dependent adhesion'). E-cadherin is the most extensively studied member of the cadherin family. During cancer progression to an invasive state, intercellular adhesions between tumour cells are disrupted. Thus, aggressive tumour cells were hypothesized to have loss of E-cadherin. And indeed, decreased E-cadherin expression has repeatedly been shown to correlate with a loss of tumour differentiation and a poor prognosis [19, 151, 152]. This correlation has been shown for several tumour types, including prostate cancer. However, large prospective studies will have to define its potential clinical relevance in prostate cancer, as a prognostic biomarker or as a molecular target for therapy.

2.5 EZH2

The EZH2 gene (enhancer of zeste homologue 2), encoding a Polycomb-group (PcG) protein, is responsible for maintaining the silent state of genes. EZH2 mediates trimethylation of histone H3 lysine 27 (H3K27), leading to repression of transcription and thereby silencing of gene expression [38, 87]. EZH2 is upregulated in various aggressive tumours, including prostate cancer [27, 85, 151]. Furthermore, it mediates transcriptional silencing of the tumour-suppressor gene E-cadherin [31]. This demonstrates an inverse correlation between dysregulation of EZH2 and repression of E-cadherin during cancer progression. In a large prostate cancer specimen, study high EZH2 expression was strongly associated with Gleason grade, advanced pathological tumour stage, positive nodal status and early PSA recurrence [108].

In conclusion, EZH2 upregulation might play a key role in oncogenesis and progression of cancer. This makes it a promising biomarker of disease progression and a viable target for therapeutic interventions in aggressive cancers.

2.6 The Neuroendocrine Phenotype

The expression of a 'pure' neuroendocrine (NE) phenotype in small cell prostate cancer is a rare entity (<1 % of all prostate cancers); however, there is a rationale that the relative fraction of cells with an NE phenotype increases in advanced prostate cancer, especially in the setting of androgen receptor targeting resistance. Moreover, clinically, NE prostate cancers are often manifested by the presence of visceral or large soft tissue metastatic disease, a disproportionately low serum PSA relative to the overall burden of the disease and a limited response to targeting of the androgen signalling axis [2]. The biology of the disease is markedly different from adenocarcinoma of the prostate, and, therefore, treatment of this type of prostate cancer is different and prognosis is worse. Preclinical studies are beginning to shine more light on this high-risk subset of disease, although novel therapies are still needed to improve survival.

2.7 ConfirmMDx

The ConfirmMDx assay (MDxHealth, Inc.) is an epigenome-based marker test to detect hypermethylation of three genes (GSTP1, APC and RASSF1) in histopathologically normal prostate biopsy tissue. This assay is based on finding field effect changes, caused by epigenetic, cytomorphological, genetic or gene/protein expression alterations in tissues that are contiguous with cancerous tissue. It therefore complements routine histopathology and increases the sensitivity of cancer diagnosis in non-cancerous biopsy tissue. With a sensitivity of 68 % and a specificity of 64 %, it contributes to reducing false-negative results, and thereby the number of repeat biopsies can be decreased [139]. With an odds ratio of 3.17, this test was an independent, significant risk factor for prostate cancer detection up to 30 months after initial biopsy. These results were validated in cancer negative prostate biopsy core tissue samples of 350 subjects, finding a NPV of 88 % with an odds ratio of 2.69 as most significant independent predictor of biopsy outcome after 24 months [123]. This test is commercially available in the USA.

2.8 Decipher

This genomic classifier (GenomeDX Biosciences) was established out of 545 radical prostatectomy samples with median clinical data follow-up of 16.9 years. The test was developed consisting of 22 markers to predict early clinical metastasis following biochemical recurrence (a rising PSA) and achieved an area under the receiver operating characteristic curve of 0.75 (0.67–0.83) in the validation cohort, outperforming clinical variables. It was the only significant prognostic factor in multivariable analyses [58]. This test may enable clinicians to better select the best candidates for intensive multimodal therapy and spare those who can be closely monitored without initiating aggressive adjuvant treatment.

2.9 Oncotype DX

The commercially available Oncotype DX Genomic Prostate Score (GPS; Genomic Health, Inc.) is a molecular assay on prostate tissue (biopsy) samples and is based on a 17-gene expression panel to predict presence or absence of adverse pathology and may aid man with prostate cancer make more informed decisions between active surveillance and immediate treatment. This panel was constructed in a 3-phase study, consisting of a discovery prostatectomy study ($n = 441$), a biopsy study ($n = 167$) and subsequently validated in a cohort of 395 prostatectomy patients. The GPS is an independent predictor of adverse pathology in potential candidates for active surveillance when added to individual clinical parameters (age, PSA, clinical stage and biopsy Gleason score) [86].

The most recent study on the GPS included 431 men treated for very low-, low- and intermediate-risk prostate cancer. GPS was strongly associated with adverse pathology and predicted time to biochemical recurrence and time to metastases [45].

2.10 Prolaris

Another prognostic tool to aid in clinical decision-making is the commercially available cell cycle progression (CCP) test (Prolaris, Myriad Genetics, Inc.) which uses a 46-gene expression panel, consisting of 31 cell-cycle progression genes and 15 housekeeping genes. In a systematic review, including 16 relevant studies, the CCP score was associated with a risk of biochemical recurrence and disease-specific mortality for clinically localized prostate cancer patients [138]. Cuzick et al. validated this test in combination with standard clinical variables (clinical cell-cycle risk [CCR] score) as a strong independent predictor of prostate cancer death outcome for conservatively managed patients [46]. Therefore, this test can be useful for determining which patients can be safely managed conservatively.

In summary, we can conclude that a robust set of candidate prognostic biomarkers is available that can be measured by immunohistochemistry and/or molecular genetic tests. Stratification of patients based on these markers is well within reach, provided the methods and scoring systems are standardized.

3 Blood Markers

3.1 Kallikreins

3.1.1 Total PSA

In 1986, PSA was approved by the Food and Drug Administration (FDA) as a marker to monitor treatment in patients with prostate cancer, and in 1994 as a diagnostic marker. It is currently still the most widely used marker for prostate cancer.

PSA, also known as kallikrein 3 or hK3, is a serine protease that is a member of the family of glandular kallikrein-related peptidases. The genes for the glandular kallikreins are clustered at chromosome 19q133-4 and transcription of PSA is regulated by androgens [103]. The function of PSA is to liquefy seminal fluid through its action on the gel-forming proteins semenogelin and fibronectin [93].

PSA is not a *cancer*-specific marker, as it is produced by both benign and malignant prostate epithelial cells. Normally, PSA blood levels are low. A healthy prostate is surrounded by a continuous layer of basal cells and a basement membrane which prevent the high concentrations of PSA in the prostate to leak into blood. High PSA blood levels can be caused by an elevated synthesis or an increased release of PSA into blood. An elevated PSA synthesis can be a result of benign prostatic hypertrophy (BPH) and prostate manipulation [76, 98]. PSA expression, ergo PSA synthesis, is slightly *de*creased in the development and progression of prostate cancer [127]. Therefore, as is seen in prostatitis, the increased PSA blood levels in prostate cancer are assumed to be a result of an increased release of PSA into blood through the disrupted architecture of the prostate. With advancing stage of prostate cancer PSA levels can increase, but for the individual patient PSA levels do not correlate directly with clinical and pathological tumour stage.

Despite extensive research, difficulty persists in defining the optimal cut-off value for PSA. Traditionally, it was set at 4.0 ng/ml. Using this PSA cut-off provides a sensitive test, with a positive predictive value of 37 % and a negative predictive value of 91 % [25]. In other words, 75 % of men with PSA 4.0–10.0 ng/ml who undergo biopsy do not have cancer [11]. In addition, several studies showed a substantial probability of prostate cancer within the PSA interval 0–4.0 ng/ml [57, 144, 145]. The Prostate Cancer Prevention Trial (PCPT), for example, reported that 27 % of men with normal digital rectal examination (DRE) and a serum total PSA between 3.1 and 4.0 ng/ml have prostate cancer [145]. On the other hand, it has never been demonstrated that lowering the PSA cut-off affects the long-term survival in men with prostate cancer. Furthermore, this will most likely lead to a higher number of unnecessary biopsies and an increased detection of clinical insignificant prostate cancer. Other factors of influence on PSA blood level is ethnic background and the use of medication. Men from African descent have higher PSA levels than Caucasian men, even after adjusting for prostate volume [64, 114]. And men using 5α-reductase inhibitors for treatment of BPH (such as dutasteride and finasteride) will have lower PSA levels by an average of 50 % after 6 months of treatment [47, 105].

Currently, screening for prostate cancer with PSA is one of the most controversial topics in the urological literature [90]. In the Cochrane review published in 2013, screening was associated with an increased diagnosis of prostate cancer, more localized disease and less advanced prostate cancer [78]. Five randomized controlled trials, including more than 341,000 men, showed no prostate cancer-specific survival benefit as a result of screening. Although demonstrating a prostate cancer-specific survival benefit was the main objective of all these five large trials, the ERSPC was the only study that reported a significant reduction in prostate-cancer-specific mortality, in a pre-specified subgroup of men aged 55–69 years of age [135]. Moreover, screening was associated with minor and major harms such as over diagnosis and overtreatment and the impact on patients' overall quality of life is still unclear. This has led to a strong advice against population-based systematic screening.

Several studies report that PSA measured before age 50 might be indicative for the risk of developing prostate cancer years, or even decades later [94, 102]. It is also suggested that total PSA level at age 44–50 might also predict the likelihood of developing advanced prostate cancer, defined as clinical T3 or higher or metastatic disease at the time of diagnosis [150]. This, however, needs further validation before possible implementation into clinical practice.

3.1.2 Risk Calculators

To predict the potential risk of prostate cancer of an individual patient, risk calculators might be useful. Risk calculators including several predictive factors to stratify patients for prostate biopsy have been developed. Two well-known calculators that are available online are the PCPTRC 2.0 and the ERSPC risk calculator [143, 154]. The first includes serum PSA, DRE results, age, family history of prostate cancer, ethnicity and prior biopsy. The latter includes serum PSA, DRE results, TRUS findings, prior biopsy and prostate volume. The use of risk calculators allows a more individual assessment of prostate cancer risk and provides a better predictive accuracy compared to PSA alone [136]. Since none of the calculators have clearly shown superiority relative to each other, there is no recommendation in the prostate cancer guidelines and it remains a personal decision to use one.

3.1.3 PSA Derivatives

PSA derivates have been evaluated in the attempt to enhance the diagnostic accuracy of total PSA: age-specific total PSA cut-offs, total PSA density, total PSA velocity and total PSA-doubling time. Age-specific PSA cut-off values were suggested to enhance the predictive value of PSA. The suggested cut-off values were: 40–49 years old: 2.5 ng/ml, 50–59: 3.5 ng/ml, 60–69: 4.5 ng/ml and 70–79: 6.5 ng/ml. However, the use of an age-specific total PSA cut-off is not validated and criticized for missing clinically significant cancers in older men [21].

PSA density is defined as the total serum PSA level divided by the volume of the prostate (in grams). The higher the PSA density, the higher the likelihood of harbouring clinically significant prostate cancer. A PSA density of 0.15 ng/nl/g or higher has been considered abnormal and suspicious for cancer. However, the value of this test remains controversial [95]. PSA density correlated with biopsy outcome, tumour aggressiveness and unfavourable pathological features in several studies [16, 84, 131]. However, other studies could not validate these results [26, 119]. In addition, PSA density requires transrectal ultrasound, which is time-consuming, expensive and causes patient discomfort. All together, PSA density is not widely used in clinical practice.

PSA kinetics has been extensively studied for their assumed predictive value to discriminate between benign and malignant conditions of the prostate. This includes PSA velocity, the change in PSA over time (absolute annual increase in serum PSA (ng/mL/year)), and PSA doubling time, the number of months for a certain level of PSA to increase by a factor of 2 (the exponential increase in serum PSA over time). PSA velocity and PSA doubling time may have a prognostic role in treated prostate cancer [7]. However, there is no sufficient evidence that PSA velocity or PSA doubling time has *additional* diagnostic value beyond the use of total PSA. Especially, because of background noise (prostate volume, and benign prostate hyperplasia), different intervals between PSA determinations and increase/decrease over time. Thus, there is no justification for the use of PSA kinetics in clinical decision-making before treatment in early-stage prostate cancer [160]. Recurrence after radical prostatectomy can be monitored with high sensitivity using PSA doubling time. Although currently widely used, PSA response to chemotherapy in castrate-resistant prostate cancer (CRPC) patients does not predict long-term benefit adequately. A recently published paper, however, demonstrated that a PSA decline of 30 % after 4 weeks of abiraterone treatment might be predictive for overall survival outcome [129].

3.1.4 PSA Molecular Forms

In the last decades, novel tests using molecular isoforms of PSA have been developed. PSA circulates in blood either in a stable complexed form or in an unbound 'free' form. Complexed PSA is bound to proteins: α1-antichymotrypsin (ACT), α2-macroglobulin (A2M) and α1-protease inhibitor (API). The unbound form is called freePSA (fPSA) and the free-to-total PSA ratio significantly improves differentiation between prostate cancer and benign conditions. A lower per cent free PSA (free PSA/total PSAx100) is correlated with a higher probability of finding prostate cancer on biopsy [35, 165]. The use of per cent free PSA has been approved as a diagnostic marker by the Food and Drug Administration in men with PSA levels 4.0–10.0 ng/ml. A cut-off value of 25 % is generally used. Note that free PSA is less stable than complexed PSA, causing greater analytic variability. Suboptimal blood sample handling can considerably influence free PSA levels [149].

Free PSA exists in different molecular isoforms, including pro-PSA, BPH-associated BPSA and intact free PSA [97, 110]. Several studies report significantly higher levels of pro-PSA in patients with prostate cancer, and decreased levels of BPSA and intact free PSA [33, 109, 111]. Especially [−2]proPSA (p2PSA) is associated with prostate cancer and has been demonstrated to significantly outperform the use of total PSA and per cent of fPSA alone. Moreover, p2PSA seemed to be related to the risk of aggressive disease [34, 69].

Human kallikrein 2 (hK2) and urokinase plasminogen activation (uPA) are potential future prostate cancer biomarkers that are thus far not validated. hK2 is from the same gene family as PSA but differs in its enzymatic activity [167]. Several studies have shown that the use of a combination of hK2 with free and total PSA might improve the predictive value for prostate cancer [14, 116]. hK2 might also have prognostic value [73, 128]. The serum protease uPA might be involved in tumour development and progression through degradation of the extracellular matrix [55]. The potential role of uPA as a biomarker of metastatic prostate cancer needs to be validated in large multicentre studies.

3.1.5 Prostate Health Index (PHI)

The Prostate Health Index (PHI) test is a recently approved diagnostic blood test, combining free and total PSA and the (−2) pro PSA isoform (p2PSA), and is calculated using the following formula: $([-2]\text{proPSA/free PSA}) \times \sqrt{\text{PSA}}$. In other words, men are more at risk of having significant PCa when they have a higher total PSA and p2 PSA and a lower fPSA [101]. PHI is now commercially available and has been approved by the US Food and Drug Administration for use in the 4.0–10 ng/ml PSA range to reduce the number of unnecessary prostate biopsies in PSA-tested men [34]. The PHI test may also have a role in monitoring men under active surveillance [99]. Its clinical impact is, as yet undetermined, given the slight net benefit for clinical decision-making [63].

3.1.6 The 4K Score

The 4 and K score test (OPKO Health, Inc.) combines the measurement of four prostate-specific kallikreins in blood with clinical information in an algorithm that calculates the probability of significant (Gleason score ≥7) prostate cancer before biopsy. This panel of four kallikrein proteins, including human kallikrein-related peptidase 2 (hK2), and total, free and intact PSA, has been studied in blood samples of pre-biopsy patients in multiple cohorts. The four-kallikrein model was able to predict the biopsy outcome more accurately than total PSA and age alone [159]. Parekh et al. showed in a cohort of 1012 men scheduled for prostate biopsy a good diagnostic performance (AUC: 0.82) in detecting significant prostate cancer [121]. A direct head-to-head comparison between the 4 and K score and phi demonstrated similarly improved discrimination when predicting prostate cancer and high-grade prostate cancer [118].

3.2 MicroRNAs

The discovery of microRNAs (miRNA) in 2004 was a revolutionary step in understanding the mechanisms regulating gene expression and function [37, 75]. Subsequently, it was reported that miRNAs play an important role in cancer by initiating carcinogenesis and driving progression [44].

miRNAs are small endogenous non-coding RNAs, up to 22 nucleotides long, which regulate gene expression post-transcriptionally. miRNAs bind to complementary sequences within messenger RNAs (mRNA) to alter their translation by inhibiting their translation or inducing the cleavage of specific target mRNAs [12]. In most cases, miRNAs 'fine-tune' protein expression (only a modest reduction of the target mRNA concentration) [13]. Occasionally, it causes upregulation or complete destruction of the target mRNA [13, 30, 70].

miRNAs are known to regulate common cellular targeted pathways (intracellular signalling, DNA repair and cellular adhesion/migration) [20, 65, 83], androgen signalling [96, 130, 161] and apoptosis avoidance [120, 140]. Substantial clinical research has been done into the possible use of miRNAs as diagnostic, prognostic and predictive markers for prostate cancer; however, results are somehow controversial [59]. Yet, miRNAs are promising potential biomarkers and novel therapeutic targets for prostate cancer; however, further studies to translate and validate the role of miRNAs in clinical prostate cancer management are needed.

3.3 Circulating Tumour Cells

The importance of circulating tumour cells (CTCs) was already acknowledged in 1869 by Thomas Ashworth, an Australian physician who observed CTCs microscopically [112]. Only recent advances in technology facilitate a reliable method for the detection of CTC in blood. The presence of CTCs in blood proved to be associated with overall survival in patients with metastatic breast [42, 43], colorectal [40, 41] and prostate cancer [49, 133].

In castration resistant prostate cancer (CRPC), the number of CTCs before and after treatment is an independent predictor of survival. This is a strong predictor both as a continuous variable as when using discrete cut-off values (≥5 CTC/7.5 ml of blood vs. <5 CTC) [48, 49, 133]. Post-treatment CTC number showed to be a stronger prognostic factor for survival than a 50 % decline in PSA (AUC: 0.87 vs. 0.62). CTCs (CellSearch) are approved by the Food and Drug Administration as a prognostic biomarker to monitor disease status in patients with metastatic breast, colorectal and prostate cancer. Currently, CTCs have been incorporated as an exploratory end point in several phase II and III trials [4]. In a phase III trial of docetaxel with or without atrasentan for CRPC patients, baseline CTC count (<5 CTCs or ≥5 CTCs) proved to be significantly associated with overall survival [66]. Future studies should provide more evidence at this point before CTCs can be implemented as a tool to redirect and optimize patient therapy.

A recent development in CTCs molecular profiling is the detection of androgen-receptor splice variant 7 messenger RNA (AR-V7) in CTCs of CRPC patients as a potential predictive biomarker. Antonarakis et al. were able to detect AR-V7 in CTCs in 39 % and 19 % of patients treated with enzalutamide and abiraterone, respectively. AR-V7-positive patients had lower PSA response rates, shorter PSA progression-free survival, clinical or radiographic progression-free survival and overall survival compared to AR-V7-negative patients [6]. The detection of AR-V7 in CTCs may therefore be associated with resistance to enzalutamide and abiraterone; however, clinical validation in large prospective studies is required.

4 Urine Markers

4.1 PCA3

In 1999, Bussemakers et al. first identified and characterized the differential display clone 3 (DD3, later called PCA3) gene, to date one of the most prostate cancer–specific genes [29]. PCA3 is non-coding RNA and located on chromosome 9q21-22. Its function is unknown. PCA3 is highly overexpressed in prostate tumours compared to adjacent benign prostate tissues, on average between 70- and 80-fold. An upregulation is seen in 95 % of the primary prostate tumours and no PCA3 expression is found in non-prostate tissue (i.e., benign and malignant tissues from breast, cervix, endometrium, ovary and testis; cell lines originating from bladder, kidney and ovarian cancer) [29].

In the initial PCA3 studies, a real-time RT-PCR analysis was used for the quantification of PCA3 messenger RNA (mRNA) in prostate tissue. Later, Hessels et al. developed a dual-time resolved fluorescence (TRF)-based RT-PCR assay to detect PCA3 mRNA in urinary sediments after digital rectal examination (DRE) [77]. A urine test provides a non-invasive method to obtain prostate (cancer) cells, which makes it suitable for clinical purposes. A DRE is performed to mobilize prostatic cells towards the prostatic urethra, which are flushed out with the first voided urine. A prostate massage is obsolete and causes needless patient discomfort, as a regular DRE sheds enough cells into urine for analysis. In 2006, the Progensa PCA3 test was introduced, a transcription-mediated amplification (TMA) assay [68]. This assay is also performed on first voided urine samples after DRE, but it is a simpler, faster and sensitive enough method compared to the initial RT-PCR-based assay, therefore, more viable for widespread clinical implementation. The PCA3 score is the ratio of PCA3:PSA mRNAs multiplied by 1000. The Progensa PCA3 test is commercially available and Conformité Européenne (CE)-approved since November 2006 to aid in the decision to take initial or repeat biopsies and it gained US Food and Drug Administration (FDA) approval in 2012 as an aid tool for decision-making in the repeat biopsy setting, with a cut-off value of 25.

The clinical utility of PCA3 and its additional predictive value beyond PSA has been extensively studied. PCA3 has been validated as a reliable predictor of prostate cancer at initial or repeat biopsy [50, 53, 72, 77, 106]. Currently, a cut-off value of 35 is used, resulting in a sensitivity of 47–68 % and a specificity of 56–80 % in the Western population [54]. However, the optimal cut-off value is subject to debate. Several studies indicate that a cut-off value of 20 or 25 might be preferable, missing less prostate cancers and still preventing a considerable amount of prostate biopsies [50]. Several studies demonstrated improved predictive accuracy integrating PCA3 into a multivariate model consisting of established prostate cancer risk factors (age, PSA, DRE, prostate volume and biopsy history) [5, 39]. The use of this PCA3-based nomogram has been validated, providing a novel tool for clinical decision-making [10]. Wei et al. incorporated PCA3 into the PCPT Risk Calculator (age, race, PSA, DRE, prior biopsy and family history) in a cohort consisting of 859 men and they found an increased accuracy of predicting high-grade prostate cancer (Gleason ≥ 7) from 0.74 for the PCPT alone to 0.78 for PCPT plus PCA3 in the initial biopsy setting [163]. A direct comparison of PCA3 with PHI and the 4 and K score added to a base model with clinical parameters showed no statistically significant differences in predictive accuracy [142, 158]. Another recent study comparing PCA3 and PHI found that the addition of PCA3 and PHI to the Epstein or PRIAS models improved their prognostic performance for insignificant prostate cancer [31].

It was hypothesized that PCA3 might be associated with more aggressive cancer. This was based on the theory that aggressive prostate cancer cells are more invasive and would therefore more easily shed into the prostatic ductal system after DRE [155]. However, to date, the prognostic value of PCA3 is considered to be limited. Some studies found a correlation of PCA3 with Gleason score [50, 72, 115], but this is contradicted by a range of other studies that show no (additional) predictive value for Gleason score [9, 79, 125, 155]. As concluded by Auprich et al., the clinical value of PCA3 to predict aggressive prostate cancer at radical prostatectomy seems to be marginal at best [9]. PCA3 has been shown, however, as a valuable predictor of tumour volume and insignificance of prostate cancer [9, 72, 125]. Data on predictive value for extracapsular extension are conflicting [9, 72, 164] and PCA3 currently has no role in risk assessment during active surveillance protocols [100].

4.2 TMPRSS2-ERG

For a complete description of the gene fusion TMPRSS2-ERG, see Sect. 2.1. In summary, TMPRSS2-ERG is a fusion of TMPRSS2 (the androgen-regulated trans-membrane protease, serine 2) to Ets family genes (oncogenic transcription factors). Oncogene ERG is the most commonly involved Ets family member in gene fusion. It occurs in approximately half of Caucasian prostate cancer patients.

A publication in 2006 showed the feasibility to detect TMPRSS2-ERG fusion transcripts noninvasively in urinary sediments obtained after DRE using an RT-PCR-based research assay [89]. Since then, extensive research has been performed on the clinical applicability of this urine test. A sensitivity of 37 % and specificity of 93 % to predict prostate cancer was reported, resulting in a positive predictive value of 94 % [78].

4.3 PCA3 and TMPRSS2-ERG Marker Panel

Given the tumour heterogeneity in prostate cancer, the use of a panel of biomarkers may provide the best diagnostic accuracy. Hessels et al. evaluated the combination of PCA3 with TMPRSS2-ERG fusion transcripts detected in the urine, showing an improved sensitivity of 73 %, compared to 62 % for PCA3 alone, without compromising the specificity for detecting prostate cancer [78]. Two recent studies demonstrated the enhanced predictive value of PCA3 combined with TMPRSS2-ERG and respectively the ERSPC and PCPT risk calculator, which may result in a reduction in the number of unnecessary prostate biopsies [87, 140]. Tomlins et al. incorporated both prostate cancer-specific urine markers in a multivariate risk calculator with PSA to improve the predictive accuracy of prostate cancer and high-grade prostate cancer upon biopsy. A combined test, the Mi-Prostate Score (University of Michigan Health System) is currently available to provide individualized risk estimates [146].

4.4 SelectMDx

The most recent development in urinary prostate cancer biomarkers is the development of the SelectMDx test (MDx Health, Inc.). In 2015 Leyten et al. described the identification of a novel urinary gene panel for the early diagnosis of prostate cancer [91]. The combination of the genes HOXC6, TDRD1 and DLX1 had the highest accuracy to predict high-grade prostate cancer (Gleason $\geq$ 7) in biopsies, outperforming PCA3 and PSA with an AUC of 0.77 versus 0.68 and 0.72, respectively. This gene panel (without TDRD1) was validated in a large cohort study and demonstrated an AUC of 0.90 in combination with the PCPT risk calculator [156]. Based on these data, the SelectMDx test has been developed as a commercially available test to be used as a risk score to identify men at risk for harbouring high-grade prostate cancer

5 Future Perspectives

In the worldwide search for novel diagnostic and prognostic biomarkers for prostate cancer, many tumour markers have been proposed. The number of articles published on this subject has increased substantially in the last decade. Although various novel markers have been implemented in daily practice (SelectMDx, PHI, 4 and K score, PCA3, TMPRSS2-ERG, MiPS, ConfirmMDx, Decipher, Oncotype DX, Prolaris and CTCs), PSA currently remains the mostly used biomarker in both diagnostics and follow-up of prostate cancer. Many published results on novel prostate cancer biomarkers appear not reproducible in subsequent studies and thus will never attain the FDA-approved status (Table 2).

Table 2 Different stadia of biomarker research

Stadia of biomarker research	Examples of markers in prostate cancer
1. Exploratory, no intended-use cohort	microRNA, uPA, EPCA-1, EPCA-2, etc.
2. Research use-only assay, evaluated retrospectively	hK2, PTEN, Ki-67, EZH2, E-Cadherin
3. Research use-only assay, evaluated prospectively	TMPRSS2-ERG, AR-V7
4. Commercially available tests	PSA, phi, 4 and K score, PCA3, MiPS, SelectMDx, ConfirmMDx, Decipher, Oncotype Dx, Prolaris, Circulating tumour cells

Where a double-blind randomized placebo controlled trial is the gold standard for therapeutic studies, biomarker studies are not regulated by clear guidelines. These studies often suffer poor study design, lack methodological quality and standardized assays, and information on key elements of design and analysis are often not reported. To improve the quality of diagnostic studies, the STARD (*STA*ndards for *R*eporting of *D*iagnostic accuracy) statement was developed by a group of scientists and editors in 2003 and updated in 2015 [23, 24]. It consists of a checklist of 30 items and a flow diagram that authors can use to ensure that all relevant information is present. In addition, the REMARK guidelines (Reporting Recommendations for Tumor Marker Prognostic Studies) were published in 2005 [107]. These are guidelines for transparent and complete reporting of studies, so that poor studies can be better identified. These initiatives are important steps forward in improving the quality of tumour marker studies, but further improvement of future studies is warranted.

Other future improvement includes the use of a secured database with audit trail, so that results cannot be manipulated after analysis. Validation of a potential novel biomarker should only be approved after multiple prospective studies with an 'intended-use' cohort. Furthermore, it should be kept in mind that it is not sufficient to show that a potential novel biomarker is statistically significant in multivariate analysis; it should improve the predictive accuracy of the multivariate model. In conclusion, future biomarker studies should meet the STARD criteria and should be reported in compliance with the REMARK guidelines.

So, many new biomarkers are ready for 'prime time', yet it needs carefully designed studies to test the exact clinical positioning. Clinical implementation of biomarkers in prostate cancer can be divided into three stages. The first stage focuses on the prediction of biopsy outcome and patient selection before biopsy. Once the decision to take a biopsy has been taken, the man becomes a patient, with or without prostate cancer. This is a tough challenge since the man with indolent cancer should not be bothered with a biopsy, yet the ones in the low PSA ranges with aggressive disease should be identified. Once prostate cancer is diagnosed, we should better predict the prognosis and therapy need/response. Therefore, various tissue-based biomarker tests are available to aid in decision-making (stage 2). At the time a patient develops recurrent disease after treatment with curative intent or a patient is diagnosed with metastatic disease, biomarkers can be helpful to predict treatment response and biomarkers can serve as a surrogate marker for overall survival (stage 3). Commercially available tests in these three stages are illustrated in Fig. 1.

The major challenge in prostate cancer biomarkers is to implement those markers which make a significant contribution to clinical decision-making. Since prostate cancer is a heterogeneous disease, focus should be on a panel of biomarkers. Moreover, to establish an individualized and personalized approach for the diagnosis and treatment of prostate cancer, biomarker panels should be incorporated with relevant clinical parameters and other valuable modalities (i.e., imaging) into a personal risk stratification. Novel markers for decision-making in therapy response are promising; however, they are still in an early stage of validation.

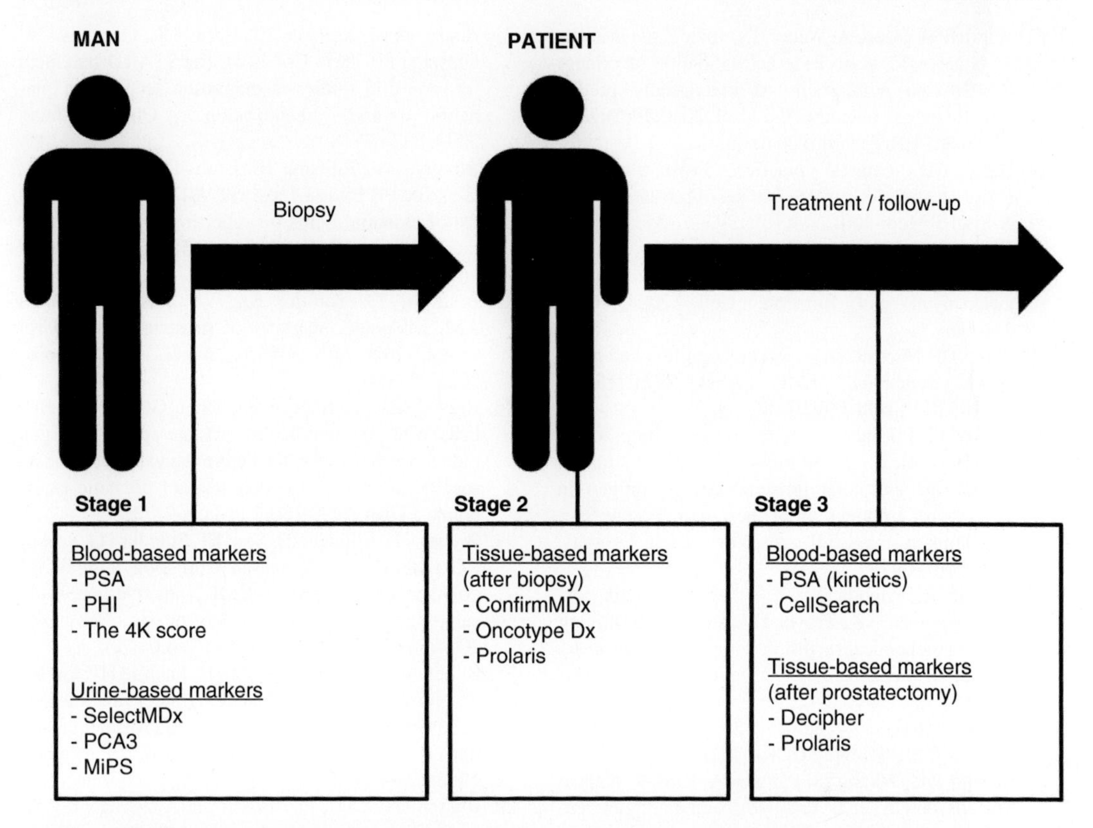

Fig. 1 Commercially available tests to be deployed during the three stages of clinical decision-making

References

1. Aaltomaa S, Lipponen P, Vesalainen S, Ala-Opas M, Eskelinen M, Syrjanen K. Value of Ki-67 immunolabelling as a prognostic factor in prostate cancer. Eur Urol. 1997;32(4):410–5.
2. Aggarwal R, Zhang T, Small EJ, Armstrong AJ. Neuroendocrine prostate cancer: subtypes, biology, and clinical outcomes. J Natl Compr Canc Netw. 2014;12(5):719–26.
3. Anai S, Goodison S, Shiverick K, Iczkowski K, Tanaka M, Rosser CJ. Combination of PTEN gene therapy and radiation inhibits the growth of human prostate cancer xenografts. Hum Gene Ther. 2006;17(10):975–84. doi:10.1089/hum.2006.17.975.
4. Ang JE, Olmos D, de Bono JS. CYP17 blockade by abiraterone: further evidence for frequent continued hormone-dependence in castration-resistant prostate cancer. Br J Cancer. 2009;100(5):671–5. doi:10.1038/sj.bjc.6604904.
5. Ankerst DP, Groskopf J, Day JR, Blase A, Rittenhouse H, Pollock BH, et al. Predicting prostate cancer risk through incorporation of prostate cancer gene 3. J Urol. 2008;180(4):1303–8. doi:10.1016/j.juro.2008.06.038; discussion 8.
6. Antonarakis ES, Lu C, Wang H, Luber B, Nakazawa M, Roeser JC, et al. AR-V7 and resistance to enzalutamide and abiraterone in prostate cancer. N Engl J Med. 2014;371(11):1028–38. doi:10.1056/NEJMoa1315815.
7. Arlen PM, Bianco F, Dahut WL, D'Amico A, Figg WD, Freedland SJ, et al. Prostate Specific Antigen Working Group guidelines on prostate specific antigen doubling time. J Urol. 2008;179(6):2181–5. doi:10.1016/j.juro.2008.01.099; discussion 5–6.
8. Attard G, Clark J, Ambroisine L, Mills IG, Fisher G, Flohr P, et al. Heterogeneity and clinical significance of ETV1 translocations in human prostate cancer. Br J Cancer. 2008;99(2):314–20. doi:10.1038/sj.bjc.6604472.
9. Auprich M, Chun FK, Ward JF, Pummer K, Babaian R, Augustin H, et al. Critical assessment of preoperative urinary prostate cancer antigen 3 on the accuracy of prostate cancer staging. Eur Urol. 2011;59(1):96–105. doi:10.1016/j.eururo.2010.10.024.

10. Auprich M, Haese A, Walz J, Pummer K, de la Taille A, Graefen M, et al. External validation of urinary PCA3-based nomograms to individually predict prostate biopsy outcome. Eur Urol. 2010;58(5):727–32. doi:10.1016/j.eururo.2010.06.038.
11. Barry MJ. Clinical practice. Prostate-specific-antigen testing for early diagnosis of prostate cancer. N Engl J Med. 2001;344(18):1373–7. doi:10.1056/NEJM200105033441806.
12. Bartel DP. MicroRNAs: genomics, biogenesis, mechanism, and function. Cell. 2004;116(2): 281–97.
13. Bartel DP. MicroRNAs: target recognition and regulatory functions. Cell. 2009;136(2):215–33. doi:10.1016/j.cell.2009.01.002.
14. Becker C, Piironen T, Pettersson K, Hugosson J, Lilja H. Clinical value of human glandular kallikrein 2 and free and total prostate-specific antigen in serum from a population of men with prostate-specific antigen levels 3.0 ng/mL or greater. Urology. 2000;55(5):694–9.
15. Bedolla R, Prihoda TJ, Kreisberg JI, Malik SN, Krishnegowda NK, Troyer DA, et al. Determining risk of biochemical recurrence in prostate cancer by immunohistochemical detection of PTEN expression and Akt activation. Clin Cancer Res Off J Am Assoc Cancer Res. 2007;13(13):3860–7. doi:10.1158/1078-0432.CCR-07-0091.
16. Benson MC, Whang IS, Pantuck A, Ring K, Kaplan SA, Olsson CA, et al. Prostate specific antigen density: a means of distinguishing benign prostatic hypertrophy and prostate cancer. J Urol. 1992;147(3 Pt 2):815–6.
17. Bettencourt MC, Bauer JJ, Sesterhenn IA, Mostofi FK, McLeod DG, Moul JW. Ki-67 expression is a prognostic marker of prostate cancer recurrence after radical prostatectomy. J Urol. 1996;156(3):1064–8.
18. Biomarkers Definitions Working Group. Biomarkers and surrogate endpoints: preferred definitions and conceptual framework. Clin Pharmacol Ther. 2001;69(3):89–95. doi:10.1067/mcp.2001.113989.
19. Birchmeier W, Behrens J. Cadherin expression in carcinomas: role in the formation of cell junctions and the prevention of invasiveness. Biochim Biophys Acta. 1994;1198(1):11–26.
20. Bonci D, Coppola V, Musumeci M, Addario A, Giuffrida R, Memeo L, et al. The miR-15a-miR-16-1 cluster controls prostate cancer by targeting multiple oncogenic activities. Nat Med. 2008;14(11):1271–7. doi:10.1038/nm.1880.
21. Borer JG, Sherman J, Solomon MC, Plawker MW, Macchia RJ. Age specific prostate specific antigen reference ranges: population specific. J Urol. 1998;159(2):444–8.
22. Borre M, Bentzen SM, Nerstrom B, Overgaard J. Tumor cell proliferation and survival in patients with prostate cancer followed expectantly. J Urol. 1998;159(5):1609–14.doi:10.1097/00005392-199805000-00054.
23. Bossuyt PM, Reitsma JB, Bruns DE, Gatsonis CA, Glasziou PP, Irwig LM, et al. The STARD statement for reporting studies of diagnostic accuracy: explanation and elaboration. Clin Chem. 2003;49(1):7–18.
24. Bossuyt PM, Reitsma JB, Bruns DE, Gatsonis CA, Glasziou PP, Irwig L, et al. STARD 2015: an updated list of essential items for reporting diagnostic accuracy studies. BMJ. 2015;351:h5527. doi:10.1136/bmj.h5527.
25. Bradford TJ, Tomlins SA, Wang X, Chinnaiyan AM. Molecular markers of prostate cancer. Urol Oncol. 2006;24(6):538–51. doi:10.1016/j.urolonc.2006.07.004.
26. Brawer MK, Aramburu EA, Chen GL, Preston SD, Ellis WJ. The inability of prostate specific antigen index to enhance the predictive the value of prostate specific antigen in the diagnosis of prostatic carcinoma. J Urol. 1993;150(2 Pt 1):369–73.
27. Breuer RH, Snijders PJ, Smit EF, Sutedja TG, Sewalt RG, Otte AP, et al. Increased expression of the EZH2 polycomb group gene in BMI-1-positive neoplastic cells during bronchial carcinogenesis. Neoplasia. 2004;6(6):736–43. doi:10.1593/neo.04160.
28. Bubendorf L, Sauter G, Moch H, Schmid HP, Gasser TC, Jordan P, et al. Ki67 labelling index: an independent predictor of progression in prostate cancer treated by radical prostatectomy. J Pathol. 1996;178(4):437–41.
29. Bussemakers MJ, van Bokhoven A, Verhaegh GW, Smit FP, Karthaus HF, Schalken JA, et al. DD3: a new prostate-specific gene, highly overexpressed in prostate cancer. Cancer Res. 1999;59(23):5975–9.
30. Calin GA, Liu CG, Sevignani C, Ferracin M, Felli N, Dumitru CD, et al. MicroRNA profiling reveals distinct signatures in B cell chronic lymphocytic leukemias. Proc Natl Acad Sci U S A. 2004;101(32):11755–60. doi:10.1073/pnas.0404432101.
31. Cantiello F, Russo GI, Cicione A, Ferro M, Cimino S, Favilla V, et al. PHI and PCA3 improve the prognostic performance of PRIAS and Epstein criteria in predicting insignificant prostate cancer in men eligible for active surveillance. World J Urol. 2015. doi:10.1007/s00345-015-1643-z.
32. Cao Q, Yu J, Dhanasekaran SM, Kim JH, Mani RS, Tomlins SA, et al. Repression of E-cadherin by the polycomb group protein EZH2 in cancer. Oncogene. 2008;27(58):7274–84. doi:10.1038/onc.2008.333.
33. Catalona WJ, Bartsch G, Rittenhouse HG, Evans CL, Linton HJ, Amirkhan A, et al. Serum pro prostate specific antigen improves cancer detection compared to free and complexed prostate specific antigen in men with prostate specific antigen 2 to 4 ng/ml. J Urol. 2003;170(6 Pt 1):2181–5.
34. Catalona WJ, Partin AW, Sanda MG, Wei JT, Klee GG, Bangma CH, et al. A multicenter study of [−2] pro-prostate specific antigen combined with prostate specific antigen and free prostate specific antigen for prostate cancer detection in the 2.0 to 10.0 ng/ml

prostate specific antigen range. J Urol. 2011;185(5):1650–5. doi:10.1016/j.juro.2010.12.032.

35. Catalona WJ, Partin AW, Slawin KM, Brawer MK, Flanigan RC, Patel A, et al. Use of the percentage of free prostate-specific antigen to enhance differentiation of prostate cancer from benign prostatic disease: a prospective multicenter clinical trial. JAMA. 1998;279(19):1542–7.
36. Cattoretti G, Becker MH, Key G, Duchrow M, Schluter C, Galle J, et al. Monoclonal antibodies against recombinant parts of the Ki-67 antigen (MIB 1 and MIB 3) detect proliferating cells in microwave-processed formalin-fixed paraffin sections. J Pathol. 1992;168(4):357–63. doi:10.1002/path.1711680404.
37. Chen K, Rajewsky N. The evolution of gene regulation by transcription factors and microRNAs. Nat Rev Genet. 2007;8(2):93–103. doi:10.1038/nrg1990.
38. Chen H, Tu SW, Hsieh JT. Down-regulation of human DAB2IP gene expression mediated by polycomb Ezh2 complex and histone deacetylase in prostate cancer. J Biol Chem. 2005;280(23):22437–44. doi:10.1074/jbc.M501379200.
39. Chun FK, de la Taille A, van Poppel H, Marberger M, Stenzl A, Mulders PF, et al. Prostate cancer gene 3 (PCA3): development and internal validation of a novel biopsy nomogram. Eur Urol. 2009;56(4):659–67. doi:10.1016/j.eururo.2009.03.029.
40. Cohen SJ, Punt CJ, Iannotti N, Saidman BH, Sabbath KD, Gabrail NY, et al. Relationship of circulating tumor cells to tumor response, progression-free survival, and overall survival in patients with metastatic colorectal cancer. J Clin Oncol Off J Am Soc Clin Oncol. 2008;26(19):3213–21. doi:10.1200/JCO.2007.15.8923.
41. Cohen SJ, Punt CJ, Iannotti N, Saidman BH, Sabbath KD, Gabrail NY, et al. Prognostic significance of circulating tumor cells in patients with metastatic colorectal cancer. Ann Oncol Off J Eur Soc Med Oncol/ESMO. 2009;20(7):1223–9. doi:10.1093/annonc/mdn786.
42. Cristofanilli M, Budd GT, Ellis MJ, Stopeck A, Matera J, Miller MC, et al. Circulating tumor cells, disease progression, and survival in metastatic breast cancer. N Engl J Med. 2004;351(8):781–91. doi:10.1056/NEJMoa040766.
43. Cristofanilli M, Hayes DF, Budd GT, Ellis MJ, Stopeck A, Reuben JM, et al. Circulating tumor cells: a novel prognostic factor for newly diagnosed metastatic breast cancer. J Clin Oncol Off J Am Soc Clin Oncol. 2005;23(7):1420–30. doi:10.1200/JCO.2005.08.140.
44. Croce CM. Causes and consequences of microRNA dysregulation in cancer. Nat Rev Genet. 2009;10(10):704–14. doi:10.1038/nrg2634.
45. Cullen J, Rosner IL, Brand TC, Zhang N, Tsiatis AC, Moncur J, et al. A biopsy-based 17-gene genomic prostate score predicts recurrence after radical prostatectomy and adverse surgical pathology in a racially diverse population of men with clinically low- and intermediate-risk prostate cancer. Eur Urol. 2015;68(1):123–31. doi:10.1016/j.eururo.2014.11.030.
46. Cuzick J, Stone S, Fisher G, Yang ZH, North BV, Berney DM, et al. Validation of an RNA cell cycle progression score for predicting death from prostate cancer in a conservatively managed needle biopsy cohort. Br J Cancer. 2015;113(3):382–9. doi:10.1038/bjc.2015.223.
47. D'Amico AV, Roehrborn CG. Effect of 1 mg/day finasteride on concentrations of serum prostate-specific antigen in men with androgenic alopecia: a randomised controlled trial. Lancet Oncol. 2007;8(1):21–5. doi:10.1016/S1470-2045(06)70981-0.
48. Danila DC, Heller G, Gignac GA, Gonzalez-Espinoza R, Anand A, Tanaka E, et al. Circulating tumor cell number and prognosis in progressive castration-resistant prostate cancer. Clin Cancer Res Off J Am Assoc Cancer Res. 2007;13(23):7053–8. doi:10.1158/1078-0432.CCR-07-1506.
49. de Bono JS, Scher HI, Montgomery RB, Parker C, Miller MC, Tissing H, et al. Circulating tumor cells predict survival benefit from treatment in metastatic castration-resistant prostate cancer. Clin Cancer Res Off J Am Assoc Cancer Res. 2008;14(19):6302–9. doi:10.1158/1078-0432.CCR-08-0872.
50. de la Taille A, Irani J, Graefen M, Chun F, de Reijke T, Kil P, et al. Clinical evaluation of the PCA3 assay in guiding initial biopsy decisions. J Urol. 2011;185(6):2119–25. doi:10.1016/j.juro.2011.01.075.
51. Deininger M, Buchdunger E, Druker BJ. The development of imatinib as a therapeutic agent for chronic myeloid leukemia. Blood. 2005;105(7):2640–53. doi:10.1182/blood-2004-08-3097.
52. Demichelis F, Fall K, Perner S, Andren O, Schmidt F, Setlur SR, et al. TMPRSS2:ERG gene fusion associated with lethal prostate cancer in a watchful waiting cohort. Oncogene. 2007;26(31):4596–9. doi:10.1038/sj.onc.1210237.
53. Deras IL, Aubin SM, Blase A, Day JR, Koo S, Partin AW, et al. PCA3: a molecular urine assay for predicting prostate biopsy outcome. J Urol. 2008;179(4):1587–92. doi:10.1016/j.juro.2007.11.038.
54. Dijkstra S, Leyten GH, Jannink SA, de Jong H, Mulders PF, van Oort IM, et al. KLK3, PCA3, and TMPRSS2-ERG expression in the peripheral blood mononuclear cell fraction from castration-resistant prostate cancer patients and response to docetaxel treatment. Prostate. 2014;74(12):1222–30. doi:10.1002/pros.22839.
55. Duffy MJ. Urokinase-type plasminogen activator: a potent marker of metastatic potential in human cancers. Biochem Soc Trans. 2002;30(2):207–10. 10.1042/.
56. Eeles R, Goh C, Castro E, Bancroft E, Guy M, Al Olama AA, et al. The genetic epidemiology of prostate cancer and its clinical implications. Nat Rev Urol. 2014;11(1):18–31. doi:10.1038/nrurol.2013.266.
57. Efstathiou JA, Chen MH, Catalona WJ, McLeod DG, Carroll PR, Moul JW, et al. Prostate-specific

antigen-based serial screening may decrease prostate cancer-specific mortality. Urology. 2006;68(2):342–7. doi:10.1016/j.urology.2006.02.030.
58. Erho N, Crisan A, Vergara IA, Mitra AP, Ghadessi M, Buerki C, et al. Discovery and validation of a prostate cancer genomic classifier that predicts early metastasis following radical prostatectomy. PLoS One. 2013;8(6):e66855. doi:10.1371/journal.pone.0066855.
59. Fabris L, Ceder Y, Chinnaiyan AM, Jenster GW, Sorensen KD, Tomlins S, et al. The potential of microRNAs as prostate cancer biomarkers. Eur Urol. 2016. doi:10.1016/j.eururo.2015.12.054.
60. Ferraldeschi R, Nava Rodrigues D, Riisnaes R, Miranda S, Figueiredo I, Rescigno P, et al. PTEN protein loss and clinical outcome from castration-resistant prostate cancer treated with abiraterone acetate. Eur Urol. 2015;67(4):795–802. doi:10.1016/j.eururo.2014.10.027.
61. FitzGerald LM, Agalliu I, Johnson K, Miller MA, Kwon EM, Hurtado-Coll A, et al. Association of TMPRSS2-ERG gene fusion with clinical characteristics and outcomes: results from a population-based study of prostate cancer. BMC Cancer. 2008;8:230. doi:10.1186/1471-2407-8-230.
62. Font-Tello A, Juanpere N, de Muga S, Lorenzo M, Lorente JA, Fumado L, et al. Association of ERG and TMPRSS2-ERG with grade, stage, and prognosis of prostate cancer is dependent on their expression levels. Prostate. 2015;75(11):1216–26. doi:10.1002/pros.23004.
63. Fossati N, Buffi NM, Haese A, Stephan C, Larcher A, McNicholas T, et al. Preoperative prostate-specific antigen isoform p2PSA and its derivatives, %p2PSA and prostate health index, predict pathologic outcomes in patients undergoing radical prostatectomy for prostate cancer: results from a multicentric European prospective study. Eur Urol. 2015;68(1):132–8. doi:10.1016/j.eururo.2014.07.034.
64. Fowler Jr JE, Bigler SA, Kilambi NK, Land SA. Relationships between prostate-specific antigen and prostate volume in black and white men with benign prostate biopsies. Urology. 1999;53(6):1175–8.
65. Galardi S, Mercatelli N, Giorda E, Massalini S, Frajese GV, Ciafre SA, et al. miR-221 and miR-222 expression affects the proliferation potential of human prostate carcinoma cell lines by targeting p27Kip1. J Biol Chem. 2007;282(32):23716–24. doi:10.1074/jbc.M701805200.
66. Goldkorn A, Ely B, Quinn DI, Tangen CM, Fink LM, Xu T, et al. Circulating tumor cell counts are prognostic of overall survival in SWOG S0421: a phase III trial of docetaxel with or without atrasentan for metastatic castration-resistant prostate cancer. J Clin Oncol Off J Am Soc Clin Oncol. 2014;32(11):1136–42. doi:10.1200/JCO.2013.51.7417.
67. Gopalan A, Leversha MA, Satagopan JM, Zhou Q, Al-Ahmadie HA, Fine SW, et al. TMPRSS2-ERG gene fusion is not associated with outcome in patients treated by prostatectomy. Cancer Res. 2009;69(4):1400–6. doi:10.1158/0008-5472.CAN-08-2467.
68. Groskopf J, Aubin SM, Deras IL, Blase A, Bodrug S, Clark C, et al. APTIMA PCA3 molecular urine test: development of a method to aid in the diagnosis of prostate cancer. Clin Chem. 2006;52(6):1089–95. doi:10.1373/clinchem.2005.063289.
69. Guazzoni G, Nava L, Lazzeri M, Scattoni V, Lughezzani G, Maccagnano C, et al. Prostate-specific antigen (PSA) isoform p2PSA significantly improves the prediction of prostate cancer at initial extended prostate biopsies in patients with total PSA between 2.0 and 10 ng/ml: results of a prospective study in a clinical setting. Eur Urol. 2011;60(2):214–22. doi:10.1016/j.eururo.2011.03.052.
70. Guo H, Ingolia NT, Weissman JS, Bartel DP. Mammalian microRNAs predominantly act to decrease target mRNA levels. Nature. 2010;466(7308):835–40. doi:10.1038/nature09267.
71. Gutman AB, Gutman EB. An "acid" phosphatase occurring in the serum of patients with metastasizing carcinoma of the prostate gland. J Clin Invest. 1938;17(4):473–8. doi:10.1172/JCI100974.
72. Haese A, de la Taille A, van Poppel H, Marberger M, Stenzl A, Mulders PF, et al. Clinical utility of the PCA3 urine assay in European men scheduled for repeat biopsy. Eur Urol. 2008;54(5):1081–8. doi:10.1016/j.eururo.2008.06.071.
73. Haese A, Graefen M, Steuber T, Becker C, Pettersson K, Piironen T, et al. Human glandular kallikrein 2 levels in serum for discrimination of pathologically organ-confined from locally-advanced prostate cancer in total PSA-levels below 10 ng/ml. Prostate. 2001;49(2):101–9.
74. Han B, Mehra R, Dhanasekaran SM, Yu J, Menon A, Lonigro RJ, et al. A fluorescence in situ hybridization screen for E26 transformation-specific aberrations: identification of DDX5-ETV4 fusion protein in prostate cancer. Cancer Res. 2008;68(18):7629–37. doi:10.1158/0008-5472.CAN-08-2014.
75. He L, Hannon GJ. MicroRNAs: small RNAs with a big role in gene regulation. Nat Rev Genet. 2004;5(7):522–31. doi:10.1038/nrg1379.
76. Herrala AM, Porvari KS, Kyllonen AP, Vihko PT. Comparison of human prostate specific glandular kallikrein 2 and prostate specific antigen gene expression in prostate with gene amplification and overexpression of prostate specific glandular kallikrein 2 in tumor tissue. Cancer. 2001;92(12):2975–84.
77. Hessels D, Klein Gunnewiek JM, van Oort I, Karthaus HF, van Leenders GJ, van Balken B, et al. DD3(PCA3)-based molecular urine analysis for the diagnosis of prostate cancer. Eur Urol. 2003;44(1):8–15; discussion –6.
78. Hessels D, Smit FP, Verhaegh GW, Witjes JA, Cornel EB, Schalken JA. Detection of TMPRSS2-ERG fusion transcripts and prostate cancer antigen 3 in urinary sediments may improve diagnosis of prostate cancer. Clin Cancer Res Off J Am Assoc Cancer Res.

2007;13(17):5103–8. doi:10.1158/1078-0432.CCR-07-0700.
79. Hessels D, van Gils MP, van Hooij O, Jannink SA, Witjes JA, Verhaegh GW, et al. Predictive value of PCA3 in urinary sediments in determining clinicopathological characteristics of prostate cancer. Prostate. 2010;70(1):10–6. doi:10.1002/pros.21032.
80. Huang H, Cheville JC, Pan Y, Roche PC, Schmidt LJ, Tindall DJ. PTEN induces chemosensitivity in PTEN-mutated prostate cancer cells by suppression of Bcl-2 expression. J Biol Chem. 2001;276(42):38830–6. doi:10.1074/jbc.M103632200.
81. Ilic D, Neuberger MM, Djulbegovic M, Dahm P. Screening for prostate cancer. Cochrane Database Syst Rev. 2013;1:CD004720. doi:10.1002/14651858.CD004720.pub3.
82. Ioannidis JP, Castaldi P, Evangelou E. A compendium of genome-wide associations for cancer: critical synopsis and reappraisal. J Natl Cancer Inst. 2010;102(12):846–58. doi:10.1093/jnci/djq173.
83. Josson S, Sung SY, Lao K, Chung LW, Johnstone PA. Radiation modulation of microRNA in prostate cancer cell lines. Prostate. 2008;68(15):1599–606. doi:10.1002/pros.20827.
84. Karazanashvili G, Abrahamsson PA. Prostate specific antigen and human glandular kallikrein 2 in early detection of prostate cancer. J Urol. 2003;169(2):445–57. doi:10.1097/01.ju.0000047085.42539.1c.
85. Kleer CG, Cao Q, Varambally S, Shen R, Ota I, Tomlins SA, et al. EZH2 is a marker of aggressive breast cancer and promotes neoplastic transformation of breast epithelial cells. Proc Natl Acad Sci U S A. 2003;100(20):11606–11. doi:10.1073/pnas.1933744100.
86. Klein EA, Yousefi K, Haddad Z, Choeurng V, Buerki C, Stephenson AJ, et al. A genomic classifier improves prediction of metastatic disease within 5 years after surgery in node-negative high-risk prostate cancer patients managed by radical prostatectomy without adjuvant therapy. Eur Urol. 2015;67(4):778–86. doi:10.1016/j.eururo.2014.10.036.
87. Koyanagi M, Baguet A, Martens J, Margueron R, Jenuwein T, Bix M. EZH2 and histone 3 trimethyl lysine 27 associated with Il4 and Il13 gene silencing in Th1 cells. J Biol Chem. 2005;280(36):31470–7. doi:10.1074/jbc.M504766200.
88. Kumaresan K, Kakkar N, Verma A, Mandal AK, Singh SK, Joshi K. Diagnostic utility of alpha-methylacyl CoA racemase (P504S) & HMWCK in morphologically difficult prostate cancer. Diagn Pathol. 2010;5:83. doi:10.1186/1746-1596-5-83.
89. Laxman B, Tomlins SA, Mehra R, Morris DS, Wang L, Helgeson BE, et al. Noninvasive detection of TMPRSS2:ERG fusion transcripts in the urine of men with prostate cancer. Neoplasia. 2006;8(10):885–8. doi:10.1593/neo.06625.
90. Leyten GH, Hessels D, Jannink SA, Smit FP, de Jong H, Cornel EB, et al. Prospective multicentre evaluation of PCA3 and TMPRSS2-ERG gene fusions as diagnostic and prognostic urinary biomarkers for prostate cancer. Eur Urol. 2014;65(3):534–42. doi:10.1016/j.eururo.2012.11.014.
91. Leyten GH, Hessels D, Smit FP, Jannink SA, de Jong H, Melchers WJ, et al. Identification of a candidate gene panel for the early diagnosis of prostate cancer. Clin Cancer Res Off J Am Assoc Cancer Res. 2015;21(13):3061–70. doi:10.1158/1078-0432.CCR-14-3334.
92. Li J, Yen C, Liaw D, Podsypanina K, Bose S, Wang SI, et al. PTEN, a putative protein tyrosine phosphatase gene mutated in human brain, breast, and prostate cancer. Science. 1997;275(5308):1943–7.
93. Lilja H. A kallikrein-like serine protease in prostatic fluid cleaves the predominant seminal vesicle protein. J Clin Invest. 1985;76(5):1899–903. doi:10.1172/JCI112185.
94. Lilja H, Ulmert D, Bjork T, Becker C, Serio AM, Nilsson JA, et al. Long-term prediction of prostate cancer up to 25 years before diagnosis of prostate cancer using prostate kallikreins measured at age 44 to 50 years. J Clin Oncol Off J Am Soc Clin Oncol. 2007;25(4):431–6. doi:10.1200/JCO.2006.06.9351.
95. Lilja H, Ulmert D, Vickers AJ. Prostate-specific antigen and prostate cancer: prediction, detection and monitoring. Nat Rev Cancer. 2008;8(4):268–78. doi:10.1038/nrc2351.
96. Lin SL, Chiang A, Chang D, Ying SY. Loss of mir-146a function in hormone-refractory prostate cancer. RNA. 2008;14(3):417–24. doi:10.1261/rna.874808.
97. Linton HJ, Marks LS, Millar LS, Knott CL, Rittenhouse HG, Mikolajczyk SD. Benign prostate-specific antigen (BPSA) in serum is increased in benign prostate disease. Clin Chem. 2003;49(2):253–9.
98. Lintula S, Stenman J, Bjartell A, Nordling S, Stenman UH. Relative concentrations of hK2/PSA mRNA in benign and malignant prostatic tissue. Prostate. 2005;63(4):324–9. doi:10.1002/pros.20194.
99. Loeb S. Guideline of guidelines: prostate cancer screening. BJU Int. 2014;114(3):323–5. doi:10.1111/bju.12854.
100. Loeb S, Bruinsma SM, Nicholson J, Briganti A, Pickles T, Kakehi Y, et al. Active surveillance for prostate cancer: a systematic review of clinicopathologic variables and biomarkers for risk stratification. Eur Urol. 2015;67(4):619–26. doi:10.1016/j.eururo.2014.10.010.
101. Loeb S, Catalona WJ. The Prostate Health Index: a new test for the detection of prostate cancer. Ther Adv Urol. 2014;6(2):74–7. doi:10.1177/1756287213513488.
102. Loeb S, Roehl KA, Antenor JA, Catalona WJ, Suarez BK, Nadler RB. Baseline prostate-specific antigen compared with median prostate-specific antigen for age group as predictor of prostate cancer risk in men younger than 60 years old. Urology. 2006;67(2):316–20. doi:10.1016/j.urology.2005.08.040.
103. Lundwall A, Clauss A, Olsson AY. Evolution of kallikrein-related peptidases in mammals and identi-

fication of a genetic locus encoding potential regulatory inhibitors. Biol Chem. 2006;387(3):243–9. doi:10.1515/BC.2006.032.

104. Magi-Galluzzi C, Tsusuki T, Elson P, Simmerman K, LaFargue C, Esgueva R, et al. TMPRSS2-ERG gene fusion prevalence and class are significantly different in prostate cancer of Caucasian, African-American and Japanese patients. Prostate. 2011;71(5):489–97. doi:10.1002/pros.21265.
105. Marks LS, Andriole GL, Fitzpatrick JM, Schulman CC, Roehrborn CG. The interpretation of serum prostate specific antigen in men receiving 5alpha-reductase inhibitors: a review and clinical recommendations. J Urol. 2006;176(3):868–74. doi:10.1016/j.juro.2006.04.024.
106. Marks LS, Fradet Y, Deras IL, Blase A, Mathis J, Aubin SM, et al. PCA3 molecular urine assay for prostate cancer in men undergoing repeat biopsy. Urology. 2007;69(3):532–5. doi:10.1016/j.urology.2006.12.014.
107. McShane LM, Altman DG, Sauerbrei W, Taube SE, Gion M, Clark GM, et al. Reporting recommendations for tumor marker prognostic studies. J Clin Oncol Off J Am Soc Clin Oncol. 2005;23(36):9067–72. doi:10.1200/JCO.2004.01.0454.
108. Melling N, Thomsen E, Tsourlakis MC, Kluth M, Hube-Magg C, Minner S, et al. Overexpression of enhancer of zeste homolog 2 (EZH2) characterizes an aggressive subset of prostate cancers and predicts patient prognosis independently from pre- and post-operatively assessed clinicopathological parameters. Carcinogenesis. 2015;36(11):1333–40. doi:10.1093/carcin/bgv137.
109. Mikolajczyk SD, Catalona WJ, Evans CL, Linton HJ, Millar LS, Marker KM, et al. Proenzyme forms of prostate-specific antigen in serum improve the detection of prostate cancer. Clin Chem. 2004;50(6):1017–25. doi:10.1373/clinchem.2003.026823.
110. Mikolajczyk SD, Grauer LS, Millar LS, Hill TM, Kumar A, Rittenhouse HG, et al. A precursor form of PSA (pPSA) is a component of the free PSA in prostate cancer serum. Urology. 1997;50(5):710–4. doi:10.1016/S0090-4295(97)00449-4.
111. Mikolajczyk SD, Millar LS, Wang TJ, Rittenhouse HG, Marks LS, Song W, et al. A precursor form of prostate-specific antigen is more highly elevated in prostate cancer compared with benign transition zone prostate tissue. Cancer Res. 2000;60(3):756–9.
112. Miller MC, Doyle GV, Terstappen LW. Significance of circulating tumor cells detected by the cell search system in patients with metastatic breast colorectal and prostate cancer. J Oncol. 2010;2010:617421. doi:10.1155/2010/617421.
113. Minner S, Enodien M, Sirma H, Luebke AM, Krohn A, Mayer PS, et al. ERG status is unrelated to PSA recurrence in radically operated prostate cancer in the absence of anti-hormonal therapy. Clin Cancer Res. 2011;17(18):5878–88.
114. Morgan TO, Jacobsen SJ, McCarthy WF, Jacobson DJ, McLeod DG, Moul JW. Age-specific reference ranges for prostate-specific antigen in black men. N Engl J Med. 1996;335(5):304–10. doi:10.1056/NEJM199608013350502.
115. Nakanishi H, Groskopf J, Fritsche HA, Bhadkamkar V, Blase A, Kumar SV, et al. PCA3 molecular urine assay correlates with prostate cancer tumor volume: implication in selecting candidates for active surveillance. J Urol. 2008;179(5):1804–9. doi:10.1016/j.juro.2008.01.013; discussion 9–10.
116. Nam RK, Diamandis EP, Toi A, Trachtenberg J, Magklara A, Scorilas A, et al. Serum human glandular kallikrein-2 protease levels predict the presence of prostate cancer among men with elevated prostate-specific antigen. J Clin Oncol Off J Am Soc Clin Oncol. 2000;18(5):1036–42.
117. Nam RK, Sugar L, Yang W, Srivastava S, Klotz LH, Yang LY, et al. Expression of the TMPRSS2:ERG fusion gene predicts cancer recurrence after surgery for localised prostate cancer. Br J Cancer. 2007;97(12):1690–5. doi:10.1038/sj.bjc.6604054.
118. Nordstrom T, Vickers A, Assel M, Lilja H, Gronberg H, Eklund M. Comparison between the four-kallikrein panel and prostate health index for predicting prostate cancer. Eur Urol. 2015;68(1):139–46. doi:10.1016/j.eururo.2014.08.010.
119. Ohori M, Dunn JK, Scardino PT. Is prostate-specific antigen density more useful than prostate-specific antigen levels in the diagnosis of prostate cancer? Urology. 1995;46(5):666–71. doi:10.1016/S0090-4295(99)80298-2.
120. Papagiannakopoulos T, Shapiro A, Kosik KS. MicroRNA-21 targets a network of key tumor-suppressive pathways in glioblastoma cells. Cancer Res. 2008;68(19):8164–72. doi:10.1158/0008-5472.CAN-08-1305.
121. Parekh DJ, Punnen S, Sjoberg DD, Asroff SW, Bailen JL, Cochran JS, et al. A multi-institutional prospective trial in the USA confirms that the 4Kscore accurately identifies men with high-grade prostate cancer. Eur Urol. 2015;68(3):464–70. doi:10.1016/j.eururo.2014.10.021.
122. Park K, Tomlins SA, Mudaliar KM, Chiu YL, Esgueva R, Mehra R, et al. Antibody-based detection of ERG rearrangement-positive prostate cancer. Neoplasia. 2010;12(7):590–8.
123. Partin AW, Van Neste L, Klein EA, Marks LS, Gee JR, Troyer DA, et al. Clinical validation of an epigenetic assay to predict negative histopathological results in repeat prostate biopsies. J Urol. 2014;192(4):1081–7. doi:10.1016/j.juro.2014.04.013.
124. Pettersson A, Graff RE, Bauer SR, Pitt MJ, Lis RT, Stack EC, et al. The TMPRSS2:ERG rearrangement, ERG expression, and prostate cancer outcomes: a cohort study and meta-analysis. Cancer Epidemiol Biomarkers Prev Publ Am Assoc Cancer Res cosponsored by the Am Soc Prev Oncol. 2012;21(9):1497–509. doi:10.1158/1055-9965.EPI-12-0042.
125. Ploussard G, Durand X, Xylinas E, Moutereau S, Radulescu C, Forgue A, et al. Prostate cancer antigen

3 score accurately predicts tumour volume and might help in selecting prostate cancer patients for active surveillance. Eur Urol. 2011;59(3):422–9. doi:10.1016/j.eururo.2010.11.044.
126. Priulla M, Calastretti A, Bruno P, Azzariti A, Paradiso A, Canti G, et al. Preferential chemosensitization of PTEN-mutated prostate cells by silencing the Akt kinase. Prostate. 2007;67(7):782–9. doi:10.1002/pros.20566.
127. Qiu SD, Young CY, Bilhartz DL, Prescott JL, Farrow GM, He WW, et al. In situ hybridization of prostate-specific antigen mRNA in human prostate. J Urol. 1990;144(6):1550–6.
128. Recker F, Kwiatkowski MK, Piironen T, Pettersson K, Lummen G, Wernli M, et al. The importance of human glandular kallikrein and its correlation with different prostate specific antigen serum forms in the detection of prostate carcinoma. Cancer. 1998;83(12):2540–7.
129. Rescigno P, Lorente D, Bianchini D, Ferraldeschi R, Kolinsky MP, Sideris S, et al. Prostate-specific antigen decline after 4 weeks of treatment with abiraterone acetate and overall survival in patients with metastatic castration-resistant prostate cancer. Eur Urol. 2016.
130. Ribas J, Ni X, Haffner M, Wentzel EA, Salmasi AH, Chowdhury WH, et al. miR-21: an androgen receptor-regulated microRNA that promotes hormone-dependent and hormone-independent prostate cancer growth. Cancer Res. 2009;69(18):7165–9. doi:10.1158/0008-5472.CAN-09-1448.
131. Rommel FM, Agusta VE, Breslin JA, Huffnagle HW, Pohl CE, Sieber PR, et al. The use of prostate specific antigen and prostate specific antigen density in the diagnosis of prostate cancer in a community based urology practice. J Urol. 1994;151(1):88–93.
132. Scalzo DA, Kallakury BV, Gaddipati RV, Sheehan CE, Keys HM, Savage D, et al. Cell proliferation rate by MIB-1 immunohistochemistry predicts postradiation recurrence in prostatic adenocarcinomas. Am J Clin Pathol. 1998;109(2):163–8.
133. Scher HI, Jia X, de Bono JS, Fleisher M, Pienta KJ, Raghavan D, et al. Circulating tumour cells as prognostic markers in progressive, castration-resistant prostate cancer: a reanalysis of IMMC38 trial data. Lancet Oncol. 2009;10(3):233–9. doi:10.1016/S1470-2045(08)70340-1.
134. Scholzen T, Gerdes J. The Ki-67 protein: from the known and the unknown. J Cell Physiol. 2000;182(3):311–22. doi:10.1002/(SICI)1097-4652(200003)182:3<311::AID-JCP1>3.0.CO;2-9.
135. Schroder FH, Hugosson J, Roobol MJ, Tammela TL, Zappa M, Nelen V, et al. Screening and prostate cancer mortality: results of the European Randomised Study of Screening for Prostate Cancer (ERSPC) at 13 years of follow-up. Lancet. 2014;384(9959):2027–35.
136. Schroder F, Kattan MW. The comparability of models for predicting the risk of a positive prostate biopsy with prostate-specific antigen alone: a systematic review. Eur Urol. 2008;54(2):274–90. doi:10.1016/j.eururo.2008.05.022.
137. Shen MM, Abate-Shen C. Pten inactivation and the emergence of androgen-independent prostate cancer. Cancer Res. 2007;67(14):6535–8. doi:10.1158/0008-5472.CAN-07-1271.
138. Sommariva S, Tarricone R, Lazzeri M, Ricciardi W, Montorsi F. Prognostic value of the cell cycle progression score in patients with prostate cancer: a systematic review and meta-analysis. Eur Urol. 2016;69(1):107–15. doi:10.1016/j.eururo.2014.11.038.
139. Stewart GD, Van Neste L, Delvenne P, Delree P, Delga A, McNeill SA, et al. Clinical utility of an epigenetic assay to detect occult prostate cancer in histopathologically negative biopsies: results of the MATLOC study. J Urol. 2013;189(3):1110–6. doi:10.1016/j.juro.2012.08.219.
140. Sylvestre Y, De Guire V, Querido E, Mukhopadhyay UK, Bourdeau V, Major F, et al. An E2F/miR-20a autoregulatory feedback loop. J Biol Chem. 2007;282(4):2135–43. doi:10.1074/jbc.M608939200.
141. Takeichi M. The cadherins: cell-cell adhesion molecules controlling animal morphogenesis. Development. 1988;102(4):639–55.
142. Tallon L, Luangphakdy D, Ruffion A, Colombel M, Devonec M, Champetier D, et al. Comparative evaluation of urinary PCA3 and TMPRSS2: ERG scores and serum PHI in predicting prostate cancer aggressiveness. Int J Mol Sci. 2014;15(8):13299–316. doi:10.3390/ijms150813299.
143. Thompson IM, Ankerst DP, Chi C, Goodman PJ, Tangen CM, Lucia MS, et al. Assessing prostate cancer risk: results from the Prostate Cancer Prevention Trial. J Natl Cancer Inst. 2006;98(8):529–34. doi:10.1093/jnci/djj131.
144. Thompson IM, Ankerst DP, Chi C, Lucia MS, Goodman PJ, Crowley JJ, et al. Operating characteristics of prostate-specific antigen in men with an initial PSA level of 3.0 ng/ml or lower. JAMA. 2005;294(1):66–70. doi:10.1001/jama.294.1.66.
145. Thompson IM, Pauler DK, Goodman PJ, Tangen CM, Lucia MS, Parnes HL, et al. Prevalence of prostate cancer among men with a prostate-specific antigen level<or =4.0 ng per milliliter. N Engl J Med. 2004;350(22):2239–46. doi:10.1056/NEJMoa031918.
146. Tomlins SA, Day JR, Lonigro RJ, Hovelson DH, Siddiqui J, Kunju LP, et al. Urine TMPRSS2:ERG plus PCA3 for individualized prostate cancer risk assessment. Eur Urol. 2015. doi:10.1016/j.eururo.2015.04.039.
147. Tomlins SA, Mehra R, Rhodes DR, Smith LR, Roulston D, Helgeson BE, et al. TMPRSS2:ETV4 gene fusions define a third molecular subtype of prostate cancer. Cancer Res. 2006;66(7):3396–400. doi:10.1158/0008-5472.CAN-06-0168.
148. Tomlins SA, Rhodes DR, Perner S, Dhanasekaran SM, Mehra R, Sun XW, et al. Recurrent fusion of

TMPRSS2 and ETS transcription factor genes in prostate cancer. Science. 2005;310(5748):644–8. doi:10.1126/science.1117679.
149. Ulmert D, Becker C, Nilsson JA, Piironen T, Bjork T, Hugosson J, et al. Reproducibility and accuracy of measurements of free and total prostate-specific antigen in serum vs plasma after long-term storage at −20 degrees C. Clin Chem. 2006;52(2):235–9. doi:10.1373/clinchem.2005.050641.
150. Ulmert D, Cronin AM, Bjork T, O'Brien MF, Scardino PT, Eastham JA, et al. Prostate-specific antigen at or before age 50 as a predictor of advanced prostate cancer diagnosed up to 25 years later: a case–control study. BMC Med. 2008;6:6. doi:10.1186/1741-7015-6-6.
151. Umbas R, Isaacs WB, Bringuier PP, Xue Y, Debruyne FM, Schalken JA. Relation between aberrant alpha-catenin expression and loss of E-cadherin function in prostate cancer. Int J Cancer. 1997;74(4):374–7.
152. Umbas R, Schalken JA, Aalders TW, Carter BS, Karthaus HF, Schaafsma HE, et al. Expression of the cellular adhesion molecule E-cadherin is reduced or absent in high-grade prostate cancer. Cancer Res. 1992;52(18):5104–9.
153. Uzoh CC, Perks CM, Bahl A, Holly JM, Sugiono M, Persad RA. PTEN-mediated pathways and their association with treatment-resistant prostate cancer. BJU Int. 2009;104(4):556–61. doi:10.1111/j.1464-410X.2009.08411.x.
154. van den Bergh RC, Roobol MJ, Wolters T, van Leeuwen PJ, Schroder FH. The Prostate Cancer Prevention Trial and European Randomized Study of Screening for Prostate Cancer risk calculators indicating a positive prostate biopsy: a comparison. BJU Int. 2008;102(9):1068–73. doi:10.1111/j.1464-410X.2008.07940.x.
155. van Gils MP, Hessels D, de Kaa CA H-v, Witjes JA, Jansen CF, Mulders PF, et al. Detailed analysis of histopathological parameters in radical prostatectomy specimens and PCA3 urine test results. Prostate. 2008;68(11):1215–22. doi:10.1002/pros.20781.
156. van Neste L, Hendriks RJ, Dijkstra S, Trooskens G, Cornel EB, Jannink SA, et al. Detection of high-grade prostate cancer using a urinary molecular biomarker-based risk score. Eur Urol. 2016. In press.
157. Varambally S, Dhanasekaran SM, Zhou M, Barrette TR, Kumar-Sinha C, Sanda MG, et al. The polycomb group protein EZH2 is involved in progression of prostate cancer. Nature. 2002;419(6907):624–9. doi:10.1038/nature01075.
158. Vedder MM, de Bekker-Grob EW, Lilja HG, Vickers AJ, van Leenders GJ, Steyerberg EW, et al. The added value of percentage of free to total prostate-specific antigen, PCA3, and a kallikrein panel to the ERSPC risk calculator for prostate cancer in prescreened men. Eur Urol. 2014;66(6):1109–15. doi:10.1016/j.eururo.2014.08.011.
159. Vickers AJ, Cronin AM, Aus G, Pihl CG, Becker C, Pettersson K, et al. A panel of kallikrein markers can reduce unnecessary biopsy for prostate cancer: data from the European Randomized Study of Prostate Cancer Screening in Goteborg, Sweden. BMC Med. 2008;6:19. doi:10.1186/1741-7015-6-19.
160. Vickers AJ, Savage C, O'Brien MF, Lilja H. Systematic review of pretreatment prostate-specific antigen velocity and doubling time as predictors for prostate cancer. J Clin Oncol Off J Am Soc Clin Oncol. 2009;27(3):398–403. doi:10.1200/JCO.2008.18.1685.
161. Waltering KK, Porkka KP, Jalava SE, Urbanucci A, Kohonen PJ, Latonen LM, et al. Androgen regulation of micro-RNAs in prostate cancer. Prostate. 2011;71(6):604–14. doi:10.1002/pros.21276.
162. Wang J, Cai Y, Ren C, Ittmann M. Expression of variant TMPRSS2/ERG fusion messenger RNAs is associated with aggressive prostate cancer. Cancer Res. 2006;66(17):8347–51. doi:10.1158/0008-5472.CAN-06-1966.
163. Wei JT, Feng Z, Partin AW, Brown E, Thompson I, Sokoll L, et al. Can urinary PCA3 supplement PSA in the early detection of prostate cancer? J Clin Oncol Off J Am Soc Clin Oncol. 2014;32(36):4066–72. doi:10.1200/JCO.2013.52.8505.
164. Whitman EJ, Groskopf J, Ali A, Chen Y, Blase A, Furusato B, et al. PCA3 score before radical prostatectomy predicts extracapsular extension and tumor volume. J Urol. 2008;180(5):1975–8. doi:10.1016/j.juro.2008.07.060; discussion 8–9.
165. Woodrum DL, Brawer MK, Partin AW, Catalona WJ, Southwick PC. Interpretation of free prostate specific antigen clinical research studies for the detection of prostate cancer. J Urol. 1998;159(1):5–12.
166. Wu Z, McRoberts KS, Theodorescu D. The role of PTEN in prostate cancer cell tropism to the bone micro-environment. Carcinogenesis. 2007;28(7):1393–400. doi:10.1093/carcin/bgm050.
167. Yousef GM, Diamandis EP. The new human tissue kallikrein gene family: structure, function, and association to disease. Endocr Rev. 2001;22(2):184–204. doi:10.1210/edrv.22.2.0424.

The Clinical Genomics of Prostate Cancer

Michael Fraser, Theo van der Kwast, Paul C. Boutros, and Robert G. Bristow

1 Key Genetic Changes in the Development of Prostate Cancer

Several recent reports have evaluated the mutational landscape of localized primary prostate cancer and have identified recurrent molecular features that typify this disease cohort. The primary characteristic of most localized PCa is a relative paucity of driver single nucleotide variants (SNVs or mutations) relative to other tumor types. This is to be contrasted with an increased occurrence of somatic genomic rearrangements, including: gene copy number aberrations (CNAs), small insertions/deletions (InDels), translocations, and gene fusions (see Fig. 1).

M. Fraser
Princess Margaret Cancer Centre,
Toronto, ON, Canada

T. van der Kwast
Princess Margaret Cancer Centre,
Toronto, ON, Canada

Departments of Laboratory Medicine and Pathology,
University of Toronto, Toronto, ON, Canada

P.C. Boutros
Ontario Institute for Cancer Research,
Toronto, ON, Canada

Bioinformatics and Computing, University of
Toronto, Toronto, ON, Canada

R.G. Bristow (✉)
Princess Margaret Cancer Centre,
Toronto, ON, Canada
e-mail: rob.bristow@rmp.uhn.on.ca

Radiation Oncology, University of Toronto,
Toronto, ON, Canada

Recent whole-genome and whole-exome sequencing studies have identified recurrent somatic mutations in SPOP, which encodes the Speckle Type BTB/POZ Protein [1–4]. SPOP is the most commonly mutated gene in localized disease with ~10 % of cases harboring such alterations. Mutation of SPOP has been implicated in dysregulation of several proteins implicated in tumorigenesis and epithelial cell invasion and genomic instability [5, 6]. Other recurrently mutated genes include TP53, FOXA1, MED12, and ATM, although the recurrence rate remains very low (i.e., <5 % of cases overall).

In contrast, several genomic rearrangements are highly recurrent in localized PCa. Approximately 50 % of PCa harbor a fusion between the 5' region of the androgen-responsive TMPRSS2 gene and the coding region of the ERG oncogene [7] (see Fig. 2). This fusion results either from an intergenic deletion on chromosome 21 between the TMPRSS2 and ERG loci (termed "Edel"), in which the 5' region of the ERG gene is deleted, or, less commonly, from the translocation of the 5' ERG region elsewhere in the nucleus (termed "Esplit"). Fusion of other ETS-family oncogenes (e.g., ETV1, ETV4, ETV5, ELK4) to both TMPRSS2 and other androgen-responsive

M. Bolla, H. van Poppel (eds.), *Management of Prostate Cancer*,
DOI 10.1007/978-3-319-42769-0_6

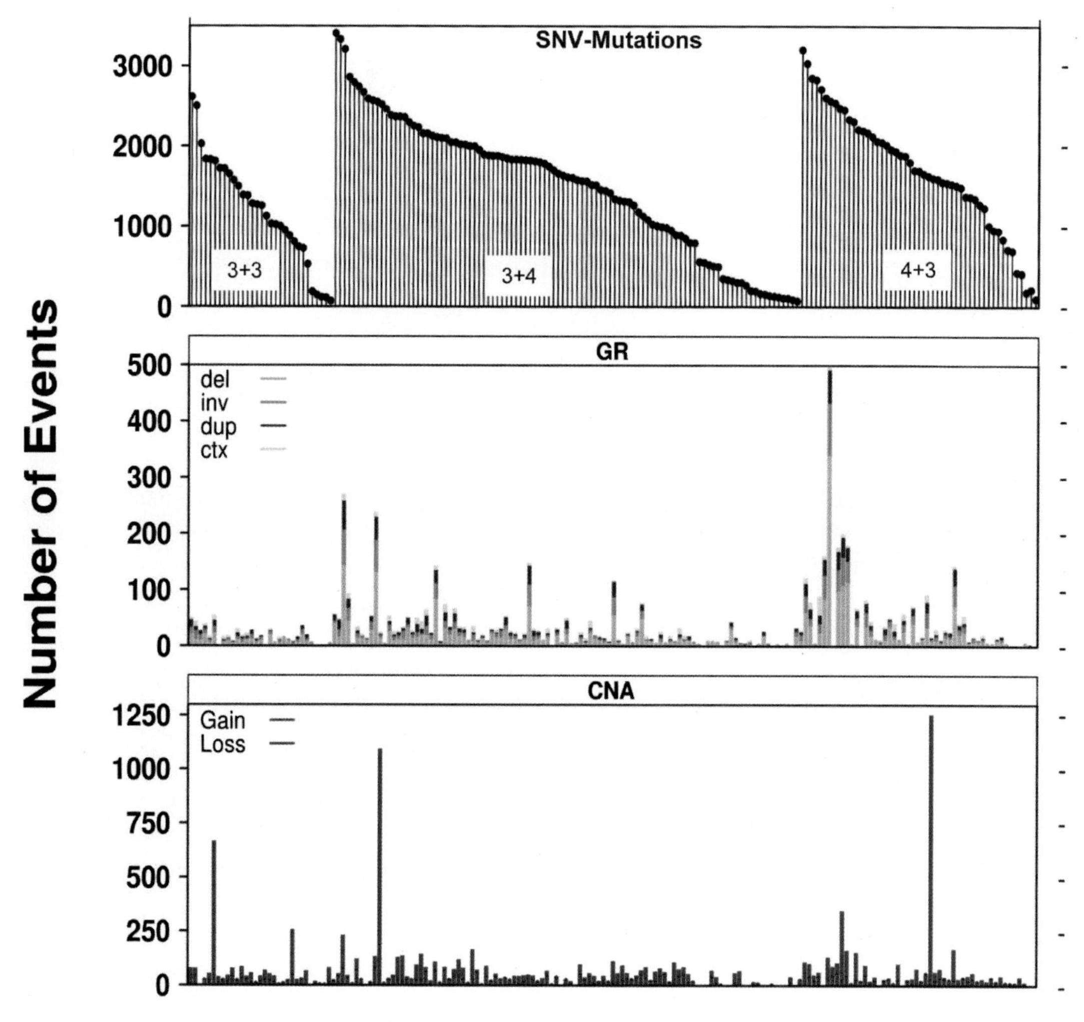

Fig. 1 The Genomics of Localized Prostate Cancer: Shown are plots of single nucleotide variants (SNVs; also called tumor mutations), gene rearrangements (GR) and copy number alteration (CNA) for localized prostate cancer with Gleason score 6 (3+3) or 7 (3+4 versus 4+3). All three indices (SNV, GR, CNA) vary within, and between, patients with different Gleason scores (Boutros, Bristow and Fraser; unpublished)

5' fusion partners (SLC45A3, KLK2, and others) is observed in a further ~20 of localized PCa, such that ~70 % of all PCa harbor an ETS fusion gene product. Clonal analyses have determined that TMPRSS2: ERG fusion is a very early event in prostate tumorigenesis, although its precise prognostic value remains unclear [8].

Recurrent gene copy number aberrations (CNAs) are also frequently observed in PCa. Frequent amplifications (2p, 8q, 15p, and chr7) and deletions (10q, 8p, 16q, 17p) are highly recurrent, and are associated with gain or loss of established oncogenes and tumor suppressors including MYC, TP53, CHD1, CDH1, NKX3-1, RB1, BRCA2, RET, and others. Several individual CNAs have been shown to be negative prognostic factors for early biochemical (i.e., PSA) and metastatic relapse for localized PCa [9–13], and CNA-based multigene signatures are even more prognostic for early biochemical relapse following either radiotherapy or radical prostatectomy [14].

PCa is also associated with several types of localized hypermutation, including chromothripsis, kataegis, and chromoplexy. Kataegis

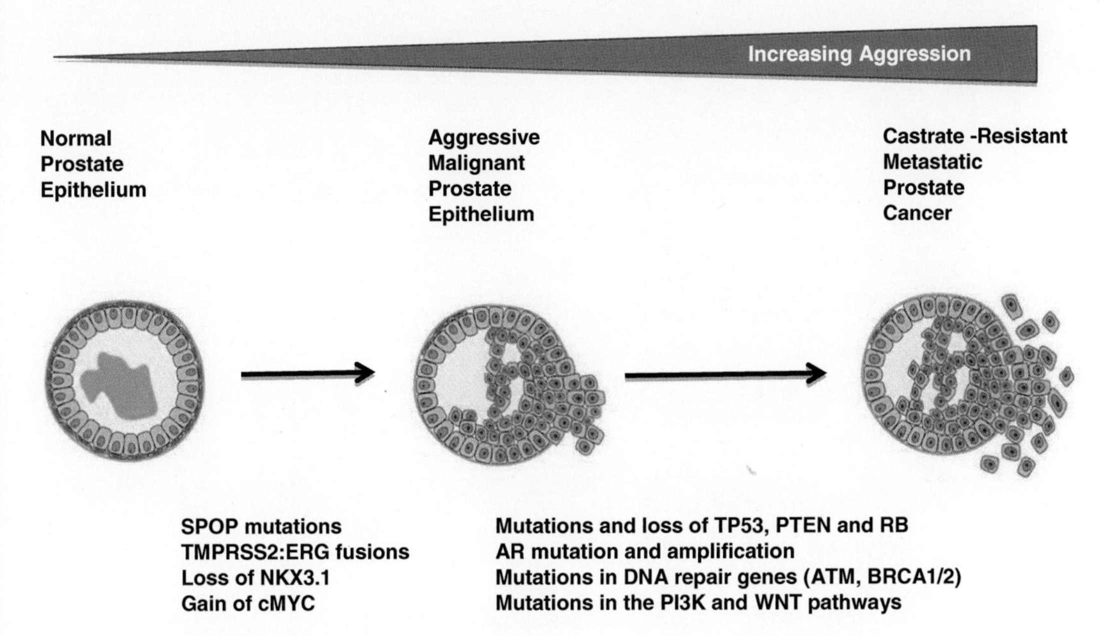

Fig. 2 Genetic Pathways of Progression in Prostate Cancer

is defined by the presence of regional substitution mutation clusters, typically C>T transitions, which was originally characterized in a panel of 21 breast cancers [15]. Kataegis occurs in one fifth of localized Gleason 6/7 PCa, and is associated with elevated Gleason grade and overall genomic instability. Chromoplexy is a unique form of hypermutation in which multiple genomic rearrangements occur in two or more chromosomes, creating a set of tandem rearrangements that disrupt multiple cancer genes simultaneously, representing a form of "punctuated evolution" for PCa genomes [3]. This pattern leads to catastrophic and random fragmentation [16]. While the precise mechanism underlying chromothripsis is unknown, the process is associated with particular molecular hallmarks, including TP53 tumor suppressor gene mutations and the presence of highly localized structural rearrangements (i.e., few chromosomes and specific chromosomal regions, therein). Approximately 20 % of localized Gleason 6/7 PCa show strong evidence of having undergone chromothripsis which is associated with deletion of a variety of tumor suppressor genes.

2 Genetic Heterogeneity and Prostate Cancer

Tumor heterogeneity can exist in many forms in prostate cancer and each may have unique genetic elements associated with it (see Fig. 3). Furthermore, these cancers emerge from an ongoing evolutionary process in which clonal adaption and selection can take place within a heterogeneous tumor microenvironment. This can lead to both multifocality and multiclonality and drive the potential for metastases and prostate cancer cancer-related death. Prostate cancers are therefore multifocal cancers that can contain clonal subpopulations and genomic abnormalities that link carcinogenesis to tumor progression. As such, there exists both intra- and interpatient genetic heterogeneity, within and between patients, even when such patients have similar clinical characteristics (e.g., PSA, Gleason score, TNM staging).

It is important to note that major differences in genomics are present across multiple foci within a prostate gland that are not accounted for by differential pathology alone (see Fig. 4). Indeed, multifocal tumors can be heterogeneous for

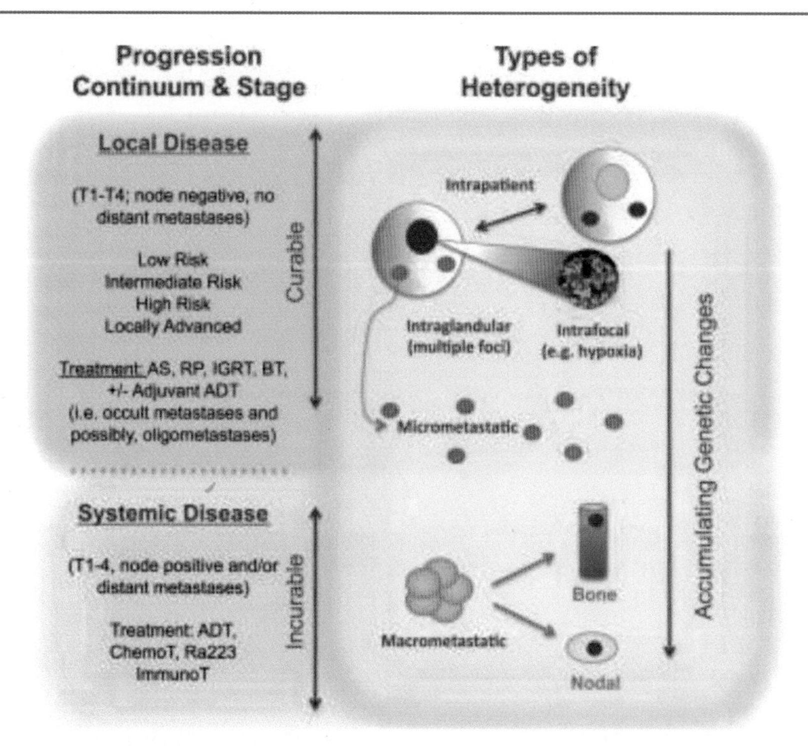

Fig. 3 Sources of heterogeneity in prostate cancer. Interpatient heterogeneity exists throughout the progression from localized, potentially curable disease to incurable, castration-resistant disease and may be related to both interfocal and intrafocal factors (Reproduced from Fraser et al. *Urol Oncol*. 2015 Feb;33(2):85–94)

SNVs (tumor mutations), CNAs (gains or losses of gene alleles) and GRs. Furthermore, using multiple samples from areas of both cancer and morphologically normal tissue within the same prostate, it has been observed that mutations can already be present in morphologically normal tissue reflecting the earliest signs of clonal expansion. This supports the hypothesis that abnormal mutational and genomic processes occurring within the gland act as "field effects" and form the basis for prostate carcinogenesis and tumor progression [17, 18].

The TMPRSS2: ERG fusion, which drives ERG overexpression, is generally considered a very early event in prostate carcinogenesis and is already present in a proportion of the high-grade prostatic intraepithelial neoplasia (an established precursor lesion of CaP) [19]. This explains why most CaP foci show a homogeneous expression of ERG consistent with their independent clonal origin, whereas the fusion can vary between foci, even within a single prostate (Fig. 4). By contrast, PTEN deletions are considered a later step in CaP progression associated with greater heterogeneity in individual CaP foci (Figs. 3, 4, and 5) [20].

Another type of genetic heterogeneity exists between the primary tumor and associated metastases. Specific genomic changes can be shared between primary and metastatic disease [19]. Using patient-matched primary/metastatic tumors, several studies have shown that anatomically distinct tumor metastases can be derived from a single progenitor clone [20–22]. Furthermore, metastasis-to-metastasis spread can be common through monoclonal or multiclonal seeding between metastatic sites[23]. This is accompanied by inaction of tumor suppressor genes (e.g., p53, PTEN) and mutations in androgen receptor signaling genes. Although distant bone metastasis is the most common pattern of prostate cancer spread, a subset of tumors gain the ability to spread to soft tissues; the differential genomics between these two states is poorly understood.

Taken together, the aforementioned data begin to help explain the relatively large disparity in clinical outcomes for patients with clinically

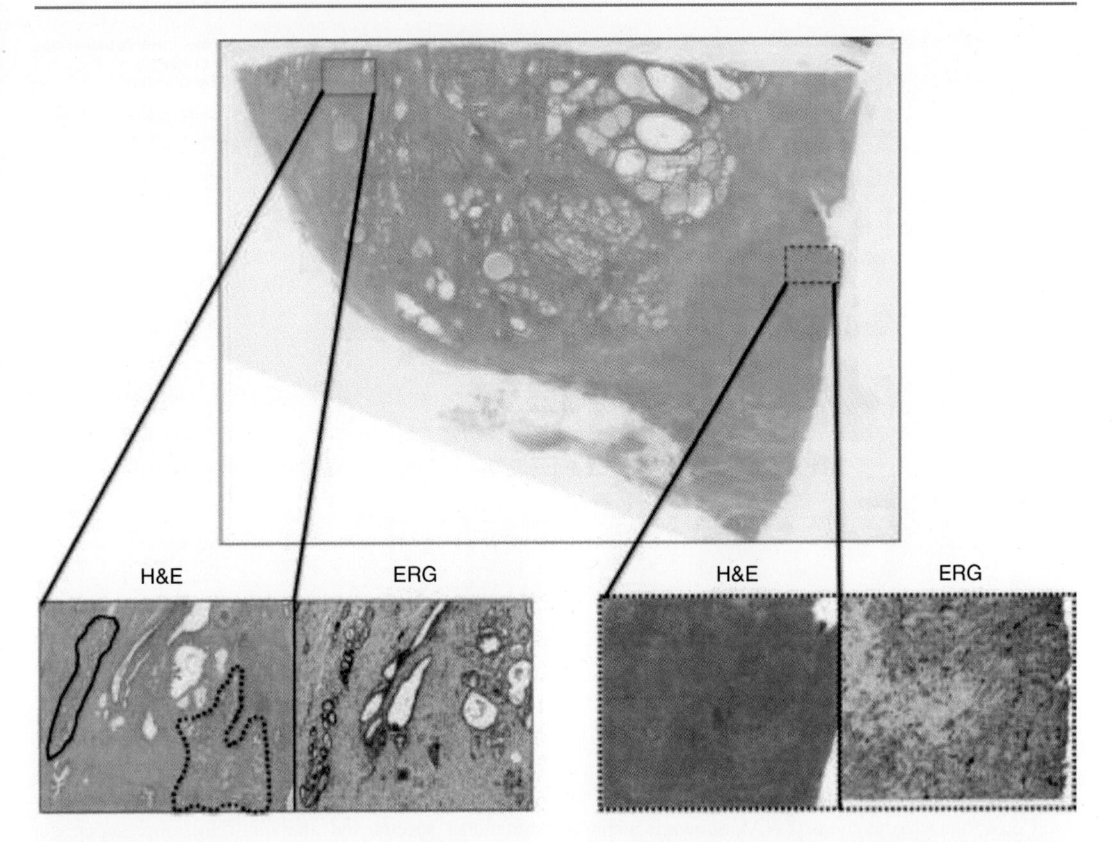

Fig. 4 Intraglandular heterogeneity of ERG fusions. Overexpression of ERG (as a consequence of androgen-driven ERG fusions) can be detected by immunohistochemical staining, and ERG fusions are believed to be early events in prostate tumorigenesis. However, ERG fusion status displays spatial heterogeneity. A single disease focus (see blowout of H&E and ERG IHC; *left panels*) may display heterogeneous ERG staining, which may (or may not) be related to the status of a distinct tumor focus within the same prostate. *H&E* hematoxylin and eosin, *IHC* immunohistochemistry (Reproduced from Fraser et al. *Urol Oncol.* 2015 Feb;33(2):85–94)

identical stage of disease. This has recently been underscored in other cancer types (e.g., renal cancer), in which single-needle biopsies did not adequately account for the uneven distribution of alterations throughout the genetically heterogeneous tumor [24]. Finally, a contribution to heterogeneity and genomic instability by tumor-adjacent prostate stroma [25] is unclear.

3 Localized vs. Metastatic Castration-Resistant Prostate Cancer (mCRPC)

Despite the use of the clinical prognostic factors of Gleason score, pretreatment PSA, and TNM staging, a substantial fraction of men with localized prostate cancer will fail primary curative treatment. This leads to the development of local and/or distant metastases and necessitates systemic treatment with androgen deprivation therapies (ADT; such as LHRH agonists or anti-androgens). While patients generally respond to ADT, this response is temporary, and incurable androgen-independent disease eventually develops. Whole genome and whole exome sequencing studies have characterized the common molecular aberrations associated with prostate cancer. These studies have confirmed that the development of castration resistance following androgen deprivation therapy (ADT) for recurrent or primary metastatic disease is associated with clonal selection and adaption; this alters the molecular landscape of these tumors. As such,

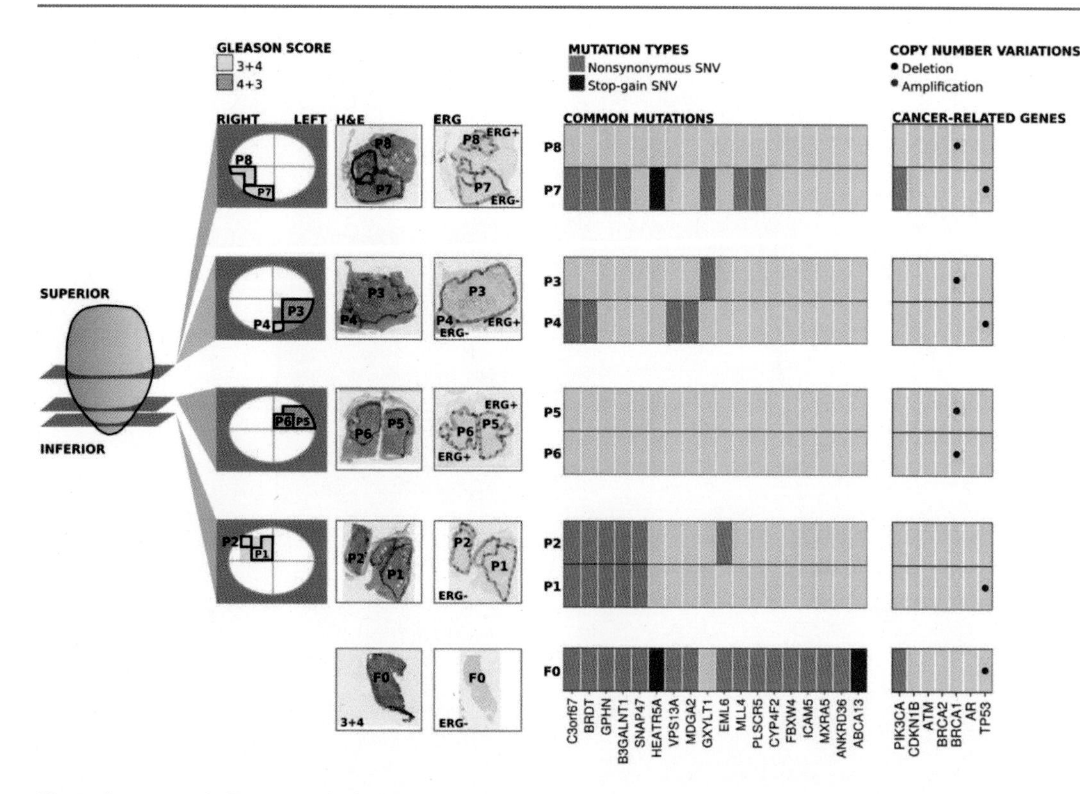

Fig. 5 Intraprostatic Heterogeneity in Mutations (SNVs) and Copy Number Alterations (CNA). Shown is a single prostate from which foci of Gleason score 7 and varying ERG status were analyzed for SNVs and CNAs. For each unique focus (based on prostatic locale and ERG status), mutational spectra and alterations in tumor suppressor genes can vary greatly (Reproduced from Boutros et al. *Nat Genet.* 2015 Jul;47(7):736–45)

metastatic, castration-resistant prostate cancer (mCRPC) represents a unique molecular and genetic disease relative to primary, hormone-naive CaP (see Figs. 1 and 2).

A major defining molecular characteristic of most localized CaP is the relative paucity of single nucleotide variants (SNVs). Observed genome-wide somatic SNV (mutation) rates vary from 0.5 to 1.0/Mb within localized, low-/intermediate risk disease CaP [1–3]. In contrast, mCRPC shows a substantially elevated median exomic SNV rate, relative to localized CaP (4.4/Mb) [26], with some tumors showing nearly 50 SNVs/Mb. This likely results from clonal selection and adaption during ADT, as well as from mutation of genes such as *MLH1* and *MSH2*, resulting in defective mismatch repair and the acquisition of a mutator phenotype. Other mutations in DNA repair are also acquired during mCRPC including the BRCA1, BRCA2, and ATM genes. This can in turn confer a "Brca-ness" in 20–30 % of mCRPC tumors which are deficient in the homologous recombination (HR) pathway: a pathway normally involved in the DNA strand break repair [26]. However, mCRPC tumors with these unique repair defects may be particularly sensitive to drugs such as PARP inhibitors, which preferentially kill HR-defective cells through synthetic lethality [27].

Similarly, localized CaP is associated with very few recurrent driver SNVs in coding regions of the genome. In a meta-analysis of 458 localized Gleason score 6 and 7 CaP, the most frequently mutated gene was *SPOP*, with an overall SNV rate of ~8.3 %. Other recurrent SNVs include *TP53*, *FOXA1*, *MED12*, *MUC16*, and *ATM*. In a broader (but overlapping) clinical cohort of 333 patients with localized disease, additional significantly mutated genes included *CDKN1B*, *BRAF*, *HRAS*, *AKT1*, *CTNNB1*, and

ZMYM3 [1]. While the overall recurrence of these SNVs was statistically significant, only one gene (*SPOP*) was mutated in >10 % of cases. This contrasts markedly with mCRPC, in which recurrent driver SNVs, while still rare relative to many solid tumor types, are far more prevalent than in localized disease. Several established driver genes, in addition to those identified in localized disease, harbor SNVs at >10 % frequency (e.g., *TP53* – 38 %, *AR* – 18 %, *FOXA1* – 11 %) [26].

Similarly, there are striking differences in gene rearrangements and fusions between localized CaP and mCRPC, the most notable of which is the occurrence of amplification of the androgen receptor (*AR*) gene. In localized CaP, *AR* amplification is rare with less than 1 % of patients showing AR amplification or mutation [1]. In contrast, *AR* is amplified in >50 % of mCRPC [26], underlying the androgen-independent growth of these tumors. Similarly, *PTEN* and *RB1* gene deletions are enriched in mCRPC at greater than 25 % when compared to localized disease.

In contrast, many driver CNA and gene rearrangements, such as *MYC* amplification, *NKX3-1* deletions, and *ETS* family gene fusions such as *TMPRSS2*: *ERG* are frequently observed in both localized CaP and mCRPC. This suggests that these events are early truncal events, occurring primarily during prostate tumorigenesis rather than during ADT-driven selection.

This hypothesis is supported by recent work by Gundem and colleagues, who systematically assessed the relative genomics of 51 tumor foci from 10 mCRPC, including the primary tumor and multiple metastases per patient. This work provides important insights into the evolution of metastatic prostate cancer, and demonstrates that metastases can be either monoclonal or polyclonal (i.e., "metastases of metastases"). Importantly, Gundem and colleagues showed that *TMPRSS2*: *ERG* fusions are present in the primary tumor of 6/6 fusion-positive mCRPC patients [23], consistent with previous work showing that TMPRSS2: ERG fusion is an early event in tumorigenesis. Similarly, *MYC* amplification occurred in the primary tumor in all 3 patients harboring this CNA. In contrast, *AR* amplification was observed in 8/10 mCRPC patients, with 7/8 of these events observed in one or more metastatic foci but not in the primary tumor.

4 Tumor and Blood Genetic Biomarkers and Predicting Patient Outcome

There is a need to develop biomarkers of clinical outcome based on intrinsic PCa tumor biology in order to inform precision medicine-based treatments. Several groups have identified RNA-based prognostic signatures for various cohorts of men with CaP (see Table 1). Klein and colleagues identified a 17 gene RNA expression signature from prostate biopsies that was prognostic of high grade disease in prostatectomy specimens [28], which was also prognostic of biochemical (PSA) recurrence (BCR) across National Comprehensive Cancer Network (NCCN)/D'Amico risk groups. Similarly, Cuzick and colleagues defined a 31 gene RNA expression signature of cell cycle-related genes (CCP) that was prognostic of BCR following radical prostatectomy and of prostate cancer-specific mortality (PCSM) in a separate validation cohort of conservatively managed localized CaP [29, 30]. This signature was subsequently validated in patients who underwent external beam radiotherapy (EBRT), in which the CCP score was prognostic for BCR and for PCSM at 10 years posttreatment [31]. Other RNA signatures have been shown to be prognostic for BCR, metastatic failure, PCSM, and/or overall survival [32–36].

On the contrary, very few DNA-based prognostic signatures have been identified in CaP. Taylor and colleagues identified six DNA CNA-based disease clusters in localized CaP, which were prognostic for BCR in a cohort of 168 men treated with radical prostatectomy [19]. The same group subsequently showed that CNA burden (i.e., percentage genome alteration; PGA) was prognostic for both biochemical and metastatic failure after radical prostatectomy in both the initial 168 men as well as a separate 104-patient cohort [37]. This was independent of

Table 1 Genomic prognostic biomarkers based on RNA expression or alterations in DNA (copy number alterations)

Signature	Details	Signature development cohort	Outcomes predicted	Validation in separate cohorts (yes/no)	Evaluated in other treatment modality cohorts
GenomeDx	A 22-gene RNA expression signature	Postsurgery recurrence	M, PCSS, and OS	Yes (2 cohorts)	No
Cell cycle progression (CCP)	A 31 -gene RNA expression signature	Postsurgery recurrence Post-TURP recurrence	BCR and PCSS	Yes (3 cohorts)	Yes (conservatively managed and radiotherapy)
Taylor et al.	A 6 CNV-based clusters	Postsurgery recurrence	BCR	No	No
Ding et al.	A 4-gene signature	Postsurgery recurrence	BCR and LM	Yes (1 cohort)	No
Massachusetts General Hospital	A 32-gene RNA expression signature	Postsurgery recurrence	BCR and M	Yes (1 cohort)	No

Reproduced from Fraser et al. *Urol Oncol.* 2015 Feb;33(2):85–94
TURP transurethral resection of the prostate, *BCR* biochemical recurrence, *M* metastases, *LM* lethal metastases, *PCSS* prostate cancer-specific survival, *OS* overall survival

the clinical prognostic variables of Gleason score, TNM stage, and serum PSA. Importantly, PGA was also prognostic of BCR in patients with Gleason 7 disease, a cohort of patients with highly heterogeneous clinical outcomes in which improved risk stratification is urgently required.

A similar CNA-based approach yielded unique clusters prognostic for BCR in men following either radical prostatectomy or EBRT for low/intermediate risk CaP [14], and validated PGA as a prognostic factor in three independent cohorts (EBRT and radical prostatectomy cohorts). Using a random forest model trained on our EBRT patient cohort, we identified a 100-locus genomic signature that was strongly prognostic of 5-year biochemical and metastatic failure across NCCN risk groups. Furthermore, this signature was prognostic of early biochemical failure (i.e., <18 months posttreatment), which is a surrogate for PCSM [38]. Furthermore, the prognostic utility of the signature was increased when another prognostic factor, that of intraglandular tumor hypoxia, was integrated into the analysis. Patients with both genetic instability and intratumoral hypoxia had only a 50 % chance of up-front biochemical control following surgery or radiotherapy (see Fig. 5). Other studies have suggested that certain DNA repair gene alterations, such as gains in the nibrin (NBN) gene, may be selectively predictive for radiotherapy outcome (versus no effect in surgical patients) and if validated could help decision making for the use of one local therapy versus another [9]. Newer signatures will no doubt be multimodal. They will use multiple DNA, RNA, and methylation indices to improve the precision of individual prognostication and treatment (Fig. 6).

Other genetic bioassays interrogate circulating tumor cells (CTCs), exosomes, or circulating tumor DNA (ctDNA). Pretreatment detection of androgen receptor splice variant-7 (AR-V7) in CTCs or ctDNA from men with mCRPC is a biomarker that may be associated with resistance to abiraterone and enzalutamide, but not to docetaxol [39, 40]. Other ctDNA changes that may be predictive of enzalutamide resistance include loss of the RB and DNA repair function or mutations in the PI3K pathway [41]. Finally, targeted proteomics with computational biology can be used to derive signatures that predict extraprostatic extension from expressed prostatic secretions in urine [42]. It may be that adding computationally guided proteomics to blood-borne genomic tests will discover highly accurate and relatively noninvasive biomarkers.

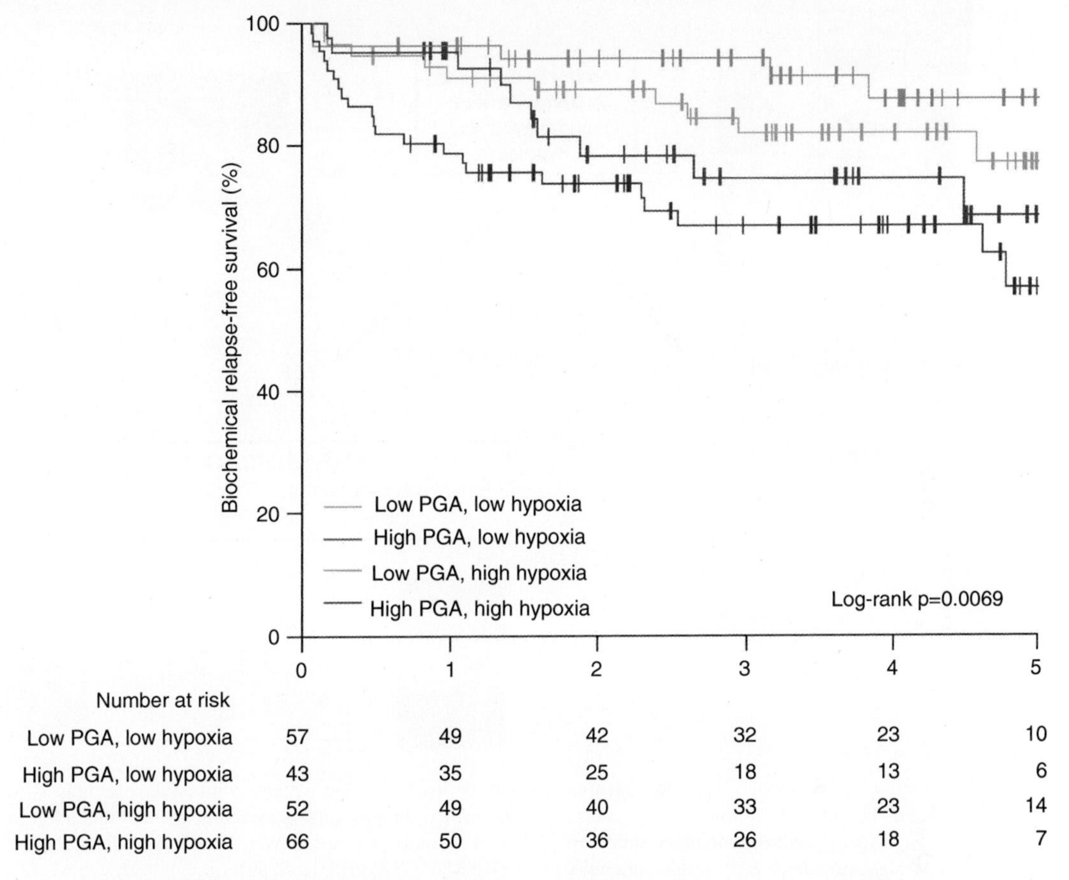

Fig. 6 Kaplan-Meier Plots for Biochemical Relapse in Localized Prostate Cancer Based on Percent Genomic Instability (PGA) and/or Intratumoral Hypoxia. Patients with both increased genetic instability (e.g., high PGA) and high levels of tumor hypoxia (based on an RNA signature of hypoxia-related genes) fare the worse after radical prostatectomy with close to 50 % of men relapsing at 5 years (Reproduced from Lalonde et al. *Lancet Oncol.* 2014 Dec;15(13):1521–32)

5 Key Outstanding Issues

Although the clinical prognostic factors of T category, serum PSA, and GS can accurately stratify populations of men with CaP into broad groups with respect to risk of disease progression, it is clear that a more robust understanding of genomics and tumor heterogeneity is required to accurately assess the development of aggressive localized disease and mCRPC. Such approaches are required to facilitate personalized medicine for CaP. For example, although the use of active surveillance protocols has drastically reduced the number of low-risk patients who are treated unnecessarily, up to one-third of these men will ultimately transit into higher-risk disease. Genomic biomarkers are being developed to increase precision for the triaging of patients to active surveillance.

Similarly, 30–40 % of men who present with potentially curable intermediate-risk disease will recur, despite radical local therapy. In both of these scenarios, it is currently not possible to accurately determine which men have more aggressive disease than suggested by the current clinical parameters. Likewise, the finding of mutations that lead to potential use of targeted therapeutic agents depends not only on the presence of "actionable" mutations but also on whether these mutations are present in the disease focus that is destined to metastasize in order that such treatments affect outcome. As such, genomic

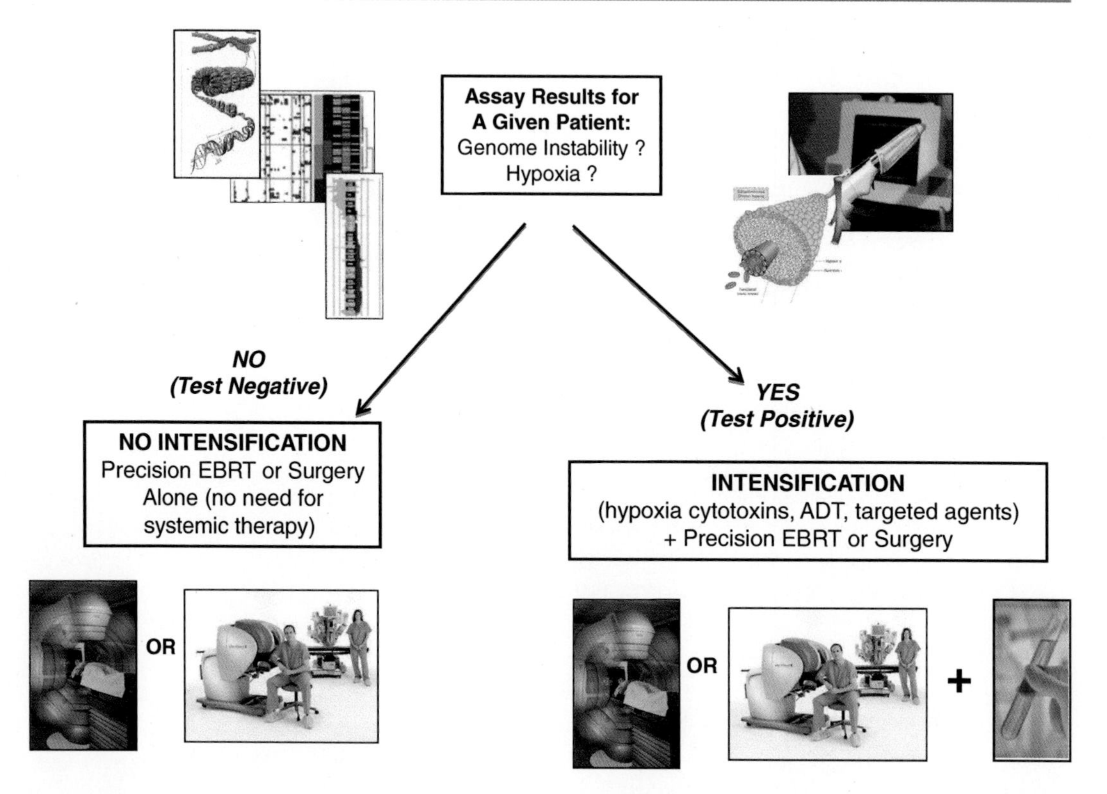

Fig. 7 The Utility of Genomic Tests for Treatment Intensification of De-intensification. Initial assays of genetic instability when combined with other indices (e.g. tumor hypoxia status, mutations, copy number alterations) can be used to triage patients with adverse prognosis to intensified therapies using systemic agents in addition to local therapies (Adapted from Berlin et al. *Br J Radiol.* 2014 Mar;87(1035):20130753)

signatures have the potential to pull patients out of otherwise clinically-homogeneous cohorts and offer intensification or de-intensification strategies (see Fig. 7).

The recent development of whole-genome sequencing technologies using submicrogram quantities of DNA has opened up new avenues of research. Genomic assessments are now able to sample the in situ heterogeneity within diagnostic biopsies or within multiple foci at final pathology following prostatectomy. It remains to be proven whether blood-based (DNA, RNA, or protein) assays can be used as a less invasive test to conclusively capture information on the most aggressive clones within the prostate to drive treatment. This could also help with the problem whereby sampling of the prostate gland at initial biopsy leads to inaccurate inappropriate clinical staging, as evidenced by the relatively high frequency of pathological "upstaging" in radical prostatectomy specimens. Such tests will be judged by their relative clinical utility and cost against current prognostic factors.

References

1. Cancer Genome Atlas Research N. The molecular taxonomy of primary prostate cancer. Cell. 2015; 163(4):1011–25. doi:10.1016/j.cell.2015.10.025.
2. Barbieri CE, Baca SC, Lawrence MS, Demichelis F, Blattner M, Theurillat JP, White TA, Stojanov P, Van Allen E, Stransky N, Nickerson E, Chae SS, Boysen G, Auclair D, Onofrio RC, Park K, Kitabayashi N, MacDonald TY, Sheikh K, Vuong T, Guiducci C, Cibulskis K, Sivachenko A, Carter SL, Saksena G, Voet D, Hussain WM, Ramos AH, Winckler W, Redman MC, Ardlie K, Tewari AK, Mosquera JM, Rupp N, Wild PJ, Moch H, Morrissey C, Nelson PS, Kantoff PW, Gabriel SB, Golub TR, Meyerson M, Lander ES, Getz G, Rubin MA, Garraway LA. Exome sequencing identifies recurrent SPOP, FOXA1 and

MED12 mutations in prostate cancer. Nat Genet. 2012;44(6):685–9. doi:10.1038/ng.2279.
3. Baca SC, Prandi D, Lawrence MS, Mosquera JM, Romanel A, Drier Y, Park K, Kitabayashi N, MacDonald TY, Ghandi M, Van Allen E, Kryukov GV, Sboner A, Theurillat JP, Soong TD, Nickerson E, Auclair D, Tewari A, Beltran H, Onofrio RC, Boysen G, Guiducci C, Barbieri CE, Cibulskis K, Sivachenko A, Carter SL, Saksena G, Voet D, Ramos AH, Winckler W, Cipicchio M, Ardlie K, Kantoff PW, Berger MF, Gabriel SB, Golub TR, Meyerson M, Lander ES, Elemento O, Getz G, Demichelis F, Rubin MA, Garraway LA. Punctuated evolution of prostate cancer genomes. Cell. 2013;153(3):666–77. doi:10.1016/j.cell.2013.03.021.
4. Weischenfeldt J, Simon R, Feuerbach L, Schlangen K, Weichenhan D, Minner S, Wuttig D, Warnatz HJ, Stehr H, Rausch T, Jager N, Gu L, Bogatyrova O, Stutz AM, Claus R, Eils J, Eils R, Gerhauser C, Huang PH, Hutter B, Kabbe R, Lawerenz C, Radomski S, Bartholomae CC, Falth M, Gade S, Schmidt M, Amschler N, Hass T, Galal R, Gjoni J, Kuner R, Baer C, Masser S, von Kalle C, Zichner T, Benes V, Raeder B, Mader M, Amstislavskiy V, Avci M, Lehrach H, Parkhomchuk D, Sultan M, Burkhardt L, Graefen M, Huland H, Kluth M, Krohn A, Sirma H, Stumm L, Steurer S, Grupp K, Sultmann H, Sauter G, Plass C, Brors B, Yaspo ML, Korbel JO, Schlomm T. Integrative genomic analyses reveal an androgen-driven somatic alteration landscape in early-onset prostate cancer. Cancer Cell. 2013;23(2):159–70. doi:10.1016/j.ccr.2013.01.002.
5. Theurillat JP, Udeshi ND, Errington WJ, Svinkina T, Baca SC, Pop M, Wild PJ, Blattner M, Groner AC, Rubin MA, Moch H, Prive GG, Carr SA, Garraway LA. Prostate cancer. Ubiquitylome analysis identifies dysregulation of effector substrates in SPOP-mutant prostate cancer. Science. 2014;346(6205):85–9. doi:10.1126/science.1250255.
6. Boysen G, Barbieri CE, Prandi D, Blattner M, Chae SS, Dahija A, Nataraj S, Huang D, Marotz C, Xu L, Huang J, Lecca P, Chhangawala S, Liu D, Zhou P, Sboner A, de Bono JS, Demichelis F, Houvras Y, Rubin MA. SPOP mutation leads to genomic instability in prostate cancer. Elife. 2015; 4. doi:10.7554/eLife.09207.
7. Tomlins SA, Rhodes DR, Perner S, Dhanasekaran SM, Mehra R, Sun XW, Varambally S, Cao X, Tchinda J, Kuefer R, Lee C, Montie JE, Shah RB, Pienta KJ, Rubin MA, Chinnaiyan AM. Recurrent fusion of TMPRSS2 and ETS transcription factor genes in prostate cancer. Science. 2005;310(5748):644–8. doi:10.1126/science.1117679.
8. Sowalsky AG, Ye H, Bubley GJ, Balk SP. Clonal progression of prostate cancers from Gleason grade 3 to grade 4. Cancer Res. 2013;73(3):1050–5. doi:10.1158/0008-5472.CAN-12-2799.
9. Berlin A, Lalonde E, Sykes J, Zafarana G, Chu KC, Ramnarine VR, Ishkanian A, Sendorek DH, Pasic I, Lam WL, Jurisica I, van der Kwast T, Milosevic M, Boutros PC, Bristow RG. NBN gain is predictive for adverse outcome following image-guided radiotherapy for localized prostate cancer. Oncotarget. 2014;5(22):11081–90. doi:10.18632/oncotarget.2404.
10. Zafarana G, Ishkanian AS, Malloff CA, Locke JA, Sykes J, Thoms J, Lam WL, Squire JA, Yoshimoto M, Ramnarine VR, Meng A, Ahmed O, Jurisica I, Milosevic M, Pintilie M, van der Kwast T, Bristow RG. Copy number alterations of c-MYC and PTEN are prognostic factors for relapse after prostate cancer radiotherapy. Cancer. 2012;118(16):4053–62. doi:10.1002/cncr.26729.
11. Locke JA, Zafarana G, Malloff CA, Lam WL, Sykes J, Pintilie M, Ramnarine VR, Meng A, Ahmed O, Jurisica I, Guns ET, van der Kwast T, Milosevic M, Bristow RG. Allelic loss of the loci containing the androgen synthesis gene, StAR, is prognostic for relapse in intermediate-risk prostate cancer. Prostate. 2012;72(12):1295–305. doi:10.1002/pros.22478.
12. Locke JA, Zafarana G, Ishkanian AS, Milosevic M, Thoms J, Have CL, Malloff CA, Lam WL, Squire JA, Pintilie M, Sykes J, Ramnarine VR, Meng A, Ahmed O, Jurisica I, van der Kwast T, Bristow RG. NKX3.1 haploinsufficiency is prognostic for prostate cancer relapse following surgery or image-guided radiotherapy. Clin Cancer Res. 2012;18(1):308–16. doi:10.1158/1078-0432.CCR-11-2147.
13. Ishkanian AS, Zafarana G, Thoms J, Bristow RG. Array CGH as a potential predictor of radiocurability in intermediate risk prostate cancer. Acta Oncol. 2010;49(7):888–94. doi:10.3109/0284186X.2010.499371.
14. Lalonde E, Ishkanian AS, Sykes J, Fraser M, Ross-Adams H, Erho N, Dunning MJ, Halim S, Lamb AD, Moon NC, Zafarana G, Warren AY, Meng X, Thoms J, Grzadkowski MR, Berlin A, Have CL, Ramnarine VR, Yao CQ, Malloff CA, Lam LL, Xie H, Harding NJ, Mak DY, Chu KC, Chong LC, Sendorek DH, P'ng C, Collins CC, Squire JA, Jurisica I, Cooper C, Eeles R, Pintilie M, Dal Pra A, Davicioni E, Lam WL, Milosevic M, Neal DE, van der Kwast T, Boutros PC, Bristow RG. Tumour genomic and microenvironmental heterogeneity for integrated prediction of 5-year biochemical recurrence of prostate cancer: a retrospective cohort study. Lancet Oncol. 2014;15(13):1521–32. doi:10.1016/S1470-2045(14)71021-6.
15. Nik-Zainal S, Alexandrov LB, Wedge DC, Van Loo P, Greenman CD, Raine K, Jones D, Hinton J, Marshall J, Stebbings LA, Menzies A, Martin S, Leung K, Chen L, Leroy C, Ramakrishna M, Rance R, Lau KW, Mudie LJ, Varela I, McBride DJ, Bignell GR, Cooke SL, Shlien A, Gamble J, Whitmore I, Maddison M, Tarpey PS, Davies HR, Papaemmanuil E, Stephens PJ, McLaren S, Butler AP, Teague JW, Jonsson G, Garber JE, Silver D, Miron P, Fatima A, Boyault S, Langerod A, Tutt A, Martens JW, Aparicio SA, Borg A, Salomon AV, Thomas G, Borresen-Dale AL, Richardson AL, Neuberger MS, Futreal PA, Campbell PJ, Stratton MR,

Breast Cancer Working Group of the International Cancer Genome Consortium. Mutational processes molding the genomes of 21 breast cancers. Cell. 2012;149(5):979–93. doi:10.1016/j.cell.2012.04.024.
16. Stephens PJ, Greenman CD, Fu B, Yang F, Bignell GR, Mudie LJ, Pleasance ED, Lau KW, Beare D, Stebbings LA, McLaren S, Lin ML, McBride DJ, Varela I, Nik-Zainal S, Leroy C, Jia M, Menzies A, Butler AP, Teague JW, Quail MA, Burton J, Swerdlow H, Carter NP, Morsberger LA, Iacobuzio-Donahue C, Follows GA, Green AR, Flanagan AM, Stratton MR, Futreal PA, Campbell PJ. Massive genomic rearrangement acquired in a single catastrophic event during cancer development. Cell. 2011;144(1):27–40. doi:10.1016/j.cell.2010.11.055.
17. Cooper CS, Eeles R, Wedge DC, Van Loo P, Gundem G, Alexandrov LB, Kremeyer B, Butler A, Lynch AG, Camacho N, Massie CE, Kay J, Luxton HJ, Edwards S, Kote-Jarai Z, Dennis N, Merson S, Leongamornlert D, Zamora J, Corbishley C, Thomas S, Nik-Zainal S, Ramakrishna M, O'Meara S, Matthews L, Clark J, Hurst R, Mithen R, Bristow RG, Boutros PC, Fraser M, Cooke S, Raine K, Jones D, Menzies A, Stebbings L, Hinton J, Teague J, McLaren S, Mudie L, Hardy C, Anderson E, Joseph O, Goody V, Robinson B, Maddison M, Gamble S, Greenman C, Berney D, Hazell S, Livni N, Group IP, Fisher C, Ogden C, Kumar P, Thompson A, Woodhouse C, Nicol D, Mayer E, Dudderidge T, Shah NC, Gnanapragasam V, Voet T, Campbell P, Futreal A, Easton D, Warren AY, Foster CS, Stratton MR, Whitaker HC, McDermott U, Brewer DS, Neal DE. Analysis of the genetic phylogeny of multifocal prostate cancer identifies multiple independent clonal expansions in neoplastic and morphologically normal prostate tissue. Nat Genet. 2015;47(4):367–72. doi:10.1038/ng.3221.
18. Boutros PC, Fraser M, Harding NJ, de Borja R, Trudel D, Lalonde E, Meng A, Hennings-Yeomans PH, McPherson A, Sabelnykova VY, Zia A, Fox NS, Livingstone J, Shiah YJ, Wang J, Beck TA, Have CL, Chong T, Sam M, Johns J, Timms L, Buchner N, Wong A, Watson JD, Simmons TT, P'ng C, Zafarana G, Nguyen F, Luo X, Chu KC, Prokopec SD, Sykes J, Dal Pra A, Berlin A, Brown A, Chan-Seng-Yue MA, Yousif F, Denroche RE, Chong LC, Chen GM, Jung E, Fung C, Starmans MH, Chen H, Govind SK, Hawley J, D'Costa A, Pintilie M, Waggott D, Hach F, Lambin P, Muthuswamy LB, Cooper C, Eeles R, Neal D, Tetu B, Sahinalp C, Stein LD, Fleshner N, Shah SP, Collins CC, Hudson TJ, McPherson JD, van der Kwast T, Bristow RG. Spatial genomic heterogeneity within localized, multifocal prostate cancer. Nat Genet. 2015;47(7):736–45. doi:10.1038/ng.3315.
19. Taylor BS, Schultz N, Hieronymus H, Gopalan A, Xiao Y, Carver BS, Arora VK, Kaushik P, Cerami E, Reva B, Antipin Y, Mitsiades N, Landers T, Dolgalev I, Major JE, Wilson M, Socci ND, Lash AE, Heguy A, Eastham JA, Scher HI, Reuter VE, Scardino PT, Sander C, Sawyers CL, Gerald WL. Integrative genomic profiling of human prostate cancer. Cancer Cell. 2010;18(1):11–22. doi:10.1016/j.ccr.2010.05.026.
20. Liu W, Laitinen S, Khan S, Vihinen M, Kowalski J, Yu G, Chen L, Ewing CM, Eisenberger MA, Carducci MA, Nelson WG, Yegnasubramanian S, Luo J, Wang Y, Xu J, Isaacs WB, Visakorpi T, Bova GS. Copy number analysis indicates monoclonal origin of lethal metastatic prostate cancer. Nat Med. 2009;15(5):559–65. doi:10.1038/nm.1944.
21. Mehra R, Tomlins SA, Yu J, Cao X, Wang L, Menon A, Rubin MA, Pienta KJ, Shah RB, Chinnaiyan AM. Characterization of TMPRSS2-ETS gene aberrations in androgen-independent metastatic prostate cancer. Cancer Res. 2008;68(10):3584–90. doi:10.1158/0008-5472.CAN-07-6154.
22. Aryee MJ, Liu W, Engelmann JC, Nuhn P, Gurel M, Haffner MC, Esopi D, Irizarry RA, Getzenberg RH, Nelson WG, Luo J, Xu J, Isaacs WB, Bova GS, Yegnasubramanian S. DNA methylation alterations exhibit intraindividual stability and interindividual heterogeneity in prostate cancer metastases. Sci Transl Med. 2013;5(169):169ra110. doi:10.1126/scitranslmed.3005211.
23. Gundem G, Van Loo P, Kremeyer B, Alexandrov LB, Tubio JM, Papaemmanuil E, Brewer DS, Kallio HM, Hognas G, Annala M, Kivinummi K, Goody V, Latimer C, O'Meara S, Dawson KJ, Isaacs W, Emmert-Buck MR, Nykter M, Foster C, Kote-Jarai Z, Easton D, Whitaker HC, Neal DE, Cooper CS, Eeles RA, Visakorpi T, Campbell PJ, McDermott U, Wedge DC, Bova GS, ICGC Prostate UK Group. The evolutionary history of lethal metastatic prostate cancer. Nature. 2015;520(7547):353–7. doi:10.1038/nature14347.
24. Gerlinger M, Rowan AJ, Horswell S, Larkin J, Endesfelder D, Gronroos E, Martinez P, Matthews N, Stewart A, Tarpey P, Varela I, Phillimore B, Begum S, McDonald NQ, Butler A, Jones D, Raine K, Latimer C, Santos CR, Nohadani M, Eklund AC, Spencer-Dene B, Clark G, Pickering L, Stamp G, Gore M, Szallasi Z, Downward J, Futreal PA, Swanton C. Intratumor heterogeneity and branched evolution revealed by multiregion sequencing. N Engl J Med. 2012;366(10):883–92. doi:10.1056/NEJMoa1113205.
25. Joshua AM, Vukovic B, Braude I, Hussein S, Zielenska M, Srigley J, Evans A, Squire JA. Telomere attrition in isolated high-grade prostatic intraepithelial neoplasia and surrounding stroma is predictive of prostate cancer. Neoplasia. 2007;9(1):81–9.
26. Robinson D, Van Allen EM, Wu YM, Schultz N, Lonigro RJ, Mosquera JM, Montgomery B, Taplin ME, Pritchard CC, Attard G, Beltran H, Abida W, Bradley RK, Vinson J, Cao X, Vats P, Kunju LP, Hussain M, Feng FY, Tomlins SA, Cooney KA, Smith DC, Brennan C, Siddiqui J, Mehra R, Chen Y, Rathkopf DE, Morris MJ, Solomon SB, Durack JC, Reuter VE, Gopalan A, Gao J, Loda M, Lis RT, Bowden M, Balk SP, Gaviola G, Sougnez C, Gupta

M, Yu EY, Mostaghel EA, Cheng HH, Mulcahy H, True LD, Plymate SR, Dvinge H, Ferraldeschi R, Flohr P, Miranda S, Zafeiriou Z, Tunariu N, Mateo J, Perez-Lopez R, Demichelis F, Robinson BD, Schiffman M, Nanus DM, Tagawa ST, Sigaras A, Eng KW, Elemento O, Sboner A, Heath EI, Scher HI, Pienta KJ, Kantoff P, de Bono JS, Rubin MA, Nelson PS, Garraway LA, Sawyers CL, Chinnaiyan AM. Integrative clinical genomics of advanced prostate cancer. Cell. 2015;161(5):1215–28. doi:10.1016/j.cell.2015.05.001.
27. Mateo J, Carreira S, Sandhu S, Miranda S, Mossop H, Perez-Lopez R, Nava Rodrigues D, Robinson D, Omlin A, Tunariu N, Boysen G, Porta N, Flohr P, Gillman A, Figueiredo I, Paulding C, Seed G, Jain S, Ralph C, Protheroe A, Hussain S, Jones R, Elliott T, McGovern U, Bianchini D, Goodall J, Zafeiriou Z, Williamson CT, Ferraldeschi R, Riisnaes R, Ebbs B, Fowler G, Roda D, Yuan W, Wu YM, Cao X, Brough R, Pemberton H, A'Hern R, Swain A, Kunju LP, Eeles R, Attard G, Lord CJ, Ashworth A, Rubin MA, Knudsen KE, Feng FY, Chinnaiyan AM, Hall E, de Bono JS. DNA-Repair Defects and Olaparib in Metastatic Prostate Cancer. N Engl J Med. 2015;373(18):1697–708. doi:10.1056/NEJMoa1506859.
28. Klein EA, Cooperberg MR, Magi-Galluzzi C, Simko JP, Falzarano SM, Maddala T, Chan JM, Li J, Cowan JE, Tsiatis AC, Cherbavaz DB, Pelham RJ, Tenggara-Hunter I, Baehner FL, Knezevic D, Febbo PG, Shak S, Kattan MW, Lee M, Carroll PR. A 17-gene assay to predict prostate cancer aggressiveness in the context of Gleason grade heterogeneity, tumor multifocality, and biopsy undersampling. Eur Urol. 2014;66(3):550–60. doi:10.1016/j.eururo.2014.05.004.
29. Cuzick J, Swanson GP, Fisher G, Brothman AR, Berney DM, Reid JE, Mesher D, Speights VO, Stankiewicz E, Foster CS, Moller H, Scardino P, Warren JD, Park J, Younus A, Flake 2nd DD, Wagner S, Gutin A, Lanchbury JS, Stone S, Transatlantic Prostate G. Prognostic value of an RNA expression signature derived from cell cycle proliferation genes in patients with prostate cancer: a retrospective study. Lancet Oncol. 2011;12(3):245–55. doi:10.1016/S1470-2045(10)70295-3.
30. Cuzick J, Berney DM, Fisher G, Mesher D, Moller H, Reid JE, Perry M, Park J, Younus A, Gutin A, Foster CS, Scardino P, Lanchbury JS, Stone S, Transatlantic Prostate G. Prognostic value of a cell cycle progression signature for prostate cancer death in a conservatively managed needle biopsy cohort. Br J Cancer. 2012;106(6):1095–9. doi:10.1038/bjc.2012.39.
31. Freedland SJ, Gerber L, Reid J, Welbourn W, Tikishvili E, Park J, Younus A, Gutin A, Sangale Z, Lanchbury JS, Salama JK, Stone S. Prognostic utility of cell cycle progression score in men with prostate cancer after primary external beam radiation therapy. Int J Radiat Oncol Biol Phys. 2013;86(5):848–53. doi:10.1016/j.ijrobp.2013.04.043.
32. Erho N, Crisan A, Vergara IA, Mitra AP, Ghadessi M, Buerki C, Bergstralh EJ, Kollmeyer T, Fink S, Haddad Z, Zimmermann B, Sierocinski T, Ballman KV, Triche TJ, Black PC, Karnes RJ, Klee G, Davicioni E, Jenkins RB. Discovery and validation of a prostate cancer genomic classifier that predicts early metastasis following radical prostatectomy. PLoS One. 2013;8(6), e66855. doi:10.1371/journal.pone.0066855.
33. Cooperberg MR, Simko JP, Cowan JE, Reid JE, Djalilvand A, Bhatnagar S, Gutin A, Lanchbury JS, Swanson GP, Stone S, Carroll PR. Validation of a cell-cycle progression gene panel to improve risk stratification in a contemporary prostatectomy cohort. J Clin Oncol Off J Am Soc Clin Oncol. 2013;31(11):1428–34. doi:10.1200/JCO.2012.46.4396.
34. Karnes RJ, Bergstralh EJ, Davicioni E, Ghadessi M, Buerki C, Mitra AP, Crisan A, Erho N, Vergara IA, Lam LL, Carlson R, Thompson DJ, Haddad Z, Zimmermann B, Sierocinski T, Triche TJ, Kollmeyer T, Ballman KV, Black PC, Klee GG, Jenkins RB. Validation of a genomic classifier that predicts metastasis following radical prostatectomy in an at risk patient population. J Urol. 2013;190(6):2047–53. doi:10.1016/j.juro.2013.06.017.
35. Wu CL, Schroeder BE, Ma XJ, Cutie CJ, Wu S, Salunga R, Zhang Y, Kattan MW, Schnabel CA, Erlander MG, McDougal WS. Development and validation of a 32-gene prognostic index for prostate cancer progression. Proc Natl Acad Sci U S A. 2013;110(15):6121–6. doi:10.1073/pnas.1215870110.
36. Ding Z, Wu CJ, Chu GC, Xiao Y, Ho D, Zhang J, Perry SR, Labrot ES, Wu X, Lis R, Hoshida Y, Hiller D, Hu B, Jiang S, Zheng H, Stegh AH, Scott KL, Signoretti S, Bardeesy N, Wang YA, Hill DE, Golub TR, Stampfer MJ, Wong WH, Loda M, Mucci L, Chin L, DePinho RA. SMAD4-dependent barrier constrains prostate cancer growth and metastatic progression. Nature. 2011;470(7333):269–73. doi:10.1038/nature09677.
37. Hieronymus H, Schultz N, Gopalan A, Carver BS, Chang MT, Xiao Y, Heguy A, Huberman K, Bernstein M, Assel M, Murali R, Vickers A, Scardino PT, Sander C, Reuter V, Taylor BS, Sawyers CL. Copy number alteration burden predicts prostate cancer relapse. Proc Natl Acad Sci U S A. 2014;111(30):11139–44. doi:10.1073/pnas.1411446111.
38. Buyyounouski MK, Pickles T, Kestin LL, Allison R, Williams SG. Validating the interval to biochemical failure for the identification of potentially lethal prostate cancer. J Clin Oncol Off J Am Soc Clin Oncol. 2012;30(15):1857–63. doi:10.1200/JCO.2011.35.1924.
39. Nakazawa M, Lu C, Chen Y, Paller CJ, Carducci MA, Eisenberger MA, Luo J, Antonarakis ES. Serial blood-based analysis of AR-V7 in men with advanced prostate cancer. Ann Oncol Off J Europ Soc Med Oncol/ESMO. 2015;26(9):1859–65. doi:10.1093/annonc/mdv282.
40. Azad AA, Volik SV, Wyatt AW, Haegert A, Le Bihan S, Bell RH, Anderson SA, McConeghy B, Shukin R, Bazov J, Youngren J, Paris P, Thomas G, Small EJ, Wang

Y, Gleave ME, Collins CC, Chi KN. Androgen receptor gene aberrations in circulating cell-free DNA: biomarkers of therapeutic resistance in castration-resistant prostate cancer. Clin Cancer Res. 2015;21(10):2315–24. doi:10.1158/1078-0432.CCR-14-2666.

41. Wyatt AW, Azad AA, Volik SV, Annala M, Beja K, McConeghy B, Haegert A, Warner EW, Mo F, Brahmbhatt S, Shukin R, Le Bihan S, Gleave ME, Nykter M, Collins CC, Chi KN. Genomic alterations in cell-free DNA and enzalutamide resistance in castration-resistant prostate cancer. JAMA oncol. 2016. doi:10.1001/jamaoncol.2016.0494.
42. Kim Y, Jeon J, Mejia S, Yao CQ, Ignatchenko V, Nyalwidhe JO, Gramolini AO, Lance RS, Troyer DA, Drake RR, Boutros PC, Semmes OJ, Kislinger T. Targeted proteomics identifies liquid-biopsy signatures for extracapsular prostate cancer. Nat Commun. 2016;7:11906. doi:10.1038/ncomms11906.

Prostate Cancer Imaging: An Ongoing Change of Paradigm

Olivier Rouvière and Jean Champagnac

For decades, accurate detection of prostate cancer foci within the gland has been considered impossible. As a result, protocols of systematically distributed prostate biopsies have been used to investigate patients with clinical suspicion of prostate cancer, and radiologic investigations have been limited to the evaluation of the extraglandular extension of the cancer. Since the end of the 2000s, a new paradigm is emerging. With the advent of new functional pulse sequences, magnetic resonance imaging (MRI) has been shown to accurately detect prostate cancer foci within the gland and to provide information on their individual aggressiveness. These new imaging possibilities have coincided with new clinical needs of tumor detection related, for example, to the advent of active surveillance protocols or salvage therapies for local recurrences. The imaging landscape of prostate cancer is thus rapidly changing. If imaging is still used as a staging method, it is increasingly used to detect the cancer foci before biopsy and help evaluate their aggressiveness.

1 Local Staging

Curative treatment is most likely when the tumor is confined within the gland (stage ≤T2c). Accurate assessment of extracapsular extension (ECE, stage pT3a) or seminal vesicle invasion (SVI, stage pT3b) is therefore of utmost importance for patient management. Although digital rectal examination (DRE), the number and sites of positive biopsy, the tumor grade, and the prostate-specific antigen (PSA) level may give information on the tumor stage, there is a need for an imaging method that could directly show the tumor extension beyond the capsule or into the seminal vesicles.

1.1 Transrectal Ultrasound

Despite its good specificity in assessing ECE and SVI, transrectal ultrasound (TRUS) is limited by

O. Rouvière (✉)
Hospices Civils de Lyon, Department of Urinary and Vascular Radiology, Hôpital Edouard Herriot, Lyon F-69437, France

Université de Lyon, Lyon F-69003, France

Inserm, U1032, LabTau, Lyon F-69003, France

service d'imagerie, pavillon B, Hôpital Edouard Herriot, 5 place d'Arsonval, 69437 Lyon, France

Université Lyon 1, faculté de médecine Lyon Est, Lyon F-69003, France
e-mail: olivier.rouviere@netcourrier.com

J. Champagnac
Hospices Civils de Lyon, Department of Urinary and Vascular Radiology, Hôpital Edouard Herriot, Lyon F-69437, France

Université de Lyon, Lyon F-69003, France

Université Lyon 1, faculté de médecine Lyon Est, Lyon F-69003, France

M. Bolla, H. van Poppel (eds.), *Management of Prostate Cancer*,
DOI 10.1007/978-3-319-42769-0_7

its poor sensitivity (4–68 %) and its tendency to understage prostate cancer [1–3]. It may even not be superior to that of DRE [4]. Even if 3D-TRUS, color Doppler, and contrast agents may help in local staging [5, 6], all TRUS techniques are largely operator-dependent and cannot differentiate between T2 and T3 tumors with sufficient accuracy to be recommended for routine staging.

1.2 Magnetic Resonance Imaging

A large number of studies have evaluated MRI accuracy in prostate cancer local staging. Most of them used an endorectal coil and 1.5 T scanners. Although diagnostic criteria varied from one author to another, MRI sensitivity was found to be moderate, for EEC (22–82 %) as for SVI (0–71 %). Its specificity seemed better and fell in the 60–100 % range. A recent meta-analysis pooling the data of 75 studies (9796 patients) reported a sensitivity and a specificity of, respectively, 0.57 (95 % confidence interval (CI): 0.49–0.64) and 0.91 (95 % CI: 0.88–0.93) for ECE (45 studies, 5681 patients), 0.58 (95 % CI: 0.47–0.68) and 0.96 (95 % CI: 0.95–0.97) for SVI (34 studies, 5677 patients), and 0.61 (95 % CI: 0.54–0.67) and 0.88 (95 % CI: 0.85–0.91) for overall stage T3 detection (38 studies, 4001 patients) [7]. Another one focused on studies reporting results obtained at 1.5 T with an endorectal coil and published after 2008. Seven series were included (603 patients). Median sensitivity and specificity were, respectively, 0.49 and 0.82 for ECE, 0.45 and 0.96 for SVI and 0.6 and 0.58 for T3 detection [8].

Several factors influence MRI performances. The most important one is probably the degree of extracapsular invasion. MRI sensitivity is poor for detecting microscopic invasion. It improves as the radial length of extension increases. In one series, the EEC detection rate was 14 % when the radial length of extension was <1 mm and 100 % when it was >3 mm [9]. In another study using the Epstein classification for capsular penetration [10], MR sensitivity, specificity and accuracy for detecting pT3 stages were, respectively, 40 %, 95 %, and 76 % for focal (i.e. microscopic) invasions and 62 %, 95 %, and 88 % for extended invasions [11].

The use of the endorectal coil improves staging accuracy at 1.5 T, as shown by two studies that found accuracies of 77–83 % for combined endorectal and external coils versus 59–68 % for external coils alone [12, 13].

The diagnosis of EEC and SVI is mostly made on T2-weighted images. Dynamic contrast-enhanced imaging used in combination with T2-weighted imaging may improve local staging, at least for less-experienced readers [14, 15]. High-field strength allows high-resolution T2-weighted imaging [16] and results obtained at 3 T seem better than those obtained at 1.5 T [17, 18]

Even if MRI performances in local staging are not perfect, it may improve the prediction of the pathological stage when combined to clinical data [19, 20].

Given its low sensitivity to microscopic invasion, MRI is not recommended in the local staging of low-risk patients but may be useful in selected patients with intermediate to high risk cancers [21].

2 Evaluation of Nodal Invasion and Distant Metastases

2.1 Lymph Node Metastases

Prostate cancer drainage patterns are complex, and the sentinel node concept barely applicable. Pelvic lymph node dissection (PLND) misses up to 40 % of positive lymph nodes (LN) that are located outside the routine surgical template. Even extended PLND has not a perfect sensitivity and is associated to substantial morbidity. An imaging method that could accurately spot positive LN is therefore needed [22].

CT and conventional MRI are widely used for detection of LN invasion, and yet their accuracy is poor. They rely only on morphologic criteria (size, shape, internal architecture) the sensitivity of which is suboptimal. The size range of normal LN varies within different anatomical regions.

Although there is no clear consensus, it is usually recommended to use a 6–8 mm threshold for LN short-axis in the pelvis. Unfortunately, up to 68 % of invaded LN have a short-axis diameter smaller than 5 mm [22, 23]. As a result, up to 70 % of positive LN may be missed by conventional CT or MRI. Because some inflammatory benign LN may be enlarged, the specificity of CT and MRI is also suboptimal.

Diffusion-weighted imaging (DWI) may improve morphologic assessment of LN. In a prospective study of 120 patients with normal-sized LN evaluated by three readers, Thoeny et al. found a per-patient sensitivity and specificity of 64–79 % and 79–85 %, respectively [24]. However, when expressed on a LN region basis, sensitivity of detection with DWI remains low (18.8–56 %) and not superior to ^{11}C-Choline PET/CT or even to CT [25, 26].

Ultrasmall superparamagnetic particles of iron oxide (USPIO) can be used as lymphotropic contrast agent. They have been reported to improve sensitivity of detection of malignant pelvic LN from 35.4 % with conventional MRI to 90.5 % [27]. However, PLND was limited in this study, and the false negative rate may have been underestimated. In a more recent prospective multicentric study of 375 patients, MR lymphography (MRL) using USPIO had a sensitivity and specificity of 82 % and 93 %, respectively, as compared to PLND. In the same study, CT had a sensitivity and specificity of 34 % and 97 %, respectively [28]. Despite these good results, MRL is limited by the lack of availability of USPIO.

One group recently combined DWI and MRL in 75 patients who underwent extended PLND. Twenty percent of the patients had LN invasion at pathology. Combined MRI was interpreted by 3 readers. On a per-patient basis, sensitivity and specificity were 65–75 % and 93–96 %, respectively. Yet, 25–35 % of patients with positive LN were still incorrectly diagnosed as negative [29].

Thus, despite recent improvements due to DWI and the use of USPIO, detection of LN invasion remains limited, and negative imaging studies cannot completely rule out LN metastases.

2.2 Bone Metastases

Classically, bone metastases are detected by ^{99m}Tc-bone scan (BS), and plain radiographs and CT are used to investigate equivocal bone scan findings.

MRI has an enhanced sensitivity for the early detection of neoplastic invasion of the bone marrow. It may combine conventional anatomic (usually T1-weighted images) and diffusion-weighted images. It may cover the whole skeleton (so-called whole-body MRI) or be limited to the axial skeleton (i.e., the spine and the pelvis) to shorten the examination time, because most metastases involve the axial skeleton [30]. Both whole-body and axial MRI have been proven to be more sensitive that bone scan and targeted radiographs [31–33] and equally effective than ^{11}C-Choline PET/CT [34] in detecting bone metastases in patients with high-risk prostate cancer. Whole-body MRI may be more sensitive and more specific than combined bone scan, targeted radiographs and abdomino-pelvic CT [35].

2.3 Towards Earlier Detection of Metastases and Better Assessment of Treatment Response ?

PET/CT- and MR-based techniques are more sensitive than standard work-up (BS and abdomino-pelvic CT) to detect bone metastases and, to a lesser extent, LN metastases (Fig. 1). The availability of these techniques raises the question whether earlier detection of metastases could lead to better patient outcome.

This is clearly the case in patients with local recurrence and fit enough to undergo a local salvage treatment. Salvage treatments are indeed associated with substantial morbidity [36]. Better discrimination of infraclinic metastases could obviate M1 patients being exposed to the useless morbidity of salvage treatments.

The benefit of earlier detection of metastases in asymptomatic high-risk patients or patients with castrate-resistant prostate cancer is less clear, but warrants careful assessment in the current context of apparition of numerous new systemic treatments [30].

The apparition of new lesions on BS remains the only recognized criteria for bone lesion response evaluation. However, the availability of new imaging biomarkers derived from MRI (as for example the apparent diffusion coefficient of metastases) or PET/CT [37] will probably change patient management in the near future and new imaging modalities will probably be extensively used to assess response to new systemic treatments.

3 Pretherapeutic Tumor Mapping: A New Paradigm

Usually, the diagnosis of prostate cancer is suggested by abnormal or rising PSA level, or by an abnormal digital rectal examination, which triggers further evaluation, typically with TRUS-guided sextant biopsies. Prostate biopsy findings are also widely used to estimate the tumor volume (number of positive samples and length of tumor invasion in each positive core) and aggressiveness (Gleason score of the tumor detected at biopsy).

However, this approach has some limitations. First, using PSA as a screening tool leads to a substantial number of unnecessary biopsies in patients with no cancer or with indolent cancer that do not need immediate treatment. Currently, overdetection rates are estimated to be between 27 and 56 % [38]. Second, a negative set of biopsies does not rule out the presence of cancer. Among the patients with negative 10–12-core biopsy schemes, 17–21 % have cancer at repeat biopsy [39, 40]. Thus, urologists with patients with persistent abnormal PSA level and negative biopsies face a dilemma: when to repeat biopsy and when to stop biopsying? Third, although PSA level and biopsy findings correlate positively with clinical stage, tumor volume, and histologic grade, they are of limited value in predicting tumor burden and aggressiveness in individual patients [38].

To overcome these difficulties, some authors proposed to further increase the number of samples taken either transrectally or using a perineal template to improve 3D registration of the cores location (so-called saturation biopsies). This approach can rule out prostate cancer and offers a better estimation of the tumor volume and Gleason score [41]. However, it is associated with increased cost and morbidity and increased risk of overdiagnosing microscopic tumor foci that do not need treatment [42, 43].

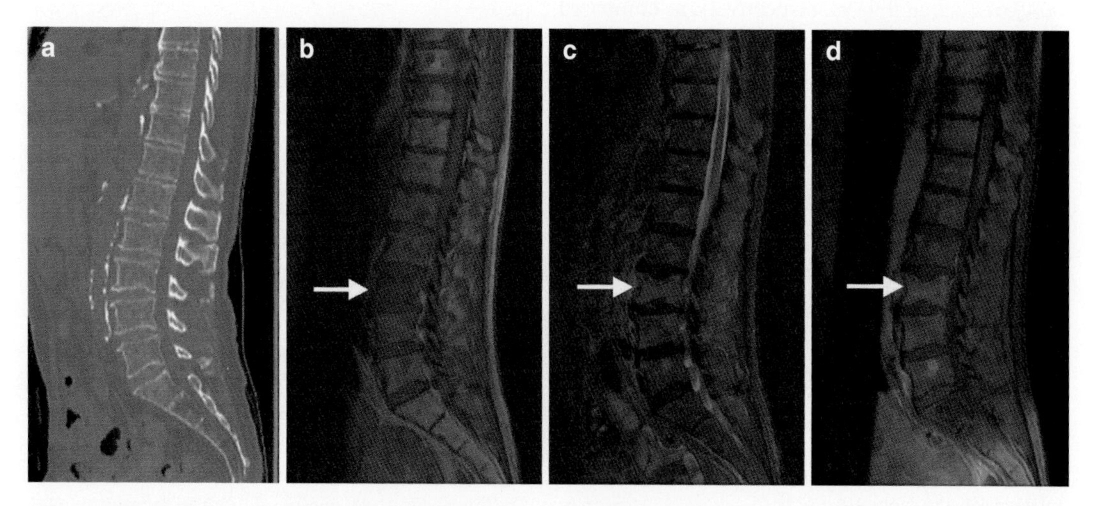

Fig. 1 Images obtained in a patient with history of radiotherapy for prostate cancer and apparition of recent back pain. Computed tomography showed no metastases (**a**). MRI of the spine showed multiple focal lesions appearing hypointense on T1-weighted images (**b**), hyperintense on T2-weighted images (**c**), with enhancement after injection of gadolinium chelates (**d**). Intervertebral discs are spared

Another option would be to develop an imaging method that could accurately distinguish prostate cancer from normal glands.

3.1 Multiparametric MRI

As a stand-alone, T2-weighted imaging has shown disappointing results in tumor detection, with moderate sensitivity (25–60 %) and many causes of false positives (prostatitis, glandular atrophy, fibrosis, etc.) [9, 44–46]. New imaging modalities such as MR spectroscopy (MRS), DWI, and dynamic contrast-enhanced (DCE) imaging have improved tumor diagnosis by allowing functional assessment [46–49]. Because they image different physiological process, they provide potentially independent information, and their combination can further improve cancer diagnosis [50, 51]. It is now recommended to perform a so-called multiparametric MRI (mpMRI) of the prostate, combining T2-weighted imaging and at least two different functional modalities [52].

3.1.1 Comparison to Radical Prostatectomy Specimens

Comparisons to prostatectomy specimens have shown that mpMRI could detect aggressive (Gleason ≥7) cancer with excellent sensitivity. However, detection rates are much smaller for Gleason 6 cancers that tend to have a signal close to that of normal glands [53–55]. Another factor impacting tumor detection is the histological architecture, with dense tumors more easily detected than sparse tumors [53, 56].

At our institution, we started in 2008 a database collecting precise correlation between MR images and prostatectomy specimens. Patients were imaged either at 1.5 T ($n=71$) or 3 T ($n=104$). Images were reviewed by 2 independent radiologists and compared to histological findings. On a series of 175 consecutive patients, the detection rates for tumors of <0.5 cc, 0.5–2 cc and >2 cc were 21–29 %, 43–54 %, and 67–75 % for Gleason ≤6 cancers, 63 %, 82–88 %, and 97 % for Gleason 7 cancers and 80 %, 93 %, and 100 % for Gleason ≥8 cancers, respectively. Results were not significantly influenced by the field strength [53].

3.1.2 The Role of mpMRI Before Biopsy

Because mpMRI can detect aggressive cancer with high sensitivity and has a tendency to miss well-differentiated tumor foci, one may argue that obtaining a prostate mpMRI before each biopsy procedure could altogether solve the issue of underdiagnosis (by orienting biopsies towards areas with aggressive tumors) and overdiagnosis (by obviating unnecessary biopsies that may randomly detect quiescent cancer foci) (Figs. 2 and 3). This raises

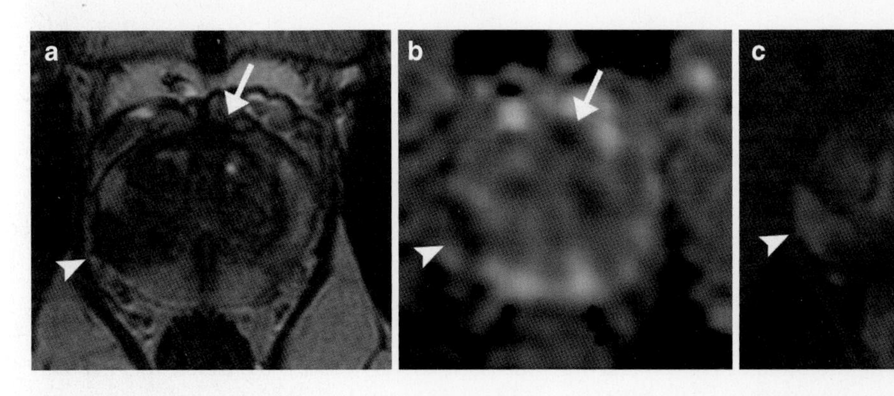

Fig. 2 Images obtained in a 67 year-old man with rising PSA (7.43 ng/ml) and systematic biopsy showing Gleason 7 cancer in the right base and midgland (two positive cores out of 12). Multiparametric MRI showed a nodule of the right base and midgland appearing as hypointense on T2-weighted imaging (**a**, *arrowhead*) and on apparent diffusion coefficient map (**b**, *arrowhead*) and showing early enhancement on dynamic contrast-enhanced imaging (**c**, *arrowhead*). The PIRADS score of the nodule was 5/5. T2-weighted imaging showed a marked extracapsular extension (**a**, *arrowhead*). Also note another tumor (PIRADS score of 5/5) in the anterior horn of the left peripheral zone (**a**–**c**, *arrow*). The patient was treated with radiotherapy and hormonotherapy

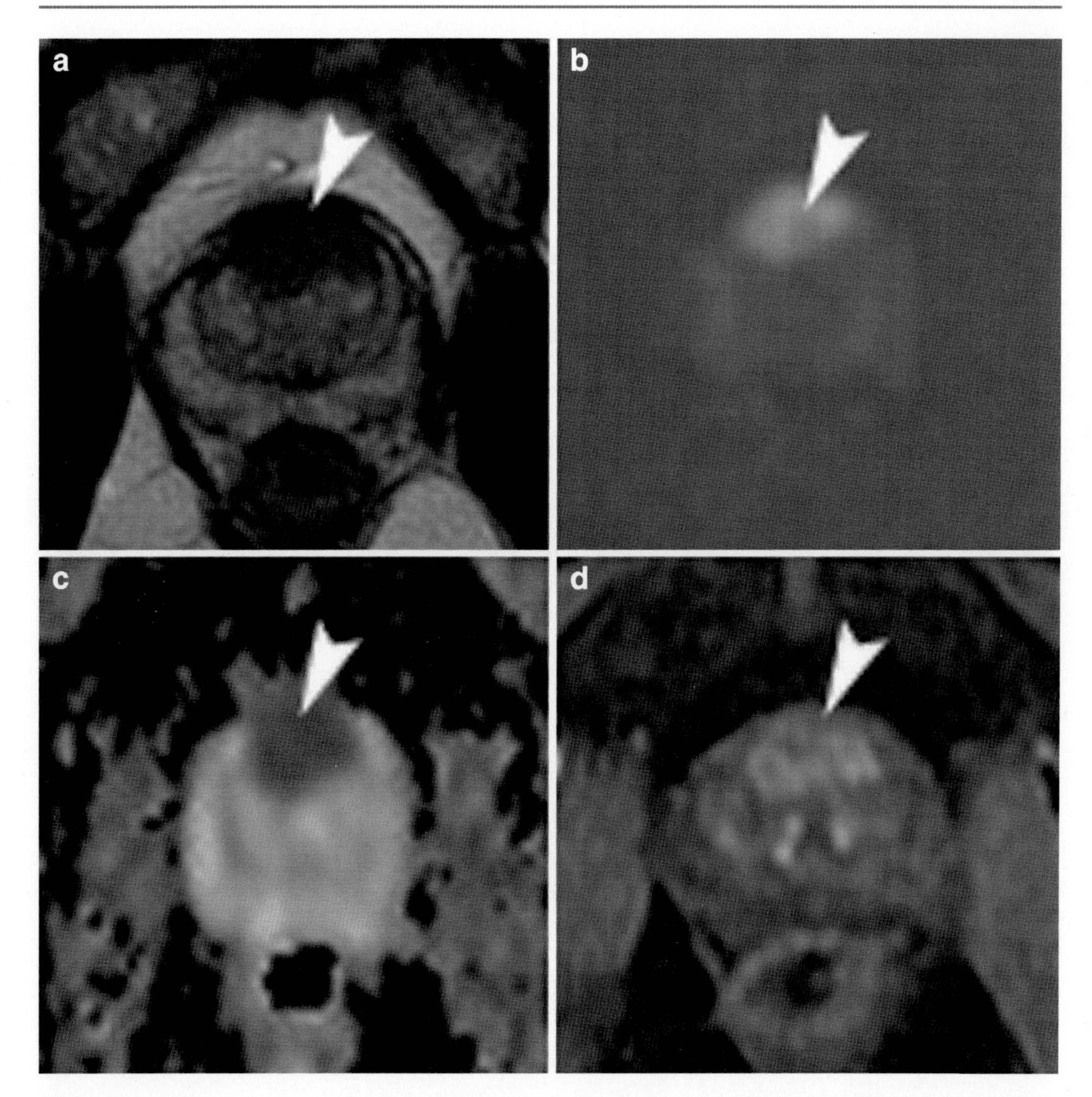

Fig. 3 Images obtained in a 67 year-old man with rising PSA (11.58 ng/ml). Systematic biopsies showed a Gleason 6 cancer (one positive core out of 12, on 3 mm). Multiparametric MRI showed a typical anterior tumor (PIRADS score of 5/5) appearing as hypointense on T2-weighted imaging (**a**, *arrowhead*), with restriction of diffusion on native diffusion-weighted images (**b**, *arrowhead*; b-value of 2000 s/mm^2) and on apparent diffusion coefficient map (**c**, *arrowhead*), and showing early enhancement on dynamic contrast-enhanced imaging (**d**, *arrowhead*). Targeted biopsies showed a Gleason 7 cancer

two different questions: the added value of targeted biopsies based on mpMRI findings (TBx) and the negative predictive value (NPV) of mpMRI for aggressive cancers. Unfortunately, the answers are not as simple as it appears. The diagnostic performance of a given test is indeed highly influenced by the population in which it is tested, and particularly by the prevalence of the disease in this population. Comparisons to prostatectomy specimens are useful to assess the cancer foci that may be missed by mpMRI. However, they are insufficient to evaluate its added value or its NPV in other populations such as the population of candidates to prostate biopsy. It is therefore mandatory to evaluate mpMRI in each specific population, before one can define its role in the future.

The Added Value of TBx in Patients with No History of Prostate Cancer

In a recent meta-analysis [57], TBx had a higher detection rate of clinically significant prostate cancer compared to systematic biopsy (sensitivity of 0.91 [95% confidence interval (CI), 0.87–0.94] versus 0.76 [95 % CI, 0.64–0.84]) and a lower rate of detection of insignificant prostate cancer (sensitivity of 0.44 [95% CI, 0.26–0.64] versus 0.83 [95% CI, 0.77–0.87]). However, the added value of TBx in detecting clinically significant prostate cancer was marked in the subgroup of patients with previous negative biopsies (relative sensitivity of 1.54 [95 % CI, 1.05–2.57]) but not in the subgroup of biopsy-naïve patients (relative sensitivity of 1.10 [95 % CI, 1.00–1.22]). There was a trend for TBx to detect less clinically insignificant cancers in both subgroups (relative sensitivity of 0.82 [95 % CI, 0.03–21.4] and 0.51 [95 % CI, 0.25–1.04], respectively), but the difference was not significant. Another systematic review also concluded that Tbx improved detection rates in the repeat biopsy setting, but not at initial biopsy [58]. These results can be explained by the fact that the proportion of tumors in locations easily missed by systematic biopsies (e.g., anterior tumors) is higher in the repeat biopsy setting. The impact of prebiopsy mpMRI is therefore easier to demonstrate in this population.

Therefore, it seems clear that mpMRI findings can sensitize repeat biopsy and it is now recommended by the European Association of Urology to obtain a prostate mpMRI before repeat biopsy [21]. The precise role of mpMRI in biopsy-naïve patients remains to be defined.

One recent meta-analysis studied the diagnostic yield of TBx using MR/US fusion software in a mixed population of biopsy-naïve patients and candidates to repeat biopsy. Tbx detected a median of 9.1% additional clinically significant cancers (range, 5–16.2%) that were missed by standard biopsy alone. In contrast, standard biopsies detected a median of 2.1% (range, 0–12.4%) additional clinically significant cancers that were missed by MRI-TRUS fusion biopsies. However, if the study using transperineal mapping biopsies is removed, then the standard biopsy is only a TRUS biopsy approach, the range stood at 0–7% [59].

Meta-analyses are limited by substantial heterogeneity among studies, particularly concerning patient inclusion criteria, definition of clinically significant, and targeted and systematic biopsy protocols. Prospective controlled trials are needed to confirm meta-analyses' findings. Prospective randomized trials in biopsy-naïve patients gave contradictory results [60–62]. Several other multicentric controlled studies are currently ongoing and should be published in the next 2 years.

The Negative Predictive Value of mpMRI in Patients with No History of Prostate Cancer

Whether the NPV of mpMRI is good enough to be used as a triage test to obviate unnecessary biopsy remains a difficult question. The NPV for exclusion of significant disease before prostate biopsy ranges from 63 to 98% [63], but expert centers repeatedly reported values over 90% [59, 64, 65]. However, reported results are impaired by substantial differences in definition of clinically significant cancer and negative mpMRI that preclude any definitive conclusion. It would also be interesting to evaluate if clinical (DRE) or biochemical (PSA level kinetics, PSA density, etc.) data could be used to further rule out clinically significant cancer in addition to mpMRI results. Unfortunately, there are no clear data on this topic yet.

3.1.3 The Role of mpMRI in Active Surveillance

MpMRI can significantly predict the presence of aggressive cancers in patients suitable for active surveillance (AS) but treated by radical prostatectomy (RP) [66]. At the start of AS, a positive mpMRI significantly predicts the presence of aggressive cancer at repeat biopsy [57]. However, there is a need for well-designed prospective multicentric studies to definitively assess the added value of TBx as compared to systematic biopsy at the start of AS. The role of mpMRI during the follow-up period of AS remains unclear. There are currently no validated radiological criteria of progression that could to trigger follow-up biopsy.

3.1.4 The Issue of the Scoring Systems and the Interreader Variability

MpMRI remains difficult to interpret. Between 40 and 75 % of focal lesions visible at mpMRI are benign [53, 67]. Therefore, it is crucial that the radiologist assesses the risk of malignancy of all visible prostate lesions. However, besides typical cancers appearing as nodules with unambiguous, marked, signal abnormalities on all MR sequences, mpMRI often shows focal abnormalities with various shapes, subtle signal changes, or discrepant results on the different MR sequences (e.g., marked signal abnormality on one sequence and normal appearance on another). The high number of possible combinations of shapes and signal abnormalities on the different MR sequences and the difficulty in interpreting them may discouraged some radiologists. Consequently, the good results reported in specialized centers are not always reproduced in daily routine.

Because it is impossible to definitively characterize as malignant or benign all focal lesions in the prostate, some authors have recommended using a 5-level suspicion score (1: definitely benign; 2: probably benign; 3: equivocal; 4: probably malignant; and 5: definitely malignant) [68]. This so-called Likert score is subjective, and there are no objective criteria to assign a given score to a given lesion. Nonetheless, it summarizes the doubts (or certainties) of the radiologist and many studies found that the Likert score was a highly significant predictor not only of the malignant nature of prostate lesions but also of their aggressiveness [53, 65, 69–71]. Unsurprisingly, the global interreader agreement of the Likert score is only moderate, even if it can be good among experienced readers [69, 71, 72].

To overcome this difficulty, several groups have proposed semiobjective scores, using better defined features to assign a given score to a given lesion [67, 73, 74]. In an effort to standardize prostate mpMRI interpretation, the European Society of Urogenital Radiology endorsed in 2012 the Prostate Imaging Reporting and Data System (PIRADS) [52] that assigns a 5-level score to T2w, DWI and DCE images, rendering an overall sum ranging from 3 to 15. This so-called PIRADS V1 score was a significant predictor of malignancy, but it failed to improve interreader agreement as compared to the Likert score [69, 71, 75]. The PIRADS V1 score was updated in 2015. The new PIRADS V2 score [76] was shown to be a significant predictor of malignancy [77], but may not improve interreader agreement [78]. It is therefore likely that the PIRADS scoring system will be further amended in the future.

Another option to assist inexperienced radiologists would be to develop quantitative models that could predict the nature (or the aggressiveness) of focal lesions. Promising results have been obtained by computer-aided systems [79, 80], but on a limited number of patients. Quantitative approaches in MR imaging are intrinsically limited by the large number of sources of variability in quantitative measurements across imagers from different manufacturers, making it difficult to define robust diagnostic thresholds. Nonetheless, recent works suggest that simple quantitative models may be robust enough to accurately characterize prostate lesions on images from different manufacturers [81, 82]. This may become a fruitful approach in the future.

3.1.5 Detection of Local Recurrences After Radiotherapy or Radical Prostatectomy

Local recurrences after radiotherapy (RT) can be treated by salvages procedures such as prostatectomy, high-intensity focused ultrasound ablation, cryotherapy, or brachytherapy. Whenever possible focal therapy is recommended to decrease the morbidity of these salvage procedures [36, 83]. As a result, it becomes important to localize local recurrences as precisely as possible to select patients fit for salvage focal ablation. Several groups have found that mpMRI could detect and localize post-RT local recurrences with excellent accuracy [84–86], and mpMRI will probably be increasingly used in the future to guide biopsies in patients with biochemical failure.

Most patients with biochemical failure after RP undergo salvage RT without imaging, because biopsies of the prostatectomy bed have a poor sensitivity, even with TRUS guidance. As a result, salvage RT delivers a uniform dose (classically 66 Gy) to the prostatectomy bed. This "blind" RT is more efficient when performed at PSA levels <0.5–1 ng/mL. Several studies reported that mpMRI could detect local recurrences in the prostatectomy bed with sensitivities and specificities of 84–88 % and 89–100 %, respectively. However, the mean PSA level in these studies was 0.8–1.9 ng/mL, which is higher than the 0.5 ng/mL threshold usually used for salvage RT [36]. Recently, two studies evaluated mpMRI in patients with PSA level <0.5 ng/mL. One found a sensitivity of only 13 % in men with PSA level <0.3 ng/mL [87], while the other reported a sensitivity of 86 % in patients with PSA level <0.4 ng/mL [88]. Therefore, it remains to be seen whether MRI is able to correctly detect local recurrences in patients with PSA level <0.5 ng/mL. If this is the case, a stereotaxic boost to the recurrence site could be applied during salvage RT.

3.2 Transrectal Ultrasound and Ultrasound-Based Methods

3.2.1 Gray-Scale Ultrasound and Doppler

Approximately 60 % of prostate cancers are hypoechoic, limiting gray-scale ultrasound (GSU) sensitivity. GSU is also limited by a high rate of false positive findings. Color or Power-Doppler can show larger feeding vessels associated to tumors [89], but its additional value as compared to GSU remains unclear [90, 91].

3.2.2 Computerized Ultrasound

Computerized ultrasound (Histoscanning™) uses computer-aided analysis to quantify tissue disorganization induced by malignant processes. Despite promising initial results [92], it achieved poor prediction of positive biopsies on larger studies, and the combination of HistoScanning™ and conventional ultrasound achieved lower detection rates than systematic biopsy [93]. Its use is therefore not recommended.

3.2.3 Contrast-Enhanced Ultrasound

Contrast-enhanced ultrasound (CEUS) uses gas-filled microbubbles administered intravenously during ultrasound imaging. Microbubbles act as additional reflectors into the bloodstream. Because their size is comparable to that of erythrocytes, they pass the capillaries and can therefore show microvasculature, as opposed to color or power-Doppler that show only large feeding vessels. It is important to understand that microbubbles stay within the vessels unlike gadolinium chelates that leak through tumor capillaries and accumulate within the interstitium. As a result, CEUS enhancement of prostate cancers is due to increased microvasculature, while enhancement at DCE MRI is due to increased permeability of tumor capillaries. Therefore, tissue enhancement observed at CEUS is different to that observed at DCE MRI and one must not think that CEUS is an ultrasound equivalent to DCE MRI [89, 94].

Several ultrasound contrast agents have been used, the main ones being Levovist™ (Schering, Berlin, Germany) and Sonovue™ (Bracco, Milan, Italy). At first, contrast agents were used in combination with Color or Power Doppler. However, Doppler imaging uses relatively high energy levels that may destroy a large proportion of the microbubbles before they reach the neovasculature of the tumors. Recently contrast-specific imaging modes became available. They use low-energy ultrasound pulses that prevent premature bursting of the microbubbles. They can also differentiate between the nonlinear signals reflected by the microbubbles and the linear signals from the tissue, allowing superior spatial and temporal resolution [89, 94].

Comparisons to RP specimens showed sensitivities of 41–69 % and specificities of 33–95 % for CEUS [89, 95–97]. A recent meta-analysis combing results of 16 studies over a 13-year period (14 studies comparing CEUS to biopsy findings and 2 to RP findings) reported a sensitivity of 0.70 (95 % CI, 0.68–0.73), a specificity of 0.74 (95 % CI, 0.72–0.75), a positive predictive value (PPV) of 0.59 (95 % CI, 0.56–0.61), a NPV of 0.82 (95 % CI, 0.81–0.84), respectively. However, there was significant between-study heterogeneity and the conclusion of the authors was that biopsy based on CEUS findings could not replace systematic biopsy [98].

CEUS has two main limitations. First, the diagnostic criteria for cancer are not standardized. Interpretation of images remains visual, features associated with malignancy being asymmetrical enhancement, increased focal enhancement or asymmetry of intraprostatic vessels. This may induce large interobserver variability [89]. Quantitative assessment is currently under development and may improve accuracy of cancer detection and user dependency of the technique [99]. Second, recording inflow and outflow takes time (1–2 min) and only one plane can be evaluated per intravenous bolus. An interval of 3–5 min is required to allow sufficient clearance of the bubbles. Ideally, endorectal probes allowing 3D repetitive imaging (so-called 4D probes) would be necessary to image the entire gland during the first-pass of a single bolus. These probes are not currently available. Until then, CEUS will be limited to academic and research centers.

3.2.4 Elastographic Techniques

It is well known that prostate cancer is harder than normal tissue. Thus, elastographic techniques may be of interest to detect and localize prostate cancer foci. There are two main types of elastographic techniques: strain elastography (SE) and shear-wave elastography (SWE).

In SE, a quasi-static compression is applied to the prostate through the endorectal probe. Stiffer tissues are less affected than softer tissues and the amount of deformation (strain) is displayed in the form of a color overlay. Many studies have evaluated SE findings to RP specimens. A recent meta-analysis of 7 series (508 patients) reported a pooled sensitivity and specificity of 0.72 (95 % CI: 0.70–0.74) and 0.76 (95 % CI: 0.74–0.78), respectively [100]. Another meta-analysis combing the results of series comparing SE findings to targeted biopsies findings reported a pooled sensitivity and specificity of 0.62 (95 % CI: 0.55–0.68) and 0.79 (95 % CI: 0.74–0.84), suggesting that biopsies targeted to SE abnormalities could be a valuable addition to systematic biopsy [101]. However, SE has two limitations: first, the need for free-hand compression induces considerable user dependency. Second, color maps are automatically scaled between the hardest and the softest tissue in the image field. As a result, this technique provides only data on the relative stiffness of the points in the image field, but does not provide measurements of absolute stiffness [89].

In SWE, shear waves are induced in the prostate using the acoustic radiation force produced by a focused ultrasound beam. Shear waves velocity is then measured. Since shear waves propagate faster in stiffer tissue, a quantitative assessment of tissue stiffness can be obtained by measuring the velocity of shear waves. Thus, SWE has, at least in theory, two main advantages over SE. It is a quantitative technique and it does not need free-hand compression and therefore may be less operator-dependent. Only a few studies have evaluated prostate SWE [102–106]. A recent study of 184 patients who underwent SWE before systematic biopsy reported that the optimal stiffness threshold for differentiating malignant from benign tissue in PZ was 35 kPa. Using this cutoff, SWE sensitivity and specificity in PZ at per-sextant analysis were, respectively, 0.96 (95 CI: 0.95–0.97) and 0.85 (95 % CI: 0.83–0.87). These results are very promising (Fig. 4).

However, one must be aware of some limitations of the technique. Even if SWE is probably less operator dependent than SE, prostate apparent stiffness measured at SWE increases with the amount of pressure applied by the endorectal probe, especially in the PZ. This is particularly marked in the posteromedian part of PZ that is the closest to the endorectal probe. As a result benign PZ appears stiffer in the paramedian part of PZ than in its lateral part [104]. At our institution, we performed SWE in axial and sagittal planes before RP in 30 patients. At multivariate analysis, measured stiffness was significantly influenced by three factors: the nature of tissues (cancers were stiffer than benign tissue), the imaging plane (all tissue classes were stiffer on sagittal than on axial images), and the location within the gland (all tissue classes were stiffer in TZ than in PZ, and in median PZ than in lateral PZ). In routine, SWE may still need experience (not to apply too much pressure on the probe) and different stiffness thresholds to diagnose cancer

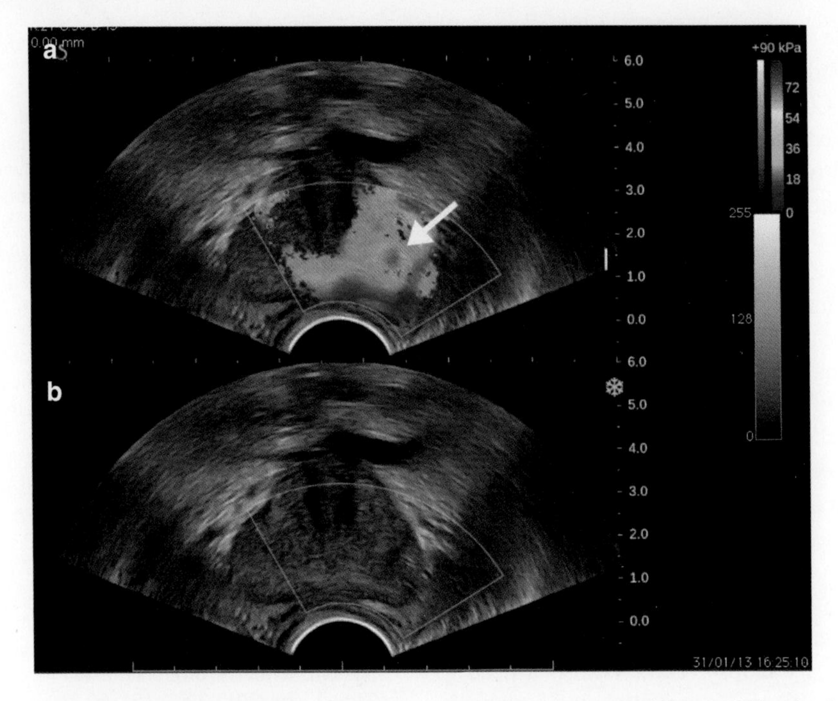

Fig. 4 Axial shear-wave elastography (SWE; **a**) and corresponding gray scale image (**b**) obtained in a 55 year-old patient with rising PSA (8 ng/ml). SWE image showed an area with increased stiffness within the left base (**a**, *arrow*). Biopsy showed a Gleason 6 cancer

in TZ, median PZ and lateral PZ, and in axial and sagittal images (unpublished results).

3.2.5 Towards Multiparametric Ultrasound?

Because the previously discussed new ultrasound-based techniques image different physiological processes, there results may not be correlated, and hence it may be possible to combine them to improve cancer detection at TRUS. Little has been published so far on this so-called multiparametric ultrasound [89].

Several studies showed that combining several techniques could increase cancer detection sensitivity [107–109]. For example, Xie et al. compared the results of a 10-biopsy scheme with GSU, power Doppler and CEUS. GSU was positive in 51 % of cancer sites, power Doppler in 48 % and CEUS in 73 %, while the combination was positive in 82 % [109]. These results show that all cancer foci are not detected by the same modality. However, combining only positive modalities increases sensitivity and NPV at the expense of specificity and PPV.

Another strategy would be to choose one modality to detect abnormal areas and a second one to further characterize these areas. This will improve specificity and PPV at the expense of sensitivity and NPV. In a study of 100 patients imaged with SE and CEUS before prostatectomy, SE was found to have a sensitivity and specificity of 0.49 and 0.74, respectively. If CEUS was used to characterize SE lesions, the PPV increased from 0.65 to 0.90 [110]. In our experience, using optimized stiffness thresholds for median and lateral PZ, SWE could correctly diagnosed as benign 25–33 % of benign hypoechoic lesions (unpublished data).

Ultimately, a better balance between sensitivity and specificity could be obtained by introducing a Likert-type score, as for mpMRI [89]. To our knowledge, such a score has not been evaluated yet.

Conclusion

Little progress has been made over the last 10 years in local staging of prostate cancer. MRI remains the best imaging technique, but because of its low sensitivity, its use is limited to moderate and high-risk patients.

If Choline PET/CT has dramatically improved the early detection of metastases, MR-derived techniques have also shown excellent accuracy in detection of bone metastases and to a lesser extent of LN metastases. However, long acquisition times remain a limitation for whole-body MRI.

Over the last years, mpMRI has made tremendous progress in the detection and localization of clinically significant prostate cancer. The challenges for the coming years will be to better define the populations in which mpMRI positive findings may help sensitize the detection of aggressive cancer at biopsy and, even more importantly, the populations in which a negative mpMRI (alone or in combination with biochemical and clinical data) may avoid unnecessary biopsy. There is also a need to improve interreader agreement that will probably be achieved through continuous refinements of scoring systems and maybe through the development of quantitative models robust enough to provide accurate characterization of prostate lesion across MR scanners from different manufacturers.

To date, the ultrasound techniques cannot match the results of mpMRI in prostate cancer detection, at least as stand-alone. Combinations of new ultrasound techniques are currently assessed, but it is too soon to determine if a multiparametric ultrasound approach will challenge mpMRI.

References

1. el-Gabry EA, Halpern EJ, Strup SE, Gomella LG. Imaging prostate cancer: current and future applications. Oncology (Williston Park). 2001;15(3):325–36; discussion 39–42.
2. Bates TS, Gillatt DA, Cavanagh PM, Speakman M. A comparison of endorectal magnetic resonance imaging and transrectal ultrasonography in the local staging of prostate cancer with histopathological correlation. Br J Urol. 1997;79(6):927–32.
3. May F, Treumann T, Dettmar P, Hartung R, Breul J. Limited value of endorectal magnetic resonance imaging and transrectal ultrasonography in the staging of clinically localized prostate cancer. BJU Int. 2001;87(1):66–9.
4. McSherry SA, Levy F, Schiebler ML, Keefe B, Dent GA, Mohler JL. Preoperative prediction of pathological tumor volume and stage in clinically localized prostate cancer: comparison of digital rectal examination, transrectal ultrasonography and magnetic resonance imaging. J Urol. 1991;146(1):85–9.
5. Mitterberger M, Pinggera GM, Pallwein L, et al. The value of three-dimensional transrectal ultrasonography in staging prostate cancer. BJU Int. 2007;100(1):47–50.
6. Sauvain JL, Palascak P, Bourscheid D, et al. Value of power doppler and 3D vascular sonography as a method for diagnosis and staging of prostate cancer. Eur Urol. 2003;44(1):21–30; discussion –1.
7. de Rooij M, Hamoen EH, Witjes JA, Barentsz JO, Rovers MM. Accuracy of magnetic resonance imaging for local staging of prostate cancer: a diagnostic meta-analysis. Eur Urol. 2015;70(2):233–45.
8. Silva RC, Sasse AD, Matheus WE, Ferreira U. Magnetic resonance image in the diagnosis and evaluation of extra-prostatic extension and involvement of seminal vesicles of prostate cancer: a systematic review of literature and meta-analysis. Int Braz J Urol. 2013;39(2):155–66.
9. Jager GJ, Ruijter ET, van de Kaa CA, et al. Local staging of prostate cancer with endorectal MR imaging: correlation with histopathology. AJR Am J Roentgenol. 1996;166(4):845–52.
10. Epstein JI, Carmichael MJ, Pizov G, Walsh PC. Influence of capsular penetration on progression following radical prostatectomy: a study of 196 cases with long-term followup. J Urol. 1993;150(1):135–41.
11. Cornud F, Flam T, Chauveinc L, et al. Extraprostatic spread of clinically localized prostate cancer: factors predictive of pT3 tumor and of positive endorectal MR imaging examination results. Radiology. 2002;224(1):203–10.
12. Hricak H, White S, Vigneron D, et al. Carcinoma of the prostate gland: MR imaging with pelvic phased-array coils versus integrated endorectal--pelvic phased-array coils. Radiology. 1994;193(3):703–9.
13. Futterer JJ, Engelbrecht MR, Jager GJ, et al. Prostate cancer: comparison of local staging accuracy of pelvic phased-array coil alone versus integrated endorectal-pelvic phased-array coils. Local staging accuracy of prostate cancer using endorectal coil MR imaging. Eur Radiol. 2007;17(4):1055–65.
14. Futterer JJ, Engelbrecht MR, Huisman HJ, et al. Staging prostate cancer with dynamic contrast-enhanced endorectal MR imaging prior to radical prostatectomy: experienced versus less experienced readers. Radiology. 2005;237(2):541–9.
15. Bloch BN, Furman-Haran E, Helbich TH, et al. Prostate cancer: accurate determination of extracapsular extension with high-spatial-resolution dynamic contrast-enhanced and T2-weighted MR imaging--initial results. Radiology. 2007;245(1):176–85.

16. Futterer JJ, Scheenen TW, Huisman HJ, et al. Initial experience of 3 tesla endorectal coil magnetic resonance imaging and 1H-spectroscopic imaging of the prostate. Invest Radiol. 2004;39(11):671–80.
17. Futterer JJ, Heijmink SW, Scheenen TW, et al. Prostate cancer: local staging at 3-T endorectal MR imaging--early experience. Radiology. 2006;238(1):184–91.
18. Heijmink SW, Futterer JJ, Hambrock T, et al. Prostate cancer: body-array versus endorectal coil MR imaging at 3 T--comparison of image quality, localization, and staging performance. Radiology. 2007;244(1):184–95.
19. Wang L, Mullerad M, Chen HN, et al. Prostate cancer: incremental value of endorectal MR imaging findings for prediction of extracapsular extension. Radiology. 2004;232(1):133–9.
20. Poulakis V, Witzsch U, De Vries R, et al. Preoperative neural network using combined magnetic resonance imaging variables, prostate specific antigen and gleason score to predict prostate cancer stage. J Urol. 2004;172(4 Pt 1):1306–10.
21. Mottet N, Bellmunt J, Briers E, et al. Guidelines on prostate cancer. London: Springer Healthcare; 2016.
22. Barentsz JO, Thoeny HC. Prostate cancer: can imaging accurately diagnose lymph node involvement? Nat Rev Urol. 2015;12(6):313–5.
23. Kiss B, Thoeny HC, Studer UE. Current Status of Lymph Node Imaging in Bladder and Prostate Cancer. Urology 2016 (in press). doi: 10.1016/j.urology.2016.02.014.
24. Thoeny HC, Froehlich JM, Triantafyllou M, et al. Metastases in normal-sized pelvic lymph nodes: detection with diffusion-weighted MR imaging. Radiology. 2014;273(1):125–35.
25. Budiharto T, Joniau S, Lerut E, et al. Prospective evaluation of 11C-choline positron emission tomography/computed tomography and diffusion-weighted magnetic resonance imaging for the nodal staging of prostate cancer with a high risk of lymph node metastases. Eur Urol. 2011;60(1):125–30.
26. Heck MM, Souvatzoglou M, Retz M, et al. Prospective comparison of computed tomography, diffusion-weighted magnetic resonance imaging and [11C]choline positron emission tomography/computed tomography for preoperative lymph node staging in prostate cancer patients. Eur J Nucl Med Mol Imaging. 2014;41(4):694–701.
27. Harisinghani MG, Barentsz J, Hahn PF, et al. Noninvasive detection of clinically occult lymph-node metastases in prostate cancer. N Engl J Med. 2003;348(25):2491–9.
28. Heesakkers RA, Hovels AM, Jager GJ, et al. MRI with a lymph-node-specific contrast agent as an alternative to CT scan and lymph-node dissection in patients with prostate cancer: a prospective multicohort study. Lancet Oncol. 2008;9(9):850–6.
29. Birkhauser FD, Studer UE, Froehlich JM, et al. Combined ultrasmall superparamagnetic particles of iron oxide-enhanced and diffusion-weighted magnetic resonance imaging facilitates detection of metastases in normal-sized pelvic lymph nodes of patients with bladder and prostate cancer. Eur Urol. 2013;64(6):953–60.
30. Sartor O, Eisenberger M, Kattan MW, Tombal B, Lecouvet F. Unmet needs in the prediction and detection of metastases in prostate cancer. Oncologist. 2013;18(5):549–57.
31. Gutzeit A, Doert A, Froehlich JM, et al. Comparison of diffusion-weighted whole body MRI and skeletal scintigraphy for the detection of bone metastases in patients with prostate or breast carcinoma. Skeletal Radiol. 2010;39(4):333–43.
32. Lecouvet FE, El Mouedden J, Collette L, et al. Can whole-body magnetic resonance imaging with diffusion-weighted imaging replace Tc 99m bone scanning and computed tomography for single-step detection of metastases in patients with high-risk prostate cancer? Eur Urol. 2012;62(1):68–75.
33. Lecouvet FE, Geukens D, Stainier A, et al. Magnetic resonance imaging of the axial skeleton for detecting bone metastases in patients with high-risk prostate cancer: diagnostic and cost-effectiveness and comparison with current detection strategies. J Clin Oncol. 2007;25(22):3281–7.
34. Luboldt W, Kufer R, Blumstein N, et al. Prostate carcinoma: diffusion-weighted imaging as potential alternative to conventional MR and 11C-choline PET/CT for detection of bone metastases. Radiology. 2008;249(3):1017–25.
35. Pasoglou V, Larbi A, Collette L, et al. One-step TNM staging of high-risk prostate cancer using magnetic resonance imaging (MRI): Toward an upfront simplified "all-in-one" imaging approach? Prostate. 2013;74(5):469–77.
36. Rouviere O, Vitry T, Lyonnet D. Imaging of prostate cancer local recurrences: why and how? Eur Radiol. 2010;20(5):1254–66.
37. Lecouvet FE, Talbot JN, Messiou C, et al. Monitoring the response of bone metastases to treatment with magnetic resonance imaging and nuclear medicine techniques: a review and position statement by the European Organisation for Research and Treatment of Cancer imaging group. Eur J Cancer. 2014;50(15):2519–31.
38. Kelloff GJ, Choyke P, Coffey DS. Challenges in clinical prostate cancer: role of imaging. AJR Am J Roentgenol. 2009;192(6):1455–70.
39. Singh H, Canto EI, Shariat SF, et al. Predictors of prostate cancer after initial negative systematic 12 core biopsy. J Urol. 2004;171(5):1850–4.
40. Mian BM, Naya Y, Okihara K, Vakar-Lopez F, Troncoso P, Babaian RJ. Predictors of cancer in repeat extended multisite prostate biopsy in men with previous negative extended multisite biopsy. Urology. 2002;60(5):836–40.
41. Delongchamps NB, Haas GP. Saturation biopsies for prostate cancer: current uses and future prospects. Nat Rev Urol. 2009;6(12):645–52.
42. Giannarini G, Autorino R, di Lorenzo G. Saturation biopsy of the prostate: why saturation does not saturate. Eur Urol. 2009;56(4):619–21.

43. Ashley RA, Inman BA, Routh JC, Mynderse LA, Gettman MT, Blute ML. Reassessing the diagnostic yield of saturation biopsy of the prostate. Eur Urol. 2008;53(5):976–81.
44. Quinn SF, Franzini DA, Demlow TA, et al. MR imaging of prostate cancer with an endorectal surface coil technique: correlation with whole-mount specimens. Radiology. 1994;190(2):323–7.
45. Ikonen S, Karkkainen P, Kivisaari L, et al. Endorectal magnetic resonance imaging of prostatic cancer: comparison between fat-suppressed T2-weighted fast spin echo and three-dimensional dual-echo, steady-state sequences. Eur Radiol. 2001;11(2):236–41.
46. Girouin N, Mege-Lechevallier F, Tonina Senes A, et al. Prostate dynamic contrast-enhanced MRI with simple visual diagnostic criteria: is it reasonable? Eur Radiol. 2007;17(6):1498–509.
47. Cheikh AB, Girouin N, Colombel M, et al. Evaluation of T2-weighted and dynamic contrast-enhanced MRI in localizing prostate cancer before repeat biopsy. Eur Radiol. 2009;19(3):770–8.
48. Tan CH, Wang J, Kundra V. Diffusion weighted imaging in prostate cancer. Eur Radiol. 2011;21(3):593–603.
49. Cirillo S, Petracchini M, Della Monica P, et al. Value of endorectal MRI and MRS in patients with elevated prostate-specific antigen levels and previous negative biopsies to localize peripheral zone tumours. Clin Radiol. 2008;63(8):871–9.
50. Tanimoto A, Nakashima J, Kohno H, Shinmoto H, Kuribayashi S. Prostate cancer screening: the clinical value of diffusion-weighted imaging and dynamic MR imaging in combination with T2-weighted imaging. J Magn Reson Imaging. 2007;25(1):146–52.
51. Yoshizako T, Wada A, Hayashi T, et al. Usefulness of diffusion-weighted imaging and dynamic contrast-enhanced magnetic resonance imaging in the diagnosis of prostate transition-zone cancer. Acta Radiol. 2008;49(10):1207–13.
52. Barentsz JO, Richenberg J, Clements R, et al. ESUR prostate MR guidelines 2012. Eur Radiol. 2012;22(4):746–57.
53. Bratan F, Niaf E, Melodelima C, et al. Influence of imaging and histological factors on prostate cancer detection and localisation on multiparametric MRI: a prospective study. Eur Radiol. 2013;23(7):2019–29.
54. Turkbey B, Mani H, Shah V, et al. Multiparametric 3T prostate magnetic resonance imaging to detect cancer: histopathological correlation using prostatectomy specimens processed in customized magnetic resonance imaging based molds. J Urol. 2011;186(5):1818–24.
55. Turkbey B, Pinto PA, Mani H, et al. Prostate cancer: value of multiparametric MR imaging at 3 T for detection--histopathologic correlation. Radiology. 2010;255(1):89–99.
56. Rosenkrantz AB, Mendrinos S, Babb JS, Taneja SS. Prostate cancer foci detected on multiparametric magnetic resonance imaging are histologically distinct from those not detected. J Urol. 2012;187(6):2032–8.
57. Schoots IG, Petrides N, Giganti F, et al. Magnetic resonance imaging in active surveillance of prostate cancer: a systematic review. Eur Urol. 2015;67(4):627–36.
58. van Hove A, Savoie PH, Maurin C, et al. Comparison of image-guided targeted biopsies versus systematic randomized biopsies in the detection of prostate cancer: a systematic literature review of well-designed studies. World J Urol. 2014;32(4):847–58.
59. Valerio M, Donaldson I, Emberton M, et al. Detection of clinically significant prostate cancer using magnetic resonance imaging-ultrasound fusion targeted biopsy: a systematic review. Eur Urol. 2015;68(1):8–19.
60. Panebianco V, Barchetti F, Sciarra A. Multiparametric magnetic resonance imaging vs. standard care in men being evaluated for prostate cancer: a randomized study. Urol Oncol. 2015;33(1):17 e1–7.
61. Baco E, Rud E, Eri LM, et al. A randomized controlled trial to assess and compare the outcomes of two-core prostate biopsy guided by fused magnetic resonance and transrectal ultrasound images and traditional 12-core systematic biopsy. Eur Urol. 2016;69(1):149–56.
62. Park BK, Park JW, Park SY, et al. Prospective evaluation of 3-T MRI performed before initial transrectal ultrasound-guided prostate biopsy in patients with high prostate-specific antigen and no previous biopsy. AJR Am J Roentgenol. 2011;197(5):W876–81.
63. Futterer JJ, Briganti A, De Visschere P, et al. Can clinically significant prostate cancer be detected with multiparametric magnetic resonance imaging? A systematic review of the literature. Eur Urol. 2015;68(6):1045–53.
64. Siddiqui MM, Rais-Bahrami S, Turkbey B, et al. Comparison of MR/ultrasound fusion-guided biopsy with ultrasound-guided biopsy for the diagnosis of prostate cancer. JAMA. 2015;313(4):390–7.
65. Habchi H, Bratan F, Paye A, et al. Value of prostate multiparametric magnetic resonance imaging for predicting biopsy results in first or repeat biopsy. Clin Radiol. 2014;69(3):e120–8.
66. Turkbey B, Mani H, Aras O, et al. Prostate cancer: can multiparametric MR imaging help identify patients who are candidates for active surveillance? Radiology. 2013;268(1):144–52.
67. Rouviere O, Papillard M, Girouin N, et al. Is it possible to model the risk of malignancy of focal abnormalities found at prostate multiparametric MRI? Eur Radiol. 2012;22(5):1149–57.
68. Dickinson L, Ahmed HU, Allen C, et al. Magnetic resonance imaging for the detection, localisation, and characterisation of prostate cancer: recommendations from a European consensus meeting. Eur Urol. 2011;59(4):477–94.
69. Vache T, Bratan F, Mege-Lechevallier F, Roche S, Rabilloud M, Rouviere O. Characterization of prostate lesions as benign or malignant at

multiparametric MR imaging: comparison of three scoring systems in patients treated with radical prostatectomy. Radiology. 2014;272(2):446–55.
70. Costa DN, Lotan Y, Rofsky NM, et al. Assessment of prospectively assigned likert scores for targeted magnetic resonance imaging-transrectal ultrasound fusion biopsies in patients with suspected prostate cancer. J Urol. 2016;195(1):80–7.
71. Renard-Penna R, Mozer P, Cornud F, et al. Prostate imaging reporting and data system and likert scoring system: multiparametric MR imaging validation study to screen patients for initial biopsy. Radiology. 2015;275(2):458–68.
72. Rosenkrantz AB, Lim RP, Haghighi M, Somberg MB, Babb JS, Taneja SS. Comparison of interreader reproducibility of the prostate imaging reporting and data system and likert scales for evaluation of multiparametric prostate MRI. AJR Am J Roentgenol. 2013;201(4):W612–8.
73. Puech P, Rouviere O, Renard-Penna R, et al. Prostate cancer diagnosis: multiparametric MR-targeted biopsy with cognitive and transrectal US-MR fusion guidance versus systematic biopsy--prospective multicenter study. Radiology. 2013;268(2):461–9.
74. Rastinehad AR, Turkbey B, Salami SS, et al. Improving detection of clinically significant prostate cancer: magnetic resonance imaging/transrectal ultrasound fusion guided prostate biopsy. J Urol. 2013;191(6):1749–54.
75. Rosenkrantz AB, Kim S, Lim RP, et al. Prostate cancer localization using multiparametric MR imaging: comparison of prostate imaging reporting and data system (PI-RADS) and likert scales. Radiology. 2013;269(2):482–92.
76. Barentsz JO, Weinreb JC, Verma S, et al. Synopsis of the PI-RADS v2 guidelines for multiparametric prostate magnetic resonance imaging and recommendations for use. Eur Urol. 2016;69(1):41–9.
77. Vargas HA, Hotker AM, Goldman DA, et al. Updated prostate imaging reporting and data system (PIRADS v2) recommendations for the detection of clinically significant prostate cancer using multiparametric MRI: critical evaluation using whole-mount pathology as standard of reference. Eur Radiol. 2015;26(6):1606–12.
78. Muller BG, Shih JH, Sankineni S, et al. Prostate cancer: interobserver agreement and accuracy with the revised prostate imaging reporting and data system at multiparametric MR imaging. Radiology. 2015;277(3):741–50.
79. Niaf E, Lartizien C, Bratan F, et al. Prostate focal peripheral zone lesions: characterization at multiparametric MR imaging--influence of a computer-aided diagnosis system. Radiology. 2014;271(3):761–9.
80. Hambrock T, Vos PC, Hulsbergen-van de Kaa CA, Barentsz JO, Huisman HJ. Prostate cancer: computer-aided diagnosis with multiparametric 3-T MR imaging--effect on observer performance. Radiology. 2013;266(2):521–30.
81. Peng Y, Jiang Y, Antic T, Giger ML, Eggener SE, Oto A. Validation of quantitative analysis of multiparametric prostate MR images for prostate cancer detection and aggressiveness assessment: a cross-imager study. Radiology. 2014;271(2):461–71.
82. Hoang Dinh A, Melodelima C, Souchon R, et al. Quantitative analysis of prostate multiparametric MR images for detection of aggressive prostate cancer in the peripheral zone: a multiple imager study. Radiology. 2016;151406.
83. Baco E, Gelet A, Crouzet S, et al. Hemi salvage high-intensity focused ultrasound (HIFU) in unilateral radiorecurrent prostate cancer: a prospective two-centre study. BJU Int. 2014;114(4):532–40.
84. Donati OF, Jung SI, Vargas HA, et al. Multiparametric prostate MR imaging with T2-weighted, diffusion-weighted, and dynamic contrast-enhanced sequences: are all pulse sequences necessary to detect locally recurrent prostate cancer after radiation therapy? Radiology. 2013;268(2):440–50.
85. Abd-Alazeez M, Ramachandran N, Dikaios N, et al. Multiparametric MRI for detection of radiorecurrent prostate cancer: added value of apparent diffusion coefficient maps and dynamic contrast-enhanced images. Prostate Cancer Prostatic Dis. 2015;18(2):128–36.
86. Alonzo F, Melodelima C, Bratan F, et al. Detection of locally radio-recurrent prostate cancer at multiparametric MRI: can dynamic contrast-enhanced imaging be omitted? Diagn Interv Imaging. 2016;97(4):433–41.
87. Liauw SL, Pitroda SP, Eggener SE, et al. Evaluation of the prostate bed for local recurrence after radical prostatectomy using endorectal magnetic resonance imaging. Int J Radiat Oncol Biol Phys. 2013;85(2):378–84.
88. Linder BJ, Kawashima A, Woodrum DA, et al. Early localization of recurrent prostate cancer after prostatectomy by endorectal coil magnetic resonance imaging. Can J Urol. 2014;21(3):7283–9.
89. Postema A, Mischi M, de la Rosette J, Wijkstra H. Multiparametric ultrasound in the detection of prostate cancer: a systematic review. World J Urol. 2015;33(11):1651–9.
90. Halpern EJ, Strup SE. Using gray-scale and color and power Doppler sonography to detect prostatic cancer. AJR Am J Roentgenol. 2000;174(3):623–7.
91. Taverna G, Morandi G, Seveso M, et al. Colour Doppler and microbubble contrast agent ultrasonography do not improve cancer detection rate in transrectal systematic prostate biopsy sampling. BJU Int. 2011;108(11):1723–7.
92. Braeckman J, Autier P, Soviany C, et al. The accuracy of transrectal ultrasonography supplemented with computer-aided ultrasonography for detecting small prostate cancers. BJU Int. 2008;102(11):1560–5.
93. Schiffmann J, Manka L, Boehm K, et al. Controversial evidence for the use of HistoScanning in the detection of prostate cancer. World J Urol. 2015;33(12):1993–9.
94. Correas JM, Bridal L, Lesavre A, Mejean A, Claudon M, Helenon O. Ultrasound contrast agents:

properties, principles of action, tolerance, and artifacts. Eur Radiol. 2001;11(8):1316–28.
95. Seitz M, Gratzke C, Schlenker B, et al. Contrast-enhanced transrectal ultrasound (CE-TRUS) with cadence-contrast pulse sequence (CPS) technology for the identification of prostate cancer. Urol Oncol. 2011;29(3):295–301.
96. Halpern EJ, McCue PA, Aksnes AK, Hagen EK, Frauscher F, Gomella LG. Contrast-enhanced US of the prostate with Sonazoid: comparison with whole-mount prostatectomy specimens in 12 patients. Radiology. 2002;222(2):361–6.
97. Matsumoto K, Nakagawa K, Hashiguchi A, et al. Contrast-enhanced ultrasonography of the prostate with Sonazoid. Jpn J Clin Oncol. 2010;40(11):1099–104.
98. Li Y, Tang J, Fei X, Gao Y. Diagnostic performance of contrast enhanced ultrasound in patients with prostate cancer: a meta-analysis. Acad Radiol. 2013;20(2):156–64.
99. Postema AW, Frinking PJ, Smeenge M, et al. Dynamic contrast-enhanced ultrasound parametric imaging for the detection of prostate cancer. BJU Int. 2016;117(4):598–603.
100. Zhang B, Ma X, Zhan W, et al. Real-time elastography in the diagnosis of patients suspected of having prostate cancer: a meta-analysis. Ultrasound Med Biol. 2014;40(7):1400–7.
101. Teng J, Chen M, Gao Y, Yao Y, Chen L, Xu D. Transrectal sonoelastography in the detection of prostate cancers: a meta-analysis. BJU Int. 2012;110(11 Pt B):E614–20.
102. Barr RG, Memo R, Schaub CR. Shear wave ultrasound elastography of the prostate: initial results. Ultrasound Q. 2012;28(1):13–20.
103. Ahmad S, Cao R, Varghese T, Bidaut L, Nabi G. Transrectal quantitative shear wave elastography in the detection and characterisation of prostate cancer. Surg Endosc. 2013;27(9):3280–7.
104. Woo S, Kim SY, Cho JY, Kim SH. Shear wave elastography for detection of prostate cancer: a preliminary study. Korean J Radiol. 2014;15(3):346–55.
105. Correas JM, Tissier AM, Khairoune A, et al. Prostate cancer: diagnostic performance of real-time shear-wave elastography. Radiology. 2015;275(1):280–9.
106. Woo S, Kim SY, Lee MS, Cho JY, Kim SH. Shear wave elastography assessment in the prostate: an intraobserver reproducibility study. Clin Imaging. 2015;39(3):484–7.
107. Aigner F, Schafer G, Steiner E, et al. Value of enhanced transrectal ultrasound targeted biopsy for prostate cancer diagnosis: a retrospective data analysis. World J Urol. 2012;30(3):341–6.
108. Nelson ED, Slotoroff CB, Gomella LG, Halpern EJ. Targeted biopsy of the prostate: the impact of color Doppler imaging and elastography on prostate cancer detection and Gleason score. Urology. 2007;70(6):1136–40.
109. Xie SW, Li HL, Du J, et al. Contrast-enhanced ultrasonography with contrast-tuned imaging technology for the detection of prostate cancer: comparison with conventional ultrasonography. BJU Int. 2012;109(11):1620–6.
110. Brock M, Eggert T, Palisaar RJ, et al. Multiparametric ultrasound of the prostate: adding contrast enhanced ultrasound to real-time elastography to detect histopathologically confirmed cancer. J Urol. 2013;189(1):93–8.

Nuclear Medicine (Bone Scan, Choline and PSMA PET/CT)

Karolien E. Goffin and Wouter Everaerts

1 Bone Scan

1.1 Role of Bone Scan in M-Staging of Prostate Cancer

Bone scan (BS) is the most widely used method for evaluating bone metastases of prostate cancer (PCa). Knowledge of the number and the pattern of bone metastases is essential to choose the correct therapy and allow proper evaluation of tumor response. The technique is based on the intravenous administration of bone seeking agents, such as Technetium-99m (^{99m}Tc)-labeled phosphonates – for example, Tc-99m methylene diphosphonate (^{99m}Tc-MDP) – which accumulate in the skeleton relative to the amount of osteoblastic activity. The osteoblastic nature of bone metastases of PCa makes a BS a sensitive technique for M-staging with a mean sensitivity value for planar BS of 79% [29], ranging from 51 to 97% [24, 32, 37, 42, 61, 67]. BS, however, suffer from a relatively low specificity (mean specificity of 59% [29], ranging from 39 to 82% [24, 32, 37, 42, 61, 67]), since also a wide variety of benign lesions, such as fractures and degenerative bone and joint changes [32], will show increased tracer uptake. The low specificity of the BS can be, in a large part, overcome by the combined acquisition of 3D functional information using single photon emission computed tomography (SPECT) and anatomical information using computed tomography (CT). Palmedo and coauthors demonstrated that the specificity to detect bone metastases in a group of 116 patients with primary PCa increased significantly from 79% using only planar BS to 94% using SPECT/CT. The use of SPECT/CT also further increased sensitivity from 93 to 97%. An example of the added value of SPECT/CT in the differential diagnosis of bone metastases is shown in Fig. 1. Furthermore, the authors report major impact on patient management with downstaging of metastatic disease in PCa group using SPECT/CT in 30% of patients. Further diagnostic imaging procedures for unclear scintigraphic findings were necessary in only 2.5% of patients [61]. Hybrid SPECT/CT systems have been implemented over the last years in most nuclear medicine and radiology departments, making SPECT/CT imaging widely available and easily accessible for the large majority of patients.

The diagnostic yield of BS is significantly influenced by PSA level, clinical stage, and Gleason score (GS) [45, 51, 55, 57, 70, 85]. In patients with low risk PCa, the rate of a positive BS is below 1% [51, 57, 85] and it increases to

K.E. Goffin (✉)
Nuclear Medicine, UZ Leuven, Leuven, Belgium
e-mail: karolien.goffin@uzleuven.be

Nuclear Medicine and Molecular Imaging, Department of Imaging and Pathology, KU Leuven, Leuven, Belgium

W. Everaerts
Urology, UZ Leuven, KU Leuven, Leuven, Belgium
e-mail: Wouter.everaerts@uzleuven.be

M. Bolla, H. van Poppel (eds.), *Management of Prostate Cancer*,
DOI 10.1007/978-3-319-42769-0_8

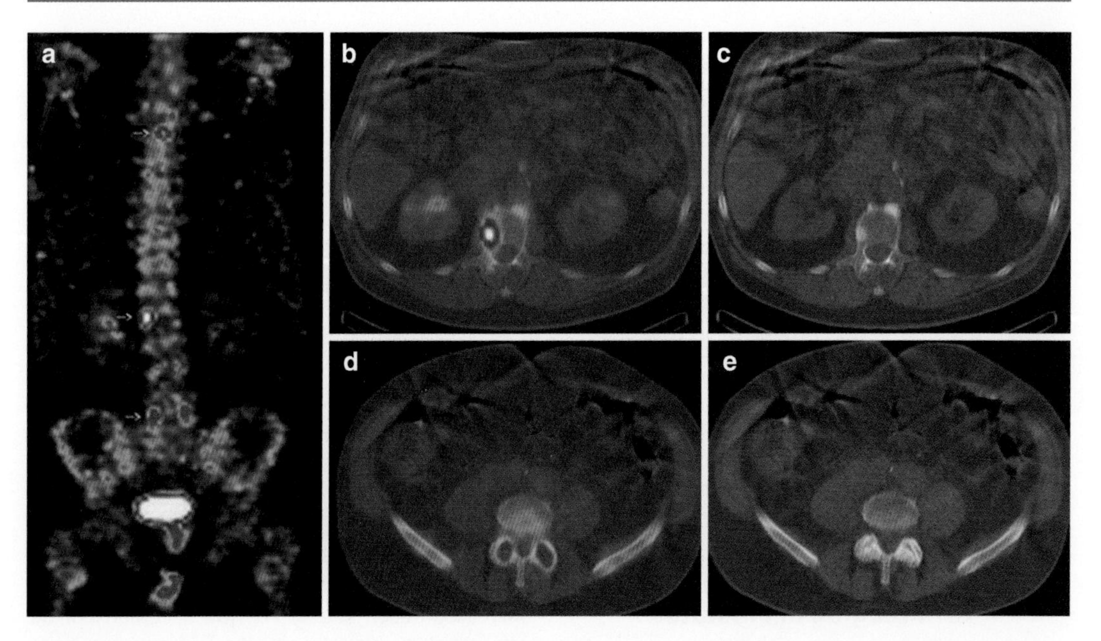

Fig. 1 Imaging in a 61-year-old patient with PCa. (**a**) Wholebody SPECT MIP image shows highly suspicious findings in thoracic vertebra 4, lumbar vertebra 1, and lumbar vertebra 5 (*arrows*). (**b–e**) SPECT-CT (**b**, **d**) and CT (**c**, **e**) show metastatic disease in lumbar vertebra 1 (**b**, **c**), and also confirmed metastatic disease in thoracic vertebra 4 (not shown). Note that metastatic disease in lumbar vertebra 1 can be precisely differentiated from the more ventrally located degenerative changes, as was also the case in thoracic vertebra 4. The lesions in lumbar vertebra 5 are seen as degenerative changes of the smaller intervertebral articulations (**d**, **e**). These images demonstrate that the extent of metastatic disease can be determined by SPECT/CT more exactly than by planar whole-body scintigraphy (Reprinted from Palmedo et al. [61])

7–38 % in patients with PSA levels of 20–50 ng/ml [51, 57]. Likewise, higher detection rates were reported in patients with stage>T3 [12, 55] and GS>8 [51, 55]. Briganti et al. showed in a large patient cohort of 853 patients with primary PCa that PSA at diagnosis, clinical stage (T2/3 vs T1c) and biopsy GS (8–10 vs. 5–6) were independent predictors of the presence of bone metastases in a multivariable logistic regression analysis [12]. Similarly, stratification of patients using the CART model into low-risk (biopsy GS≤7, cT1–T3, PSA <10 ng/ml), intermediate-risk (biopsy GS≤7, cT2/T3, PSA >10 ng/ml), and high-risk (biopsy GS >7) groups gave optimal accuracy for predicting the detection of bone metastases on BS [12].

Taken these data into account, the EAU guidelines for management of PCa state that a BS is required in patients with intermediate-risk PCa with predominantly Gleason pattern 4 and in patients with high-risk localized PCa or high-risk locally advanced PCa [55]. Bone scanning should also be performed in symptomatic patients, independent of PSA level, GS or clinical stage [1].

Apart from ^{99m}Tc-MDP bone scans, bone metastases of PCa can also be visualized using ^{18}F-fluoride positron emission tomography (PET) or PET/CT. As phosphonates, fluoride is taken up by the bone relative to the rate of bone turnover. Compared to conventional BS, ^{18}F-fluoride PET/CT shows superior sensitivity [24, 32, 67]. Poulsen et al. report sensitivity values of 51 and 93 % for BS and ^{18}F-fluoride PET/CT, respectively, in a prospective analysis of 50 men with primary PCa [67]. Uptake values of fluoride in metastatic lesions is significantly higher than in benign degenerative lesions, but values showed a wide variance and overlapping values, reducing the specificity of ^{18}F-fluoride PET/CT [59]. Semiquantitative approaches using a cutoff SUV_{max} value to differentiate degenerative joint disease from bone metastases have shown potential to increase the specificity of ^{18}F-fluoride PET/CT [56]. The availability of ^{18}F-fluoride PET/CT is however much less compared to conventional BS using SPECT/CT, especially in Europe. Moreover, the cost-effectiveness of PET/CT remains to be assessed. BS is therefore still preferred for primary M-staging of PCa on the basis of availability and cost [55].

1.2 Role of Bone Scan in Biochemical Recurrence

After treatment with curative intent (radical prostatectomy (RP) or radiotherapy (RT)), between 27 and 53 % of patients develop PSA-only or 'biochemical' recurrence [55]. The standard workup to detect PCa metastases include BS and abdominopelvic CT. The diagnostic yield of these imaging techniques is however very low in asymptomatic patients, likely due to a very small tumorburden. The probability of a positive BS was less than 5 % at PSA-values below 40 ng/ml [21]. At lower PSA values, PSA doubling time (DT) below 6 months was associated with a slightly higher rate of positive BS (26 % vs. 3 % with PSA DT greater than 6 months) [58]. Similar findings were reported by Gomez and co-authors who found a 33 % positivity rate of BS in patients with biochemical recurrence who had a mean PSA of 30.7 ng/ml [40]. The likelihood of a positive BS in patients with biochemical recurrence depends on PSA slope, PSA velocity, and trigger PSA, in a multivariate analysis: for trigger PSA levels of 10 ng/ml or less, BS was positive in only 4 % of cases [10, 26].

As in primary staging of PCa, ^{18}F-fluoride PET and PET/CT have a higher sensitivity than BS in detecting bone metastases in patients with biochemical recurrence [7]. An example of the improved sensitivity of ^{18}F-fluoride PET/CT in comparison to the BS can be seen in Fig. 2. However, ^{18}F-fluoride is limited by a relative lack of specificity and by the fact that it does not assess soft-tissue metastases [9]. ^{68}Ga-PSMA PET/CT has shown great potential to visualize bone metastases as well as local recurrence, lymph node (LN), and soft tissue metastases in patients with biochemical recurrence, even at very low PSA values [2, 28, 48], but further studies are needed to evaluate this new imaging technique.

In patients with biochemical recurrence, bone scans should performed only in patients with a PSA level >10 ng/mL, or with high PSA kinetics (PSA DT <6 months or a PSA velocity >0.5 ng/mL/month) or in patients with symptoms of bone disease [55].

1.3 Role of Bone Scan in Follow-Up

1.3.1 Follow-Up After Treatment with Curative Intent

Routine BS is not recommended in asymptomatic patients if there are no signs of biochemical relapse. In patients with bone pain or other symptoms of progression, restaging should be considered irrespective of serum PSA level [55].

1.3.2 Follow-Up During Systemic Treatment

The main objectives of imaging follow-up in patients undergoing systemic treatments are monitoring of response to treatment and guidance of modalities of palliative symptomatic treatment at the time of castration-resistant PCa (CRPC) [55]. Asymptomatic patients with a stable PSA level should not undergo imaging at regular intervals [52]. In the case of bone symptoms or PSA progression under castration, a BS might be helpful, if a treatment modification is considered. The Prostate Cancer Clinical Trials Working Group 2 has clarified the definition of BS progression as the appearance of at least two new lesions, later confirmed [72].

Apart from the visual qualitative interpretation of BS in routine clinical practice as well as in the follow-up of novel therapeutic agents in clinical trials, a more quantitative approach can be used by calculation of the BS index (BSI) [43], which offers a reproducible expression of tumor burden seen on BS, expressing it as a percentage of the total skeletal mass. On-treatment changes in BSI are a response indicator, validating the further use of BS as an imaging biomarker in metastatic CRPC [25]. These BSI scores can be generated

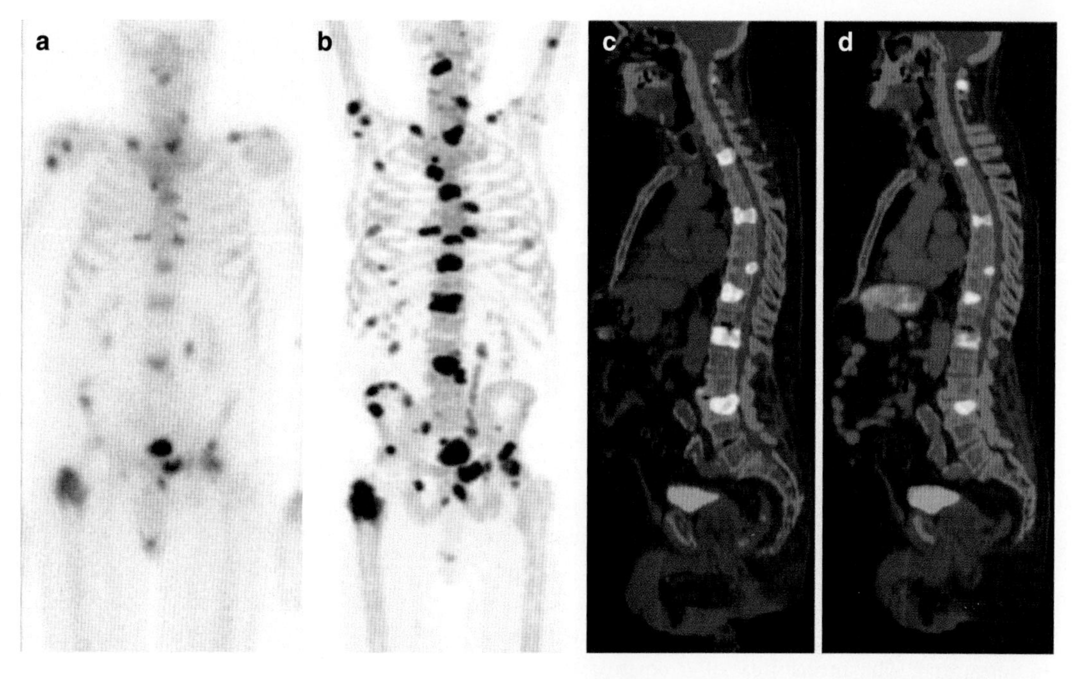

Fig. 2 Images of a patient with GS 7 (4+3) and PSA 77 ng/ml. (**a**) Whole-body bone scintigraphy (WBS) images. (**b**) [^{18}F]-sodium fluoride (NAF)-positron emission tomography (PET) images. WBS detects the major lesions; however, NAF-PET detects additional minor lesions both in the costae, spine, pelvis and extremities. (**c**) NAF PET/CT images. (**d**) [^{18}F]-fluoromethylcholine (FCH)-PET/CT. The detection of bone lesions appear to be similar between the two PET/CT scans; however, when looking at the anterior part of third lumbar vertebra, we find a benign degeneration. On FCH-PET/CT the benign lesion does not appear as a hot spot, whereas it does on NAF-PET/CT (Reprinted from Poulsen et al. [67])

fully automatically, reducing turnaround time and eliminating operator-dependent subjectivity. The technique however remains to be validated in routine clinical practice and clinical trials [79].

2 Choline PET/CT

^{18}F-fluorodeoxyglucose (FDG) PET imaging is a well-established tool in diagnosis, staging and therapy monitoring in many tumor types. PCa however lacks FDG avidity, motivating the development and implementation of alternative metabolic tracers, such as choline-based PET tracers. Increased choline uptake in PCa cells may be explained by increased cell proliferation in tumors and by upregulation of choline kinase in cancer cells. The uptake of radiolabelled choline in PCa therefore represents the rate of tumor cell proliferation [11]. Three choline-based PET tracers are being used, namely, carbon-11 (^{11}C)-choline, ^{18}F-methylcholine, and ^{18}F-ethylcholine. These three radiotracers exhibit a somewhat different biodistribution due to slight chemical differences. Their diagnostic performance is however overall similar [16, 82].

2.1 Role of Choline PET/CT in Primary Staging of PCa

The detection rate of choline PET/CT in primary staging of PCa ranges from 11 to 100 %, depending on the extent of image analysis [30]. When only intraprostatic primary cancer is being evaluated, detection rate varies between 31 and 100 % [8, 83], while lower values are reported when looking at LN metastases (11–93 %) [15, 23] or bone metastases (29 %) [31]. These differences may in part be explained by disease stage and GS. An example of a positive choline PET/CT at primary LN staging is shown in Fig. 3.

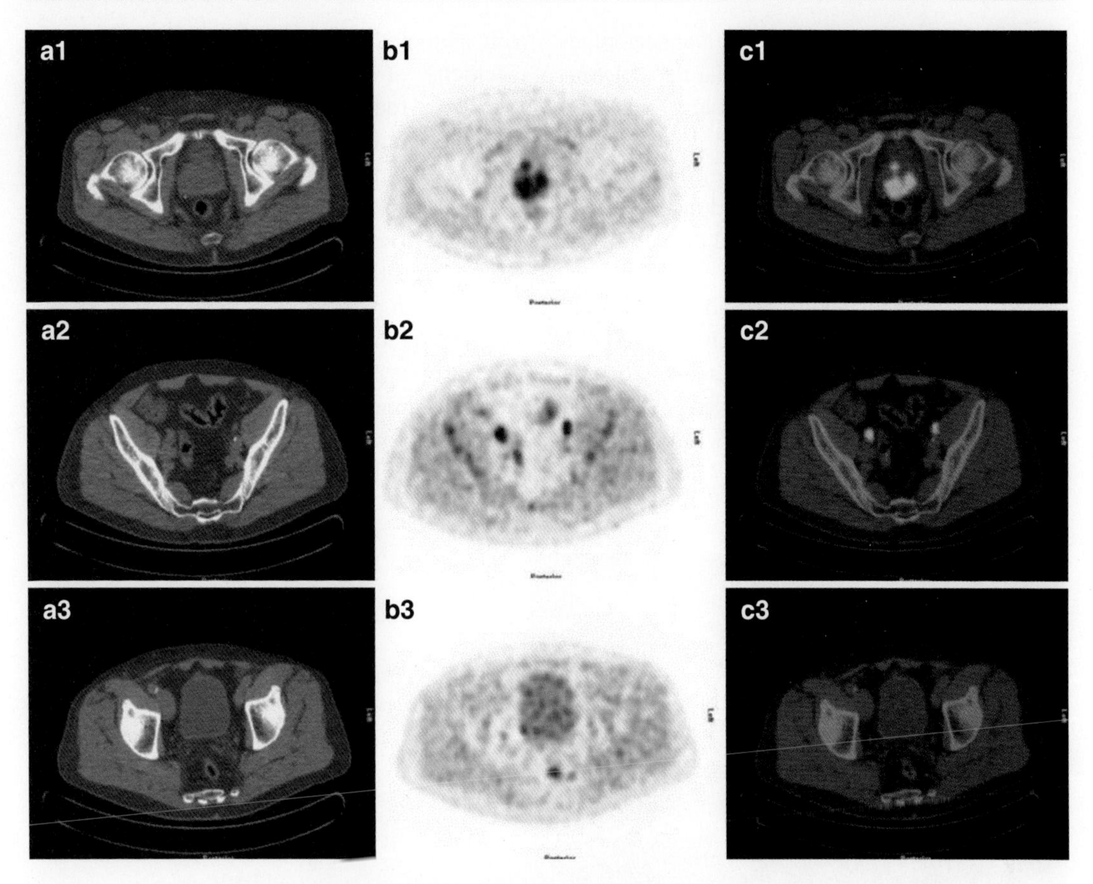

Fig. 3 A 71-year-old patient with biopsy-proven PCa, initial PSA 193 ng/ml, referred for [^{18}F] choline PET/CT for primary staging. [^{18}F] choline PET/CT revealed advanced disease (primary PCa, iliacal and pararectal LN metastases) (**a** 1–3) CT scan, (**b** 1–3) PET scan, (**c** 1–3) PET/CT fused images (Reprinted from Schwarzenböck et al. [74])

Compared to histopathology, choline PET/CT has a pooled sensitivity of 62 % and specificity of 92 % for detection of LN metastases [81], but these values range between 19 and 90 % for sensitivity [15, 23, 41] and between 88and 98 % for specificity [23, 66]. This large variation is related to inhomogeneous populations included in the different studies, with variable numbers of patients with low-, intermediate-, and high-risk PCa as well as the size of metastatic LN (micro-/ macrometastases) and technical factors such as the type of PET camera that was used [30]. In a prospective trial of 75 patients at intermediate risk of nodal involvement, the sensitivity was only 8.2 % in a region-based and 18.9 % in a patient-based analysis [15]. These low sensitivity values were caused by micrometastatic disease that was present in the majority of patients, but could not be visualized using PET-imaging at that time.

Due to the large reported variability in detection rate, sensitivity, and specificity among different studies and the lack of accurate visualization of micrometastatic disease, choline PET/CT should not be used for up-front staging of PCa at present [55].

2.2 Role of Choline PET/CT in Biochemical Recurrence

As in the setting of primary staging, accuracy of choline PET/CT remains difficult to assess in patients with biochemical recurrence because most studies are retrospective, evaluate heterogeneous populations, use nonstandardized definitions of biochemical failure, and are limited by the lack of a reliable histological gold standard [55]. Furthermore, results may be reported on a per-patient or per-lesion basis and may combine detection of local recurrences and distant metastases [13].

In a recent meta-analysis including over 2000 patients, pooled detection rate of choline PET/CT was 62 % [33]. Pooled overall sensitivity and specificity could be calculated in over 1000 patients and was 89 % and 89 %, respectively. Local relapse was detected in 27 % of patients with a pooled sensitivity of 61 % and pooled specificity of 97 %. Similar pooled detection rates were found for nodal disease (36 %) and bone metastases (25 %) [33]. An example of a positive choline PET/CT in a patient with biochemical recurrence after RP is shown in Fig. 4. Compared to conventional BS, choline PET/CT is more sensitive and can detect multiple bone metastases in patients showing a single metastasis on BS [36] and may be positive for bone metastases in up to 15 % of patients with biochemical failure after RP and negative BS [35]. The specificity of choline PET/CT is also higher than that of BS with less false positive and

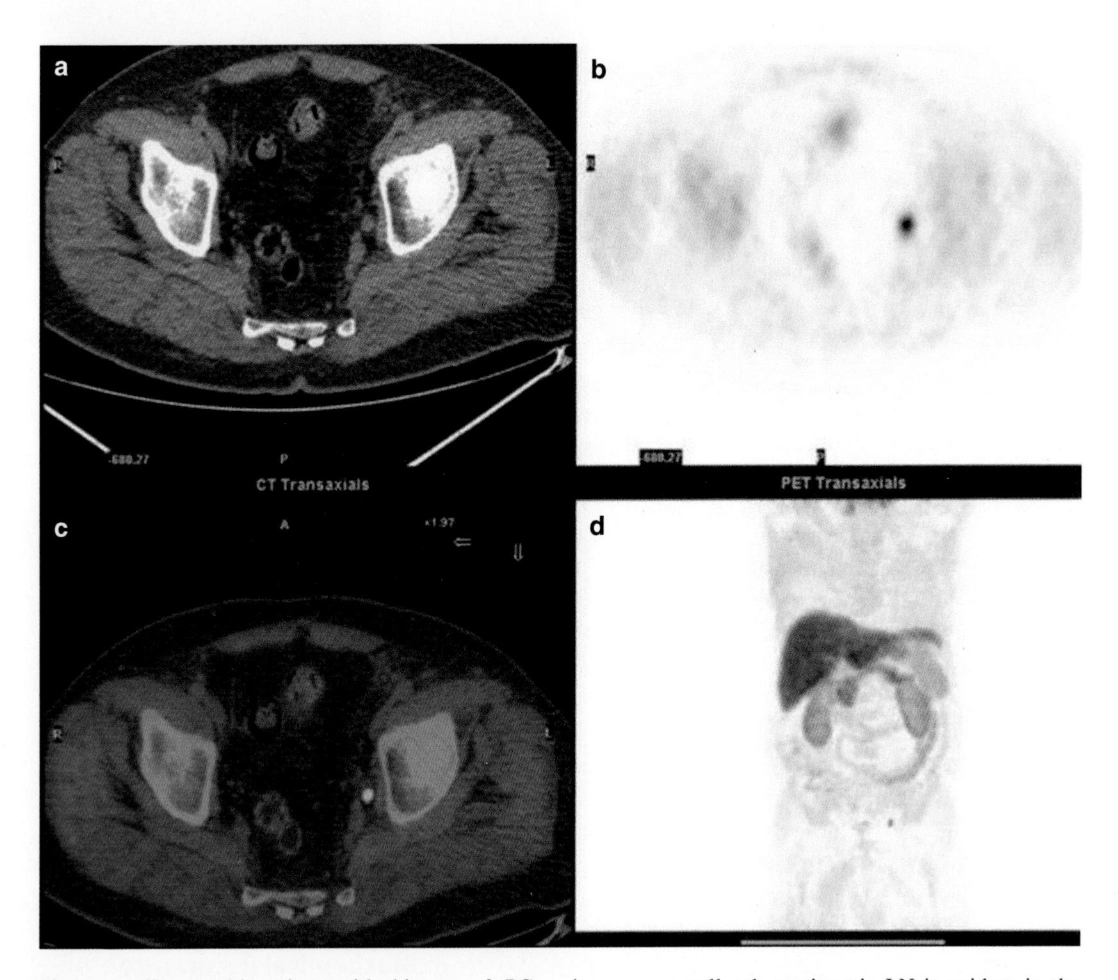

Fig. 4 A 68-year-old patient with history of PCa (T3aN1Mx). Biochemical relapse 2 years after RP. PSA = 1.3 ng/ml at the time of ^{11}C-Choline PET/CT. PSA DT = 3 months. ^{11}C-Choline PET/CT detected a single positive LN in the left iliac chain. (**a**) CT images, a small sub-centimetric LN is evident in the left iliac chain; (**b**) focal increased uptake of ^{11}C-Choline in the left iliac chain; (**c**) fused images; (**d**) MIP (Reprinted from Picchio et al. [65])

indeterminate findings [7, 9, 55]. An example of the improved sensitivity and specificity of choline PET/CT to detect bone metastases compared to BS and ^{18}F-fluoride PET/CT is shown in Fig. 2.

A number of studies have evaluated the role of choline PET/CT in LN staging in patients with biochemical failure after primary treatment, using LN dissection and histology as gold standard. Scattoni et al. performed either bilateral pelvic or both pelvic and retroperitoneal LN dissection in 21 patients with biochemical recurrence (median PSA 1.98 ng/ml), based on evidence of LN metastases on a choline PET/CT scan. About 90 % of patients with positive choline PET/CT had LN metastases at histologic evaluation. A lesion-based analysis showed that choline PET/CT had a sensitivity of 64 % and specificity of 90 %. Interestingly, the mean maximum diameter of true positive metastases was significantly larger than of false-negative ones (15.0 vs. 6.3 mm) [71]. The low sensitivity was mainly caused by the lack of detection of LN micro-metastases. Other authors, however, report much lower specificity values of below 30 % [60] with false-positive rates of 30–50 % [60, 68, 73].

It has been established extensively that the detection rate of choline PET/CT depends strongly on PSA value at the time of scanning as well as on PSA kinetics: detection rate is reported to be >50 % at a PSA level of 2 ng/ml, while it falls to <30 % at PSA levels <1 ng/ml [30]. Independent of PSA values, the detection rate of choline PET/CT is higher in case of high PSA velocity (>5 ng/ml/year) and short PSA DT (<2 or 3 months) [30]. In a recent meta-analysis, the overall pooled choline PET/CT detection rate in restaging PCa was 58 %, which increased to 65 % when PSA DT was ≤6 months and to 71 and 77 % when PSA velocity was >1 or >2 ng/(ml year), respectively. PSA DT of ≤6 months and PSA velocity >1 or >2 ng/(ml year) proved to be relevant factors in predicting the positive result of choline PET/CT [78]. Apart from PSA and PSA kinetics, also a high GS of the primary PCa (≥8) is an independent predictive variable for a positive PET/CT scan, even for low PSA levels (<1 ng/ml; detection rate: 47 %) [22]. Clinical stage at initial diagnosis of PCa [53] and ongoing androgen deprivation therapy (ADT) [18] are significant predictors of positive choline PET/CT. Due to its high cost, PET/CT cannot be recommended in all patients with PSA relapse. After RP, the optimal PSA cutoff level seems to be between 1 and 2 ng/ml [55]. After RT, the PSA cutoff level is unclear due to the lack of sufficient data and because the PSA level is more difficult to interpret due to the "physiological" amount of measurable PSA produced by the non-tumoral prostate [17, 55].

Despite these limitations, choline PET/CT has an important impact on medical management of patients with biochemical failure after primary treatment. In a retrospective analysis, 32 % of choline PET/CT scans were deemed clinically useful as defined by the ability to identify lesions not delineated using conventional imaging, thereby prompting changes in clinical management [53]. Soyka and coauthors reported a change in treatment plan due to choline PET/CT in 48 % of patients (mainly a change from palliative treatment to treatment with curative intent) [76]. Another retrospective study in 150 patients with biochemical recurrence confirmed these findings: changes in therapy after choline PET/CT were implemented in 47 % of patients, with major clinical impact in 39 % and minor clinical impact in 61 % [18]

2.3 Role of Choline PET/CT in Guiding Salvage Therapy

As choline PET/CT is able to detect metastatic disease quite accurately, it has been used to guide tailored therapies in selected patients, particularly in those showing few metastatic sites detected by choline PET/CT, i.e., oligometastatic disease.

Salvage LN dissection is a possibly curative approach in patients with LN metastases only, as detected on imaging. Scattoni et al. reported nodal involvement at histological evaluation in 90 % in patients with a positive choline PET/CT. None of the patients with a negative preoperative choline PET/CT had nodal metastases at histology. Patient-based sensitivity, specificity, positive predictive value (PPV), negative predictive value (NPV) and accuracy were therefore 64 %, 90 %, 86 %, 72 %, and 77 %, respectively [71]. Tilke et al. performed a lesion- and site-based analysis in 56 patients with positive choline PET/CT findings that underwent salvage LN dissection. LN metastases were confirmed by histology in 86 % of patients. The lesion-based analysis yielded a sensitivity, specificity, PPV and NPV of 40 %, 96 %, 76 % and 83 %, respectively. A site-based analysis yielded sensitivity, specificity, PPV and NPV of 68 %, 73 %, 81 % and 58 %, respectively. These results show that a positive choline PET/CT correctly predicts the presence of LN metastases in the majority of PCa patients with biochemical failure after RP but does not allow for localization of all metastatic LN and therefore underestimates the extent of nodal recurrence in these patients [77]. Karnes et al. applied salvage LN dissection in patients with biochemical recurrence and nodal disease detected by choline PET/CT and described good outcome results after 20 months: 58 % of patients had PSA remain less than 0.2 ng/ml, 75 % remained free of systemic progression and 96 % of the men were alive. Three-year biochemical recurrence-free, systemic progression-free, and cancer-specific survival were 46 %, 47 %, and 93 %, respectively [46]

Salvage RT of the prostatic fossa after RP has to be tailored to the patients recurrent disease: higher doses to the prostatic bed are given when local recurrence can be detected using imaging [4, 5, 75], likewise pelvic LN can be boosted to doses >60 Gy when they are suspect for malignancy based on imaging [44, 64, 84]. Indeed, choline PET/CT was found to change the extent of planning target volume (PTV) in 37 patients: 30 % of patients had a positive finding on choline PET/CT that was located outside of the prostatic fossa in 13 % of patients, causing an increase in PTV [75]. Very recently, Fodor and co-workers performed choline PET/CT-guided helical tomotherapy (HTT) of LN relapses in 81 patients with biochemical recurrence after surgery ± adjuvant/salvage RT or radical RT. With a median follow-up of 36 months, 91 % of patients presented a PSA reduction 3 months after HTT. The 3-year overall, local-relapse-free and clinical-relapse-free survival were 80 %, 90 %, and 62 %, respectively [34].

3 PSMA PET/CT

Prostate-specific membrane antigen (PSMA) is a transmembrane, 750 amino acid type II glycoprotein which is primarily expressed in normal human prostate epithelium but is upregulated in PCa, including metastatic disease. Since PSMA is expressed by virtually all PCa and its expression is further increased in poorly differentiated, metastatic and hormone-refractory PCa [38, 47], it is a very attractive target for diagnosis and staging and treatment of this disease. While malignant prostatic tissue exhibits high PSMA expression that is directly related to tumor aggressiveness [62], the presence of PSMA has also been detected in renal proximal tubules, in cells of the intestinal brush-border membrane, in rare cells in the colonic crypts, in brain, salivary glands [47] and in the neovasculature of non-prostatic, solid carcinomas (e.g., renal cell, breast, colon, pancreas, melanoma, and lung carcinoma) [19]. Its expression level is however about 1000-fold higher in PCa compared to physiologic levels found in these other tissues [38]. Recently, new PSMA-targeted imaging agents, including both new antibodies with improved imaging characteristics and small-molecule inhibitors of PSMA have been developed and extensively studied. Many of these agents are labeled with PET-radionuclides, such as fluorine-18 (^{18}F) and gallium-68 (^{68}Ga). The most frequently used PSMA-radiotracer is PSMA-HBED-CC (PSMA-11) that has been developed by the Heidelberg group [27]. Since its publication, ^{68}Ga-PSMA PET imaging has been implemented very rapidly in many nuclear medicine departments, mainly in Europe, replacing choline PET/CT imaging in the setting of biochemical recurrence. ^{68}Ga is an attractive radionuclide for PET imaging since it is produced by a tabletop ^{68}Ge/^{68}Ga generator, not requiring a cyclotron. Very recently, also a number of ^{18}F-labeled agents have been developed, of which ^{18}F-DCFPyL shows the best potential [20, 69].

3.1 PSMA PET/CT in Primary Lymph Node Staging

As described above, choline PET imaging for LN staging of patients with primary PCa is hampered by a moderate sensitivity and is therefore not recommended by current guidelines [55]. The use of PSMA PET imaging may overcome this limitation, although the findings of studies so far are somewhat contradictory. Two retrospective analyses reported sensitivities of 33 % and 66 %, and specificities of 100 % and 99 %, respectively, to detect LN metastases at patient level with histology as gold standard [14, 50]. The patients with tumor-positive LN that were missed by PSMA PET presented with PSMA-negative primary tumors or had micrometastases in single LN. Very recently, van Leeuwen et al. reported the first prospective results of primary LN staging in 30 patients with mainly high risk PCa and found a patient-based sensitivity of 64 %, specificity of 95 %, PPV of 88 % and NPV of 82 %. In a region-based analysis, sensitivity dropped to 56 %, while specificity remained high (98 %) [80]. Although these initial findings are promising, further research is needed before drawing robust conclusions. Also intraoperative guidance with PSMA ligands could be an important application of these agents in primary disease staging.

3.2 PSMA PET/CT in Staging of Recurrence PCa

In 2015, 2 large retrospective studies were published on the accuracy of PSMA PET/CT in restaging of patients with biochemical recurrence. Afshar-Oromieh et al. analyzed 319 patients and found at least one lesion suggestive of PCa in 83 % of cases [2]. Eiber et al. studied 248 patients after RP and report a detection rate of 90 % [28]. In both studies, detection rates were positively correlated to serum PSA levels: detection rates of ~50 and 58 % for PSA values <0.5 ng/ml and 58 and 73 % for PSA values from 0.5 to 1 ng/ml [2, 28]. Correlations between detection rate and other factors such as PSA DT, PSA velocity, initial GS and ongoing ADT are however not consistent between studies.

Morigi et al. compared PSMA PET/CT to choline PET/CT in 38 patients with biochemical recurrence and report higher detection rates of PSMA than of choline PET/CT at all ranges of PSA (overall 66 % vs. 32 %), with the difference being the most pronounced at PSA values below 0.5 ng/ml (50 % vs 12 %) [54]. Moreover, PSMA PET/CT had a higher overall impact on patient management. An example of the superior accuracy of PSMA PET/CT is shown in Fig. 5. Pfister et al. compared choline to PSMA PET in 38 and 28 patients, respectively, prior to salvage pelvic and/or retroperitoneal lymphadenectomy. They demonstrated a higher positive predictive value of PSMA (82 %) compared to choline imaging (79 %) in a patient based analysis. Also on a node basis, PSMA performed better than choline with higher negative predictive value (97 % vs. 89 %) and accuracy (92 % vs 82 %) [63]. Also when compared to 3D volumetric CT, PSMA PET is clearly superior: two thirds of patients with LN identified by PET were negative on contrast enhanced CT [39]. Rowe et al. prospectively compared ^{18}F-DCFPyL PET/CT to conventional imaging in 8 patients with evidence of metastatic PCa on conventional imaging, detecting 139 sites of PET positive ^{18}F-DCFPyL uptake suspect for metastatic disease, while conventional imaging only detected 45 lesions, implying that PSMA PET imaging detects a large number of suspected sites of PCa that are occult on conventional imaging [69] (Fig. 6).

Although the results of these studies are promising, especially systematic histological confirmation is still lacking. Nevertheless, rapid spread of this new technology has been observed in countries where application of PSMA-ligands for imaging is permitted, replacing choline imaging

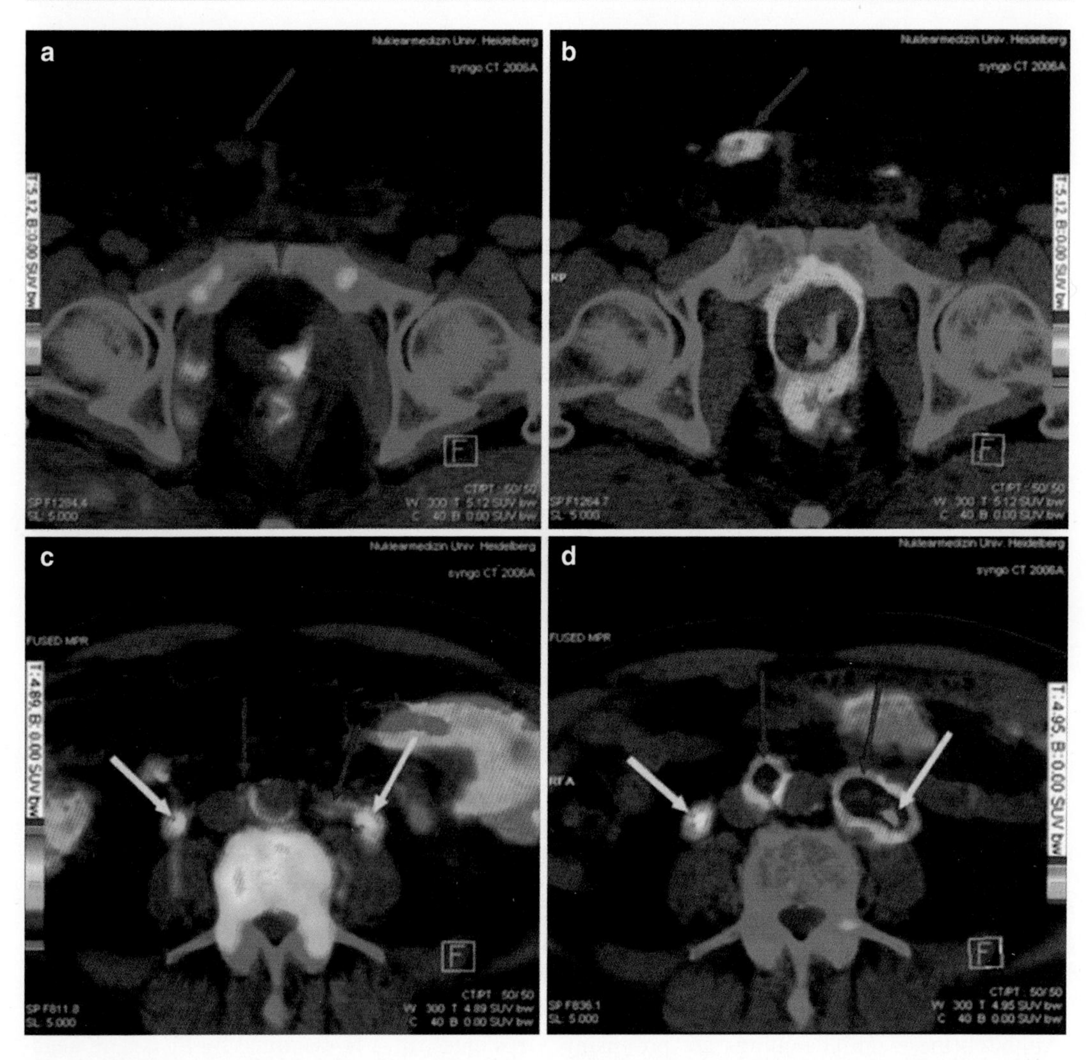

Fig. 5 Patient 1 (**a**, **b**) and patient 2 (**c**, **d**). *Red arrows* point to a nodular pelvic wall metastasis (**a**, **b**, histologically confirmed) and to small lymph nodes (**c**, **d**) which present with clearly pathological tracer uptake in ^{68}GaPSMA PET/CT (**b**, **d**) only. *Yellow arrows* point to both catheterized ureters (**c**, **d**). Patient 1 presented with a minimal PSA value (0.01 ng/ml) despite visible tumor lesions. The PSMA ligand is therefore able to detect low differentiated PC. (**a**, **c**) Fusion of ^{18}F-fluoromethylcholine PET and CT, (**b**, **d**) fusion of ^{68}Ga-PSMA PET and CT. Color scales as automatically produced by the PET/CT machine (Reprinted from Afshar-Oromieh et al. [3])

in patients with biochemical recurrence. Currently, PSMA-based imaging is however not globally available, mainly owing to regulatory issues [49].

Novel application of PSMA PET imaging could be the identification of patients with oligometastatic disease that are suitable for PSMA-radioguided surgery [49]. The high uptake of PSMA-inhibitors in CRPC means that these ligands are also good candidates for facilitating guided endo-radiotherapy in patients with metastatic PCa, such as ^{177}Lu-PSMA therapy [6]. Hereby, PSMA inhibitors could potentially be used as theranostic agents in patients with metastasic PCa, to visualize and treat these lesions at the same time.

Conclusions

Bone scan is still an important staging tool to detect bone metastases in patients with primary intermediate or high risk PCa, due to its high sensitivity, low price and wide availability. The implementation of hybrid SPECT/CT systems improves the specificity of this technique and reduces the number of additional exams due to inconclusive bone scan findings.

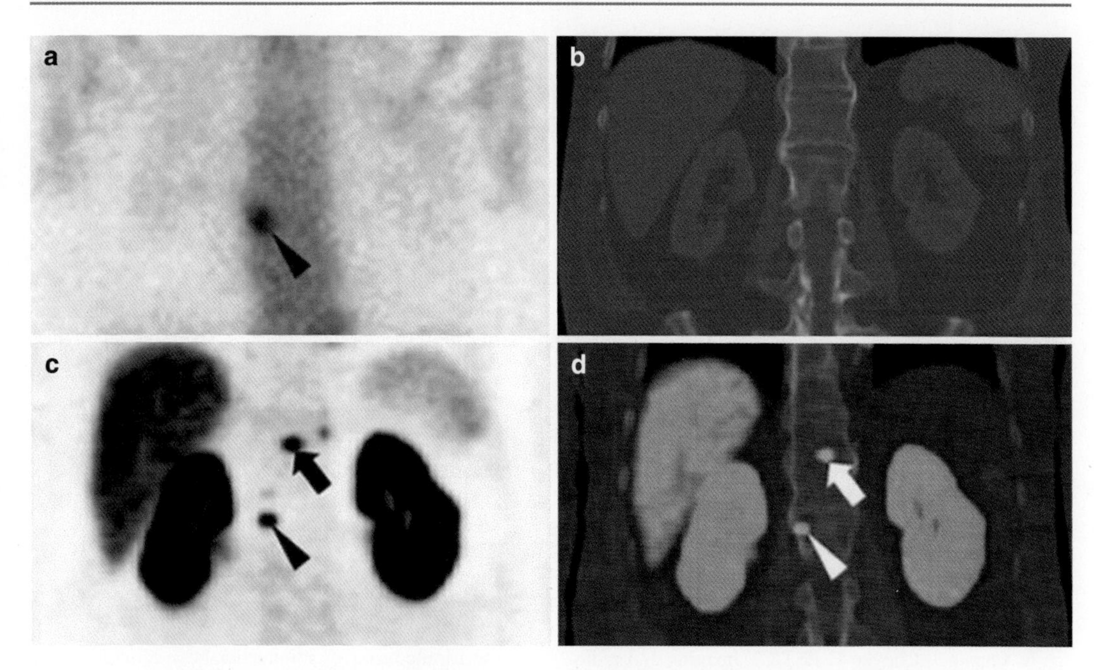

Fig. 6 (**a**) Anterior planar bone scan; (**b**) coronal contrast enhanced CT; (**c**) coronal [^{18}F] DCFPyL PET; and (**d**) coronal [^{18}F] DCFPyL PET/CT images from a patient with multiple sites of presumed metastatic disease. Uptake in the left anterior L2 vertebral body (*arrowheads*) is clearly visible on [^{18}F] DCFPyL PET and BS but occult on CT. An additional site of uptake seen on [^{18}F] DCFPyL PET in T12 vertebral body (*arrows*) is not seen on BS or CECT. Of note, there is also subtle [^{18}F] DCFPyL PET uptake also seen in L1 and in a small retrocrural lymph node (Reprinted from Rowe et al. [69])

^{18}F fluoride PET is more sensitive, but also lacks specificity and is not as widely available. Choline PET/CT is not recommended for primary LN staging but is a very useful imaging technique in patients with biochemical recurrence, guiding salvage treatments. In this setting, PSMA-based PET imaging has however shown clear superiority and a greater impact on patient management, but large homogenous patient series with histological validation are still lacking. PSMA PET imaging may also proof useful in primary LN staging and to guide salvage treatment or radionuclide therapy in patients with metastatic PCa.

References

1. Abuzallouf S, Dayes I, Lukka H. Baseline staging of newly diagnosed prostate cancer: a summary of the literature. J Urol. 2004;171:2122–7.
2. Afshar-Oromieh A, Avtzi E, Giesel FL, Holland-Letz T, Linhart HG, Eder M, Eisenhut M, Boxler S, Hadaschik BA, Kratochwil C, Weichert W, Kopka K, Debus J, Haberkorn U. The diagnostic value of PET/CT imaging with the (68)Ga-labelled PSMA ligand HBED-CC in the diagnosis of recurrent prostate cancer. Eur J Nucl Med Mol Imaging. 2015;42:197–209.
3. Afshar-Oromieh A, Zechmann CM, Malcher A, Eder M, Eisenhut M, Linhart HG, Holland-Letz T, Hadaschik BA, Giesel FL, Debus J, Haberkorn U. Comparison of PET imaging with a 68Ga-labelled PSMA ligand and 18F-choline-based PET/CT for the diagnosis of recurrent prostate cancer. Eur J Nucl Med Mol Imaging. 2014;41:11–20.
4. Alongi F, Comito T, Villa E, Lopci E, Cristina I, Mancosu P, Navarria P, Liardo RL, Tomatis S, Chiti A, Scorsetti M. What is the role of [11C]choline PET/CT in decision making strategy before post-operative salvage radiation therapy in prostate cancer patients? Acta Oncol. 2014;53:990–2.
5. Alongi F, Liardo RL, Iftode C, Lopci E, Villa E, Comito T, Tozzi A, Navarria P, Ascolese AM, Mancosu P, Tomatis S, Bellorofonte C, Arturo C, Scorsetti M. 11C choline PET guided salvage radiotherapy with volumetric modulation arc therapy and hypofractionation for recurrent prostate cancer after HIFU failure: preliminary results of tolerability and acute toxicity. Technol Cancer Res Treat. 2014;13:395–401.
6. Baum RP, Kulkarni HR, Schuchardt C, Singh A, Wirtz M, Wiessalla S, Schottelius M, Mueller D, Klette I, Wester HJ. Lutetium-177 PSMA radioligand

therapy of metastatic castration-resistant prostate cancer: safety and efficacy. J Nucl Med. 2016;57:1006.
7. Beer AJ, Eiber M, Souvatzoglou M, Schwaiger M, Krause BJ. Radionuclide and hybrid imaging of recurrent prostate cancer. Lancet Oncol. 2011;12:181–91.
8. Beheshti M, Imamovic L, Broinger G, Vali R, Waldenberger P, Stoiber F, Nader M, Gruy B, Janetschek G, Langsteger W. 18F choline PET/CT in the preoperative staging of prostate cancer in patients with intermediate or high risk of extracapsular disease: a prospective study of 130 patients. Radiology. 2010;254:925–33.
9. Beheshti M, Vali R, Waldenberger P, Fitz F, Nader M, Loidl W, Broinger G, Stoiber F, Foglman I, Langsteger W. Detection of bone metastases in patients with prostate cancer by 18F fluorocholine and 18F fluoride PET-CT: a comparative study. Eur J Nucl Med Mol Imaging. 2008;35:1766–74.
10. Beresford MJ, Gillatt D, Benson RJ, Ajithkumar T. A systematic review of the role of imaging before salvage radiotherapy for post-prostatectomy biochemical recurrence. Clin Oncol (R Coll Radiol). 2010;22:46–55.
11. Bouchelouche K, Tagawa ST, Goldsmith SJ, Turkbey B, Capala J, Choyke P. PET/CT imaging and radioimmunotherapy of prostate cancer. Semin Nucl Med. 2011;41:29–44.
12. Briganti A, Passoni N, Ferrari M, Capitanio U, Suardi N, Gallina A, DA Pozzo LF, Picchio M, DI Girolamo V, Salonia A, Gianolli L, Messa C, Rigatti P, Montorsi F. When to perform bone scan in patients with newly diagnosed prostate cancer: external validation of the currently available guidelines and proposal of a novel risk stratification tool. Eur Urol. 2010;57:551–8.
13. Brogsitter C, Zophel K, Kotzerke J. 18F-Choline, 11C-choline and 11C-acetate PET/CT: comparative analysis for imaging prostate cancer patients. Eur J Nucl Med Mol Imaging. 2013;40 Suppl 1:S18–27.
14. Budaus L, Leyh-Bannurah SR, Salomon G, Michl U, Heinzer H, Huland H, Graefen M, Steuber T, Rosenbaum C. Initial experience of (68)Ga-PSMA PET/CT imaging in high-risk prostate cancer patients prior to radical prostatectomy. Eur Urol. 2016;69:393–6.
15. Budiharto T, Joniau S, Lerut E, Van Den Bergh L, Mottaghy F, Deroose CM, Oyen R, Ameye F, Bogaerts K, Haustermans K, Van Poppel H. Prospective evaluation of 11C-choline positron emission tomography/computed tomography and diffusion-weighted magnetic resonance imaging for the nodal staging of prostate cancer with a high risk of lymph node metastases. Eur Urol. 2011;60:125–30.
16. Calabria F, Gallo G, Schillaci O, Cascini GL. Biodistribution, imaging protocols and diagnostic accuracy of PET with tracers of lipogenesis in imaging prostate cancer: a comparison between 11C-choline, 18FFluoroethylcholine and 18F-methylcholine. Curr Pharm Des. 2015;21:4738–47.
17. Calabria F, Rubello D, Schillaci O. The optimal timing to perform 18F/11C-choline PET/CT in patients with suspicion of relapse of prostate cancer: trigger PSA versus PSA velocity and PSA doubling time. Int J Biol Markers. 2014;29:e423–30.
18. Ceci F, Herrmann K, Castellucci P, Graziani T, Bluemel C, Schiavina R, Vollmer C, Droll S, Brunocilla E, Mazzarotto R, Buck AK, Fanti S. Impact of 11C-choline PET/CT on clinical decision making in recurrent prostate cancer: results from a retrospective two-centre trial. Eur J Nucl Med Mol Imaging. 2014;41:2222–31.
19. Chang SS, Reuter VE, Heston WD, Bander NH, Grauer LS, Gaudin PB. Five different anti-prostate-specific membrane antigen (PSMA) antibodies confirm PSMA expression in tumor-associated neovasculature. Cancer Res. 1999;59:3192–8.
20. Chen Y, Pullambhatla M, Foss CA, Byun Y, Nimmagadda S, Senthamizhchelvan S, Sgouros G, Mease RC, Pomper MG. 2-(3-{1-Carboxy-5-[(6-[18F]fluoro-pyridine-3-carbonyl)-amino]-pentyl}-ureido)-pen tanedioic acid, [18F]DCFPyL, a PSMA-based PET imaging agent for prostate cancer. Clin Cancer Res. 2011;17:7645–53.
21. Cher ML, Bianco Jr FJ, Lam JS, Davis LP, Grignon DJ, Sakr WA, Banerjee M, Pontes JE, Wood Jr DP. Limited role of radionuclide bone scintigraphy in patients with prostate specific antigen elevations after radical prostatectomy. J Urol. 1998;160:1387–91.
22. Cimitan M, Evangelista L, Hodolic M, Mariani G, Baseric T, Bodanza V, Saladini G, Volterrani D, Cervino AR, Gregianin M, Puccini G, Guidoccio F, Fettich J, Borsatti E. Gleason score at diagnosis predicts the rate of detection of 18F-choline PET/CT performed when biochemical evidence indicates recurrence of prostate cancer: experience with 1,000 patients. J Nucl Med. 2015;56:209–15.
23. Contractor K, Challapalli A, Barwick T, Winkler M, Hellawell G, Hazell S, Tomasi G, Al-Nahhas A, Mapelli P, Kenny LM, Tadrous P, Coombes RC, Aboagye EO, Mangar S. Use of [11C]choline PET-CT as a noninvasive method for detecting pelvic lymph node status from prostate cancer and relationship with choline kinase expression. Clin Cancer Res. 2011;17:7673–83.
24. Damle NA, Bal C, Bandopadhyaya GP, Kumar L, Kumar P, Malhotra A, Lata S. The role of 18F-fluoride PET-CT in the detection of bone metastases in patients with breast, lung and prostate carcinoma: a comparison with FDG PET/CT and 99mTc-MDP bone scan. Jpn J Radiol. 2013;31:262–9.
25. Dennis ER, Jia X, Mezheritskiy IS, Stephenson RD, Schoder H, Fox JJ, Heller G, Scher HI, Larson SM, Morris MJ. Bone scan index: a quantitative treatment response biomarker for castration-resistant metastatic prostate cancer. J Clin Oncol. 2012;30:519–24.
26. Dotan ZA, Bianco Jr FJ, Rabbani F, Eastham JA, Fearn P, Scher HI, Kelly KW, Chen HN, Schoder H, Hricak H, Scardino PT, Kattan MW. Pattern of prostate-specific antigen (PSA) failure dictates the probability of a positive bone scan in patients with an increasing PSA after radical prostatectomy. J Clin Oncol. 2005;23:1962–8.

27. Eder M, Schafer M, Bauder-Wust U, Hull WE, Wangler C, Mier W, Haberkorn U, Eisenhut M. 68Ga-complex lipophilicity and the targeting property of a urea-based PSMA inhibitor for PET imaging. Bioconjug Chem. 2012;23:688–97.
28. Eiber M, Maurer T, Souvatzoglou M, Beer AJ, Ruffani A, Haller B, Graner FP, Kubler H, Haberhorn U, Eisenhut M, Wester HJ, Gschwend JE, Schwaiger M. Evaluation of hybrid 68Ga-PSMA ligand PET/CT in 248 patients with biochemical recurrence after radical prostatectomy. J Nucl Med. 2015;56:668–74.
29. Evangelista L, Bertoldo F, Boccardo F, Conti G, Menchi I, Mungai F, Ricardi U, Bombardieri E. Diagnostic imaging to detect and evaluate response to therapy in bone metastases from prostate cancer: current modalities and new horizons. Eur J Nucl Med Mol Imaging. 2016;43:1546.
30. Evangelista L, Briganti A, Fanti S, Joniau S, Reske S, Schiavina R, Stief C, Thalmann GN, Picchio M. New clinical indications for F/C-choline, new tracers for positron emission tomography and a promising hybrid device for prostate cancer staging: a systematic review of the literature. Eur Urol. 2016;70:161.
31. Evangelista L, Cimitan M, Zattoni F, Guttilla A, Saladini G. Comparison between conventional imaging (abdominal-pelvic computed tomography and bone scan) and [(18)F]choline positron emission tomography/computed tomography imaging for the initial staging of patients with intermediate- tohigh-risk prostate cancer: a retrospective analysis. Scand J Urol. 2015;49:345–53.
32. Even-Sapir E, Metser U, Mishani E, Lievshitz G, Lerman H, Leibovitch I. The detection of bone metastases in patients with high-risk prostate cancer: 99mTc-MDP Planar bone scintigraphy, single- and multi-field-of-view SPECT, 18F-fluoride PET, and 18F-fluoride PET/CT. J Nucl Med. 2006;47:287–97.
33. Fanti S, Minozzi S, Castellucci P, Balduzzi S, Herrmann K, Krause BJ, Oyen W, Chiti A. PET/CT with (11)C-choline for evaluation of prostate cancer patients with biochemical recurrence: meta-analysis and critical review of available data. Eur J Nucl Med Mol Imaging. 2016;43:55–69.
34. Fodor A, Berardi G, Fiorino C, Picchio M, Busnardo E, Kirienko M, Incerti E, Dell'oca I, Cozzarini C, Mangili P, Pasetti M, Calandrino R, Gianolli L, DI Muzio NG. Toxicity and efficacy of salvage 11C-Choline PET/CT-guided radiation therapy in patients with prostate cancer lymph nodal recurrence. BJU Int. 2016. doi:10.1111/bju.13510.
35. Fuccio C, Castellucci P, Schiavina R, Guidalotti PL, Gavaruzzi G, Montini GC, Nanni C, Marzola MC, Rubello D, Fanti S. Role of 11C-choline PET/CT in the re-staging of prostate cancer patients with biochemical relapse and negative results at bone scintigraphy. Eur J Radiol. 2012;81:e893–6.
36. Fuccio C, Castellucci P, Schiavina R, Santi I, Allegri V, Pettinato V, Boschi S, Martorana G, Al-Nahhas A, Rubello D, Fanti S. Role of 11C-choline PET/CT in the restaging of prostate cancer patients showing a single lesion on bone scintigraphy. Ann Nucl Med. 2010;24:485–92.
37. Garcia JR, Moreno C, Valls E, Cozar P, Bassa P, Soler M, Alvarez-Moro FJ, Moragas M, Riera E. Diagnostic performance of bone scintigraphy and (11)C-Choline PET/CT in the detection of bone metastases in patients with biochemical recurrence of prostate cancer. Rev Esp Med Nucl Imagen Mol. 2015;34:155–61.
38. Ghosh A, Heston WD. Tumor target prostate specific membrane antigen (PSMA) and its regulation in prostate cancer. J Cell Biochem. 2004;91:528–39.
39. Giesel FL, Fiedler H, Stefanova M, Sterzing F, Rius M, Kopka K, Moltz JH, Afshar-Oromieh A, Choyke PL, Haberkorn U, Kratochwil C. PSMA PET/CT with Glu-urea-Lys-(Ahx)-[(6)(8)Ga(HBED-CC)] versus 3D CT volumetric lymph node assessment in recurrent prostate cancer. Eur J Nucl Med Mol Imaging. 2015;42:1794–800.
40. Gomez P, Manoharan M, Kim SS, Soloway MS. Radionuclide bone scintigraphy in patients with biochemical recurrence after radical prostatectomy: when is it indicated? BJU Int. 2004;94:299–302.
41. Heck MM, Souvatzoglou M, Retz M, Nawroth R, Kubler H, Maurer T, Thalgott M, Gramer BM, Weirich G, Rondak IC, Rummeny EJ, Schwaiger M, Gschwend JE, Krause B, Eiber M. Prospective comparison of computed tomography, diffusion-weighted magnetic resonance imaging and [11C]choline positron emission tomography/computed tomography for preoperative lymph node staging in prostate cancer patients. Eur J Nucl Med Mol Imaging. 2014;41:694–701.
42. Iagaru A, Mittra E, Dick DW, Gambhir SS. Prospective evaluation of (99m)Tc MDP scintigraphy, (18)F NaF PET/CT, and (18)F FDG PET/CT for detection of skeletal metastases. Mol Imaging Biol. 2012;14:252–9.
43. Imbriaco M, Larson SM, Yeung HW, Mawlawi OR, Erdi Y, Venkatraman ES, SCHER HI. A new parameter for measuring metastatic bone involvement by prostate cancer: the Bone Scan Index. Clin Cancer Res. 1998;4:1765–72.
44. Incerti E, Fodor A, Mapelli P, Fiorino C, Alongi P, Kirienko M, Giovacchini G, Busnardo E, Gianolli L, DI Muzio N, Picchio M. Radiation treatment of lymph node recurrence from prostate cancer: is 11C-choline PET/CT predictive of survival outcomes? J Nucl Med. 2015;56:1836–42.
45. Jacobson AF. Association of prostate-specific antigen levels and patterns of benign and malignant uptake detected. on bone scintigraphy in patients with newly diagnosed prostate carcinoma. Nucl Med Commun. 2000;21:617–22.
46. Karnes RJ, Murphy CR, Bergstralh EJ, Dimonte G, Cheville JC, Lowe VJ, Mynderse LA, Kwon ED. Salvage lymph node dissection for prostate cancer nodal recurrence detected by 11C-choline positron emission tomography/computerized tomography. J Urol. 2015;193:111–6.
47. Kinoshita Y, Kuratsukuri K, Landas S, Imaida K, Rovito Jr PM, Wang CY, Haas GP. Expression of pros-

tate-specific membrane antigen in normal and malignant human tissues. World J Surg. 2006;30:628–36.
48. Lavalaye J, Kaldeway P, Van Melick HH. Diffuse bone metastases on Ga-PSMA PET-CT in a patient with prostate cancer and normal bone scan. Eur J Nucl Med Mol Imaging. 2016;43:1563.
49. Maurer T, Eiber M, Schwaiger M, Gschwend JE. Current use of PSMA-PET in prostate cancer management. Nat Rev Urol. 2016;13:226–35.
50. Maurer T, Gschwend JE, Rauscher I, Souvatzoglou M, Haller B, Weirich G, Wester HJ, Heck M, Kubler H, Beer AJ, Schwaiger M, Eiber M. Diagnostic efficacy of (68)gallium-PSMA positron emission tomography compared to conventional imaging for lymph node staging of 130 consecutive patients with intermediate to high risk prostate cancer. J Urol. 2016;195:1436–43.
51. Mcarthur C, Mclaughlin G, Meddings RN. Changing the referral criteria for bone scan in newly diagnosed prostate cancer patients. Br J Radiol. 2012;85:390–4.
52. Miller PD, Eardley I, Kirby RS. Prostate specific antigen and bone scan correlation in the staging and monitoring of patients with prostatic cancer. Br J Urol. 1992;70:295–8.
53. Mitchell CR, Lowe VJ, RANGEL LJ, Hung JC, Kwon ED, Karnes RJ. Operational characteristics of (11)c-choline positron emission tomography/computerized tomography for prostate cancer with biochemical recurrence after initial treatment. J Urol. 2013;189:1308–13.
54. Morigi JJ, Stricker PD, Van Leeuwen PJ, Tang R, HO B, Nguyen Q, Hruby G, Fogarty G, Jagavkar R, Kneebone A, Hickey A, Fanti S, Tarlinton L, Emmett L. Prospective comparison of 18F-fluoromethylcholine versus 68Ga-PSMA PET/CT in prostate cancer patients who have rising PSA after curative treatment and are being considered for targeted therapy. J Nucl Med. 2015;56:1185–90.
55. Mottet N, Bellmunt J, Briers E, Van den Bergh RCN, Bolla M, Van Casteren NJ, Conford P, Culine S, Joniau S, Lam T, Mason MD, Matveev V, Van der Poel H, Van der Kwast TH, Rouviere O, Wiegel T. Guidelines on prostate cancer. EAU Guidelines. European Association of Urology. 2015.
56. Muzahir S, Jeraj R, Liu G, Hall LT, Rio AM, Perk T, Jaskowiak C, Perlman SB. Differentiation of metastatic vs degenerative joint disease using semi-quantitative analysis with (18)F-NaF PET/CT in castrate resistant prostate cancer patients. Am J Nucl Med Mol Imaging. 2015;5:162–8.
57. O'sullivan JM, Norman AR, Cook GJ, Fisher C, Dearnaley DP. Broadening the criteria for avoiding staging bone scans in prostate cancer: a retrospective study of patients at the Royal Marsden Hospital. BJU Int. 2003;92:685–9.
58. Okotie OT, Aronson WJ, Wieder JA, Liao Y, Dorey F, De K. J, Freedland SJ. Predictors of metastatic disease in men with biochemical failure following radical prostatectomy. J Urol. 2004;171:2260–4.
59. Oldan JD, Hawkins AS, Chin BB. (18)F sodium fluoride PET/CT in patients with prostate cancer: quantification of normal tissues, benign degenerative lesions, and malignant lesions. World J Nucl Med. 2016;15:102–8.
60. Osmonov DK, Heimann D, Janssen I, Aksenov A, Kalz A, Juenemann KP. Sensitivity and specificity of PET/CT regarding the detection of lymph node metastases in prostate cancer recurrence. Springerplus. 2014;3:340.
61. Palmedo H, Marx C, Ebert A, Kreft B, Ko Y, Turler A, Vorreuther R, Gohring U, Schild HH, Gerhardt T, Poge U, Ezziddin S, Biersack HJ, Ahmadzadehfar H. Whole-body SPECT/CT for bone scintigraphy: diagnostic value and effect on patient management in oncological patients. Eur J Nucl Med Mol Imaging. 2014;41:59–67.
62. Perner S, Hofer MD, Kim R, Shah RB, Li H, Moller P, Hautmann RE, Gschwend JE, Kuefer R, Rubin MA. Prostate-specific membrane antigen expression as a predictor of prostate cancer progression. Hum Pathol. 2007;38:696–701.
63. Pfister D, Porres D, Heidenreich A, Heidegger I, Knuechel R, Steib F, Behrendt FF, Verburg FA. Detection of recurrent prostate cancer lesions before salvage lymphadenectomy is more accurate with Ga-PSMA-HBED-CC than with F-Fluoroethylcholine PET/CT. Eur J Nucl Med Mol Imaging. 2016;43:1410.
64. Picchio M, Berardi G, Fodor A, Busnardo E, Crivellaro C, Giovacchini G, Fiorino C, Kirienko M, Incerti E, Messa C, Gianolli L, DI Muzio N. (11)C-Choline PET/CT as a guide to radiation treatment planning of lymph-node relapses in prostate cancer patients. Eur J Nucl Med Mol Imaging. 2014;41:1270–9.
65. Picchio M, Castellucci P. Clinical indications of C-choline PET/CT in prostate cancer patients with biochemical relapse. Theranostics. 2012;2:313–7.
66. Poulsen MH, Bouchelouche K, Hoilund-Carlsen PF, Petersen H, Gerke O, Steffansen SI, Marcussen N, Svolgaard N, Vach W, Geertsen U, Walter S. [18F] fluoromethylcholine (FCH) positron emission tomography/computed tomography (PET/CT) for lymph node staging of prostate cancer: a prospective study of 210 patients. BJU Int. 2012;110:1666–71.
67. Poulsen MH, Petersen H, Hoilund-Carlsen PF, Jakobsen JS, Gerke O, Karstoft J, Steffansen SI, Walter S. Spine metastases in prostate cancer: comparison of technetium-99m-MDP whole-body bone scintigraphy, [(18) F]choline positron emission tomography(PET)/computed tomography (CT) and [(18) F]NaF PET/CT. BJU Int. 2014;114:818–23.
68. Rinnab L, Mottaghy FM, Simon J, Volkmer BG, DE Petriconi R, Hautmann RE, Wittbrodt M, Egghart G, Moeller P, Blumstein N, Reske S, Kuefer R. [11C] Choline PET/CT for targeted salvage lymph node dissection in patients with biochemical recurrence after primary curative therapy for prostate cancer. Preliminary results of a prospective study. Urol Int. 2008;81:191–7.

69. Rowe SP, Macura KJ, Mena E, Blackford AL, Nadal R, Antonarakis ES, Eisenberger M, Carducci M, Fan H, Dannals RF, Chen Y, Mease RC, Szabo Z, Pomper MG, Cho SY. PSMA-based [(18)F]DCFPyL PET/CT is superior to conventional imaging for lesion detection in patients with metastatic prostate cancer. Mol Imaging Biol. 2016;18:411–9.
70. Rydh A, Tomic R, Tavelin B, Hietala SO, Damber JE. Predictive value of prostate-specific antigen, tumour stage and tumour grade for the outcome of bone scintigraphy in patients with newly diagnosed prostate cancer. Scand J Urol Nephrol. 1999;33:89–93.
71. Scattoni V, Picchio M, Suardi N, Messa C, Freschi M, Roscigno M, Da Pozzo L, Bocciardi A, Rigatti P, Fazio F. Detection of lymph-node metastases with integrated [11C]choline PET/CT in patients with PSA failure after radical retropubic prostatectomy: results confirmed by open pelvic-retroperitoneal lymphadenectomy. Eur Urol. 2007;52:423–9.
72. Scher HI, Halabi S, Tannock I, Morris M, Sternberg CN, Carducci MA, Eisenberger MA, Higano C, Bubley GJ, Dreicer R, Petrylak D, Kantoff P, Basch E, kelly WK, Figg WD, Small EJ, Beer TM, Wilding G, Martin A, Hussain M. Design and end points of clinical trials for patients with progressive prostate cancer and castrate levels of testosterone: recommendations of the Prostate Cancer Clinical Trials Working Group. J Clin Oncol. 2008;26:1148–59.
73. Schilling D, Schlemmer HP, Wagner PH, Bottcher P, Merseburger AS, Aschoff P, Bares R, Pfannenberg C, Ganswindt U, Corvin S, Stenzl A. Histological verification of 11C-choline-positron emission/computed tomography-positive lymph nodes in patients with biochemical failure after treatment for localized prostate cancer. BJU Int. 2008;102:446–51.
74. Schwarzenbock S, Souvatzoglou M, Krause BJ. Choline PET and PET/CT in primary diagnosis and staging of prostate cancer. Theranostics. 2012;2:318–30.
75. Souvatzoglou M, Krause BJ, Purschel A, Thamm R, Schuster T, Buck AK, Zimmermann F, Molls M, Schwaiger M, Geinitz H. Influence of (11)C-choline PET/CT on the treatment planning for salvage radiation therapy in patients with biochemical recurrence of prostate cancer. Radiother Oncol. 2011;99:193–200.
76. Soyka JD, Muster MA, Schmid DT, Seifert B, Schick U, Miralbell R, Jorcano S, Zaugg K, Seifert HH, Veit-Haibach P, Strobel K, Schaefer NG, Husarik DB, Hany TF. Clinical impact of 18F-choline PET/CT in patients with recurrent prostate cancer. Eur J Nucl Med Mol Imaging. 2012;39:936–43.
77. Tilki D, Reich O, Graser A, Hacker M, Silchinger J, Becker AJ, Khoder W, Bartenstein P, Stief CG, Loidl W, Seitz M. 18F-Fluoroethylcholine PET/CT identifies lymph node metastasis in patients with prostate-specific antigen failure after radical prostatectomy but underestimates its extent. Eur Urol. 2013;63:792–6.
78. Treglia G, Ceriani L, Sadeghi R, Giovacchini G, Giovanella L. Relationship between prostate-specific antigen kinetics and detection rate of radiolabelled choline PET/CT in restaging prostate cancer patients: a meta-analysis. Clin Chem Lab Med. 2014;52:725–33.
79. Ulmert D, Kaboteh R, Fox JJ, Savage C, Evans MJ, Lilja H, Abrahamsson PA, Bjork T, Gerdtsson A, Bjartell A, Gjertsson P, Hoglund P, Lomsky M, Ohlsson M, Richter J, Sadik M, Morris MJ, Scher HI, Sjostrand K, Yu A, Suurküla M, Edenbrandt L, Larson SM. A novel automated platform for quantifying the extent of skeletal tumour involvement in prostate cancer patients using the Bone Scan Index. Eur Urol. 2012;62:78–84.
80. Van Leeuwen PJ, Emmett L, Ho B, Delprado W, Ting F, Nguyen Q, Stricker P. Prospective evaluation of 68Gallium-PSMA positron emission tomography/computerized tomography for preoperative lymph node staging in prostate cancer. BJU Int. 2016. [epub ahead of print] 10.1111/bju.13540
81. Von Eyben FE, Kairemo K. Meta-analysis of (11) C-choline and (18)F-choline PET/CT for management of patients with prostate cancer. Nucl Med Commun. 2014;35:221–30.
82. von Eyben FE, Kairemo K. Acquisition with C-choline and F-fluorocholine PET/CT for patients with biochemical recurrence of prostate cancer: a systematic review and meta-analysis. Ann Nucl Med. 2016;30:385.
83. Watanabe H, Kanematsu M, Kondo H, Kako N, Yamamoto N, Yamada T, Goshima S, Hoshi H, Bae KT. Preoperative detection of prostate cancer: a comparison with 11C-choline PET, 18F-fluorodeoxyglucose PET and MR imaging. J Magn Reson Imaging. 2010;31:1151–6.
84. Wurschmidt F, Petersen C, Wahl A, Dahle J, Kretschmer M. [18F]fluoroethylcholine-PET/CT imaging for radiation treatment planning of recurrent and primary prostate cancer with dose escalation to PET/CT-positive lymph nodes. Radiat Oncol. 2011;6:44.
85. Zacho HD, Barsi T, Mortensen JC, Mogensen MK, Bertelsen H, Josephsen N, Petersen LJ. Prospective multicenter study of bone scintigraphy in consecutive patients with newly diagnosed prostate cancer. Clin Nucl Med. 2014;39:26–31.

Diagnosis, Clinical Workup, and TNM Classification

Jean-Luc Descotes

1 Introduction

Prostate cancer is the second most common cancer in men worldwide. Most information concerning clinical presentation are available with analysis of countries databases (SEER database for United states) [1]; SEER database points out sociodemographic differences in screening and treatments in the world and the lack on the risk profile of patients with localized prostate cancer in the United States which represents the current clinical presentation of patients in countries where PSA screening has been developed.

So, taking into account therapeutic decisions with our patients, description of contemporary tools used for diagnosis and classifications are a major issue for prostate cancer.

In 2016, prostate cancer diagnosis still remains on digital rectal examination (DRE), PSA blood test and prostate biopsies with description of the Gleason score (GS).

Improvements in prostate imaging, especially with multiparametric MRI (mp MRI), and recent marketed blood, urine, or tissue markers, will probably, in a short future, modify our approach of this cancer and optimize our clinical workup.

J.-L. Descotes
Department of Urology and Renal Transplantation, CHU de GRENOBLE, La Tronche, France
e-mail: JLDescotes@chu-grenoble.fr

Our goals for diagnosis and clinical workup are as follows:

- First to diagnose patients with "aggressive" cancers
- Second to better define and limit if possible unnecessary biopsies in patients with very low risk lesions
- Third to characterize the extend of the tumor, its aggressiveness, and the burden of disease in order to determine the appropriate treatment for the good patient

The important literature with regard to over diagnosis that may result in over treatments, the heterogeneity of the disease, and the diversity of treatments highlight the fact that clinicians need to rely their decisions on competitive risk factors, analysis of comorbidities, and risk classifications.

2 Initial Diagnosis of Prostate Cancer

2.1 Digital Rectal Examination (DRE)

While rectal prostate palpation is carried out on a systematic way to evaluate benign prostate hyperplasia (BPH) and voiding dysfunction in male, its performance for the initial detection of cancer and local staging is limited.

M. Bolla, H. van Poppel (eds.), *Management of Prostate Cancer*,
DOI 10.1007/978-3-319-42769-0_9

For initial detection, most of cancers detected when screening PSA program is used have normal DRE. However, palpation of irregularity or nodule during DRE still remains an indication for prostate biopsy regardless of the level of PSA. When DRE is suspect and PSA level ≤2 ng/ml, the positive predictive value for cancer varies from 5 to 30 % [2].

Subjectivity of DRE when assigning clinical abnormality and its drawback in staging led initially to extensive prescription of transrectal ultrasound evaluation of the prostate gland (TRUS).

Unfortunately, TRUS is not helpful to confirm that clinical abnormality is associated with prostate cancer lesion; thus, TRUS should not be prescribed to detect cancer.

Compared to ultrasound, other imaging modalities like multiparametric MRI (mp MRI) is a promising modality for the diagnosis of prostate cancer, more accurate, and fusion of these imaging modalities (TRUS/ mp MRI) will improve our performance for prostate cancer early detection.

2.2 Role of PSA in Diagnosis

In the evolving landscape of tumor markers, PSA remains the cornerstone of biological test for cancer detection. PSA level is associated with advanced pathology. Unfortunately, PSA is organ specific and not prostate cancer specific, and this explains the overlap in PSA levels between benign pathologies, BPH, prostatitis and prostate cancer [3]. Then, fluctuation may occur for patient on repeated dosage and PSA level is affected by 5α-reductase, statin medication, and should be evaluated in reference to man's age and his general health.

Therefore, stratifying prostate cancer risk to indicate prostate biopsy with PSA level alone is difficult and the widespread adoption of PSA screening has resulted in a significant stage migration toward early disease when PSA level is below 10 ng/ml. Tacking account low specificity demonstrated for patients with PSA >4 ng and <10 ng/ml, many of these men have no evidence of cancer on biopsy.

Table 1 Risk of prostate cancer in relation to low PSA (PCPT study)

PSA level (ng/ml)	Risk of cancer (%)	Risk of aggressive cancer ≥7 (%)
0–0.5	6.6	0.8
0.6–1	10.1	1.0
1.1–2	17	2.0
2.1–3	23.9	4.6
3.1–4	26.9	6.7

However, the PCPT trial showed that 5–26 % of cancers have a PSA below 4 ng/ml (Table 1).

Considering the potential morbidity of biopsies which increases with the number of cores, and anticoagulant treatments, several utilization of PSA and PSA derivatives (PSA density, PSA velocity, PSA doubling time, free to total PSA ratio) have been widely used to improve the diagnosis performance of this blood test and clarify indications for biopsy [4].

- Free PSA is the noncomplexed form of PSA and has several molecular forms (nicked, intact, and pro PSA). In proportion to total PSA, free PSA is lower in men with prostate cancer and f PSA/t PSA ratio is suspicious for cancer when the report is <10–15 %, especially when the volume of the prostate is <30 ml; this ratio improves the specificity of t PSA between 4 and 10 ng/ml, but to our knowledge, no study justifies its prescription for a first round of screening.
- PSA density (PSA/prostate volume) is suggestive of prostate cancer when the value is greater than 0.15 ng/ml, but errors in prostate volume measurement limit its utility for an individual patient.
- PSA velocity >2 ng/ml/year and PSA doubling time (PSA DT) are associated with shorter time to death, high Gleason score, and an advanced pathology, but measurements do not provide a clear additional value for prostate cancer detection [5].

As none of these tests are completely accurate, new biomarkers, more specific and sensitive for the detection of aggressive cancers are clearly needed.

2.3 Additional Markers

This subject is widely discussed by J. Schalken in this book.

Today, to improve prostate diagnosis, 2 blood tests (PHI and 4K score) and one urinary test (PCA3) are commercially available and have been evaluated.

2.3.1 Prostate Heath Index (PHI)

PHI is a mathematical formula combining PSA isoforms: (-2)pro PSA/fPSA × t PSA1/2.

This marker was FDA approved in 2012 after a multicenter study published by WJ Catalona showing that an increasing PHI level was associated with a 4.7-fold increased risk of prostate cancer and a 1.61 risk of aggressive disease on biopsy (GS ≥ 7) [6].

Several studies have evaluated the performance of PHI for biopsy indication. Compared to t PSA, f PSA/t PSA [7], in a prospective multicenter study of 658 patients enrolled with normal DRE and PSA between 2 and 10 ng/ml, reported a clinical impact of PHI.Compared to other markers, PHI had the highest AUC on receiver operat ing characteristic analysis (0.708) and a greater predictive accuracy for clinically significant prostate cancer, higher than its individual component (PSA, f PSA/t PSA, and [-2]pro PSA).

Compared to PSA, [-2] pro PSA and free PSA, Loeb concluded that PHI improves detection of clinically significant cancer and claimed that, for men with PSA 2–10 ng/ml, at a 90 % sensitivity cutoff, using a score of 28.6, PHI will fail to detect 10.1 % of clinically significant cancer, 4, 8 % cancers with GS 3+4 or greater and avoid approximately 30 % of biopsies in men with benign or insignificant disease. This conclusion was considered inaccurate by N Shah considering that significant cancer is based on prostatectomy specimen rather than biopsy grade.

Other authors, after analysis of the PROMETHEUS database (PRO-PSA Multi European Study Group) recently confirmed that PHI may correlate with pathologic cancer feature and could discriminate indolent from cancer with GS ≥ 7, but the gain in accuracy promoted by PHI was low for the prediction of pT3 disease and moderate for Gleason score (3 % vs. 6 %) [8].

In a recent review [9], pointed out PHI score for predicting greater risk of clinically significant disease on biopsy and adverse prostatectomy outcome; he suggested that this test could help monitoring patients on active surveillance.

2.3.2 4K Score

4-Kallikrein (4K) panel (tPSA, % free PSA, intact free PSA, and hk2) is a new biomarker proposed to improve detection of aggressive prostate cancers (GS ≥ 7) before a first set of biopsy or after a first negative biopsy evaluation.

This marker was first evaluated retrospectively on the screen population of the ERSPC study [10]. The review of different studies done on the ERSPC population showed that 4K increases detection of high grade cancer and the AUC between 0.03 and 0.11. According to the cohorts, 2.5–12 % of high grade cancer were missed [11]. This test was then validated in a prospective multi-institutional study conducted in United States on 1370 men. 26 investigators compared the 4K score with the PCPT RC 2.0 risk calculator and showed that 4K was superior to predict Gleason 7 or more with an AUC of 0.82 versus 0.74 ($p < 0.0001$). With a cutoff of 9 %, this test could reduce the number of prostate biopsies performed for indolent cancer up to 41 % and delayed diagnosis of GS ≥ 7 for 24 men (2.4 %) including 2 patients with Gleason 4+4 or higher. With a cutoff of 15 %, this test could reduce the number of prostate biopsies performed for indolent cancer up to 58 % and delayed diagnosis of GS ≥ 7 for 48 men (4.7 %) [12].

Comparison between 4K and PHI was published after a 531 population men study done in Stockholm country with PSA 3–15 ng/ml. Both of them reduced the number of unnecessary biopsies and improved discrimination when predicting high grade cancer. Head-to-head evaluation of 4K score and PHI was similar in term of reduced number of biopsies and missed cancer and the authors could not explain the poorer results of 4K compared to previously reported results leading to questions about calibration of these biochemical analysis [13].

2.3.3 The Urine PCA3

Described by Bussemakers and colleagues in 1999, a urinary biomarker, Differential Display Code 3 characterized as a noncoding RNA highly specific for prostate cancer detectable in urine sediments obtain after prostatic massage. Progensa PCA3 assay was developed and then use in clinical practice.

PCA3 assay should not be used for patients who are taking medication known to affect serum PSA levels such as finasteride, dutasteride, and leuprorelin. The effect of these medications on PCA3 gene expression has not yet been evaluated.

PCA3 was initially used after a first negative biopsy and studies have shown PCA3 to be independent to age, prostate volume and to improve diagnosis compared to PSA, but the assessment of pathologically advanced or aggressive PCa was not improved using PCA3 [14]. International recommendations suggest performing this test to determine whether repeat biopsy is need after an initially negative biopsy and a score less than 20 seem to rule out the risk of aggressive cancer on repeated biopsy but its “clinical effectiveness for this purpose is uncertain” (Guidelines EAU 2016).

2.4 Nomograms and Multivariable Prediction Models

Several risk calculators have been developed in order to guide the clinician for biopsy decision. Many of prostate risk calculators are accessible online [15]. However, most of nomograms are based on old cohorts of patients and do not take account new techniques of biopsy and recent pathologic grading pattern.

PCPT risk calculator was posted on line in 2006 by Thompson to distinguish low grade versus high grade disease (GS > 7) and updated first in 2014 incorporating prostate volume, AUA symptom score and number of biopsy cores, but these modifications offered only modest improvements to the standard PCPT risk calculators [16].

This recalibration of the PCPTRC based on an institution analysis was recently published [17] and is available on line at myprostatecancerrisk.com. It accommodates missing values of DRE, family history or prior biopsy; the accuracy of PCPTRC tool seems better and despite of cost the authors suggest that this tool should allow institution to customize their practice.

Nevertheless, in clinical practice, nomogram utilization among urologists seems low despite their accessibility on line.

To Sum Up

For early detection of prostate cancer, DRE and tPSA remain the goal standard; PSA density, free/t PSA ratio can help the clinician to inform his patient about prostate cancer risk and using nomograms can help these men after an inform consent, to decide whether or not to perform a prostate biopsy.

Today, three tests are commercially available to predict individual risk of cancer (PHI and PCA3) and high grade cancer on biopsy (4K). So far, none of the biomarkers can be used systematically to counsel an individual patient on the need to perform a prostate biopsy to rule out prostate cancer.

Tomorrow, with the rapidly evolving field of genomics and genetics, individual risk and personalized indications for prostate biopsy will certainly occur.

2.5 Radiological Initial Diagnosis with mp MRI

To optimize prostate detection of high risk prostate cancer, clinician needs to improve sampling efficiency by targeting images specific of cancer.

These are the goals of mp MRI (cf Chap. 7, Pr O Rouvière in this book), and targeted biopsies with or without MRI/US fusion devices.

Today, mp MRI, which includes T2 weighted imaging, diffusion weighted imaging (DWI) with apparent diffusion coefficient (ADC), and dynamic intravenous contrast-enhanced imaging (DCE), is the only radiologic tool performed for the detection of suspicious lesions and local extension evaluation of prostate cancer (Fig. 1).

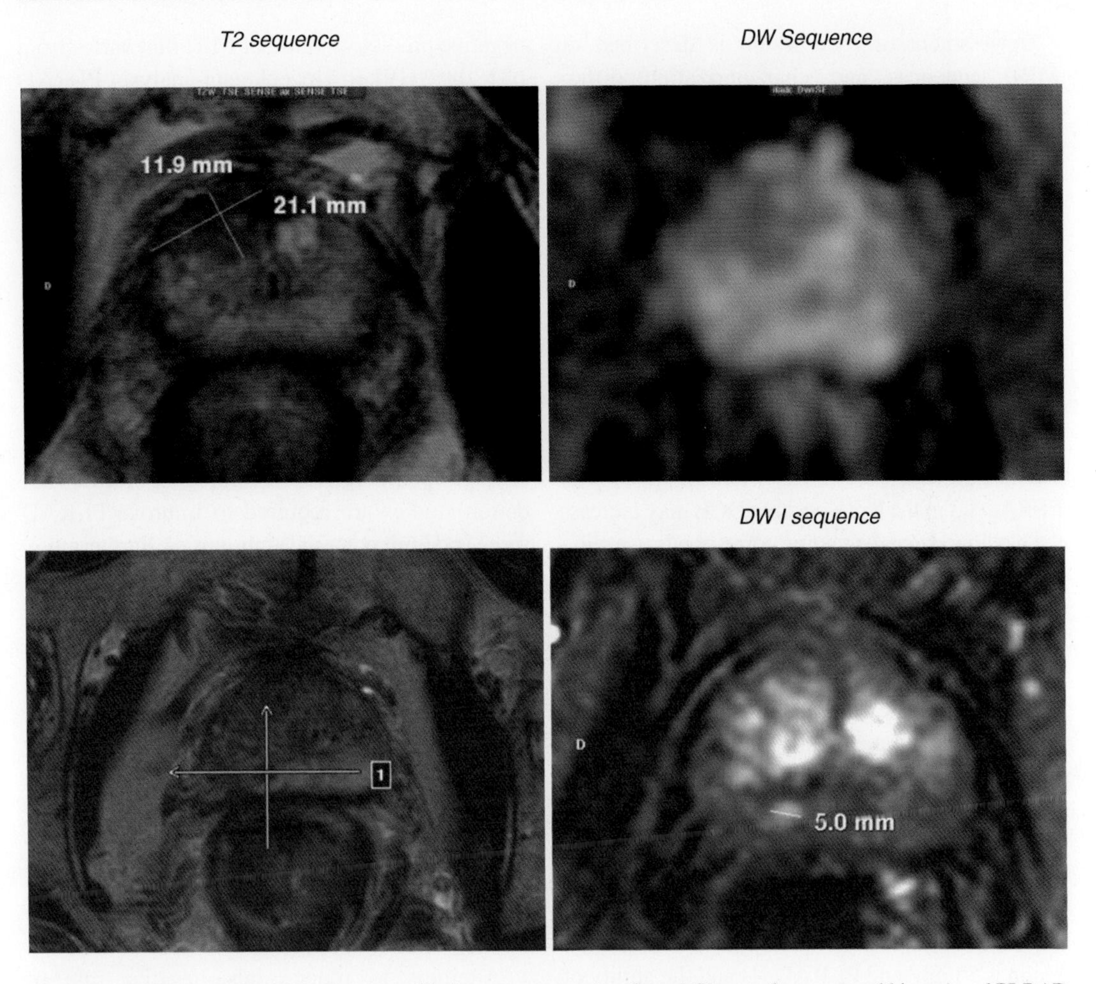

Fig. 1 Mp MRI and PI-RAD 5 anterolateral lesion on prostate (confirmed Gleason 8 on targeted biopsy) and PI-RAD 4 posterior lesion

Magnet machines allowing high "b value" and rapid scan times for dynamic sequences acquisition give optimal functional and anatomical information on prostate, and PI-RAD V2 assessment (Prostate Imaging and Reporting and Data System) already describe in chapter is helpful to standardize interpretation of prostate MR imaging and estimate the risk of significant cancer. An online atlas of findings and cases is also being developed as a learning and reference tool (http://www.acr.org/Quality-Safety/Resources/PIRADS).

PI-RAD V2 is described below intended to standardize reporting of MRI findings only and each lesion should be evaluated using a 5 point scale based on T2W, DCE, and DWI sequences [18].

- PI-RADS 1 – Very low (clinically significant cancer is highly unlikely to be present)
- PI-RADS 2 – Low (clinically significant cancer is unlikely to be present)
- PI-RADS 3 – Intermediate (the presence of clinically significant cancer is equivocal around 23 %)
- PI-RADS 4 – High (clinically significant cancer is likely to be present in 75 %)
- PI-RADS 5 – Very high (clinically significant cancer is highly likely to be present almost in 100 %)

Assessment of each lesion is described on MRI sequences and characterization differs between peripheral and transitional zone only for T2W images (Tables 2 and 3).

As shown in the Table 4, DCE plays a minor role in determining PI-RADS Assessment Category. The absence of early enhancement within a lesion usually adds little information, and diffuse enhancement not localized to a specific T2W or DWI abnormality can be seen in the setting of prostatitis. Moreover, DCE does not contribute to the overall assessment when the finding has a low (PI-RADS 1 or 2) or high (PI-RADS 4 or 5) likelihood of clinically significant cancer. However, when DWI is PI-RADS 3 in the PZ, a positive DCE may increase the likelihood that the finding corresponds to a clinically significant cancer and may upgrade the Assessment Category to PI-RADS (Table 5).

Likewise when T2W is PI-RAD 3 in the transition zone, DWI may increase the likelihood that the findings corresponds to a clinically significant cancer and may update the assessment to PI-RADS 4 (Table 6).

Indeed accuracy and performance of mp MRI depends on different factors, the volume and Gleason score of the lesion and the expertise of the radiologist. Basically, detection rate of lesions GS $\geq$ 7 is around 85 % when the volume of the lesion is >1 cm^3 and PI-RAD > 3 and the ability of mp MRI to rule out nonsignificant prostate cancer has to be considered taking into account the negative predictive value of MRI that varies from 63 to 98 % [19]. In a recent meta-analysis, PI-RAD V2 showed sensitivity of 0.78 (95 % confidence interval (CI) 0.70–0.84) and specificity of 0.79 (95 % CI 0.68–0.86) for prostate detection, with negative predictive values ranging from 0.58 to 0.95. Sensitivity analysis revealed pooled sensitivity of 0.82 (95 % CI 0.72–0.89) and specificity of 0.82 (95 % CI 0.67–0.92) in studies with the correct use of score [20]. This variability point out the fact that the performance of mp MRI is clearly depending on methodology, expertise of the radiologist and justify a close collaboration between urologist pathologist and radiologist. Indeed, validation studies are required to improve PI-RAD score and limit potential ambiguities. Furthermore, a lot of work is needed to compare the radiologic lesion to prostatectomy specimens in order to target and personalize treatments because MRI frequently under estimates cancer volume.

2.6 Prostate Biopsies

2.6.1 Random Biopsy

Twelve random biopsies performed under TRUS remains the gold standard procedure for prostate cancer detection.

Attempts to reduce false-negative rate of TRUS-randomized biopsies by saturated biopsies with transperineal approach, or by adding anterior

Table 2 Assessment for T2W is described below and differs between PZ and TZ

Score	Peripheral zone (PZ)	Transition zone (TZ)
1	Uniform hyperintense signal intensity (normal)	Homogeneous intermediate signal intensity (normal)
2	Linear or wedge-shaped hypointensity or diffuse mild hypointensity, usually indistinct margin	Circumscribed hypointense or heterogeneous encapsulated nodule(s) (BPH)
3	Heterogeneous signal intensity or noncircumscribed, rounded, moderate hypointensity Includes others that do not qualify as 2, 4, or 5	Heterogeneous signal intensity with obscured margins Includes others that do not qualify as 2, 4, or 5
4	Circumscribed, homogenous moderate hypointense focus/mass confined to prostate and <1.5 cm in greatest dimension	Lenticlularor noncircumscribed, homogeneous, moderately hypointense, and <1.5 cm in greatest dimension
5	Same as 4 but ≥1.5 cm in greatest dimension or definite extraprostatic extension/invasive behavior	Same as 4, but ≥ 1.5 cm in greatest dimension or definite extraprostatic extension/invasive behavior

Table 3 Assessment for DWI is identical for PZ and TZ

Score	Peripheral zone (PZ) or transition zone (TZ)
1	No abnormality (i.e., normal) on ADC and high b-value DWI
2	Indistinct hypointense on ADC
3	Focal mildly/moderately hypointense on ADC and isointense/mildly hyperintense on high b-value DWI
4	Focal markedly hypontense on ADC and markedly hyperintense on high b-value DWI; <1.5 cm in greatest dimension
5	Same as 4 but ≥1.5 cm in greatest dimension or definite extraprostatic extension/invasive behavior

Table 4 Assessment for DCE is simplified

Score	Peripheral zone (PZ) or transition zone (TZ)
(−)	No early enhancement, or diffuse enhancement not corresponding to a focal finding on T2 and/or DWI or focal enhancement corresponding to a lesion demonstrating features of BPH on T2WI
(+)	Focal, and earlier than or contemporaneously with enhancement of adjacent normal prostatic tissues, and corresponds to suspicious finding on T2W and/or DWI

Table 5 PI-RADS assessment category for the peripherical zone

	T2W	DCE	PIRAD
1	Any	Any	1
2	Any	Any	2
3	Any	–	3
		+	4
4	Any	Any	4
5	Any	Any	5
Any indicates 1–5			

Table 6 PI-RADS assessment category for transition zone

DWI	T2W	DCE	PIRAD
Any	1	Any	1
Any	2	Any	2
≤4	3	Any	3
5		Any	4
Any	4	Any	4
Any	5	Any	5
Any indicates 1–5			

and apical sampling were not very conclusive. Today, the role of perineal biopsies is discussed controversially since there is no statistically evidence of benefit compared to TRUS (guidelines EAU 2014). Transperineal approach is associated with a higher rate of acute urinary retention and it usually needs for general anesthesia. Detection rate is quite equivalent to transrectal approach, but the risk of sepsis is minimal, especially when saturated biopsies are performed [21]. Results of other clinical studies were marginally successful pointing out the interest of mp MRI and targeted biopsies on suspicious lesion defined on PI-RAD.

2.6.2 Targeted Biopsies

While MRI was initially applied to local staging after biopsy, literature is now gaining attention for the detection of suspicious lesions, leading to targeted biopsies. The advantage of targeted biopsies is clearly important for anterior lesions which represent up to 30 % of cancer because random TRUS biopsy performance is limited by little access to those lesions.

Prospective series have shown that mp MRI targeted biopsies can improve the detection of clinically significant tumors based on the percentage of positive core, and detection of more aggressive tumors on Gleason score (GS). Centers using targeted biopsy, either with cognitive or fusion devices, report more accuracy with a 90 % NPV if biopsy targets PI-RAD > 3 lesions [22].

A recent meta-analysis of MRI targeted biopsy confirms that this approach may enhance diagnostic of significant cancer compared to standard transrectal ultrasound guided biopsy Significant improvement was noted in a subgroup of men with negative first setting of biopsies and for anterior lesions or transition cancers which are more easily detected and sampled with targeted biopsies [23].

Repeat biopsy is then more efficient with an overall cancer detection rate between 38 and 76 % according to PI-RAD 3, 4, or 5 with clearly a better detection of anterior lesions. Despite methodological flaws of targeted biopsy (physician may be influenced by mp MRI findings and look for hypo echogenic lesions during biopsies), this report of 1926 men with positive MRI showed a prevalence of prostate cancer of 59 %. Targeted biopsies seem to improve significant cancer detection rate by 20 % compared to TRUS biopsies (sensitivity 0.91, vs. 0.76) and decrease detection rate of insignificant cancer (sensitivity 0.56 vs. 0.83).

Therefore, for the EAU guidelines, mp MRI could be recommended after a first set of negative biopsies in patients with persistent elevated PSA or abnormal DRE with a level 1 A of evidence.

On the opposite, the role for mp MRI before a first set of biopsies in order to replace random by targeted biopsies raises economical questions and today is not recommended until further evaluation and clear results on prospective studies [24,25].

Literature also highlights the fact that TRUS biopsies in MRI-negative men indicated significant cancer in 10–15 % of cases. Therefore, today, protocols including mp MRI before biopsy combine systematic randomized biopsies and 2 or 3 sampling or MRI lesions PIRAD >3 or ≥3.

To conclude, clinical studies need also to integrate additional value of biology and new biomarkers with mp MRI, either to inform the patient to perform a mp MRI before a second set of biopsies, or to influence the decision for a second set of biopsies if mp MRI is negative. Medicoeconomic studies have to be carried on to determine what guidance is cost-effective (cf Guidelines NICE 2015 http://www.nice.org.uk/guidance/dg17).

3 Staging and Clinical Workup After Cancer Diagnosis

Primary treatment depends on age, local, and distant staging (lymph node metastasis evaluation), surgical risk and performance status. Clinical workup is performed to decide with the patient the best approach.

3.1 Local Staging

Local staging is essential to decide optimal treatment according to cancer localization.

For example, during radical prostatectomy, the urologist has to choose before surgery the best plane for his dissection. Extrafascial approach and wide dissection of the prostate are associated with an increased risk of sexual and continence side effects, while intrafascial dissection exposes to positive surgical margins. Being able to accurately diagnose the extra prostatic extension and the limits of the tumor are essential to adapt surgical decisions.

Rectal Examination for Local Staging Literature has suggested that errors in clinical staging are common, and intra observer variability of DRE may lead to misinterpretation of real staging but can detect more aggressive cancer more selectively [26].

Radiological Evaluation
Unfortunately, studies have not shown TRUS to be superior to DRE for local staging of prostate cancer and TRUS is unable to detect focal extra prostatic extension and mp MRI gives better results and is considered the gold standard.

For local staging, mp MRI is indicated at least 6 weeks after biopsies to minimize artifacts induced by hemorrhages post punctures. A meta-analysis reported by De Rooij analyzed the role of MRI for staging. For ECE (45 studies, 5681 patients), SVI (34 studies, 5677 patients), and overall stage T3 detection (38 studies, 4001 patients) showed sensitivity and specificity of 0.57 (95 % confidence interval [CI] 0.49–0.64) and 0.91 (95 % CI 0.88–0.93), 0.58 (95 % CI 0.47–0.68) and 0.96 (95 % CI 0.95–0.97), and 0.61 (95 % CI 0.54–0.67) and 0.88 (95 % CI 0.85–0.91), respectively [20]. Accuracy of mp MRI remains very poor for the detection of microscopic capsular extension. Sensitivity for ECE detection increases with the radius of extension and 3Tesla mp MRI could be added to nomograms to improve the prediction of pathological T3a disease, while for low risk patients, MRI is not very helpful (Fig. 2).

Consequently, given its low sensitivity for focal (microscopic) extraprostatic extension in the European Association of Urology guidelines

2016, mp MRI "is not recommended for local staging in low-risk patients." However, mp MRI can still be useful for treatment planning in selected low-risk patients and in the NCCN guidelines 2016 mp MRI "can be used in the staging and characterization of prostate cancer."

3.2 Lymph Node staging

Although nomograms can be helpful in predicting lymph node metastasis risk, CT or MRI can be considered as standard imaging modalities for the assessment of lymph node extension for patients with intermediate or high risk prostate cancer or when nomogram indicate a probability of lymph node involvement ≥10 %. Number, shape, and size of lymph nodes (diameter 8–12 mm in short axis) are analyzed, but the sensitivity of these radiological investigation varies from 20 to 60 % according to the diameter threshold and micrometastases are often undetected. Thus, extended lymphadenectomy according to initial risk factors and nomograms remains the standard of care for lymph node assessment.

More recently, choline PET/CT which combine anatomical and functional imaging was introduced. ^{18}F-choline and ^{11}C-choline were evaluated via a meta-analysis for initial lymph node staging [27]. Many of the authors underlined a high false-negative rate in relation to the small dimension of a lymph node. However, some reported a similar PPV for 18 F-choline PET/CT in lymph nodes both <5 mm and >5 mm

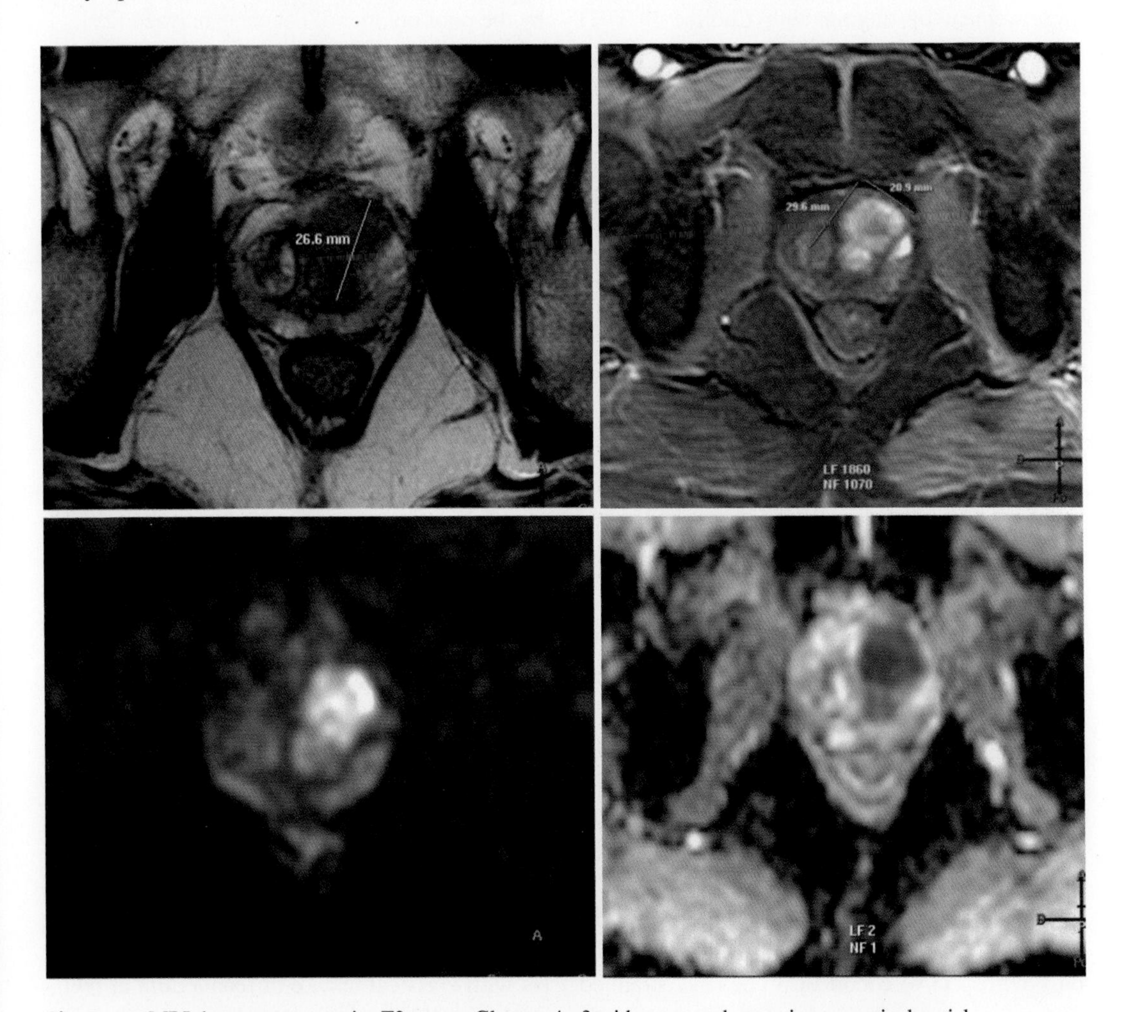

Fig. 2 mp MRI demonstrate anterior T3 cancer Gleason 4 + 3 with suspected extension to seminal vesicle

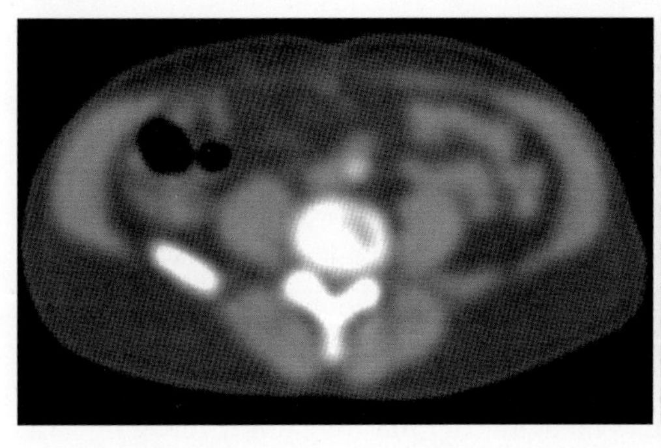
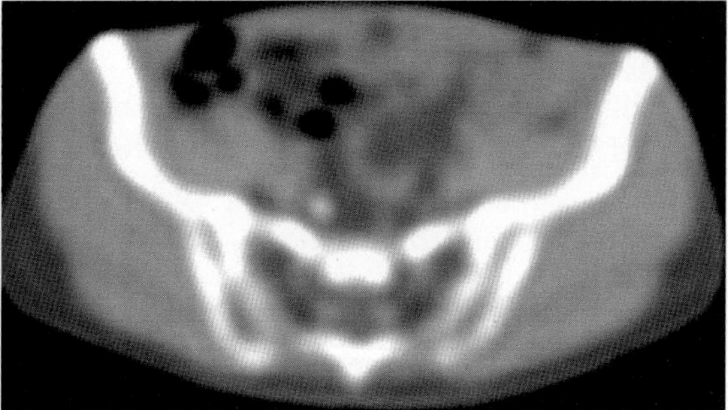

Fig. 3 Suspected lymph node on 18 F-choline TEP (confirmed during lymphadenectomy)

in diameter (PPVs = 82 %), suggesting that the FP rate can be reduced by acquiring delayed images rather than early images [28] (Fig. 3).

In a recent review, the authors report an improvement of staging with Choline PET/CT compared to anatomical imaging with a sensitivity for lymph node detection up to 69.2 (95 % Cl : 39.9–58.4 %) with a good specificity of 95 % (95%Cl : 92–97.1 %), but these studies are limited by the poor number of patients analyzed [29].

					PET or PET/CT		Comparative imaging	
Author	Year	Nb Pts	RFA	Comparative imaging	Se (%)	Sp (%)	Se (%)	Sp (%)
Budiharto	2011	36	11 C-choline	DWI- MRI	9.4	99.7	18.8	97.6
Heck	2014	33	11 C-choline	DWI- MRI	57.1	89.5	57.1	78.9
Pinaquy	2015	47	11 C-choline	DWI- MRI	78	94	33	91
Evangelista	2015	48	18 F-choline	BS or CT	LN: 69.2 B: 100	92.3 86.4	CT : 46.2 BS : 90	92.3 77.2

Diagnostic accuracies of PET/CT and conventional imaging in staging prostate cancer
From Ref. [29] Evangelista 2016
BS bone scan, *RFA* radiopharmaceutical agent

However, medicoeconomic studies are missing, and today, choline PET/CT has a limited place for initial staging and is more useful after local treatment to evaluate PSA recurrence, looking for lymph nodes extension or recurrence outside the pelvic field.

Due to limitations of choline PET, other innovative PET tracers like Ga68-PSMA represent a new emerging and promising challenge for prostate cancer lymph node imaging. PSMA is a membrane glycoprotein that is characterized and clinically validated as a marker of prostate cancer expressed in high grade tumors [30]. Different types of radiotracers have been developed because a large number of ligands are available [29]. Budaus et al. [31], on a retrospective cohort of 30 patients stratified after prostatectomy by nodal status reported with Ga68_PSMA a PPV of 100 % and a NPV of 69.2 %. These results were influenced by lymph node metastasis size. Indeed, we have to wait for new data comparing 68 Ga-PSMA findings and histological assessment to confirm these preliminary promising results.

3.3 Distant Bone Metastasis

X-ray for bone metastatic lesion is out of date compared to other imaging investigation.

Technetium scintigraphy, despite a poor performance unless PSA >20 ng/ml, remains the gold standard for the detection of bone metastasis with classical uptake of technetium at metastatic sites [32].

The NCCN guidelines suggest that bone scan should be performed in men who meet any of the following criteria: clinical T1 disease and PSA >20, clinical T2 disease and PSA >10, Gleason score 8, clinical T3 or T4 disease, or symptoms suggestive of metastases.

CT is also widely used for evaluating bone metastasis in spite of low specificity which increases with PSA level. When metastasis avec evoked, MRI optimizes morphologic evaluation of help determining bone fracture and neurological risk [33].

3.4 PSA Relapse and Detection of Local Recurrence After Curative Treatment

When biochemical recurrence occurs, hormonotherapy is often the first option to treat the patient. However, radiologic investigation is important and may change our management, especially if we find an isolated recurrence in the prostate or in a lymph node and even a unique metastasis. Then according to the radiological target, it is possible to discuss in a multidisciplinary board the opportunity of salvage treatments.

3.4.1 Rectal Examination and Clinical Workup

After radical prostatectomy, biological recurrence is determined by PSA level >0.2 ng/ml.

At these low level of PSA, DRE is usually negative and unable to detect local recurrence and taking account clinical modifications of rectal examination created by these treatments, DRE is of a little help for identifying recurrence. However, rectal examination is essential to analyze rectal flexibility and discuss patient management and treatment.

After external radiotherapy or brachytherapy, biological recurrence is defined by Phoenix criteria: PSA level over Nadir + 2 ng/ml and 3 consecutive elevations.

When patients treated initially by EBRT experience biochemical recurrence are suitable for another local treatment, it may be reasonable to rule out local recurrence with mp MRI according to initial staging of the disease and comorbidities of the patient. When T2 and DCE show abnormalities, the cancer rate detection is important and TRUS biopsies can be performed to confirm the diagnosis.

If iterative irradiation is decided, on a clinical point of view, complete local evaluation including uretrocystoscopy and rectoscopy should be considered to explore and anticipate side effects of retreatment (rectorragies and hematuria) especially in this elderly population susceptible to need anticoagulant medication for cardiovascular or neurological diseases. Distant metastasis have also to be rule out with anatomical and TEP metabolic exploration.

3.4.2 PET/CT

While (FDG) PET scanning is of limited utility with suspected recurrent prostate cancer, PET choline has been studied in restaging and results were compared with classical imaging by Evangelista [29].

					PET or PET/CT		Comparative imaging	
Author	Year	Nb Pts	RFA	Comparative imaging	Se (%)	Sp (%)	Se (%)	Sp (%)
Richter	2010	42	11 C- Choline	FDG	61	100	31	100
Picchio	2012	78	11 C- Choline	BS	89	98–100	70–100	75–100
Van Den Berg	2012	49	11 C- Choline	MRI	77.4	44.9	33.5	94.6
Panebianco	2012	84	18 F- Choline	MRI	A: 62 B: 92	50 33	92 94	75 100

Diagnostic accuracies of PET/CT and conventional imaging in restaging prostate cancer
From Ref. [29] Evangelista 2016
RFA radiopharmaceutical agent

Sensitivity depends on the cutoff of PSA, but two different factors increase the likelihood of positive PET : PSA > 2 ng/ml PSA DT < 6 months [34].

^{68}Ga-PSMA PET/CT has also demonstrated promising results and might be a better tracer than choline for detection of lymph node metastasis. It was reported that 68Ga-PSMA tracer is able to detect a significant uptake in more than 60 % of recurrent prostate cancer patients with a PSA less than 1 ng/ml and in more than 80 % in those with a PSA higher than 2 ng/ml. On a short cohort of 17 patients with PET-positive nodal oligometastatic lesion treated by extensive salvage lymphadenectomy, Hijazi et al. [35] reported 2 false-positive nodes and one negative node in the obturator fossa.

Choline PET was also compared versus ^{68}Ga-PSMA in patients with rising PSA after curative treatment in 38 patients. The mean PSA level was 1.74 ± 2.54 ng/ml. The scan result was negative for both tracers in 32 %. However, ^{68}Ga-PSMA demonstrated a higher detection rate compare to choline. These promising results are very preliminary and have to be confirmed [36] and this radiotracer, highly specific for prostate cancer, could be used without delay in biochemical recurrence.

PSA level	Choline detection	PSMA detection
0.5 ng/ml	12.5 %	50 %
0.5–2 ng/ml	31 %	69 %
2 ng/ml	57 %	86 %

4 Classifications

It is important to differentiate between the clinical and pathological staging of prostate cancer. Clinical staging and pathological staging are defined by the American Joint Committee on Cancer.

These classifications represent the cornerstone of all guidelines for treatment decisions and follow-up of patients. They should be used widely.

4.1 Clinical TNM Staging of Prostate Cancer

Primary tumor (T)	Regional lymph nodes (N)	Distant metastasis (M)
cTx : Primary tumor cannot be assessed	Nx : Regional lymph nodes not sampled	M0 : No distant metastasis
cT0 : No evidence of tumor	N0 : No positive regional lymph node	M1 : Distant metastasis
cT1 : Clinical unapparent tumor neither palpable nor visible by imaging	N1 : Metastases in regional lymph nodes	M1a : Non regional lymph node(s)

Primary tumor (T)	Regional lymph nodes (N)	Distant metastasis (M)
cT1a : Tumor incidental histological finding in less than 5 % of tissue resected		M1b : Bone(s)
cT1b : Tumor incidental histological finding in more than 5 % of tissue resected		M1c : Other site(s) with or without bone disease
cT1c : Tumor identified by needle biopsy (e.g., because of elevated PSA)		
cT2 : Tumor confined within the gland		
cT2a : Tumor involves one half of one lobe or less		
cT2b : Tumor involves more than one half of one lobe but not both lobes		
cT2c : Tumor involves both lobes		
cT3 : Tumor extends through the prostate capsule		
cT3a : Extracapsular extension (unilateral or bilateral)		
cT3b : Tumor invades seminal vesicle(s)		
cT4 : Tumor is fixed or invades adjacent structures other than seminal vesicles such as rectum, bladder, levator muscles, and/or pelvic wall		

Note that tumor found in one or both lobes by needle biopsy but not palpable or visible by imaging is classified as T1c
Laterality does not affect the N classification
When more than one site of metastasis is present, the most advanced category should be used

4.2 Pathologic TNM Staging

Pathologic stage (T)	Regional lymp nodes (pN)	Distant metastasis (M)
pT2 : Organ confined	Nx : Regional lymph nodes not assessed	M0 : No distant metastasis
pT2a : Unilateral, one half of one side or less	N0 : No regional lymph node metastases	M1 : Distant metastasis
pT2b : Unilateral, involving more than one half of one side but not both sides	N1 : Metastasis in regional lymph nodes	M1a : Non regional lymph node(s)
pT2c : Bilateral disease		M1b : Bone(s)
pT3 : Extraprostatic extension		M1c : Other site(s) with or without bone disease
pT3a : Extracapsular extension or microscopic invasion of bladder neck		
pT3b : Seminal vesicle invasion		
pT4 : Invasion of rectum, levator muscles, and/or pelvic wall		

Invasion to the prostatic apex, or into (but not beyond) the prostate capsule is not classified a pT3, but as pT2

The regional lymph nodes are the nodes of the true pelvis, which essentially are the pelvic nodes below the bifurcation of the common iliac arteries

4.3 Prognostic risk group classification

4.3.1 D'Amico Classification

The D'Amico classification based on DRE, PSA level, and Gleason score is used all over the world to classify patients with prostate cancer.

Low risk	Intermediate risk	High risk	
PSA < 10 ng/ml and GS < 7 and cT1-T2a	PSA 10–20 ng/ml or GS 7 or cT2b	PSA > 20 ng/ml or GS > 7 or cT2c	any PSA any GS cT3 T4 or cN+
Localized			Locally advanced

4.3.2 EAU Classification

The European Association of Urology guidelines is based on three groups :

Low risk	Intermediate risk	High risk
PSA < 10 ng/ml and GS < 7 and cT1	PSA 10–20 ng/ml or GS 7 or cT2b – *T2c*	PSA > 20 ng/ml or GS 8–10 or ≥ cT3a

4.3.3 NCCN Classification

The NCCN clinical practice guideline classification and staging is also design to help clinician to determine an individual patient risk and adapt treatment or active surveillance according to sub classifications.

Major interest was focused on low risk prostate cancer because screening programs had increased the number of these patients. While active surveillance (AS) is recommended to reduce overtreatments in patients with D'Amico low risk group, criteria to stratify in this group candidates for surveillance are needed because these patients do not have homogeneous histology after radical prostatectomy.

Taking account this heterogeneity, several studies propose to differentiate between low risk and very low risk patients.

Likewise, the treatment of intermediate and high risk patients is also controversial due to the heterogeneity of the patients and the necessity of multimodal treatments.

For the Prostate Cancer International Research Group, active surveillance include a biopsy GS ≤ 6, a PSA level ≤ 10 ng/ml, a PSA density ≤0.2 ng/mL/cm^3, and no more than 2 positive cores.

In the NCCN classification, version 1.2014, low risk tumors are divided according to the results of the biopsies into very low and low risk groups. For cT2c tumors, they are considered intermediate as opposed to high risk in D'Amico.

	Very low	Low	Intermediate	High	Locally advanced	Metastatic
Clinical stage	T1c	T1-T2 a	T2b- *T2c* or	T3a or	T3b – T4	Any T, N1 Any T, N, M1
Gleason score	≤6	≤6	=7 or	8–10 or		
PSA ng/ml	<10	<10	10–20	>20		
Cores results	*Fewer than 3 prostate biopsy cores positive, less than 50 % of cancer in each core*					
PSA d ng/ml/g	*<0.15*					

The NCCN.org Classification.

4.3.4 Other Classifications

Other factors have been described to dichotomize low risk group patient like the level of PSA (<6.7 ng/ml versus >6.7 and <10), and patient age >69 years that could be more likely to harbor either intermediate or high risk characteristic at final prostatectomy [37].

To stratify patients discuss in a multidisciplinary approach and set up treatments, risk group classifications or scores have been described. As examples,

- CAPRA-S score is use to assess disease risk and improve the prediction of outcome after radical prostatectomy [38]. Capra-S score is calculated combining 6 variables: PSA, surgical margins, seminal vesicle invasion, GS, extracapsular extension, lymph node involvement. Capra score identified 3 groups of risk : low risk patients with Capra <3; intermediate between 3 and 5 and high risk group with a score from 6 to 10 .
- Zumsteg described a new classification system for therapeutic decisions making with intermediate risk prostate cancer patients undergoing dose escaladed external beam radiation therapy. Dint suggests modifications of NCCN risk groups according to pathologic results of radical prostatectomy in low risk patients after analysis of 14,902 patients from the SEER database. On multivariate analysis, low risk patients with ≥50 % PCB have similar risk of pathologic high risk specimen define by pT3a-T4 or GS>7 than favorable intermediate disease and this concerns almost one in five patients of this group [39].
- On a large multicentric cohort of 1360 consecutive high risk patients treated with prostatectomy at eight European tertiary centers, Joniau et al. [40] propose also a stratification for high risk cancers with a dichotomization using PSA ≤ 20 ng/ml and >20, GS 2-7 versus 8-10, cT1 2 versus T3 T4 . He showed that 3 groups could be stratified according to cancer specific survival : good prognostic group with only one defavorable factor, intermediate sub group with 2 risk factors (PSA>20 ng/ml and cT3 T4) and poor prognostic subgroup with all 3 defavorable factors.

All these sub classification can be helpful for counseling patients and decide treatments or surveillance modalities, and in the future, tissue based genomic tools could also help stratifying intermediate and high risk patients and evaluate the natural history of prostate cancers.

Conclusion

Clinical guidelines are increasingly being used in the world to promote high quality evidence patient care and critical analysis of literature. Clearly recent classifications changed to consider heterogeneity of prostate cancers.

We need, to improve our clinical decisions, new tools helping us in a real time for prediction of aggressive cancer. Biomarkers, recent modalities of anatomical and metabolic imaging techniques, appear to be particularly important in men with high risk disease when a multidisciplinary approach is necessary to improve the outcome of these men with personalize medicine.

References

1. Mahmood U, Levy LB, Nguyen PL, et al. Current clinical presentation and treatment of localized prostate cancer in the united states. J Urol. 2014;192(6):1650–6.
2. Loeb S, Catalona WJ. What is the role of digital rectal examination in men undergoing serial screening of serum PSA levels? Nat Clin Pract Urol. 2009;6(2):68–9.
3. Stamey TA, Mitchell Caldwell M, Mcneal JE, et al. The prostate specific antigen era in the United States is over for prostate cancer: what happened in the last 20 years? J Urol. 2004;172(4):1297–301.

4. Roddam AW, Duffy MJ, Hamdy FC. Use of prostate-specific antigen (PSA) isoforms for the detection of prostate cancer in men with a PSA level of 2–10 ng/ml: systematic review and meta-analysis. Eur Urol. 2005;48(3):386–99.
5. Mottet N, Bellmunt J, Briers E, et al. Prostate cancer guideline EAU ESTRO SIOG. Eur Urol. 2016. in press.
6. Catalona WJ, Partin AW, Sanda MG, et al. A multicenter study of [−2]Pro-prostate specific antigen combined with prostate specific antigen and free prostate specific antigen for prostate cancer detection in the 2.0 to 10.0 ng/ml prostate specific antigen range. J Urol. 2011;185(5):1650–5.
7. Loeb S, Sanda MG, Dennis L, et al. The prostate health index selectively identifies clinically significant prostate cancer stacy. J Urol. 2015;193:1163–9.
8. Fossati N, Buffi NM, Haese A, et al. Preoperative prostate-specific antigen isoform p2PSA and its derivatives, %p2PSA and prostate health index, predict pathologic outcomes in patients undergoing radical prostatectomy for prostate cancer: results from a multicentric European prospective study. Eur Urol. 2015;68(1):132–8.
9. Lepor A, Catalona WJ, Loeb S. The prostate health index: its utility in prostate cancer detection : review article. Urol Clin North Am. 2016;43(1):1–6.
10. Vedder MM, De Bekker-Grob EW, Lilja HG, et al. The added value of percentage of free to total prostate-specific antigen, PCA3, and a kallikrein panel to the ERSPC risk calculator for prostate cancer in prescreened men. Eur Urol. 2014;66(6):1109–15.
11. McDonald ML, Parsons JK. 4-Kallikrein test and Kallikrein markers in prostate screening. M L. Urol Clin North Am. 2016;43:39–46.
12. Parekha DJ, Punnena S, Sjobergb DD, et al. A multi-institutional prospective trial in the USA confirms that the 4Kscore accurately identifies men with high-grade prostate cancer. Eur Urol. 2015;68:464–70.
13. Nordström T, Vickers A, Assel M, Lilja H, et al. Comparaison between the four-kallikrein panel and prostate health index for predicting prostate cancer. Eur Urol. 2015;68:139–46.
14. Auprich M, Chun FKH, Ward JF, et al. Critical assessment of preoperative urinary prostate cancer antigen 3 on the accuracy of prostate cancer staging. Eur Urol. 2011;59(1):96–105.
15. Roobol MJ, Zhu X, Schröder FH, et al. A calculator for prostate cancer risk 4 years after an initially negative screen: findings from ERSPC Rotterdam. Eur Urol. 2013;63(4):627–33.
16. Ankerst DP, Cathee Till C, Andreas Boeck A, et al. The impact of prostate volume, number of biopsy cores and American urological association symptom score on the sensitivity of cancer detection using the prostate cancer prevention trial risk calculator. J Urol. 2013;190(1):70–6.
17. Thompson IM, Vickers AJ, Strobl AN, et al. The next generation of clinical decision making tools: development of a real-time prediction tool for outcome of prostate biopsy in response to a continuously evolving prostate cancer landscape. J Urol. 2015;194(1):58–64.
18. Weinreb JC, Barentsz JO, Choyke PL, et al. PI-RADS prostate imaging – reporting and data system: 2015, version 2. Eur Urol. 2016;69(1):16–40.
19. Fütterer JJ, Briganti A, De Visschere P, et al. Can clinically significant prostate cancer be detected with multiparametric magnetic resonance imaging? a systematic review of the literature. Eur Urol. 2015;68(6):1045–53.
20. De Rooij M, Hamoen EH, Witjes A, et al. Accuracy of magnetic resonance imaging for local staging of prostate cancer: a diagnostic meta-analysis. Eur Urol. 2016;70(2):233–45.
21. Jiang X, Zhu S, Feng G, et al. Is an initial saturation prostate biopsy scheme better than an extended scheme for detection of prostate cancer? a systematic review and meta-analysis. Eur Urol. 2013;63(6):1031–9.
22. Barry Delongchamps N, Lefevre A, Bouazza M, et al. Detection of significant prostate cancer with magnetic resonance targeted biopsies : should transrectal ultrasound-magnetic resonance imaging fusion guided biopsies alone be a standard of care? J Urol. 2015;193:1198–204.
23. Baco E, Rud E, Ukimura O, et al. Effect of targeted biopsy guided by elastic image fusion of MRI with 3D-TRUS on diagnosis of anterior prostate cancer. Urol Oncol. 2014;32:1300–7.
24. Baco E, Rud E, Eri LM, et al. A randomized controlled trial to assess and compare the outcomes of two-core prostate biopsy guided by fused magnetic resonance and transrectal ultrasound images and traditional 12-core systematic biopsy. Eur Urol. 2016;69(1):149–56.
25. Schoots G, Roobol MJ, Nieboer D, et al. Magnetic resonance imaging–targeted biopsy may enhance the diagnostic accuracy of significant prostate cancer detection compared to standard transrectal ultrasound-guided biopsy: a systematic review and meta-analysis. Eur Urol. 2015;68(3):438–50.
26. Gosselaar C, Kranse R, Roobol MJ. The inter observer variability of digital rectal examination in a large randomized trial for the screening of prostate cancer. Prostate. 2008;68:985–93.
27. Evangelista L, Guttilla A, Zattoni F, et al. Utility of choline positron emission tomography/computed tomography for lymph node involvement identification in intermediate- to high-risk prostate cancer: a systematic literature review and meta-analysis. Eur Urol. 2013;63(6):1040–8.
28. Beheshti M, Imamovic L, Broiger G, et al. 18F choline PET/CT in the preoperative staging of prostate cancer in patients with intermediate or high risk of extracapsular disease: a prospective study of 130 patients. Radiology. 2010;254:925–33.
29. Evangelista L, Briganti A, Fanti S, et al. New clinical indications for ^{18}F/^{11}C-choline, new tracers for positron

emission tomography and a promising hybrid device for prostate cancer staging: a systematic review of the literature. Eur Urol. 2016;70(1):161–75.
30. Afshar-Oromieh A, Avtzi E, Giesel FL, et al. The diagnostic value of PET/CT imaging with the 68Ga-labelled PSMA ligant HBED-CC in the diagnosis of recurrent prostate cancer. Eur J Nucl Med Mol Imaging. 2015;42:197–209.
31. Budäus L, Leyh-Bannurah S-R, Salomon G, et al. Initial experience of 68Ga-PSMA PET/CT imaging in high-risk prostate cancer patients prior to radical prostatectomy. Eur Urol. 2016;69(3):393–6.
32. Langsteger W, et al. Imaging of bone metastasis in prostate cancer: an update. Q J Nucl Med Mod Imaging. 2012;56:447.
33. Lecouvet FE, Geukens D, Stainier A, et al. Magnetic resonance imaging of the axial skeleton for detecting bone metastases in patients with high-risk prostate cancer: diagnostic and cost-effectiveness and comparison with current detection strategies. J Clin Oncol. 2007;25(22):3281.
34. Ceci F, Castellucci P, Graziani T, et al. PET/computed tomography in the individualization of treatment of prostate cancer. PET Clin. 2015;10(4):487–94.
35. Hijazi S, Meller B, Leitsmann C, et al. Pelvic lymph node dissection for nodal oligometastatic prostate cancer detected by 68Ga-PSMA-positron emission tomography/computerized tomography. Prostate. 2015;75(16):1934–40.
36. Morigi JJ, Stricker PD, van Leeuwen PJ, et al. Prospective comparison of 18F-fluoromethylcholine versus 68Ga-PSMA PET/CT in prostate cancer patients Who have rising PSA after curative treatment and are being considered for targeted therapy. J Nucl Med. 2015;56(8):1185–90.
37. Gandaglia G, Schiffmann J, Schlomm T, et al. Identification of pathologically favorable disease in intermediate-risk prostate cancer patients: implications for active surveillance candidates selection. Prostate. 2015;75(13):1484–91.
38. Punnen S, Freedland SJ, Presti JC, et al. Multi-institutional validation of the CAPRA-S score to predict disease recurrence and mortality after radical prostatectomy. Eur Urol. 2014;2014(65):1171–7.
39. Zumsteg ZS, Spratt DE, Pei I, et al. A new risk classification system for therapeutic decision making with intermediate-risk prostate cancer patients undergoing dose-escalated external-beam radiation therapy. Eur Urol. 2013;64:895–902.
40. Joniau S, Briganti A, Gontero P, et al. Stratification of high-risk prostate cancer into prognostic categories: a European multi-institutional study, European multi-center prostate cancer clinical and translational research group (EMPaCT). Eur Urol. 2015;67:157–64.

Active Surveillance for Low Risk Prostate Cancer

Laurence Klotz

1 Introduction

The approach to favorable risk prostate cancer known as "active surveillance" was first described explicitly in 2002 [1]. This was a report of 250 patients managed with a strategy of expectant management, with serial PSA and periodic biopsy, and radical intervention advised for patients who were re-classified as higher risk. This was initiated as a prospective clinical trial, complete with informed consent, beginning in 2007. Thus, there is now 20 years of experience with this approach, which has become widely adopted around the world. In this chapter, we will summarize the biological basis for active surveillance, review the experience to date, including many lessons that have been learned, describe the current approach to active surveillance, enhanced by the use of MRI, and forecast the future directions.

2 Background

The identification of men with indolent, clinically insignificant prostate cancer began in the 1950s, when TURP became widely adopted for BPH. About 10% of men having undergoing a TURP were found to have clinically unsuspected prostate cancer; in most cases this was small volume, low-grade disease (stage T1a). A largely unremarked but remarkable consensus developed that this cancer did not warrant treatment. This is extraordinary in the context of the perception of cancer at the time as a uniformly lethal and aggressive disease. Following the advent of PSA testing around 1990, the incidence of microfocal low-grade disease increased dramatically.

The Achilles heel of screening is the overdiagnosis and overtreatment of clinically insignificant disease. At roughly the same time as PSA testing became widely available, the nerve sparing radical prosatatectomy also became popularized. The combination of increased detection and well meaning enthusiasm for surgical resection of cancer as a definitive curative therapy with less morbidity than in previous years led to a dramatic wave of radical prostatectomies. This was soon followed by an increase in radiation treatment, which was seen as less morbid.

Enthusiasm for early detection and aggressive management of most cancers so identified continued relatively unabated until 2012, when the US Preventive Services Task Force announced a

L. Klotz, MD, FRCSC, CM
Division of Urology, Sunnybrook Health Sciences Centre, 2075 Bayview Ave. #MG408, Toronto, ON M4N 3M5, Canada
e-mail: Laurence.klotz@sunnybrook.ca

M. Bolla, H. van Poppel (eds.), *Management of Prostate Cancer*,
DOI 10.1007/978-3-319-42769-0_10

Table 1 Outcomes of AS in prospective series with >100 patients

Reference	*n*	Median follow-up (months)	% treated overall; % treatment free	Overall/disease specific survival (%)	% BCR post deferred treatment
Klotz et al. (2015) [21] University of Toronto	993	92	30; 72 at 5 years	79/ 97 at 10 years	25 % (6 % overall)
Tosian et al. (2015) [22], Johns Hopkins, USA	1298	NR 60	50 % at 10 years 57 % at 15 years	69 % /99.9 % at 15 years	NR
Bul et al. (2013) [23], Multicentre, Europe	2500 2494	20	21 %	77/100 at 10 years	20 %^
Dall'Era et al. (2008) [24] UCSF	328 321	43	24; 67 at 5 years	CSS 100 %	NR
Kakehi et al. (2008) [25], Multicentre, Japan	118	36	51; 49 at 3 years	NR	NR
Roemeling et al. (2007) [26], Rotterdam Netherlands	273	41	29; 71 at 5 years	89/100 at 5 years	NR [31 % of 13 RP positive margins]
Barayan et al. (2014) [27] McGill, Canada	155 155	65	20 %	100/100	NR
Rubio-Briones et al. (2014) [28] Spain	232	36	27 %	93 % @ 5 years/99.5 %	NR
Godtman et al. (2014) [29]	439		63 %	81/99.8	14
Thomsen et al. (2013) [30] Denmark	167	40	35/60 % 5 years		
Selvadurai et al. (2014) [31] UK	471	67	30	98/99.7	12

level D recommendation against PSA screening [2], followed by recommendations regarding PSA screening by several other respected national health policy organizations. Criticism was warranted. Overdetection had resulted in a great deal of overtreatment with attendant side effects, which undermined the benefit of the cancer deaths avoided. This remains a topic of intense controversy and disagreement. (Most experts believe that PSA screening provides a mortality benefit and the cost of significant overdiagnosis; if overtreatment is avoided, the mortality benefit is compelling) [3]. However, the consequences of the USPSTF recommendation (and that of other groups) has been a steady drop in the rate of PSA testing and referral for biopsy over the last few years. In 2016, 4 years after the USPSTF recommendation, an increase in locally advanced and metastatic cancers has now been reported by several groups, along with less low-grade cancers (i.e., overdiagnosis) [4].

Where PSA testing was widely prevalent, a striking phenomenon was observed. For 5 years after testing was introduced, the annual age adjusted incidence tripled, followed by a gradual decrease. At the same time, the average volume of cancer at the time of diagnosis diminished steadily. This was a paradigmatic example of stage migration of cancer, occurring as a result of a new diagnostic test which detects cancer that was previously undiagnosed but highly prevalent. The new testing paradigm (PSA followed by a biopsy) resulted in the almost instantaneous (in epidemiologic terms) diagnosis of hundreds of thousands of men who harbored preclinical prostate cancer. As the prevalent cases were identified, treated, and "extracted" from the pool, the incidence gradually drifted back towards baseline levels, reflecting the "true" incidence of the disease.

From 1990 to 2010, more than 90 % of patients diagnosed with low risk prostate cancer by PSA and biopsy were treated radically [5]. However, following the task force recommendation, and bolstered by substantial evidence regarding the indolent nature of low-grade disease and the favorable outcome with conservative management, an increasing consensus about the value and benefit of active surveillance has emerged. The most recent available data are that the proportion of patients with low risk disease managed conservatively increased from about 10 % in 2000 to 40 % in 2013 [5].

3 The Natural History and Molecular Genetics of Low-Grade Prostate Cancer

Prostate cancer occurs as part of the aging process in all races and regions. In Caucasians and Blacks, the chance of harboring prostate cancer is approximately the same as one's age; 30 % of men in their 30s, 40 % in their 40s, and 80 % of men in their 80s [6]. Most of these are microscopic foci (<1 mm^3) and low grade. A recent autopsy study in both Japan and Russia, both countries in which PSA testing was not widely performed, found that in men who died of other causes 35 % had prostate cancer. Surprisingly, 50 % of the cancers in Japanese men >70 were Gleason score 7 or above [7]. This finding suggests that, particularly in men over 70, microfocal Gleason 3+4 might also represent "overdiagnosis."

4 Genetic Features of Low-Grade Prostate Cancer

Gleason 3 and 4 patterns the two most common histologic patterns of prostate cancer, differ profoundly in terms of their molecular characteristics. The hallmarks of cancer biology include unlimited replicative potential, sustained angiogenesis, local tissue invasion, insensitivity to antigrowth signals, metastasis, and replicative self-sufficiency, de-regulating cellular energetics, and evasion of immune destruction [8, 9]. Despite Gleason grading being based on a low power view of cellular architecture, the Gleason score has a remarkable ability to disaggregate prostate cancer between genetically normal and abnormal cells. Genetic pathways mediating apoptosis resistance, angiogenesis and the development of other pro-angiogenic factors, genes involved in regulating cellular metabolomics, and metastasis and invasion processes, are abnormal in Gleason 4 and normal in 3. The abnormality, typically, is overexpression in the case of oncogenes, and deletion or inactivation in the case of tumor suppressor genes. The profound genetic differences between most Gleason pattern 3 and pattern 4 cancers are summarized in an excellent review by Ahmed et al. [10].

Although most Gleason pattern 3 cells have relatively normal genetic characteristics, preclinical genetic changes may occur. (This is the basis for molecular biomarkers). The TMPRSS2-ERG translocation [11], and pTEN deletion [12], are common in most Gleason 4s, and are altered in about 10 % of Gleason 3 cancers. Given the limits of histologic assessment, this is not surprising. However, these isolated genetic alterations do not appear to translate into an aggressive metastatic phenotype, with rare exceptions.

4.1 Metastatic Potential of Low Risk Prostate Cancer

Prostate cancer is heterogeneous, ranging from completely indolent to extremely aggressive. Some cancers, due to lack of telomerase/VEGF/other biological machinery, may undergo spontaneous involution [13]. Several large clinical series have reported a rate of metastasis for surgically confirmed Gleason 6 (where there is no possibility of occult higher grade cancer lurking in the prostate) that approximates zero. Studies based on biopsy assessment showing low-grade cancer are limited the presence of occult higher grade cancer in about 25 % of men These are likely responsible for most of the prostate cancer deaths reported in conservative management series.

An alternative explanation for the very low rate of metastasis following surgery for Gleason 6 cancer is that the intervention is highly successful, alters the natural history of the disease, and prevents all cancer deaths. However, if Gleason 6 had even modest metastatic potential, one would have expected a few of the Gleason 6 cancers to have micro-metastasized prior to surgery, or to have a local recurrence with subsequent metastasis. This is rarely if ever observed.

One multicenter study of 24,000 men with long-term follow-up after surgery included 12,000 with surgically confirmed Gleason 6 cancer [14]. The 20-year prostate cancer mortality was 0.2 %. About 4000 of these were treated at MSKCC; of these, 1 died of prostate cancer; a pathological review of this patient revealed Gleason 4+3 disease in the primary; in other words, it was misclassified as Gleason 6 [15]. A second study of 14,000 men with surgically confirmed Gleason 6 disease found only 22 with lymph node metastases; review of these cases showed that all 22 were misclassified, and had higher grade cancer in the primary tumor. The rate of node positive disease in the 14,000 patients with no Gleason 4 or 5 disease in their prostates was therefore zero [16].

Gleason grading does not correlate perfectly with biology, although it is powerfully predictive. A recent genetic analysis of multiple metastatic sites from a patient who had extensive Gleason 4+3 pT3a N1 disease resected at age 47, and died 17 years later of metastatic CRPC, reported that the metastatic lesions appeared to derive from a microfocus of Gleason pattern 3 disease, rather than, as expected, from the high-grade cancers elsewhere in the prostate [17]. This case report is a challenge to the view that Gleason pattern 3 does not behave like a malignancy. It is fair to say in response that (a) biology is complex and not 100 % predictable; (b) this is a single case report and should be viewed in that context; and (c) it is possible that histological Gleason pattern 3, particularly when it coexists with higher grade cancer, may harbor prehistological genetic alterations that confer a more aggressive phenotype. This is the conceptual basis for genetically based predictive assays. This case should be balanced against the extensive clinical evidence supporting the absence of metastatic potential in pure Gleason pattern 3 cancers. It has been suggested that perhaps the explanation in this case is "backwards" differentiation of higher grade to lower grade cancer, as a re-differentiated clonal offspring of a cancer that had metastasized, resulting in a shared genetic phenotype [18]. Another provocative explanation is the recent observation that cancer cells shed extracellular vesicles containing biological material including mRNA, which may adversely influence the biological behavior of more favorable cancer cells in the same tumor, or elsewhere in the body [19].

Understanding that Gleason pattern 3 has little or no metastatic phenotype has altered the approach to these patients. The fundamental concept is that Gleason 6 is a risk biomarker for having significant prostate cancer, but is not a significant disease in itself. Some clinical and pathological parameters in men with Gleason 6 predict for an increase of higher grade cancer. These include volume of disease on biopsy (i.e., number of cores and extent of core involvement); PSA density; and race (higher in blacks). Thus the main significance of higher volume Gleason pattern 3 cancer is that it should prompt a vigorous search for higher grade disease, either with MRI or extended systematic biopsies, but does not warrant intervention on its own in most cases. A threshold effect of more than 8 mm of total cancer on systematic biopsy has recently been described [20]. Many studies have also reported that a PSA density >0.15 is associated with occult higher grade cancer.

Young age should not preclude offering patients active surveillance. The QOL benefits of preserving erectile function and continence are greater in young men, and the risks of second malignancies as sequelae of radiation are also greater in men with a long life expectancy. 40 % of men in their 40s harbor microfocal prostate cancer [6]. Most will never be diagnosed.

Active surveillance offers the prospect of reduced morbidity and improved quality of life, but its adoption should also result in an improvement in prostate cancer survival. How could less treatment of prostate cancer improve mortality? PSA screening has been discredited by influential groups such as the USPSTF because of their concern about the risks of overtreatment and a high number needed to treat (NNT). Active surveillance, embodying selective treatment, would result in a substantial decrease in the NNT. If widely adopted, active surveillance should eventually result in a reappraisal of the benefits of PSA screening, and a greater acceptance of its value by organizations such as the USPSTF. The result will be "rehabilitation" of PSA screening, earlier identification of those with aggressive disease, lives saved, and an overall reduction in prostate cancer mortality (compared to no screening resulting from the perceived hazards of overtreatment). How long this will take is a matter of speculation; likely it will not happen quickly.

Results of Surveillance There are now approximately 10 groups worldwide who have reported the results of prospective cohorts. These are summarized in Table 1. It is instructive to focus on two groups who represent the two philosophical boundaries of active surveillance: an inclusive approach, offering it to most patients who might benefit; and a restrictive approach, offering it to only those patients who are at exceptionally low risk of disease progression.

The Toronto group, which initiated the first active surveillance cohort in 1996, has deliberately taken an inclusive approach. This was based on the desire to include as many eligible patients as possible on a surveillance program, and to learn as much as possible about the outcome in a range of patients. The Toronto cohort of 993 patients includes 221 who are intermediate risk, either Gleason 7 or PSA >10 [21]. 38 % of these intermediate risk patients were <70 years. About 50 % of newly diagnosed patients were eligible for surveillance using these criteria.

By comparison, the Hopkins group selected only very low risk patients who fulfilled Epstein criteria (≤2 positive cores, < 50 % core involvement, and PSA density <015) [22]. Radical intervention was initiated for any increase in cancer volume above these criteria, or grade increase. This restrictive approach was driven by a desire to reduce the risk of disease progression to the minimum. About 20 % of newly diagnosed patients were eligible.

The Toronto group, with a median follow-up of 9.5 years and a range of 0.5–20 years, now has 30 patients who have progressed to metastatic disease, and 15 who have died of prostate cancer. The 15-year prostate cancer actuarial mortality is 5 %. A recent analysis of the men who developed metastatic disease revealed that the Gleason 7 patients had a dramatically increased risk of progression to metastasis over time, with a HR of 3.75 compared to Gleason 6. PSA >10 did not confer a significant increase in risk. Of the 3 % of the overall cohort who developed mets, about 2/3 of these (2 %) occurred after 5 years, representing the men who were poorly served by surveillance; it is plausible (although not necessarily true) that had they been treated at diagnosis, they might have avoided metastatic disease.

In contrast, the Hopkins group, using a restrictive approach and more aggressive intervention strategy (for volume progression) has reported a 15-year PCa mortality of 0.5 %. This remarkably low figure validates the restrictive approach.

A key point, therefore, is that surveillance is safe for the vast majority of men, particularly Gleason 6 at diagnosis. Strenuous efforts to improve surveillance by incorporating MRI and/or biomarkers are directed towards reducing the 2–3 % mortality rate, as well as to better select those patients who can avoid treatment.

These recent publications now allow us to define the risk of surveillance as a function of inclusion criteria. A more inclusive approach will allow surveillance to be offered to about half of newly diagnosed men; but the cost is 2–3 % experiencing progression to metastases at 15 years. In contrast, a restrictive approach will deny surveillance to many men who might otherwise benefit from it, but a 15-year prostate cancer mortality of <1 %. There is, likely, a middle ground of eligibility: Most Gleason 6, regardless of volume (except, perhaps, very extensive disease or very young patients, i.e., <50). Surveillance for Gleason 7 should be offered more cautiously; it is an option for older men with a life expectancy <15 years (i.e., over 70) but embodies significant risk for younger men.

Race is relevant. African Americans on AS have a higher rate of risk re-classification and PSA failure after treatment than Caucasian men, and have a higher rate of large anterior cancers [32]. Japanese men younger than 60 have a lower rate of histological "autopsy" cancer than Caucasian men. Thus the finding of low-grade prostate cancer in young Asian men is less common, and the risk of overdiagnosis may be less. However, Black and Asian patients diagnosed with low-grade prostate cancer includes men who have little or no probability of a prostate cancer related-death during their remaining lives, and active surveillance is still an appealing option for those who have been appropriately risk-stratified.

Two genetic biomarkers have recently been approved by the FDA based on their ability to predict progression in low-grade prostate cancer. These include the Oncotype DX assay (Genome Health) which identifies a panel of genes linked to a more aggressive phenotype [33], and the Prolaris assay [34] (Myriad Genetics), which looks for abnormal expression of cell cycle related genes. A number of others are in the pipline: the Mitomics assay, which identifies the presence of a functional mitochondrial DNA deletion associated with aggressive prostate cancer [35], and the Promark assay are not yet FDA approved. These tests hold the promise of interrogating the microfocus of Gleason 6 found on biopsy for molecular alterations that provide a clue to the presence of higher grade cancer elsewhere in the prostate. That the biomarkers can achieve this confirms the "social" inter-relationship of heterogeneous multifocal cancers.

These tests, performed on biopsy tissue, are a tool to predict future biological behavior based on genetic alterations in low-grade cancer cells. A patient with low-grade prostate cancer and a strongly positive (i.e., high risk) Oncotype DX or Prolaris test should have an MRI and be treated according to the results. A further area for research is to better understand how to integrate the results of genetic biomarker tests and MRI. For example, optimal management of the patient in whom results are discrepant (i.e., genetic test indicates high risk but MRI is negative) is currently unknown. False-positive and false-negative results undoubtedly occur with both diagnostic approaches, but how commonly is unknown. The potential benefit of molecular predictive assays is compelling, but further validation of their performance is needed. In particular the utility of these assays in clinical practice has not been established. How many assays are required for each patient whose treatment is changed, for each mortality avoided by more timely treatment, and for each unnecessary treatment avoided, and an economic analysis based on these estimates is an unmet need.

The benefit of surveillance compared to surgery and radiation has been modeled by several groups. A decision analysis of surveillance compared to initial treatment showed that surveillance had the highest QALE even if the relative risk of prostate cancer-specific death for initial treatment versus active surveillance was as low as 0.6 [36]. (In fact, it is almost certainly 0.95 or better at 15 years).

4.2 Active Surveillance Technique

Implementation of AS has evolved over the last 15 years. Most clinicians use some variation of serial PSA (a useful risk predictor but not a valid trigger for intervention), periodic biopsy, and more recently selective use of MRI and/or molecular biomarkers. After the initial diagnosis of Gleason 6 prostate cancer on a systematic biopsy with 10 or more cores, PSA is performed every 6 months. A confirmatory biopsy is carried out within 6–12 months of the initial diagnostic biopsy. This confirmatory biopsy should target the areas that are often missed on systematic diagnostic biopsies, specifically the anterior prostate, prostatic apex and base. If the confirmatory biopsy is either negative or confirms microfocal Gleason 3+3 disease, subsequent biopsies are performed every 3–5 years until the patient reaches age 80, or has a life expectancy <5 years because of co-morbidity. In those patients whose biopsy shows substantial volume increase, who is upgraded to Gleason 3+4 and surveillance is still desired as a management option, or whose PSA kinetics suggest more aggressive disease (usually defined as a PSA DT <3 years), multiparametric MRI, including T2-weighted image, dynamic contrast-enhanced image, and diffusion-weighted image, should be performed. Identification of an MRI target suspicious for high-grade disease should warrant a targeted biopsy; or, if the lesion is large and unequivocal, intervention.

The role of MRI in the management of men on surveillance is currently in a state of rapid evolution. Increasing availability of MRI, diffusion of expertise in interpretation of MRI, and more data on the accuracy and limitations of MRI are all influencing its use. It is probable that routine MRI will become incorporated into the management of all patients with localized prostate cancer, resulting in earlier diagnosis of those with adverse histology and a reduction in the requirement for serial biopsies. Recent studies have suggested that the negative predictive value of MRI for clinically significant cancer is greater than 90 % [37, 38]. However, MRI will fail to detect small volume (<0.5 cc) high-grade cancers. Fortunately, these are uncommon. The performance of MRI in men with early prostate cancer, and its ability to replace systematic biopsy in the diagnosis of prostate cancer and follow-up of men on surveillance is currently being evaluated by many groups, and a detailed discussion of this topic is beyond the focus of this article.

Death from prostate cancer is a relatively rare event. In the most mature surveillance cohort [22], with a median follow-up of 8 years and range of 2–18 years, the cumulative hazard ratio (or relative risk) of nonprostate cancer death was 10 times that for prostate cancer. The published literature on surveillance includes 13 prospective studies, encompassing about 5000 men [22–31]. A limitation of most studies is that the median follow-up is too short relative to the natural history of prostate cancer. For example, a pivotal Swedish study reported that the risk of prostate cancer mortality in patients managed by watchful waiting was low for many years, but tripled after 15 years of follow-up [39]. ("Watchful waiting" meant no opportunity for selective delayed intervention, whereas about 30 % of patients in the surveillance series have had radical treatment). However, a few of the prospective studies now have patients followed for more than 15 years. Table 1 summarizes the results of the 10 non-overlapping prospective series with >100 patients. Overall, about one-third of patients are eventually treated. Most series have few or no prostate cancer deaths.

PSA kinetics are now used as a guide to identify patients at higher risk, but not to drive the treatment decision. This is a shift in practice. Until multiparametric MRI became available, men on AS with poor PSA kinetics (doubling time <3 years) were offered definitive therapy. In the PRIAS multiinstitutional AS registry, 20 % of men being treated had intervention based on a PSA doubling time <3 years [24]. Poor PSA kinetics are sensitive for aggressive disease. In the Toronto series, a PSADT <3 years was associated with a HR of 3.7 for the risk of metastasis [40]. The problem with using PSA DT to drive treatment is poor specificity Vickers, in an overview of all of the studies of more than 200 patients examining the predictive value of PSA kinetics in localized prostate cancer, concluded that kinetics had no independent predictive value beyond the absolute value of PSA [41]. In a study of PSA kinetics in a large surveillance cohort, false-positive PSA triggers (doubling time <3 years, or PSA velocity >2 ng/year) occurred in 50 % of stable untreated patients, none of whom went on to progress, require treatment, or die of prostate cancer [42].

The Future Many groups are now reporting on active surveillance cohorts, and evaluating the incorporation of biomarkers, MRI, and other imaging modalities into the routine assessment of patients. The earlier introduction of more sophisticated techniques to identify the aggressive occult cancers earlier will improve the long-term outcome and enhance precision in decision making. A number of criteria should be addressed in reporting the outcome of surveillance. These include baseline demographic data (age, race); NCCN risk category; the proportion of men with biopsy Gleason score ≥7; median follow-up; the frequency of biopsy during the follow-up period; the biopsy technique, whether standard or targeted; treatment rates, metastasis rates, overall and cause specific mortality, and biochemical recurrence rates in the treated patients, at 5, 10, and 15 years. Many important research questions remain, including the role of dietary and life style interventions, and other strategies to reduce the rate of progression (i.e., statins, 5 ARIs, metformin, etc.); the marginal utility of biomarkers in the context of MRI; and how to optimally identify intermediate risk patients who can be managed safely with surveillance.

Conclusion

Active surveillance is a solution to the widely recognized problem of overtreatment of screen detected prostate cancer. Adoption of surveillance for low risk disease would reduce the number of screen detected patients needed to treat for each death avoided without substantially increasing the risk of disease mortality. Improvements in diagnostic accuracy based on genetic predictors and multiparametric MRI should reduce the need for systematic biopsies, improve the early identification of occult higher risk disease, and enhance the ability to detect patients destined to have grade progression over time. A confirmatory biopsy targeting the anterolateral horn and anterior prostate should be performed within 6–12 months. PSA should be performed every 6 months and subsequent biopsies every 3–5 years until the patient is no longer a candidate for definitive therapy. MRI is indicated for men with a grade or volume increase, or adverse PSA kinetics. Treatment should be offered for most patients with upgraded disease.

References

1. Choo R, Klotz L, Danjoux C, Morton GC, DeBoer G, Szumacher E, Fleshner N, Bunting P, Hruby G. Feasibility study: watchful waiting for localized low to intermediate grade prostate carcinoma with selective delayed intervention based on prostate specific antigen, histological and/or clinical progression. J Urol. 2002;167(4):1664–9.
2. Lin K, Croswell JM, Koenig H, Lam C, Maltz A. Prostate-specific antigen-based screening for prostate cancer: an evidence update for the U.S. Preventive Services Task Force [Internet]. Rockville: Agency for Healthcare Research and Quality (US); 2011.
3. Carlsson SV, Kattan MW. Prostate cancer: personalized risk – stratified screening or abandoning it altogether? Nat Rev Clin Oncol. 2016;13(3):140–2.
4. Barry MJ, Nelson JB. Patients present with more advanced prostate cancer since the USPSTF screening recommendations. J Urol. 2015;194(6):1534–6.
5. Tosoian JJ, Carter HB, Lepor A, Loeb S. Active surveillance for prostate cancer: current evidence and contemporary state of practice. Nat Rev Urol. 2016; 13(4):205–15.
6. Sakr WA, Grignon DJ, Crissman JD, Heilbrun LK, Cassin BJ, Pontes JJ, Haas GP. High grade prostatic intraepithelial neoplasia (HGPIN) and prostatic adenocarcinoma between the ages of 20–69: an autopsy study of 249 cases. In Vivo. 1994;8(3):439–43.
7. Zlotta AR, Egawa S, Pushkar D, Govorov A, Kimura T, Kido M, Takahashi H, Kuk C, Kovylina M, Aldaoud N, Fleshner N, Finelli A, Klotz L, Sykes J, Lockwood G, van der Kwast TH. Prevalence of prostate cancer on autopsy: cross-sectional study on unscreened Caucasian and Asian men. J Natl Cancer Inst. 2013;105(14):1050–8.
8. Hanahan D, Weinberg RA. The hallmarks of cancer. Cell. 2000;100:57–70.
9. Hanahan D, Weinberg RA. Hallmarks of cancer: the next generation. Cell. 2011;144(5):646–74.
10. Ahmed H, Emberton M. Do low-grade and low-volume prostate cancers bear the hallmarks of malignancy? Lancet Oncol. 2012;13(11):e509–17.
11. Berg KD, Vainer B, Thomsen FB, Røder MA, Gerds TA, Toft BG, Brasso K, Iversen P. ERG protein expression in diagnostic specimens is associated with increased risk of progression during active surveillance for prostate cancer. Eur Urol. 2014; 66(5):851–60.

12. Lotan TL, Carvalho FL, Peskoe SB, Hicks JL, Good J, Fedor HL, Humphreys E, Han M, Platz EA, Squire JA, De Marzo AM, Berman DM. PTEN loss is associated with upgrading of prostate cancer from biopsy to radical prostatectomy. Mod Pathol. 2015;28(1):128–37.
13. Serrano M. Cancer: a lower bar for senescence. Nature. 2010;464(7287):363–4.
14. Eggener S, Scardino P, Walsh P, et al. 20 year prostate cancer specific mortality after radical prostatectomy. J Urol. 2011;185(3):869–75.
15. Scott Eggener, personal communication.
16. Ross HM, Kryvenko ON, Cowan JE, Simko JP, Wheeler TM, Epstein JI. Do adenocarcinomas of the prostate with Gleason score (GS)<=6 have the potential to metastasize to lymph nodes? Am J Surg Pathol. 2012;36(9):1346–52.
17. Haffner M, Yegasubramanian S. The clonal origin of lethal prostate cancer. J Clin Invest. 2013;123(11):4918–22.
18. Barbieri CE, Demichelis F, Rubin MA. The lethal clone in prostate cancer: redefining the index. Eur Urol. 2014;66(3):395–7.
19. Zomer A, Maynard C, Verweij FJ, Kamermans A, Schäfer R, Beerling E, Schiffelers RM, de Wit E, Berenguer J, Ellenbroek SI, Wurdinger T, Pegtel DM, van Rheenen J. In vivo imaging reveals extracellular vesicle-mediated phenocopying of metastatic behavior. Cell. 2015;161(5):1046–57.
20. Bratt O, Folkvaljon Y, Loeb S, Klotz L, Egevad L, Stattin P. Optimizing the definition of very low risk prostate cancer. BJU Int. 2015;116(2):213–9.
21. Klotz L, Vesprini D, Sethukavalan P, Jethava V, Zhang L, Jain S, Yamamoto T, Mamedov A, Loblaw A. Long-term follow-up of a large active surveillance cohort of patients with prostate cancer. J Clin Oncol. 2015;33(3):272–7.
22. Tosoian JJ, Mamawala M, Epstein JI, Landis P, Wolf S, Trock BJ, Carter HB. Intermediate and longer-term outcomes from a prospective active-surveillance program for favorable-risk prostate cancer. J Clin Oncol. 2015;33(30):3379–85.
23. Bul M, Zhu X, Valdagni R, et al. Active surveillance for low-risk prostate cancer worldwide: the PRIAS study. Eur Urol. 2013;63:597.
24. Dall'Era MA, Konety BR, Cowan JE, Shinohara K, Stauf F, Cooperberg MR, Meng MV, Kane CJ, Perez N, Master VA, Carroll PR. Active surveillance for the management of prostate cancer in a contemporary cohort. Cancer. 2008;112(12):2664–70.
25. Kakehi Y, Kamoto T, Shiraishi T, Ogawa O, Suzukamo Y, Fukuhara S, Saito Y, Tobisu K, Kakizoe T, Shibata T, Fukuda H, Akakura K, Suzuki H, Shinohara N, Egawa S, Irie A, Sato T, Maeda O, Meguro N, Sumiyoshi Y, Suzuki T, Shimizu N, Arai Y, Terai A, Kato T, Habuchi T, Fujimoto H, Niwakawa M. Prospective evaluation of selection criteria for active surveillance in Japanese patients with stage T1cN0M0 prostate cancer. Jpn J Clin Oncol. 2008;38(2):122–8.
26. Roemeling S, Roobol MJ, de Vries SH, Wolters T, Gosselaar C, van Leenders GJ, Schröder FH. Active surveillance for prostate cancers detected in three subsequent rounds of a screening trial: characteristics, PSA doubling times, and outcome. Eur Urol. 2007;51(5):1244–50.
27. Barayan GA, Brimo F, Bégin LR, Hanley JA, Liu Z, Kassouf W, Aprikian AG, Tanguay S. Factors influencing disease progression of prostate cancer under active surveillance: a McGill university health center cohort. BJU Int. 2014;114(6b):E99–104.
28. Rubio-Briones J, Iborra I, Ramírez M, Calatrava A, Collado A, Casanova J, Domínguez-Escrig J, Gómez-Ferrer A, Ricós JV, Monrós JL, Dumont R, López-Guerrero JA, Salas D, Solsona E. Obligatory information that a patient diagnosed of prostate cancer and candidate for an active surveillance protocol must know. Actas Urol Esp. 2014;38(9):559–65.
29. Godtman RA, Holmberg E, Khatami A, Stranne J, Hugosson J. Outcome following active surveillance of men with screen-detected prostate cancer. Results from the Göteborg randomised population-based prostate cancer screening trial. Eur Urol. 2013;63(1):101–7.
30. Thomsen FB, Røder MA, Hvarness H, Iversen P, Brasso K. Active surveillance can reduce overtreatment in patients with low-risk prostate cancer. Dan Med J. 2013;60(2):A4575.
31. Selvadurai ED, Singhera M, Thomas K, Mohammed K, Woode-Amissah R, Horwich A, Huddart RA, Dearnaley DP, Parker CC. Medium-term outcomes of active surveillance for localised prostate cancer. Eur Urol. 2013;64:981–7.
32. Sundi D, Ross AE, Humphreys EB, Han M, Partin AW, Carter HB, Schaeffer EM. African American men with very low-risk prostate cancer exhibit adverse oncologic outcomes after radical prostatectomy: should active surveillance still be an option for them? J Clin Oncol. 2013;31(24):2991–7.
33. Knezevic D, Goddard AD, Natraj N, Cherbavaz DB, Clark-Langone KM, Snable J, Watson D, Falzarano SM, Magi-Galluzzi C, Klein EA, Quale C. Analytical validation of the Oncotype DX prostate cancer assay – a clinical RT-PCR assay optimized for prostate needle biopsies. BMC Genomics. 2013;14:690.
34. Cuzick J, Berney DM, Fisher G, the Transatlantic Prostate Group. Prognostic value of a cell cycle progression signature for prostate cancer death on conservatively managed needle biopsy cohort. Br J Cancer. 2012;106:1095–9.
35. Robinson K, Creed J, Reguly B, Powell C, Wittock R, Klein D, Maggrah A, Klotz L, Parr RL, Dakubo GD. Accurate prediction of repeat prostate biopsy outcomes by a mitochondrial DNA deletion assay. Prostate Cancer Prostatic Dis. 2013;16(4):398.
36. Hayes JH, Ollendorf DA, Pearson SD, Barry MJ, Kantoff PW, Stewart ST, Bhatnagar V, Sweeney CJ, Stahl JE, McMahon PM. Active surveillance compared with initial treatment for men with low-risk

prostate cancer: a decision analysis. JAMA. 2010; 304(21):2373–80.
37. Vargas HA, Akin O, Afaq A, Goldman D, Zheng J, Moskowitz CS, Shukla-Dave A, Eastham J, Scardino P, Hricak H. Magnetic resonance imaging for predicting prostate biopsy findings in patients considered for active surveillance of clinically low risk prostate cancer. J Urol. 2012;188(5):1732–8.
38. Panebianco V, Barchetti F, Sciarra A, Ciardi A, Indino EL, Papalia R, Gallucci M, Tombolini V, Gentile V, Catalano C. Multiparametric magnetic resonance imaging vs. standard care in men being evaluated for prostate cancer: a randomized study. Urol Oncol. 2015;33(1):17.e1–7.
39. Popiolek M, Rider JR, Andrén O, Andersson SO, Holmberg L, Adami HO, Johansson JE. Natural history of early, localized prostate cancer: a final report from three decades of follow-up. Eur Urol. 2013; 63(3):428–35.
40. Yamamoto T, Musunuru B, Vesprini D, Zhang L, Ghanem G, Loblaw A, Klotz L. Metastatic prostate cancer in men initially treated with active surveillance. J Urol. 2016;195(5):1409–14. pii: S0022-5347 (15)05445-2.
41. Vickers A. Systematic review of pretreatment PSA velocity and doubling time as PCA predictors. J Clin Oncol. 2008;27:398–403.
42. Loblaw A, Zhang L, Lam A, Nam R, Mamedov A, Vesprini D, Klotz L. Comparing prostate specific antigen triggers for intervention in men with stable prostate cancer on active surveillance. J Urol. 2010; 184(5):1942–6.

Open Radical Prostatectomy

Hein Van Poppel, Lorenzo Tosco, and Steven Joniau

Abbreviations

BPFS	Biochemical progression-free survival
CSS	Cancer-specific survival
DVC	Dorsal venous complex
HT	Hormone therapy
NVB	Neurovascular bundle
PCa	Prostate cancer
PCSM	Prostate cancer-specific mortality
PSA	Prostate-specific antigen
RP	Radical prostatectomy
RRP	Retropubic radical prostatectomy
RT	Radiation therapy
TRUS	Transrectal ultrasound
TURP	Transurethral resection of the prostate

1 Introduction

The surgical treatment of prostate cancer has been introduced more than a century ago. The first important series of radical prostatectomies (RPs) were performed through a perineal approach. The retropubic approach to RP was adopted in the 1940s and is now the most commonly used operative technique for the treatment of clinically localised prostate cancer (PCa). Reiner and Walsh defined the anatomy of the dorsal vein complex and the neurovascular bundles which led to improvement of the morbidity [53]. In 1983, Walsh described the technique for anatomic nerve-sparing RP [72, 73] Since the initial report of anatomic RP by Walsh et al. in 1998 [70] and refinements in the understanding of the surgical anatomy of the prostate, open retropubic radical prostatectomy (RRP) techniques have been modified and continue to evolve. Together with the widespread application of PSA testing, RP became more popular and is still in many countries the gold standard surgical procedure attempting to control localised and more recently also locally advanced prostate cancer. The goal of RP is to eradicate cancer while preserving continence and whenever possible potency [5]. Currently, RP is the only treatment for localised PCa to show a benefit for cancer-specific survival (CSS) compared with watchful waiting, as shown in a prospective, randomised study [6, 7]. In the past decade, several centres have acquired experience with laparoscopic RP and robot-assisted laparoscopic RP has been developed. At present, the available data are not sufficient to prove superiority of any surgical approach in terms of functional and oncological outcomes. Further prospective studies are warranted [3, 16]. In this chapter, we will focus on the indications of RP, our institutional experience with RRP, the surgery-related complications and review the oncological and functional results based on the available literature.

H. Van Poppel (✉) • L. Tosco • S. Joniau
Department of Urology, University Hospital, K.U. Leuven, B-3000 Leuven, Belgium
e-mail: hendrik.vanpoppel@uzleuven.be

M. Bolla, H. van Poppel (eds.), *Management of Prostate Cancer*,
DOI 10.1007/978-3-319-42769-0_11

2 Indications

RP was a common treatment for patients with low- and intermediate-risk localised PCa (cT1a-cT2b and Gleason score 2–7 and PSA ≤20 ng/mL) and life expectancy >10 years. RP was also an option for patients with T1a disease and a life expectancy >15 years or Gleason score 7 and for selected patients with low-volume high-risk localised PCa (cT3a or Gleason score 8–10 or PSA >20 ng/mL) [24]. Since the introduction of active surveillance as a management option for low-risk disease, the definition of this pathological entity has been refined. With the revision of the Gleason pattern, today patients with low-volume Gleason grade 3 + 3, Gleason score 6 are mostly not anymore treated actively. Only when the disease becomes so-called "significant" active treatment will be given. Nowadays, also low-volume Gleason 3 + 4 prostate cancer patients are offered active surveillance.

The patient's performance status and the assessment of the individual's life expectance will be important factors when advising a patient the most appropriate treatment option. Most used are the Charlson's score, the ASA score and the Frailty index. Obese patients should be carefully selected and counselled about the risk of their physical condition since the RRP procedure can be more challenging. Older patients should also be cautiously selected because of possible comorbidities (i.e. geriatric assessment) and complications such as urinary incontinence. While initially RP was offered to well-selected unilateral T3 prostate cancer patients only [68] in recent years, RP has become a treatment choice in selected patients with locally advanced and high-risk localised PCa (cT3b-T4 N0 or any T N1) in the frame of a multimodality treatment strategy [20, 33, 43], certainly in young patients [14].

3 Surgical Technique

3.1 Preoperative Measures

Before performing a RRP, it is best to wait 6–8 weeks after transrectal ultrasound (TRUS)-guided biopsy and at least 12 weeks after transurethral resection of the prostate (TURP). Both procedures cause inflammation, possible hematoma and periprostatic fibrosis, which could increase the risk of surgical complications such as rectal injury. They also make difficult the preservation of the neurovascular bundle (NVB) or the evaluation of possible extraprostatic extension. The period between TRUS biopsy and RP permits inflammatory adhesions or hematoma to resolve and gives time for further tumour staging, surgical risk assessment and patient counselling. Whether or not performing a nerve-sparing RP should be decided preoperatively taking into consideration the location, the stage, grade and size of the tumour and the results of the digital rectal examination (DRE), TRUS and nowadays multiparametric magnetic resonance imaging (mpMRI). The latter will exactly depict the tumour(s) location as well as its' clinical stage, the vicinity of the urethral sphincter or NVB and the length of the urethral sphincter. The latter can vary from only 8 mm to more than 20 mm. Patients with a shorter urethral sphincter might have a greater risk at post-operative stress urinary incontinence that might necessitate a prolonged and intense pelvic floor re-education programme.

While many groups will not advocate any bowel preparation in any patient, we believe that in patients with extensive extracapsular disease, a classical bowel preparation should be given the evening before surgery to ensure a clean and empty colon, which is important in case of a rectal injury. Before going to the operating room, patients receive subcutaneous low molecular weight heparin. For open RRP we favour a combined spinal-epidural anaesthesia, which is associated with a reduced intraoperative blood loss [51, 56] a faster recovery and a reduction in the use of opioid analgesics [55]. Other advantages are a lower incidence of pulmonary embolism and deep venous thrombosis, and optimal pain management through the epidural catheter. The latter may be used for patient-controlled analgesia for the first 24–48 h post-operatively, rendering the procedure extremely well tolerated and really comfortable for the patient.

3.2 Surgical Procedure

The patient is placed in supine position with slight hyperextension of the chest. The skin is prepared and draped in the usual way. A thick latex Foley catheter, at least 20 French is placed. Following an 8–10 cm, midline, extraperitoneal, lower abdominal incision between the umbilicus and the pubis the preperitoneal space of Retzius can be opened. By gentle cephalad retraction of the bladder and sweeping of fatty tissue, the anterior aspect of the prostate and the endopelvic fascia are exposed. The latter is cleared of all covering fat in order to visualise it, covering the levator ani muscle and allowing to later incise it under good vision, reducing the chance of entering the big thin-wall veins covering the gland.

An extended lymph node dissection is performed at this stage of the procedure in men with intermediate- and high-risk PCa [8], encompassing the external iliac nodes, the obturator fossa, the internal iliac and presacral nodes and the common iliac artery up to the crossing of the ureters [45].

The endopelvic fascia is then incised with curved scissors and the muscle fibres of the levator ani muscle are sweeped of the lateral aspect of the prostate. Dissection of the levator muscle allows full exposure of the NVBs dorsolaterally to the prostate and anterior to the rectum. Now, the puboprostatic ligaments are divided, since they have no role in urinary incontinence, in order to get a view on the apex of the prostate and the overlying DVC. An important step in RRP is to prepare the DVC with blunt dissection in front of the thick transurethral catheter, between thumb and index finger. The DVC is then controlled in a standardised way by passing a right-angled clamp just anterior to the urethra and just distal to the apex. This allows to pass a 2-0 ligature. A back-bleeding stitch is placed more cranially on the dorsal aspect of the prostate and the DVC is then divided. Any persistent oozing from the DVC can be oversewn at this stage. Haemostasis must be perfect till now so that the apex of the prostate and the urethra are now in full view. By gentle scissor dissection, very close to the urethra, the NVBs are separated from the prostatic apex. A right-angled clamp is passed underneath the urethra, leaving the NVBs posteriorly in place, and a vessel loop is placed around the urethra, allowing accurate dissection of the prostatic apex before transection of the urethra with the cold knife. At this stage, some urologists place one or more stitches to facilitate finding the urethral stump at the time of anastomosis. The apical dissection is a critical manoeuvre in the procedure because of the need for a complete resection to avoid apical positive margins and the close relation with the NVBs. After division of the recto-urethralis muscle, the posterior aspect of the prostate is bluntly dissected with the index finger. At this point of the procedure, depending on the indication of a nerve-sparing or non-nerve-sparing procedure, the NVB is either taken along with the prostate and all tissues covering the rectum are resected, or the lateral dissection is done closely to the prostate capsule, without touching the NVB. When the NVB needs to be resected for oncological reasons, the NVB is taken down with the prostate apex, and the bundle is clipped next to the urethra. Nerve-sparing surgery has a significant impact on sexual function and urinary continence and should be performed in all patients provided that excision of all tumour is not compromised. Today, it is safe to preserve one or both NVBs in most men who are candidates for RRP and it is rarely necessary to excise both of them [71]. The next step is the transection of the prostatic pedicles. The dissection is continued with clipping until the lateral aspect of the seminal vesicles is reached. At this point, the lateral aspect of the bladder neck can also be dissected already. Dissection of the seminal vesicles must be carried out very carefully in order to avoid injury to the pelvic plexus and represents a critical point for a successful nerve-sparing. The Denonvilliers fascia is divided sharply between both vasa deferentia reaching the posterior bladder wall. The vessels at the apex of the seminal vesicles are clipped and divided. At this stage, the prostate is completely mobilised posteriorly and laterally up to the bladder neck. Once the prostate has been removed, the specimen is inspected carefully for capsular incision. If an incision is found, an extra resection can be performed at the corresponding location. If there is concern about the margin on the posterolateral surface of the prostate, the NVB on that side should be excised [21, 75]. The bladder neck must be considered for either resection or preservation. The so-called bladder-neck-preserving RP is actually more an intraprostatic-urethral-preserving resection enabling the reconstruction of a neo-bladder neck. The bladder neck can be restored with a classical "tennis racket" closure and meticulous eversion of the bladder mucosa. Some surgeons have proposed a bladder neck "intussusception" with buttressing sutures lateral and posterior to the reconstructed bladder neck to hasten the early return of urinary control that would prevent passive opening of the bladder neck with filling [74]. An intravenous diuretic may be administered to help identifying the ureteral orifices and 2 tubes can be inserted temporarily, avoiding to close the urethral meatus during bladder neck reconstruction. Once the bladder neck has been reconstructed, the ureteral catheters are removed. The new bladder neck mucosa needs to be meticulously everted with several stitches in order to avoid anastomotic strictures. Haemostasis is done avoiding the use of electrocautery in the case of a nerve-sparing procedure because this could definitely damage the NVBs. The last step of the procedure is the vesico-urethral anastomosis. A Ch 14-16 Foley (silicone) catheter is brought into the new bladder neck and four anastomotic sutures are placed at 7, 5, 2 and 11 o'clock. At this point, the balloon is inflated. Careful traction on the inflated balloon catheter brings the bladder neck down to the urethral stump. The four anastomotic sutures are then tied and the bladder can be rinsed to check the anastomosis for leakage. Diuretics can be given to dilute any hematuria. Subsequently, two suction drains are placed in the pelvis and the wound is closed.

The surgical technique of a RP for locally advanced T3 cancer is obviously different from that applied in locally confined tumours. RP of locally advanced T3 PCa must include a more radical extirpation including an extensive lymph node dissection, a clean apical dissection, a broad NVB resection at least at the tumour-bearing site, a complete resection of the seminal vesicles and in many cases a resection of the bladder neck. In patients with small unilateral and non-apical T3a prostate cancer, the contralateral NVB can be spared. Absolute contraindications of the nerve-sparing procedure are the T3b tumours and the palpable lesions at the apex [57]. The bladder neck or intraprostatic urethra can usually be preserved in apical T3 tumours [27, 67]. More and more authors today report their experience with RP in clinically localised and high-risk PCa [9, 14, 19, 33, 34, 37, 42, 43, 46, 64, 69, 76].

3.3 Post-operative Care

For the first 48 h after surgery, a patient controlled analgesia (PCA) pump is used for pain control. Post-operatively, attention should be given to general status, wound control, drain volume and bowel movements. On the second post-operative day, a regular diet is offered provided that peristalsis is restored. The suction drains are taken out when daily drainage is less than 10 mL. Low molecular weight heparin that has already started the day before surgery is continued up to 1 month after the operation, to prevent thrombo-embolism. Five or six days after the operation, the patients are discharged from the hospital with a Foley catheter in place. Ten to 14 days after the operation, they return for removal of the catheter. A cystogram before withdrawal of the catheter is only carried out, if any post-operative problem has arisen that might have caused leakage. Directly after removal of the Foley catheter, pelvic floor physiotherapy is started, to regain continence as soon as possible.

3.4 Complications and Functional Results

3.4.1 Intra-operative Complications

The acute side effects of RRP are haemorrhage, rectal injury and ureteral injury. The most common intra-operative complication is haemorrhage that can occur because of a blunt lateral dissection of the lateral aspect of the prostate, because of insufficient control of the DVC, because of the presence of veins that perforate the pelvic floor or because of the nerve-sparing procedure. Bleeding is usually sufficiently managed once the dorsal vein has been divided and ligated [75] and will only rarely exceed 1000 ml. Rectal laceration is an uncommon (once in every 100–300 patients) but serious complication. It occurs during apical dissection while attempting to develop the plane between rectum and the recto-urethralis muscle or the Denonvilliers' fascia. In some cases it can be mandatory to do an omentoplasty and anal dilatation. Ureteral injury occurs during transection of the bladder neck with intravesical injury of the ureteral meatus. Therefore the ureteral catheters should be carefully inserted before restoring the bladder neck with a tennis racket closure.

3.4.2 Post-operative Complications

General post-operative complications after RP are deep venous thrombosis and pulmonary embolism. These complications should be prevented by low molecular weight heparin started the day before surgery and continued up to 1 month after the operation. Early post-operative complications include anastomotic leak, prolonged lymphatic drainage, premature accidental catheter withdrawal and recto-urethral fistula. Prolonged lymphatic drainage occurs if the pelvic cavity is not drained appropriately after surgery. The use of active suction drains is therefore advocated. They should not be taken out until they drain less than 10 ml per 24 h. The incidence of clinically important urinary fistula is very low to inexistent in open RRP. With just four anastomotic stitches only, some patients can indeed have a temporary urine leak in the suction drains but when the catheter is correctly inserted in the bladder this will, with continued active suction, spontaneously resolve in all cases. Urinary fistula can also occur after catheter blockage by blood clots from bleeding in the bladder that must be avoided by proper bladder neck reconstruction and eversion of the bladder neck mucosa. A ureteral damage can be the cause of a urine leak. Accidental early catheter withdrawal is a rare event that most often is caused by a technical defect or a damage to the balloon catheter. Recto-urethral fistula is uncommon (unless in patients that had previous radiotherapy or rectal surgery) and actually only occurs when a rectal laceration has not been recognised during surgery. When it occurs immediate colostomy is mandatory.

The late complications of RP are anastomotic strictures, urinary incontinence and erectile dysfunction. To avoid anastomotic strictures one should perform a good bladder neck reconstruction with eversion of the mucosa and avoiding making a too narrow bladder neck. Anastomotic strictures, predominantly in patients who had a previous TURP, excessive bleeding or an anastomotic leak, can often be successfully treated with a urethral dilatation. Incision of the stricture must be avoided as this may compromise urinary continence.

Urinary continence and potency are among the key concerns that men have with respect to the complications of RRP. Urinary incontinence is for most men the most disabling complication and is very difficult to predict. The reason is invariably damage to the urethral sphincter or its innervation. Men with shorter sphincters will be more prone to early stress urinary incontinence after catheter withdrawal. Pelvic floor muscle exercises after RP may improve early urinary continence (Overgärd et al. [49]). Erectile dysfunction is associated with age, pre-operative erectile function and the oncologically required degree of resection of one or two NVBs. Recovery of potency also depends on the proper selection of patients and the experience of the surgeon with performing nerve-sparing operations. After open RP, most patients will suffer a temporary reduced erectile function, but when one or two NVBs were spared, reinnervation will take about 8–9 months with further recovery over 2 years, certainly in younger men [65]. A placebo-controlled prospective study showed no statistically significant difference among patients with erectile dysfunction following bilateral nerve-sparing RP receiving nightly PD5 inhibitors and those receiving on-demand treatment in the post-operative period [44]. In another placebo-controlled prospective study nightly sildenafil administration increased the return of normal spontaneous erections [50]. Men who fail phosphodiesterase-5-inhibitors treatment for their post RRP erectile dysfunction are excellent candidates for intracavernous injection therapy. The need for penile implants after RP, which implies a full destruction of the cavernous tissue, is rather limited since most of them will do very well with intracavernous injection therapy.

3.5 Surgical Modifications to Standard Anatomic RP

During the last decades surgical modifications to standard anatomic RP have been proposed in order to improve early return of urinary continence, erectile function, or both. This became possible because of a better understanding of the surgical anatomy of the prostate. These modifications focus on the role of the bladder neck in urinary control, dissection around the seminal vesicles and placement of interposition nerve grafts when resection of the NVBs is required [75]. It has been suggested that bladder neck preservation may help in an early return of continence although its role in recovering urinary continence after RRP is controversial. Although in many studies bladder neck preservation was associated with earlier continence [1, 13, 58], the randomised study of Srougi et al. found no difference in urinary continence rates in patients in the bladder neck resection and preservation group [60]. Whether the seminal vesicle should be spared to avoid potential damage of the surrounding structures and maintain urinary continence [31] or should be removed completely to ensure cancer control [63] remains also controversial.

4 Results

4.1 Surgical Margins and Oncological Results

A study evaluating the outcome of RP in patients with unilateral T3a PCa showed that increased overall surgical experience results in improved positive surgical margin rates over time (75 % in 1987–1994, 42 % in 1995–1999 and 10.4 % in 2000–2004) [26]. When used on well-selected patients, the nerve-sparing procedure does not increase the risk of getting positive surgical margins or biochemical recurrence following RP [47]. Surgical experience influences the occurrence of surgical margins and cancer control.

Open RRP provides excellent long-term oncological outcomes for the majority of patients with clinically localised PCa. Studies showed 10-year PSA-free survival rates of >60 % and 10-year CSS rates of >94 % [23, 29, 30, 52, 54]. At present, an externally validated nomogram predicting PCa-specific mortality after RP can be used in patient counselling and clinical trial design [61]. Although still controversial, it is increasingly evident that surgery is getting a more and more prominent as initial treatment for locally advanced disease (cT3a). Several retrospective case-series including patients with cT3 disease that underwent RP monotherapy showed 5- and 10-year overall survival (OS) rates of >75 % and >60 %, respectively. The CSS after RP at 5- and 10-year follow-up varied between, respectively, 85–100 % and 57–91.6 % [19, 42, 64, 76]. In a recent study Hsu et al., evaluated the long-term outcome of 164 patients with locally advanced PCa after RP and reported a 15-year CSS of 66.3 %. Mean follow-up was 100 months [28]. Nomograms can be used for recognising patients with locally advanced or high-grade PCa most likely to benefit from surgical treatment [18, 32]. Patients with cT3 disease are overstaged 9–44 % of the time [11, 17, 25, 26, 39, 69, 76]. For these patients who have organ-confined disease but also for those who actually have pT3 disease, RP alone might result in a definitive cure. In patients with high-grade PCa, Donohue and colleagues examined the outcome of RP monotherapy and found a 5- and 10-year biochemical progression-free survival (BPFS) of 51 % and 39 %, respectively [15]. This is in agreement with rates reported in other series [36, 48, 62]. Up to one third of patients with high-grade PCa are subsequently downgraded and have better BPFS probability after RP [4, 22, 41]. In a substantial number of patients with locally advanced or high-grade PCa, RP monotherapy will not be sufficient. Therefore, multimodality treatment consisting of RP with adjuvant or salvage radiation (RT) or hormone treatment (HT) or both should be considered [33, 34].

A study evaluating the outcome of locally advanced PCa after RP showed that pathological tumour grade and node status were significant predictor factors in biochemical progression-free survival (BPFS), clinical progression-free survival (CPFS) and CSS after 100 months follow-up [28]. Another study showed that biopsy Gleason score is the strongest predictor of progression and mortality. PSA >20 ng/mL associated with biopsy Gleason score ≤7 resulted in 10-year PCa-specific mortality (PCSM) of only 5 %; when associated with biopsy Gleason score ≥8, PCSM was 35 % [59].

4.2 Functional Results

The complications associated with RP are described in an earlier section (see Sect. 3.4). Even using a standardised technique for the nerve-sparing procedure, a learning curve exists, giving better functional results for the more experienced surgeon. Short retraining in specialised centres can have a positive effect on the surgical quality. Urinary continence and erectile dysfunction rates vary among different studies. The incontinence rate after open RRP is low and is highly associated with the nerve-sparing technique [10]. Kundu et al. evaluated urinary incontinence, potency and post-operative complications in preoperatively potent men treated with RRP from 1983 to 2003 with a minimum follow-up of 18 months. They concluded that when RRP is performed by an experienced surgeon the rate of long-term incontinence after RRP is only 2–7 %. The potency rate was 76 % after bilateral nerve-sparing RRP (1,770) and 53 % after unilateral or partial nerve-sparing (64) RRP. Potency rates following bilateral versus unilateral nerve-sparing RRP were better for men <70 years (78 %% vs. 53 %; $P=0.001$) compared with those in men ≥70 years (52 % vs. 56 %; $P=0.6$). The post-operative complication rate was 9 % [35]. Another large study has reported similar rates after 18 months of follow-up [38]. One study [2] reported the return of erectile function in 1620 consecutive preoperatively potent men treated from 1992 to 2006 with nerve-sparing RP where feasible. Follow-up was minimum 6 months. Of 619 men who had a bilateral and of 178 who had a unilateral nerve-sparing RRP, 72 % and 53 %, respectively, were potent. When stratifying by age group (≤49, 50–59, 60–69 and ≥70 years) potency rates were 86 %, 76 %, 58 % and 37 %, respectively. In line with other large studies [35, 38], the authors concluded that potency rates after RRP were better in younger men [2, 65]. Recently, Löppenberg et al. have evaluated complication rates after RP at a single centre between 2003 and 2009. All 10 Martin criteria for a high quality report of complications were fulfilled. All complications that occurred within a 30-day post-operative period were graded retrospectively according to the Clavien-Dindo classification. Complications after patient discharge were captured using a non-validated questionnaire. The authors observed an acceptable overall complication rate of 27.7 % (801 of 2,893 patients). Of these complications 596 were grade I (63.2 %), 183 grade II (19.5 %), 142 grade III (15.1 %) and 15 grade IV (1.8 %). The mortality rate (grade IV) was 0.1 % (4 of 2,893). Patients of older age, those with greater prostate volume and those who had undergone simultaneous lymphadenectomy were at risk for higher grade complications (grade III or greater) [40].

For patients with cT3 disease, the morbidity is similar to that previously reported for patient with cT2 disease [76]. In a study evaluating the outcome of RP in patients with locally advanced or high-risk PCa, potency and continence rates were preserved in 60 % and 92 %, respectively. Median follow-up was 88 months [39].

Conclusion

Contemporary nerve-sparing open RRP remains the gold standard for patients with localised PCa who can be cured and who have at least a 10-year life expectancy. The increasing experience of surgeons together with better knowledge of the periprostatic anatomy and the refinements in nerve-sparing techniques has resulted in excellent oncological outcomes, decreased positive surgical margins, significantly reduced operative complications and better functional results. Most of the complications are low grade. In the hands of an experienced surgeon, incontinence rates are low. Nerve-sparing RP performed with sufficient expertise and additional phosphodiesterase-5-inhibitors or intracavernous injection therapy provide acceptable potency rates. RRP is nowadays less frequently performed in low-risk prostate cancer patients and is recommended as initial treatment for locally advanced and high-grade PCa in the frame of a multimodality treatment, including adjuvant or salvage RT, HT or a combination of both.

References

1. Abou-Elela A, Reyad I, Morsy A, Elgammal M, Bedair AS, Abdelkader M. Continence after radical prostatectomy with bladder neck preservation. Eur J Surg Oncol. 2007;33:96–101.
2. Ayyathurai R, Manoharan M, Nieder AM, Kava B, Soloway MS. Factors affecting erectile function after radical retropubic prostatectomy: results from 1620 consecutive patients. BJU Int. 2008;101:833–6.
3. Barocas DA, Salem S, Kordan Y, et al. Robotic assisted laparoscopic prostatectomy versus radical retropubic prostatectomy for clinically localized prostate cancer: comparison of short-term biochemical recurrence-free survival. J Urol. 2011;183:990–6.
4. Bastian PJ, Gonzalgo ML, Aronson WJ, et al. Clinical and pathologic outcome after radical prostatectomy for prostate cancer patients with a preoperative Gleason sum of 8 to 10. Cancer. 2006;107:1265–72.
5. Bianco Jr FJ, Scardino PT, Eastham JA. Radical prostatectomy: long-term cancer control and recovery of sexual and urinary function ("trifecta"). Urology. 2005;66:83–94.
6. Bill-Axelson A, Holmberg L, Filen F, et al. Radical prostatectomy versus watchful waiting in localized prostate cancer: the Scandinavian prostate cancer group-4 randomized trial. J Natl Cancer Inst. 2008;100:1144–54.
7. Bill-Axelson A, Holmberg L, Ruutu M, et al. Radical prostatectomy versus watchful waiting in early prostate cancer. N Engl J Med. 2011;364:1708–17.
8. Briganti A, Chun FK, Salonia A, et al. Validation of a nomogram predicting the probability of lymph node invasion based on the extent of pelvic lymphadenectomy in patients with clinically localized prostate cancer. BJU Int. 2006;98:788–93.
9. Briganti A, Karnes RJ, Gandaglia G, Spahn M, Gontero P, Tosco L, Kneitz B, et al. Natural history of surgically treated high-risk prostate cancer. Urol Oncol. 2015;33:163.e7–163.e13.
10. Burkhard FC, Kessler TM, Fleischmann A, Thalmann GN, Schumacher M, Studer UE. Nerve sparing open radical retropubic prostatectomy – does it have an impact on urinary continence? J Urol. 2006;176:189–95.
11. Carver BS, Bianco Jr FJ, Scardino PT, Eastham JA. Long-term outcome following radical prostatectomy in men with clinical stage T3 prostate cancer. J Urol. 2006;176:564–8.
12. Centemero A, Rigatti L, Giraudo D, et al. Preoperative pelvic floor muscle exercise for early continence after radical prostatectomy: a randomised controlled study. Eur Urol. 2010;57:1039–43.
13. Deliveliotis C, Protogerou V, Alargof E, Varkarakis J. Radical prostatectomy: bladder neck preservation and puboprostatic ligament sparing – effects on continence and positive margins. Urology. 2002;60:855–8.
14. Dell'Oglio P, Karnes RJ, Joniau S, Spahn M, Gontero P, Tosco L, et al. Very long-term survival patterns of young patients treated with radical prostatectomy for high-risk prostate cancer. Urol Oncol. 2016;34:234.e13–9.
15. Donohue JF, Bianco Jr FJ, Kuroiwa K, et al. Poorly differentiated prostate cancer treated with radical prostatectomy: long-term outcome and incidence of pathological downgrading. J Urol. 2006;176:991–5.
16. Ficarra V, Novara G, Artibani W, et al. Retropubic, laparoscopic, and robot-assisted radical prostatectomy: a systematic review and cumulative analysis of comparative studies. Eur Urol. 2009;55:1037–63.
17. Freedland SJ, Partin AW, Humphreys EB, Mangold LA, Walsh PC. Radical prostatectomy for clinical stage T3a disease. Cancer. 2007;109:1273–8.
18. Gallina A, Chun FK, Briganti A, et al. Development and split-sample validation of a nomogram predicting the probability of seminal vesicle invasion at radical prostatectomy. Eur Urol. 2007;52:98–105.
19. Gerber GS, Thisted RA, Chodak GW, et al. Results of radical prostatectomy in men with locally advanced prostate cancer: multi-institutional pooled analysis. Eur Urol. 1997;32:385–90.
20. Gontero P, Spahn M, Tombal B, et al. Is there a prostate-specific antigen upper limit for radical prostatectomy? BJU Int. 2011;108(7):1093–100.
21. Graefen M, Walz J, Huland H. Open retropubic nerve-sparing radical prostatectomy. Eur Urol. 2006;49:38–48.
22. Grossfeld GD, Latini DM, Lubeck DP, Mehta SS, Carroll PR. Predicting recurrence after radical

prostatectomy for patients with high risk prostate cancer. J Urol. 2003;169:157–63.
23. Han M, Partin AW, Pound CR, Epstein JI, Walsh PC. Long-term biochemical disease-free and cancer-specific survival following anatomic radical retropubic prostatectomy. The 15-year Johns Hopkins experience. Urol Clin North Am. 2001;28:555–65.
24. A. Heidenreich, PJ Bastian, J Belmunt, M Bolla, S Joniau, T Van der Kwast, M Mason, V Madveev, T Wiegel, F Zatony, N Mottet. EAU Guidelines on prostate cancer: part 1: screening, diagnosis and local treatment with curative intend 2013. Eur Urol 2014; 65: 124–137
25. Hsu CY, Joniau S, Oyen R, Roskams T, Van Poppel H. Outcome of surgery for clinical unilateral T3a prostate cancer: a single-institution experience. Eur Urol. 2007;51:121–8; discussion 8–9.
26. Hsu CY, Joniau S, Roskams T, Oyen R, Van Poppel H. Comparing results after surgery in patients with clinical unilateral T3a prostate cancer treated with or without neoadjuvant androgen-deprivation therapy. BJU Int. 2007;99:311–4.
27. Hsu CY, Joniau S, Van Poppel H. Radical prostatectomy for locally advanced prostate cancer: technical aspects of radical prostatectomy. EAU Updat Ser. 2005;3:90–7.
28. Hsu CY, Wildhagen MF, Van Poppel H, Bangma CH. Prognostic factors for and outcome of locally advanced prostate cancer after radical prostatectomy. BJU Int. 2010;105:1536–40.
29. Hull GW, Rabbani F, Abbas F, Wheeler TM, Kattan MW, Scardino PT. Cancer control with radical prostatectomy alone in 1,000 consecutive patients. J Urol. 2002;167:528–34.
30. Isbarn H, Wanner M, Salomon G, et al. Long-term data on the survival of patients with prostate cancer treated with radical prostatectomy in the prostate-specific antigen era. BJU Int. 2009;106:37–43.
31. John H, Hauri D. Seminal vesicle-sparing radical prostatectomy: a novel concept to restore early urinary continence. Urology. 2000;55:820–4.
32. Joniau S, Hsu CY, Lerut E, et al. A pretreatment table for the prediction of final histopathology after radical prostatectomy in clinical unilateral T3a prostate cancer. Eur Urol. 2007;51:388–94; discussion 95–6.
33. Joniau S, Briganti A, Gontero P, et al. Stratification of high-risk prostate cancer info prognostic categories: a European multi-institutional study. Eur Urol. 2015;67:157–64.
34. Joniau S, Spahn M, Briganti A, et al. Pretreatment tables predicting pathologic stage of locally advanced prostate cancer. Eur Urol. 2015;67:319–25.
35. Kundu SD, Roehl KA, Eggener SE, Antenor JA, Han M, Catalona WJ. Potency, continence and complications in 3,477 consecutive radical retropubic prostatectomies. J Urol. 2004;172:2227–31.
36. Lau WK, Bergstralh EJ, Blute ML, Slezak JM, Zincke H. Radical prostatectomy for pathological Gleason 8 or greater prostate cancer: influence of concomitant pathological variables. J Urol. 2002;167:117–22.
37. Lerner SE, Blute ML, Zincke H. Extended experience with radical prostatectomy for clinical stage T3 prostate cancer: outcome and contemporary morbidity. J Urol. 1995;154:1447–52.
38. Loeb S, Roehl KA, Helfand BT, Catalona WJ. Complications of open radical retropubic prostatectomy in potential candidates for active monitoring. Urology. 2008;72:887–91.
39. Loeb S, Smith ND, Roehl KA, Catalona WJ. Intermediate-term potency, continence, and survival outcomes of radical prostatectomy for clinically high-risk or locally advanced prostate cancer. Urology. 2007;69:1170–5.
40. Loppenberg B, Noldus J, Holz A, Palisaar RJ. Reporting complications after open radical retropubic prostatectomy using the Martin criteria. J Urol. 2010;184:944–8.
41. Manoharan M, Bird VG, Kim SS, Civantos F, Soloway MS. Outcome after radical prostatectomy with a pretreatment prostate biopsy Gleason score of >/=8. BJU Int. 2003;92:539–44.
42. Martinez de la Riva S, Lopez-Tomasety J, Dominguez R, Cruz E, Blanco P. Radical prostatectomy as monotherapy for locally advanced prostate cancer (T3a): 12-years follow-up. Arch Esp Urol. 2004;57:679–92.
43. Moltzahn F, Karnes J, Gontero P, Kneitz B, Tombal B, et al. Predicting prostate cancer specific outcome after radical prostatectomy among men with very high-risk cT3b/4 PCa: a multi-institutional outcome study of 266 patients. Prostate Cancer Prostatic Dis. 2015;18:31–7.
44. Montorsi F, Brock G, Lee J, et al. Effect of nightly versus on-demand vardenafil on recovery of erectile function in men following bilateral nerve-sparing radical prostatectomy. Eur Urol. 2008;54:924–31.
45. Moschini M, Fossati N, Abdollah F, Gandaglia G, Cucchiara V, et al. Determinants of long-term survival of patients with locally advanced prostate cancer: the role of extensive pelvic lymph node dissection. Prostate Cancer Prostatic Dis. 2016;19:63–7.
46. Morgan WR, Bergstralh EJ, Zincke H. Long-term evaluation of radical prostatectomy as treatment for clinical stage C (T3) prostate cancer. Urology. 1993;41:113–20.
47. Nelles JL, Freedland SJ, Presti Jr JC, et al. Impact of nerve sparing on surgical margins and biochemical recurrence: results from the SEARCH database. Prostate Cancer Prostatic Dis. 2009;12:172–6.
48. Oefelein MG, Grayhack JT, McVary KT. Survival after radical retropubic prostatectomy of men with clinically localized high grade carcinoma of the prostate. Cancer. 1995;76:2535–42.
49. Overgard M, Angelsen A, Lydersen S, Morkved S. Does physiotherapist-guided pelvic floor muscle training reduce urinary incontinence after radical prostatectomy? A randomised controlled trial. Eur Urol. 2008;54:438–48.
50. Padma-Nathan H, McCullough AR, Levine LA, et al. Randomized, double-blind, placebo-controlled study

of postoperative nightly sildenafil citrate for the prevention of erectile dysfunction after bilateral nerve-sparing radical prostatectomy. Int J Impot Res. 2008;20:479–86.

51. Peters CA, Walsh PC. Blood transfusion and anesthetic practices in radical retropubic prostatectomy. J Urol. 1985;134:81–3.
52. Porter CR, Kodama K, Gibbons RP, et al. 25-year prostate cancer control and survival outcomes: a 40-year radical prostatectomy single institution series. J Urol. 2006;176:569–74.
53. Reiner WG, Walsh PC. An anatomical approach to the surgical management of the dorsal vein and Santorini's plexus during radical retropubic surgery. J Urol. 1979;121:198–200.
54. Roehl KA, Han M, Ramos CG, Antenor JA, Catalona WJ. Cancer progression and survival rates following anatomical radical retropubic prostatectomy in 3,478 consecutive patients: long-term results. J Urol. 2004;172:910–4.
55. Salonia A, Crescenti A, Suardi N, et al. General versus spinal anesthesia in patients undergoing radical retropubic prostatectomy: results of a prospective, randomized study. Urology. 2004;64:95–100.
56. Shir Y, Raja SN, Frank SM, Brendler CB. Intraoperative blood loss during radical retropubic prostatectomy: epidural versus general anesthesia. Urology. 1995;45:993–9.
57. Sokoloff MH, Brendler CB. Indications and contraindications for nerve-sparing radical prostatectomy. Urol Clin North Am. 2001;28:535–43.
58. Soloway MS, Neulander E. Bladder-neck preservation during radical retropubic prostatectomy. Semin Urol Oncol. 2000;18:51–6.
59. Spahn M, Joniau S, Gontero P, et al. Outcome predictors of radical prostatectomy in patients with prostate specific antigen < 20ng/ml. Eur Urol. 2010;58:1–7.
60. Srougi M, Nesrallah LJ, Kauffmann JR, Nesrallah A, Leite KR. Urinary continence and pathological outcome after bladder neck preservation during radical retropubic prostatectomy: a randomized prospective trial. J Urol. 2001;165:815–8.
61. Stephenson AJ, Kattan MW, Eastham JA, et al. Prostate cancer-specific mortality after radical prostatectomy for patients treated in the prostate-specific antigen era. J Clin Oncol. 2009;27:4300–5.
62. Tefilli MV, Gheiler EL, Tiguert R, et al. Role of radical prostatectomy in patients with prostate cancer of high Gleason score. Prostate. 1999;39:60–6.
63. Theodorescu D, Lippert MC, Broder SR, Boyd JC. Early prostate-specific antigen failure following radical perineal versus retropubic prostatectomy: the importance of seminal vesicle excision. Urology. 1998;51:277–82.
64. Van den Ouden D, Hop W, Schröder F. Progression in and survival of patients with locally advanced prostate cancer (T3) treated with radical prostatectomy as monotherapy. J Urol. 1998;160:1392–7.
65. Van der Aa F, Joniau S, De Ridder D, Van Poppel H. Potency after unilateral nerve sparing surgery. Prostate Cancer Prostatic Dis. 2003;6:61–5.
66. Van Kampen M, De Weerdt W, Van Poppel H, De Ridder D, Feys H, Baert L. Effect of pelvic-floor re-education on duration and degree of incontinence after radical prostatectomy: a randomised controlled trial. Lancet. 2000;355:98–102.
67. Van Poppel H. Surgery for clinical T3 prostate cancer. Eur Urol. 2005;4:12–4.
68. Van Poppel H, Goethuys H, Callewaert P, et al. Radical prostatectomy can provide cure for well-selected clinical stage 3 prostate cancer. Eur Urol. 2000;38:372–9.
69. Van Poppel H, Vekemans K, Da Pozzo L, et al. Radical prostatectomy for locally advanced prostate cancer: results of a feasibility study (EORTC 30001). Eur J Cancer. 2006;42:1062–7.
70. Walsh PC. Anatomic radical prostatectomy: evolution of the surgical technique. J Urol. 1998;160:2418–24.
71. Walsh PC. Nerve grafts are rarely necessary and are unlikely to improve sexual function in men undergoing anatomic radical prostatectomy. Urology. 2001;57:1020–4.
72. Walsh PC, Donker PJ. Impotence following radical prostatectomy: insight into etiology and prevention. J Urol. 1982;128:492–7.
73. Walsh PC, Lepor H, Eggleston JC. Radical prostatectomy with preservation of sexual function: anatomical and pathological considerations. Prostate. 1983;4:473–85.
74. Walsh PC, Marschke PL. Intussusception of the reconstructed bladder neck leads to earlier continence after radical prostatectomy. Urology. 2002;59:934–8.
75. Walsh PC, Partin A, eds. Anatomic radical retropubic prostatectomy. In: Wein J, Kavoussi LR, Novick AC, Partin AW, Peters CA, Editors: Campbell-walsh. Urology, 9th ed. vol. 1, Chapter 97. Philadelphia: WB Saunders Co; 2007.
76. Ward JF, Slezak JM, Blute ML, Bergstralh EJ, Zincke H. Radical prostatectomy for clinically advanced (cT3) prostate cancer since the advent of prostate-specific antigen testing: 15-year outcome. BJU Int. 2005;95:751–6.

The Robotic Laparoscopic Radical Prostatectomy

Aaron Leiblich, Prasanna Sooriakumaran, and Peter Wiklund

1 From the Origins of Radical Prostatectomy to Robot Assisted Surgery

The history of surgical treatment for prostate cancer dates back to 7 April 1904, when Dr. Hugh Young, with the assistance of William Halsted, performed the world's first radical prostatectomy at Johns Hopkins Hospital, Baltimore [1]. His technique was adapted from an operation he learnt from the iconoclastic American surgeon, George Goodfellow, who developed a surgical method of prostatic enucleation via a transperineal route for the treatment of bladder outlet obstruction.

Over the course of 30 years, Young performed his operation on thousands of men with prostate cancer, teaching his method of transperineal radical prostatectomy to at least two generations of urologists trained at the Brady Urological Institute at Johns Hopkins. His operation was rapidly adopted by contemporaries and became widely disseminated throughout the United States and Europe in the first half of the twentieth century. This technique prevailed until the Irish urologist Terence Millin originated the retropubic approach for performing prostatectomy [2]. Initially, his operation was developed for the treatment of benign prostatic enlargement, but he later adapted the technique to encompass the treatment of prostate cancer.

Little progress was seen in the technique and technology of radical prostatectomy in the 40-plus years between Millin's description of a retropubic approach in 1945 and the advent of laparoscopy in the early 1990s. William Schuessler, who published the first case series of patients who had undergone laparoscopic prostatectomy, initially demonstrated the feasibility of a minimally invasive surgical approach for the treatment of prostate cancer [3]. Although this represents a landmark in the history of prostate cancer surgery, adoption of laparoscopic techniques was slow, due in part to the technical difficulty of the procedure.

The development of robotic surgical technologies in the late 1990s and early 2000s saw the most significant advance in recent years in the surgical treatment of localized prostate cancer.

A. Leiblich
Nuffield Department of Surgical Sciences, University of Oxford, Oxford, UK

P. Sooriakumaran
Nuffield Department of Surgical Sciences, University of Oxford, Oxford, UK

Department of Molecular Medicine and Surgery, Karolinska Institute, Stockholm, Sweden

P. Wiklund (✉)
Department of Molecular Medicine and Surgery, Karolinska Institute, Stockholm, Sweden
e-mail: peter.wiklund@karolinska.se

M. Bolla, H. van Poppel (eds.), *Management of Prostate Cancer*,
DOI 10.1007/978-3-319-42769-0_12

Robotic technology in surgery was initially developed by the United States Department of Defense, who foresaw applications in battlefield surgery. The translation of this technology for civilian use was largely driven by the entrepreneurial efforts of two rival American companies, Intuitive Surgical (IS), Inc and Computer Motion, Inc. Simultaneously, both companies developed robotic interfaces for use in human surgical applications, with Intuitive Surgical's da Vinci Surgical System receiving FDA approval in 2000 while approval was granted to Computer Motion's ZEUS system shortly after in 2001. In 2003, Computer Motion was merged into Intuitive Surgical, and shortly afterwards the ZEUS robot was phased out. The da Vinci System remains the most widely used surgical robotic interface worldwide.

Abbou et al. described the first reported radical prostatectomy using the da Vinci System in 2001. The operation took place in the Henri Mondor Hospital in Creteil, France, with an operative time of 7 h and a hospital stay of 4 days [4]. Soon after, robot assisted radical prostatectomy (RARP) was refined and popularized by the pioneering work of Mani Menon and his colleagues at the Vattikuti Urology Institute at Henry Ford Hospital in Detroit [5, 6]. Over the last decade, RARP has gained widespread acceptance around the world as an important advance in the surgical management of prostate cancer.

2 Surgical Techniques in Robot Assisted Laparoscopic Radical Prostatectomy

The last 10 years has seen a boom in the number of RARPs being performed around the world, with more than 80 % of all radical prostatectomies performed in the United States now being done with the aid of a robotic system [7]. The rise in popularity of robotic prostatectomy has also seen the development of a variety of different approaches to performing the operation. Although transperitoneal approaches currently predominate, robot prostatectomy may be performed via an entirely extra-peritoneal approach [8]. For the purposes of this chapter, we will restrict the discussion of technique to describing transperitoneal prostatectomy, as this is the approach employed routinely in our practice.

3 Patient Positioning and Trocar Placement

The patient is placed under general anesthesia in a supine position. The lower limbs are placed in leg supports and abducted slightly. After prepping the abdomen, genitalia and perineum and draping the patient, a 16 French two-way Foley catheter is inserted to drain the bladder. A 3–4 cm supra-umbilical incision is made in the skin and the anterior rectus sheath is exposed by blunt dissection of adipose tissue with Langenbeck retractors. A small incision is made in the sheath carefully and the peritoneum is opened either by the mini-Hassan technique or by gentle, blunt dissection with the little finger. Once the peritoneum has been opened, the camera trocar is inserted into the abdominal cavity and insufflation of CO_2 is initiated. Once the abdomen has been distended the da Vinci camera with 0° optic is inserted and the abdominal cavity is explored, with particular note taken of the presence of adhesions that may need to be dealt with. With the use of the camera, all subsequent ports are inserted into the abdominal cavity under direct vision. A right-sided 8 mm robot trocar inserted about 10 cm laterally to the umbilicus and a further 8 mm trocar is placed on the left side at the same distance from the umbilicus. An additional 8 mm robot trocar may be inserted on the left, at a distance of approximately 5–8 cm above the left anterior superior iliac spine (ASIS), although some centers choose to forego this additional port especially for cases that do not require lymph node dissection. A 12 mm assistant trocar is placed in the right side of the abdomen laterally, approximately 5–8 cm above the ASIS. Then a 5-mm assistant port is inserted between the camera and right-sided robotic trocar. The patient is then placed in the Trendelenberg position, with a tilt of 30–35°.

The surgical arm cart is then placed into position between the patient's abducted legs. The robotic and camera trocars are then docked onto the robot arms and the camera is inserted back into the abdominal cavity. The robotic instruments are then placed into the abdomen with laparoscopic control under direct vision ready for use by the console surgeon.

4 The Posterior Approach

Our favored method of performing the robotic operation is to begin by dissecting the posterior to peritoneum beneath the prostate [9], with mobilization of the paired vasa deferentia and seminal vesicles (SVs). As this step is performed prior to dropping the bladder, the working space for this portion of the operation is very favorable, improving access and efficiency. Furthermore, mobilization of the vasa and SVs at the beginning of the operation simplifies the later posterior bladder-neck dissection. To gain access to the vasa differentia, an incision is made in the peritoneum, low and in the midline. The vasa are identified and dissected out bluntly. The vasa must be confidently differentiated from ureters prior to transection. Three anatomical features permit accurate identification of the vasa: firstly, ureters are located superior and lateral to the vasa deferentia. Secondly, vasa deferentia meet in the midline, whereas ureters do not. Thirdly, seminal vesicles lie behind the vasa, but not behind ureters. Once the vasa and SVs have been dissected out, an incision is then made in Denonvilliers fascia and a plane is developed between the posterior aspect of the prostate and the rectum, again employing a technique of blunt dissection. Following this, a plane is developed anterior to where the mobilized vasa meet in the midline, essentially creating a space behind the posterior bladder neck.

5 Dropping the Bladder

After the posterior dissection is complete, the bladder is then mobilized. An incision is made with monopolar scissors in the peritoneum on the right side lateral to the union of the umbilical arteries and an avascular plane is developed, aided by the pneumoperitoneum. This space is dissected out until the endopelvic fascia is exposed and the pubis is visible superiorly. The endopelvic fascia on the left is exposed in an identical fashion. Dissecting in the midline plane between the bladder and the anterior abdominal wall completes the bladder drop.

6 Dissecting the Bladder Neck

Once the bladder has been dropped, fat may be removed from the surface of the prostate if necessary. This step is often helpful if there is a great deal of adipose tissue present and the anatomy is unclear. Next, an incision is made on each side in the already-exposed endopelvic fascia. Muscle fibers of the pelvic floor are gently teased away from the lateral margins of the prostate and the edge of the prostate is then defined. Identification of the bladder neck may be aided by manipulating the urethral catheter such that the movement of the balloon in the bladder can be detected by the console surgeon. During the bladder neck dissection, the bladder is gently retracted with the third robotic instrument arm.

The dissection begins in the midline with sharp dissection with the incision moving laterally either side to follow the contour of the bladder neck. Continued dissection in the midline will reveal a preprostatic portion of the urethra continuous with the bladder neck. Space either side of this structure is developed laterally towards the prostatic pedicles to maximize bladder neck exposure. Once the exposure is adequate an incision in the anterior bladder neck is made. The catheter, with balloon deflated, is then retrieved through this incision and can be retracted upwards by the bedside surgeon to facilitate exposure of the posterior bladder neck, which is incised in the midline with monopolar cautery by the console surgeon.

Dissection of the posterior bladder neck in the correct plane will invariably meet up with the space created posteriorly at the beginning of the operation and the mobilized vasa deferentia and seminal vesicles will be encountered. These structures can then be retrieved through the bladder neck incision using the third robotic arm and used to provide traction on the prostate.

7 Lateral Dissection and Nerve Preservation

A number of different techniques have been described to achieve the objective of nerve preservation, and although a comprehensive description of these is beyond the scope of this chapter, each method shares core principles. Once the vessels of the prostatic pedicles are controlled with hemostatic clips and are then cut, the lateral peri-prostatic fascia containing the neurovascular bundle is separated from the surface of the prostate by sharp scissor dissection. To avert thermal injury to the neurovascular bundle all dissection is performed sharply without cautery.

8 Apical Dissection

The puboprostatic ligaments are divided using monopolar scissors and then a plane is developed between the urethra and dorsal venous complex (DVC) by sharp dissection. Due to the vascularity of the DVC, minimal-to-moderate bleeding is often encountered at this step, and it can be useful to increase the pressure of the pneumoperitoneum temporarily at this point to ensure good vision is maintained (we perform most of the operation at a pressure of 12 mmHg and increase it to 18 mmHg at this stage). Once the anterior wall of the urethra is exposed, an incision is made a few millimeters distal to the apex of the prostate. Once transection of the urethra is complete, the freed specimen is placed into an endoscopic retrieval bag for removal upon completion of the anastomosis. Bleeding at the DVC is controlled at this stage by oversewing with a 3.0 V-Loc™ suture (Medtronic). This suture is barbed and has a loop at the non-needle end, avoiding the need for knot tying.

9 Urethrovesical Anastomosis

For the anastomosis, we use 3.0 V-Loc sutures. Before the anastomosis is performed, the urethra and bladder are approximated with a "Rocco stitch," a step that helps reduce traction on the urethra-sphincteric complex [10]. The anastomosis begins with approximation of the posterior wall of the urethra to the posterior bladder, with the suture taking mucosal bites of both structures. The anastomosis is continued with continuous sutures and extended anteriorly. Once the anastomosis is visibly complete, a new 16 French Foley catheter is inserted and the balloon inflated with 20 ml of water. To test the integrity of the anastomosis, the bladder is filled with 300 ml saline.

10 Specimen Removal and Wound Closure

Upon completion of the anastomosis, the robotic instruments are withdrawn and the robot undocked. The patient is then placed in a flat, horizontal position. The robot and assistant trocars are removed under direct vision and the 12 mm assistant port is closed with 3.0 PDS. The camera trocar is removed and the specimen is retrieved through the supra umbilical wound (which often needs to be enlarged at this stage). This wound is closed with 2.0 PDS, with care taken to ensure that the rectus sheath is approximated. Skin closure is achieved with 3.0 vicyl rapide.

11 Outcomes After Robot Assisted Radical Prostatectomy

Radical prostatectomy holds a reasonably unique position among cancer surgeries in that success is not based solely on favorable oncologic outcomes. In addition to undetectable PSA, surgical quality is also measured against the key functional outcomes of continence and potency. These outcomes form the so-called "trifecta" of radical prostatectomy

[11]. Therefore, in order to compare robot assisted surgery with alternative surgical approaches, these functional outcomes must be considered in addition to the oncologic outcomes.

12 Oncologic Outcomes: Robot vs. Laparoscopic vs. Open

Positive surgical margin (PSM) rates are a widely acknowledged benchmark for technical quality in radical prostatectomy. Furthermore, PSM rate is known to affect the risk of biochemical recurrence post-surgery [12]. A large study of more than 22,000 men who underwent surgery for radical prostatectomy (RP) compared the PSM rates of men who had open RP versus laparoscopic RP versus robot assisted RP [13]. The crude PSM rates were lowest for robotic RP (13.8 %), intermediate for laparoscopic RP (16.3 %) and highest for open RP (22.8 %). Even after classical adjustment, the risk of PSM remained lower after laparoscopic RP and robotic RP than after open RP (odds ratio 0.76).

Although robotic surgery is still a relatively new endeavor, and long-term data regarding oncologic outcomes are somewhat scarce, some centers are beginning to publish data showing favorable results with respect to biochemical recurrence more than 5 years after robot assisted RP. For example, biochemical recurrence–free survival (BRFS) outcomes at a single European center are reported at 87.1 %, 84.5 % and 82.6 % at 5, 7 and 9 years respectively [14]. An additional report of a cohort of nearly 500 men who underwent robotic RP demonstrates a BRFS of 73.1 % at 10 years with a cancer-specific survival (CSS) of 98.8 % over the same time frame [15]. The largest report of oncologic outcomes to date in robot assisted RP examines data from a cohort of nearly 5000 men. At 8 years this study shows a BRFS of 81 % and CSS of 99.1 % [16]. Taken together, these data indicate the effectiveness of robotic RP for conferring long-term biochemical control.

13 Continence and Sexual Function After Robot Assisted Radical Prostatectomy

The preservation of urinary continence after radical prostatectomy is a key determinant influencing patient wellbeing and maintenance of quality of life (QOL) after radical therapy for prostate cancer [17]. A large systematic review and meta-analysis examining data from more than 4000 patients was published in 2012 by Ficarra and colleagues and showed that continence rates (when using a no pad definition of continence) at 12 months after robotic RP ranged from 69 to 96 %, with a mean value of 84 % [18]. Furthermore, their analysis demonstrated statistically significant improved continence outcomes in favor of robotic prostatectomy in comparison to both laparoscopic and open surgery. Similar to open and laparoscopic techniques, increasing age, high BMI and the presence of LUTS correlated with a higher risk of incontinence following robot assisted RP.

Early potency with or without pharmacological assistance appears to be improved with robot assisted RP compared to open surgery. With bilateral extended nerve sparing, intercourse is achieved in up to 90 % of all patients [19]. In the largest meta-analysis of its kind, potency rates following nerve sparing robot assisted RP ranged from 54 to 90 % at 12 months and 63–94 % at 24 months. Furthermore, cumulative analyses demonstrated superior 12-month potency rates after robot assisted RP compared to open RP, with an odds ratio (OR) of 2.4; 95 % confidence interval: 1.46–5.43; $p = 0.02$ [20].

14 Patient Satisfaction After Robotic Assisted Radical Prostatectomy

Interestingly, a study of patient satisfaction after radical prostatectomy found that robotic RP was independently associated with more dissatisfaction and regret, with patients undergoing a robotic procedure being 3–4 times more likely to express regret than patients undergoing an open procedure [21]. The authors postulated that patients might be more likely to be regretful because of the higher expectations associated with a cutting edge procedure. Indeed, a follow up study by the same group indicates that subjecting patients to a preoperative education and counseling program can achieve high levels of satisfaction after robotic assisted RP [22].

Conclusion

The development of robotic surgical technologies has revolutionized prostate cancer surgery. The high quality of vision and the precision of instrument movement afforded by robot assistance continue to translate as favorable outcomes for patients, both oncologically and functionally. We anticipate that robotic technology will continue to progress and improve surgical quality for men undergoing radical prostatectomy.

References

1. Engel RM. Hugh Hampton Young: father of American urology. J Urol. 2003;169(2):458–64.
2. Millin T. Retropubic prostatectomy; a new extravesical technique; report of 20 cases. Lancet. 1945;2(6380):693–6.
3. Schuessler WW, et al. Laparoscopic radical prostatectomy: initial short-term experience. Urology. 1997;50(6):854–7.
4. Abbou CC, et al. Laparoscopic radical prostatectomy with a remote controlled robot. J Urol. 2001;165(6 Pt 1):1964–6.
5. Menon M, et al. Laparoscopic and robot assisted radical prostatectomy: establishment of a structured program and preliminary analysis of outcomes. J Urol. 2002;168(3):945–9.
6. Tewari A, et al. Technique of da Vinci robot-assisted anatomic radical prostatectomy. Urology. 2002;60(4):569–72.
7. Singh I, Hemal AK. Robotic-assisted radical prostatectomy in 2010. Expert Rev Anticancer Ther. 2010;10(5):671–82.
8. Gettman MT, et al. Laparoscopic radical prostatectomy: description of the extraperitoneal approach using the da Vinci robotic system. J Urol. 2003;170(2 Pt 1):416–9.
9. Nilsson AE, et al. Karolinska prostatectomy: a robot-assisted laparoscopic radical prostatectomy technique. Scand J Urol Nephrol. 2006;40(6):453–8.
10. Rocco F, et al. Restoration of posterior aspect of rhabdosphincter shortens continence time after radical retropubic prostatectomy. J Urol. 2006;175(6):2201–6.
11. Borregales LD, et al. 'Trifecta' after radical prostatectomy: is there a standard definition? BJU Int. 2013;112(1):60–7.
12. Wieder JA, Soloway MS. Incidence, etiology, location, prevention and treatment of positive surgical margins after radical prostatectomy for prostate cancer. J Urol. 1998;160(2):299–315.
13. Sooriakumaran P, et al. A multinational, multi-institutional study comparing positive surgical margin rates among 22393 open, laparoscopic, and robot-assisted radical prostatectomy patients. Eur Urol. 2014;66(3):450–6.
14. Sooriakumaran P, et al. Biochemical recurrence after robot-assisted radical prostatectomy in a European single-centre cohort with a minimum follow-up time of 5 years. Eur Urol. 2012;62(5):768–74.
15. Diaz M, et al. Oncologic outcomes at 10 years following robotic radical prostatectomy. Eur Urol. 2015;67(6):1168–76.
16. Sukumar S, et al. Oncological outcomes after robot-assisted radical prostatectomy: long-term follow-up in 4803 patients. BJU Int. 2014;114(6):824–31.
17. Bradley EB, Bissonette EA, Theodorescu D. Determinants of long-term quality of life and voiding function of patients treated with radical prostatectomy or permanent brachytherapy for prostate cancer. BJU Int. 2004;94(7):1003–9.
18. Ficarra V, et al. Systematic review and meta-analysis of studies reporting urinary continence recovery after robot-assisted radical prostatectomy. Eur Urol. 2012;62(3):405–17.
19. Kaul S, et al. Functional outcomes and oncological efficacy of Vattikuti Institute prostatectomy with Veil of Aphrodite nerve-sparing: an analysis of 154 consecutive patients. BJU Int. 2006;97(3):467–72.
20. Ficarra V, et al. Systematic review and meta-analysis of studies reporting potency rates after robot-assisted radical prostatectomy. Eur Urol. 2012;62(3):418–30.
21. Schroeck FR, et al. Satisfaction and regret after open retropubic or robot-assisted laparoscopic radical prostatectomy. Eur Urol. 2008;54(4):785–93.
22. Douaihy YE, et al. A cohort study investigating patient expectations and satisfaction outcomes in men undergoing robotic assisted radical prostatectomy. Int Urol Nephrol. 2011;43(2):405–15.

Permanent and High Dose Rate Brachytherapy (Technique, Indications, Results, Morbidity)

Ann Henry

1 Introduction

Brachytherapy (derived from the Greek word brachys meaning 'short-distance') is a form of radiation therapy where a sealed radiation source is placed directly into the body. In prostate brachytherapy, the placement of radiation sources in the gland can be permanent or temporary. Both are forms of interstitial brachytherapy, which is defined as the insertion of brachytherapy applicators or sources directly into tissue i.e. the prostate gland.

Permanent interstitial brachytherapy, also known as seed brachytherapy, involves placing small radioactive pellets into the prostate and leaving them permanently to gradually release radiation over time. After all the radiation has decayed the inactive pellets remain in the prostate gland. Permanent brachytherapy uses low dose rate (LDR) sources emitting radiation over weeks and months.

Temporary brachytherapy involves first placing needles or catheters within the prostate and, on confirmation of accurate positioning, temporarily introducing the radioactive source into the prostate. Radiation is delivered using a high dose rate (HDR) machine where actual treatment times are minutes. The radiation dose rate is very similar to that used in external beam radiotherapy. Comparisons of LDR and HDR prostate brachytherapy treatments are listed in Table 1.

Prostate brachytherapy allows safe radiation dose escalation beyond that achieved using external beam radiotherapy alone as it has greater conformity around the prostate, sparing surrounding rectum and bladder. In addition, there are fewer issues with changes in prostate position during treatment delivery. Randomized trials using both techniques demonstrate improved disease control when compared to external beam radiotherapy alone [1, 2].

2 Permanent Prostate Brachytherapy Techniques

The breakthrough in the development of modern brachytherapy was the establishment in the early 1980s of trans-rectal ultrasound (TRUS) combined with the use of a template attached to the TRUS probe to guide trans-perineal needle placement [3]. The procedure was refined by the Seattle group [4] and remains the most commonly used permanent prostate brachytherapy technique.

2.1 Patient Preparation

The procedure is often done as a day-case under general or regional anaesthesia (spinal or caudal

A. Henry
University of Leeds, Leeds, UK
e-mail: a.henry@leeds.ac.uk

M. Bolla, H. van Poppel (eds.), *Management of Prostate Cancer*,
DOI 10.1007/978-3-319-42769-0_13

Table 1 Comparison of prostate brachytherapy techniques

Low dose rate (LDR)	Permanent seeds implanted
	Uses Iodine-125 (most common), Palladium-103 or Caesium-131 isotopes
	Radiation dose delivered over weeks and months
	Acute side effects resolve over months
	Radiation protection issues for patient and carers
	Established as monotherapy for low and selected intermediate risk localized prostate cancer
	Established as a boost treatment with external beam radiation in higher risk or locally advanced prostate cancer
High dose rate (HDR)	Temporary implantation
	Ir-192 isotope introduced through implanted applicators (needles or catheters)
	Radiation dose delivered in minutes
	Treatment may need to be fractionated
	Acute side effects resolve over weeks
	No radiation protection issues for patient or carers
	Established as boost treatment with external beam radiation in higher risk or locally advanced prostate cancer
	Investigational as monotherapy (recommended only within clinical trials)

blocks). An empty rectum helps optimize TRUS images and the patient should have an enema before the procedure to clear the rectum. Once anaesthetized, the patient is placed in the lithotomy position and a Foley catheter introduced to visualize the urethra. Aerated gel (lubricating gel plus air to make small bubbles) can be used to help visualize the urethra. The scrotum is moved away from the operating field and fixed with an adhesive dressing; the perineum is then cleaned with antiseptic solution.

2.2 TRUS Volume Study

The ultrasound probe placed within the stepper unit (Fig. 1) is inserted into the rectum and positioned under the prostate. The stepping unit can make steps (generally at 5 mm transverse intervals) through the prostate acquiring an image

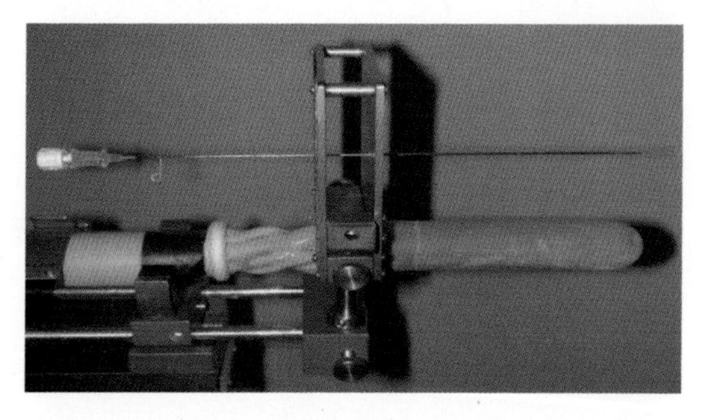

Fig. 1 Trans-rectal ultrasound (TRUS) probe placed within stepper unit allows TRUS image acquisition at 5 mm intervals from prostate base to apex. The trans-perineal template attached to the stepper unit guides accurate needle placement during the implant

dataset which is then used to contour the prostate volume and adjacent organs at risk (urethra, rectum, bladder neck, neurovascular bundles). Attached to the trans-rectal ultrasound is a perineal template. The coordinates of the template are automatically transposed over the ultrasound images of the prostate.

The prostate is positioned so that it lies centrally within the template grid with the lower border on the first row and the urethra centred on the middle row (large D). Care should be taken to ensure the prostate is not angled or rotated around its axis. Once the prostate is accurately positioned relative to the template, serial sections are taken from the base to apex at 5 mm intervals. On each section, the prostate capsule is contoured and the information analysed within a planning computer to calculate the exact number and position of seeds required for the implant (Fig. 2).

2.3 Treatment Planning and Implantation

The planning and implantation technique may follow one of the following depending on departmental preferences and experience [5]:

1. Pre-planning: A two-step procedure where there is delayed execution of the treatment plan. The TRUS pre-plan takes place a few weeks before actual implantation.

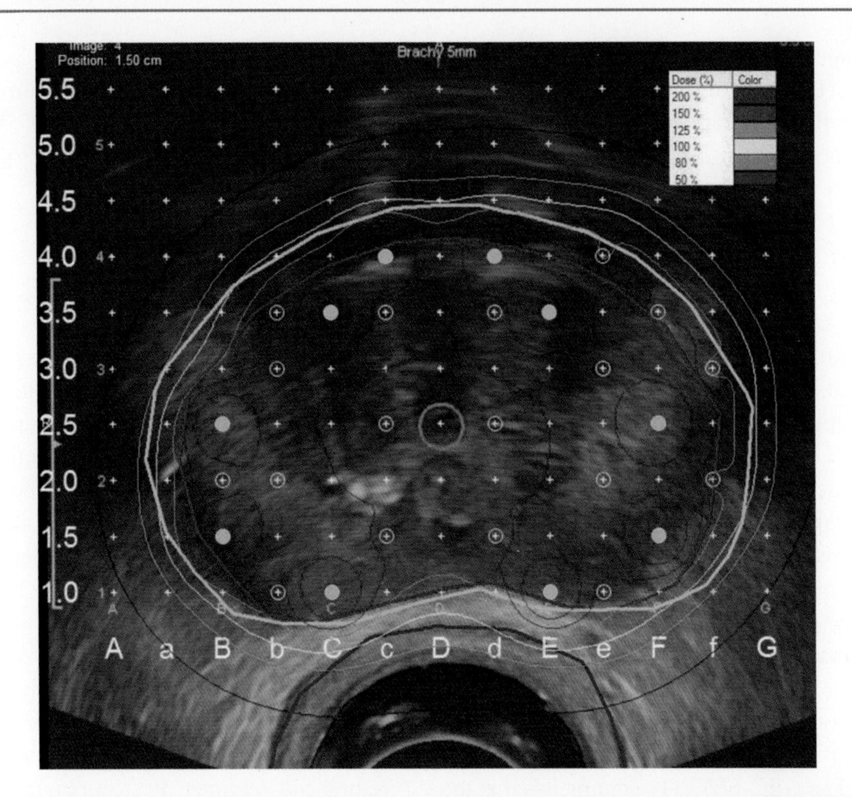

Fig. 2 TRUS prostate image with prostate capsule outlined in *red* and planned seed positions represented by *green dots*. The coordinates of the template (letters on *x*-axis and numerals on *y*-axis) are superimposed on the TRUS image to guide accurate needle placement. The varying radiation isodose lines are displayed in the key. In I-125 brachytherapy the dose (145 Gy) is prescribed to the 100 % isodose (*yellow line*) which should encompass the entire prostate with a 3 mm margin apart from posteriorly adjacent to the rectum where no margin is applied (CTV: *light blue line*)

2. Intraoperative planning: The plan is created in the operating room immediately prior to the procedure.
3. Interactive planning: Stepwise modification of the plan using computerized dose calculations that have been obtained from image-based needle-position feedback.
4. Dynamic dose calculation: Constant updating of the dose distribution using continuous seed position feedback.

Typically about 80–100 seeds will be implanted using 25–30 needles, but the precise number will depend on the prostate size/shape and the activity of the seeds. The needles are 20 cm long (18 gauge). A modified peripheral loading pattern is used where the majority of seeds are positioned adjacent to the capsule and a smaller number placed centrally but away from the urethra.

The needles are guided through the perineal skin using the template that provides the X and Y co-ordinates with the depth (Z co-ordinate) confirmed using sagittal ultrasound imaging. Seed positions are referenced to the base plane defined as where the prostate meets the bladder base. Not all needles are inserted as far as the base plane, some are inserted closer to the apex to provide seed coverage more proximally. Stranded or linked seed trains are often used as this reduces seed migration into the peri-prostatic venous circulation. A Mick applicator can be used to insert single or 'loose' seeds into gland.

The most frequently used isotope for permanent seed implantation is Iodine-125. It has a mean energy of 25 KeV with a half-life of 59.6 days. The Iodine-125 is absorbed onto a silver rod, which is encased in a titanium case. The overall size of seeds is just under 5 mm long and 1 mm in diameter. In the early years of permanent prostate brachytherapy Palladium-103 was used, citing a theoretical advantage for more rapidly growing tumours as it has a shorter half-life (i.e. higher dose rate) than Iodine-125, but with long-term follow-up no clinical advantage has been demonstrated. The prescribed dose when using Iodine-125 is 145 Gy for monotherapy and 110 Gy when used as a boost treatment with supplemental external beam radiotherapy.

Detailed GEC-ESTRO (Groupe Europeen de Curietherapie -European Society of Therapeutic Radiation Oncology) guidelines on the clinical and technical aspects of permanent prostate brachytherapy are recommended [6, 7]. The clinical target volume (CTV) is defined as the prostate gland plus a 3 mm margin in each direction. This can be constrained to the rectum posteriorly and the bladder neck cranially.

The dose distribution inside a prostate implant is highly non uniform and doses can be considerably higher than the minimum peripheral dose to the CTV. The GEC-ESTRO recommends that the following dosimetric parameters should be aimed for and recorded:

Clinical Target Volume (CTV)

- $V100_{CTV}$ (percentage of the CTV that receives the prescription dose) ≥95 %
- $V150_{CTV}$ (percentage of the CTV that receives the 150 % prescription dose) ≤50 %
- $D90_{CTV}$ (dose that covers 90 % of the CTV) > prescription dose

Rectum

- $D2cc_{rectum}$ (the minimum dose in the most irradiated 2 cc volume of the rectum) < prescription dose
- D0.1 cc_{rectum} (the minimum dose in the most irradiated 0.1 cc volume of the rectum) <200 Gy

Urethra

- $D10\%_{urethra}$ (the minimum dose in the most irradiated 10 % of the urethral volume) <150 % of prescription dose
- $D30\%_{urethra}$ (the minimum dose in the most irradiated 30 % of the urethral volume) <130 % of the prescription dose

2.4 Quality Assurance

Practice guidelines to ensure high quality training and quality assurance have been published following errors in US centres, where poor quality implants led adverse patient outcomes [8–10]. It is recommended that all patients undergo post implantation CT based dosimetry to compare the actual dose delivered to the treatment plan. If available, MR-CT fusion is a useful tool to more accurately evaluate seed placement relative to the prostate capsule (Fig. 3). The optimal timing of imaging has not been established and it can be undertaken Day 0, 1 or 2–6 weeks following the implant. Post-implant dosimetry should measure the following parameters: Prostate D90%, V100%, V150% and organ at risk doses (urethra and rectum). Post-implantation results should be reviewed and action, such as re-implantation, undertaken to compensate for sub-optimal treatment in individual patients. The impact on post-implant dosimetry of changes in personnel or implant technique should also be assessed by regular review, as a learning curve for permanent prostate brachytherapy is well described.

2.5 Radiation Protection

The low emission energy of the seeds and the ease of shielding mean that seed loading and implantation can be undertaken without the need for significantly increased radiation protection measures in the operating theatre.

Following implantation, men and their families should be given radiation protection advice both verbally and on an information card. This advice should include this information;

- Avoid close (<1 m) contact with young children and pregnant women in the first 2 months following implantation.

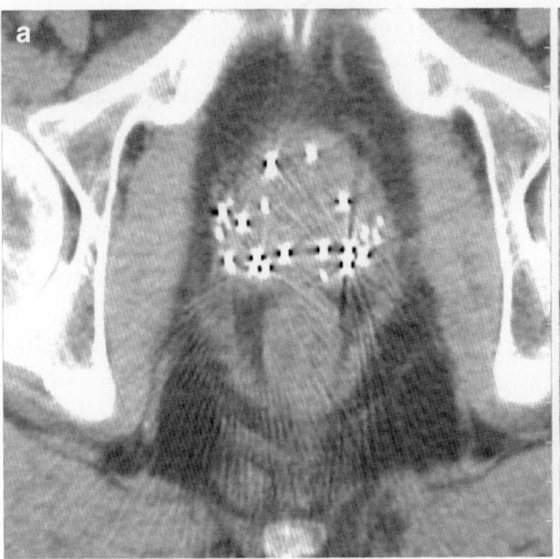

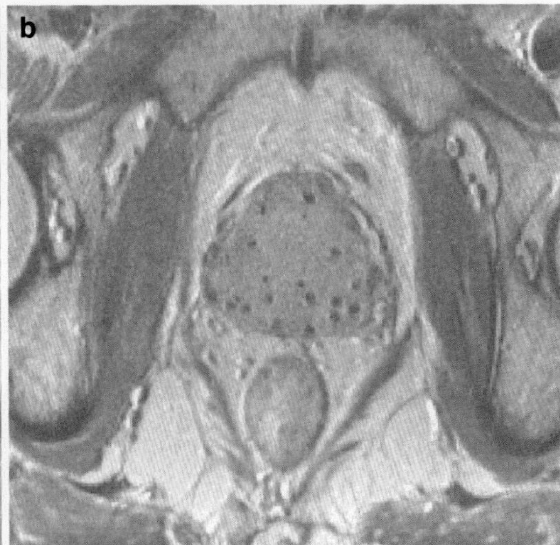

Fig. 3 Post Implant dosimetry should be undertaken in all seed brachytherapy patients to check actual dose delivered. (**a**) Pelvic CT scan demonstrating seeds within gland. (**b**) CT can be fused with MRI to aid prostate capsule identification

- Partners can safely sleep in the same bed.
- Sex can resume when comfortable after implantation but condoms should be used for the first 5 ejaculations, then flushed away.
- Should a seed be passed pick it up with a spoon or long handled tweezers and flush away.
- In the event of death within 20 months of implantation cremation is not allowed.
- Airport radiation monitors may be triggered up to 6 months after and a wallet sized information card should be carried with information for airport security staff.

3 Indications for Permanent Prostate Brachytherapy

3.1 Monotherapy in Localized Prostate Cancer

Non-metastatic prostate cancer is stratified into risk groups depending on PSA, T stage and Gleason score. In broad terms, low risk is defined as T1/T2a, PSA ≤10 ng/mL and Gleason score 6, intermediate risk as T1/2 and/or PSA 10–20 ng/mL and/or Gleason 7 and high risk as any having one of the following features T3-4, PSA >20 ng/mL or Gleason 8–10. Stratification into these risk categories helps guide treatment choices and predicts long term outcomes.

Patients with low risk localized prostate cancer (T1c-T2a, Gleason 6, <50 % core positive, PSA ≤10 ng/mL) and selected patients with low volume intermediate risk localized prostate cancer (T1c-T2a, Gleason 3+4, PSA ≤10 ng/mL, <33 % core positive) are suitable for permanent prostate brachytherapy alone (Table 2).

Men with pre-existing urinary symptoms and/or enlarged prostate glands are at high risk of acute retention of urine after brachytherapy and/or experiencing prolonged urinary symptoms. The patient completed International Prostate Symptom Score (IPSS) can be used to screen for significant pre-existing urinary symptoms with a score <9 being ideal and scores <15 acceptable [11]. A more objective measure of urinary function can be obtained from urinary flow tests. Men with peak urinary flow rates of <10 ml/s have a 30 % risk of post-implant retention and brachytherapy is generally not advised. Those with peak flow rates >20 ml/s have <10 % risk of catheterization and are good candidates for brachytherapy [12].

In patients with enlarged prostate glands (over 50 ml) it can be difficult to achieve good

Table 2 Patient selection criteria for curative permanent prostate brachytherapy as monotherapy

Inclusion criteria
Stages T1c-T2a N0 M0
Gleason 3 + 3 with < 50 % core involvement *or*
Gleason 3 + 4 with < 33 % core involvement
PSA < 10 ng/mL
Exclusion criteria
Limited overall life expectancy
Extensive TURP defect or TURP within 3–6 months
Maximal urinary flow rate (Qmax) < 10 ml/s
IPSS > 15
Gland size >50 ml (may be downsized with neo-adjuvant androgen deprivation)
Pubic arch interference
Lithotomy position or anaesthesia not possible
Rectal fistula or previous abdomino-perineal resection (APR)

implantation of the gland because the pubic arch may shield the anterior prostate. Neo-adjuvant androgen deprivation for 3–6 months before implantation can be used to downsize the gland with the greatest gland shrinkage achieved using luteinizing hormone releasing hormone (LHRH) agonists rather than anti-androgens [13]. LHRH agonists will often achieve a 30 % reduction in prostate size.

Previous trans-urethral resection of the prostate (TURP) is a relative contra-indication to prostate brachytherapy particularly if there is a large prostate defect. The presence of a significant defect makes it difficult to achieve a satisfactory dose distribution. Patients who have had a TURP a number of years before or those where a more recent narrow channel procedure has been undertaken can be considered for brachytherapy.

3.2 Boost Treatment with External Beam Radiotherapy in Intermediate and High Risk Disease

In patients with intermediate and high risk localized prostate cancer there is a significant risk of microscopic extra-capsular spread that may not be included in the high dose region of a seed implant leading to local treatment failure. In this situation brachytherapy may be combined with external beam radiotherapy to ensure an appropriate target volume is treated. External beam doses in the order of 46 Gy in 23 fractions are delivered to either prostate and seminal vesicles or whole pelvis with a boost of 110 Gy delivered to the prostate using 1–125 permanent prostate brachytherapy [2]. Neo-adjuvant and adjuvant hormone manipulation should also be considered as standard care.

4 Results for Permanent Prostate Brachytherapy

There have been no randomized trials comparing brachytherapy as monotherapy with other curative treatment modalities. Outcome data are available from a number of large cohort studies with mature follow-up [14–22]. The biochemical control for low risk patients has been reported to range from 72 to 98 % with follow-up out to 12 years. Morris et al. [22] reported the population based outcomes from British Colombia, Canada and demonstrated biochemical disease-free survival of 94 % at 10 years in low and selected intermediate risk patients. For all series, outcomes for intermediate risk patients vary from 61 to 96 % which is likely to reflect variation in patient selection.

A significant correlation has been shown between the implanted dose and recurrence rates [23]. Patients receiving a D90 (dose covering 90 % of the prostate volume) of >140 Gy had a significantly higher biochemical control rate (PSA < 1.0 ng/mL) after 4 years than patients who received less than 140 Gy (92 vs. 68 %). There is no benefit in adding neo-adjuvant or adjuvant ADT to LDR monotherapy [14].

Dose-escalated external beam radiotherapy has been compared with external beam radiotherapy followed by a LDR brachytherapy boost in intermediate-risk and high-risk patients in a recently presented randomized trial [2]. The ASCENDE-RT (Androgen Suppression Combined with Elective Nodal and Dose Escalated Radiation Therapy) multi-centre

Canadian trial compared external beam (total dose of 78 Gy) to external beam (total dose 46 Gy) followed by LDR brachytherapy boost (prescribed dose 115 Gy). With a median follow-up of 6.5 years, a significant improvement in recurrence-free survival at 7 years was found, increasing from 71 % in the dose escalated external beam alone arm to 86 % in the LDR boost arm. This was associated with a higher rate of late urinary morbidity with a 5-year cumulative Grade 3 toxicity rate of 19 % in the LDR boost arm compared to 5 % in the external beam radiotherapy alone arm [24]. Approximately 50 % of the urinary toxicity was due to urethral strictures and it is recommended that a boost dose of 110 Gy rather than 115 Gy should be used in routine practice. Care should also be taken not to over-treat the membranous urethra distal to the prostate apex when using this technique. In addition, although associated with improved recurrence-free survival, use of LDR boost had a significant negative impact on health related quality of life (HRQoL) for urinary and sexual function, general health and bodily pain [25].

5 Morbidity

5.1 Urinary Morbidity

Immediate post-implantation side effects are predominantly urinary. Irritative and obstructive urinary symptoms are very common in the first 2–3 weeks and are relieved by alpha-blocker drugs. Alpha-blockers should be commenced just before the procedure and may need to be continued for several months afterwards until urinary symptoms resolve. Regular anti-inflammatory use will help with pain and discomfort on passing urine. Acute urinary retention can occur in 10–20 % of patients and is managed by urethral catheterization. This usually resolves within 4–6 weeks but in the few patients with on-going problems intermittent self-catheterization effectively manages this symptom. In 95 % of men, urinary symptoms have resolved by 12 months. It is advisable to avoid TURP in the first 12 months, as this is associated with risks of urethral necrosis and incontinence. A narrow-channel TURP can be undertaken after this if outflow symptoms persist.

5.2 Rectal Morbidity

Rectal side effects are usually mild with a minority experiencing rectal discomfort, proctitis and rectal bleeding, which usually resolves within 12 months of treatment. There is a small risk of rectal ulceration and development of recto-prostatic fistulae (0.1–0.2 %).

5.3 Sexual Dysfunction

Erectile dysfunction develops in about 40 % of the patients after 3–5 years. The risk is less in younger men who are fully potent pre-treatment and greater in older men who may already have reduced potency. Daily sildenafil can be used prophylactically for the first 6 months following treatment to help maintain sexual function [26].

5.4 Health Related Quality of Life

It is increasingly recognized that patient outcomes measured objectively using validated health related quality of life (HRQoL) questionnaires allow measurement and comparison of how different treatment options impact the individual's life in a valid and reproducible way. The most robust information about long term HRQoL following treatment for prostate cancer is from randomized trials where groups have balanced baseline characteristics. Attempts to recruit patients into Phase III trials comparing radical prostatectomy versus permanent prostate brachytherapy have been unsuccessful as a significant proportion of informed patients feel unable to commit to a random allocation of treatment. The SPIRIT trial closed early but a comparison of HRQoL at a median of 5.2 years after treatment with either prostatectomy or brachytherapy (no neo-adjuvant hormone use) has been published [27]. This cross-sectional study assessed 168 trial eligible men 3.2–6.5 years after treatment and demonstrated those who had I-125 brachytherapy had better urinary, sexual and patient satisfaction scores than men undergoing radical prostatectomy.

Prospective longitudinal studies comparing non-randomized cohorts of patients undergoing prostatectomy, brachytherapy or external beam radiotherapy without hormone manipulation demonstrate that 3–5 years after treatment brachytherapy patients have less urinary incontinence, bowel effects and sexual dysfunction but more urinary irritative-obstructive symptoms [28–30]. There does appear to be a trend to decreased sexual function with time in brachytherapy patients, which may be related to increasing age and/or a late effect of radiation [28]. Sanda et al. included men who had neo-adjuvant hormone treatment in a multi-centre prospective longitudinal study of brachytherapy, external beam radiotherapy and radical prostatectomy [31]. The use of hormone manipulation in brachytherapy patients was associated with more sexual dysfunction and hormonal symptoms in the first 12 months after treatment but by 2 years function had returned to a level similar to that of the cohort who had brachytherapy alone.

6 Temporary High Dose Rate (HDR) Prostate Brachytherapy Techniques

6.1 Advantages of HDR Prostate Brachytherapy

Although permanent prostate brachytherapy has been the most commonly used prostate brachytherapy technique to date, temporary high dose rate (HDR) brachytherapy techniques using after-loading machines are now increasingly used. HDR is most commonly used as a boost treatment in intermediate and high risk patients combined with external beam radiotherapy.

The principal differences are:

- Applicators (needles or catheters) are inserted into the prostate ± seminal vesicles and post-implant dosimetry undertaken with no pre-plan required.
- There is more scope to treat extra-capsular and seminal vesicle disease as applicators can be placed into tissues adjacent to the prostate.
- There is more flexibility in dosimetry and the technique is less operator dependent.
- Dose is delivered in large fraction sizes and this may have a biological advantage when treating prostate cancer.
- HDR brachytherapy is a cost effective option as a single source is repeatedly used for treatments.
- Use of after-loading means minimal radiation protection issues for staff and patients.

After-loading systems were developed from the 1970s onwards as a way of reducing the radiation exposure to medical and nursing staff. After-loading involves the initial placement of a non-radioactive applicator (metal needles or plastic catheters) into the patient followed by the subsequent insertion of the radioactive isotope. Radiation is then delivered ‘remotely’ with the staff outside the room by computer control of a treatment machine inside the room. With appropriately shielded rooms this technique permits high dose-rate treatments with high activity sources. Modern HDR machines generally use a small iridium-192 source which is stepped through a series of dwell positions in all the treatment needles/catheters in turn, thereby removing the need for several sources or source trains to be present in the machine. Complex 3D dose distributions can be produced from the large combination of dwell times and positions.

6.2 Treatment Planning and Implantation

Patient preparation and positioning are identical to LDR brachytherapy. The patient undergoes general or regional anaesthesia, has a urethral catheter inserted and is placed in the lithotomy position. Trans-rectal ultra-sound is used to guide HDR applicator insertion in the same manner as LDR brachytherapy. Applicators may be hollow blind ending metal needles (re-useable) or plastic catheters (disposable). Applicators are inserted around the periphery of the prostate, generally 1 cm apart, with a small number centrally (Fig. 4). Additional applicators can be inserted into regions of gross tumour to facilitate higher dose delivery in these sub-volumes.

Once the applicators are positioned, they are held fixed within the perineal template. If multiple fractions of HDR brachytherapy are planned using the same implant, a means of fixing the perineal template to the perineum will be required. This is usually involves suturing the template to the perineum or use of an adhesive dressing.

After inserting the applicators, 3D imaging is acquired and imported into the computerized treatment planning system so that a treatment plan with dwell positions and timings for the radioactive source can be generated. Imaging with ultrasound, MR and/or CT can all be used to plan HDR treatments. There are two general approaches:

1. Trans-rectal ultrasound obtained whilst the patient remains in the lithotomy position under anaesthetic or sedation, known as real-time US guidance;
2. CT or MR images obtained following recovery from anaesthetic and transfer to the imaging department.

Real-time US imaging in theatre provides good organ definition and allows in-room treatment without the need to change patient positioning. Alternatively, CT or MRI may be used but necessitates moving the patient for imaging and subsequent treatment. In this second situation, quality assurance is essential to ensure that catheters do not move with change in patient positioning. As a minimum, the distal catheter length from the perineal template to the connecting hub should be measured and checked at each step to ensure catheters have not shifted position. If multiple HDR fractions are to be delivered using the same implant a number of hours apart imaging should be re-acquired before each fraction and treatment re-planned or catheters adjusted if clinically relevant changes are found.

Once the 3D image set (either US, CT or MR) is acquired, the following volumes for treatment planning are defined on the planning images (Fig. 5);

- Clinical target volume (CTV) including the prostate capsule plus any macroscopic

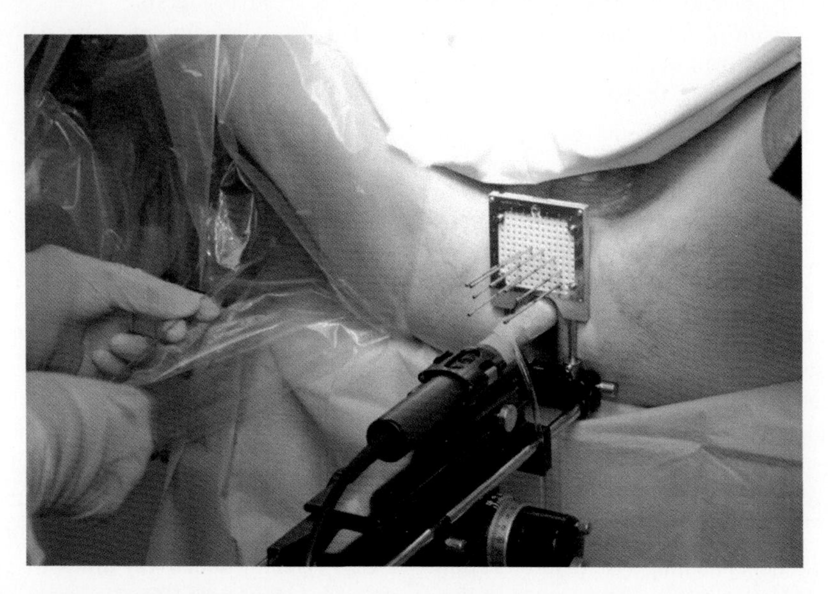

Fig. 4 Metal needles used for HDR brachytherapy inserted through trans-perineal template into the prostate gland at approximately 1 cm intervals around the periphery of the gland under trans-rectal ultrasound guidance

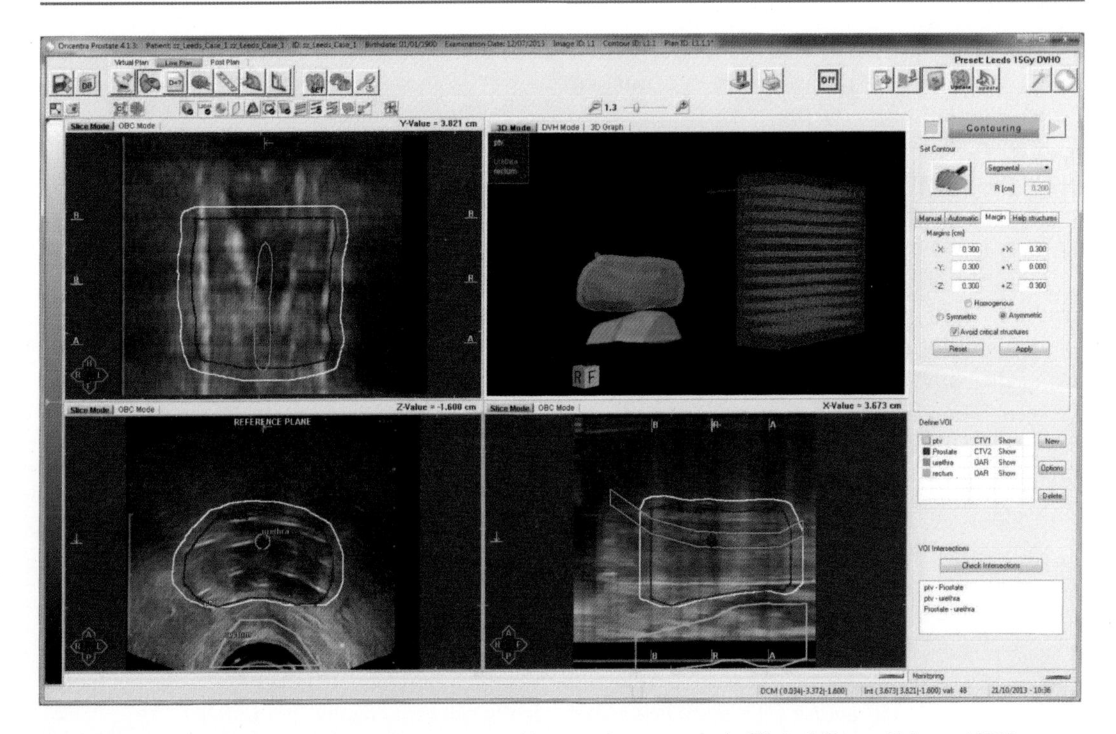

Fig. 5 Trans-rectal ultrasound images of the prostate with implanted HDR needles imported into computerised treatment planning system. Prostate (*red*), rectum (*green*) and urethra contoured. Clinical Target Volume (*CTV*) generated by expanding prostate contour

extra-capsular disease or seminal vesicle involvement identified on diagnostic images expanded by 3 mm to encompass potential microscopic disease. This is usually constrained posteriorly to the anterior rectal wall and superiorly to the bladder base;

- Gross tumour volume (GTV) may be defined, if this sub-volume is being boosted, using information from previous diagnostic imaging
- Rectum defined as outer rectal wall
- Urethra using the urethral catheter as the landmark on imaging for the urethral contour, which should extend from bladder base to 5–10 mm below the prostatic apex. Contrast such as aerated gel within the catheter will aid visualization on ultrasound
- Other adjacent organs at risk such as penile bulb, bladder neck and neurovascular bundles may be outlined (optional)

In the treatment planning system through optimization, a balance will be reached between dose to the CTV (± GTV) and the adjacent organs at risk (rectum and urethra). The prescription dose is defined as $D90_{CTV}$ i.e. the dose delivered to 90 % of the CTV. This is individualized for each patient and should be higher than the planning aim, i.e. >100 % (Fig. 6).

The heterogeneity of dose delivered using varying external beam and HDR brachytherapy schedules makes the definition of generalized maximal rectal and urethral doses difficult and the reader should refer to comprehensive guidelines [32].

There are no data available on which recommendations for constraints for penile bulb or neurovascular bundles can currently be made and detailed long term follow-up in cohorts receiving HDR brachytherapy is required.

Once treatment is planned and checked connecting tubes from the HDR treatment machine are attached to each applicator. All staff must leave the HDR treatment room and the patient is observed using remote monitors and CCTV. Treatment delivery times are generally of the order of minutes (Fig. 7).

On completion of treatment the applicators, template and urinary catheter are removed.

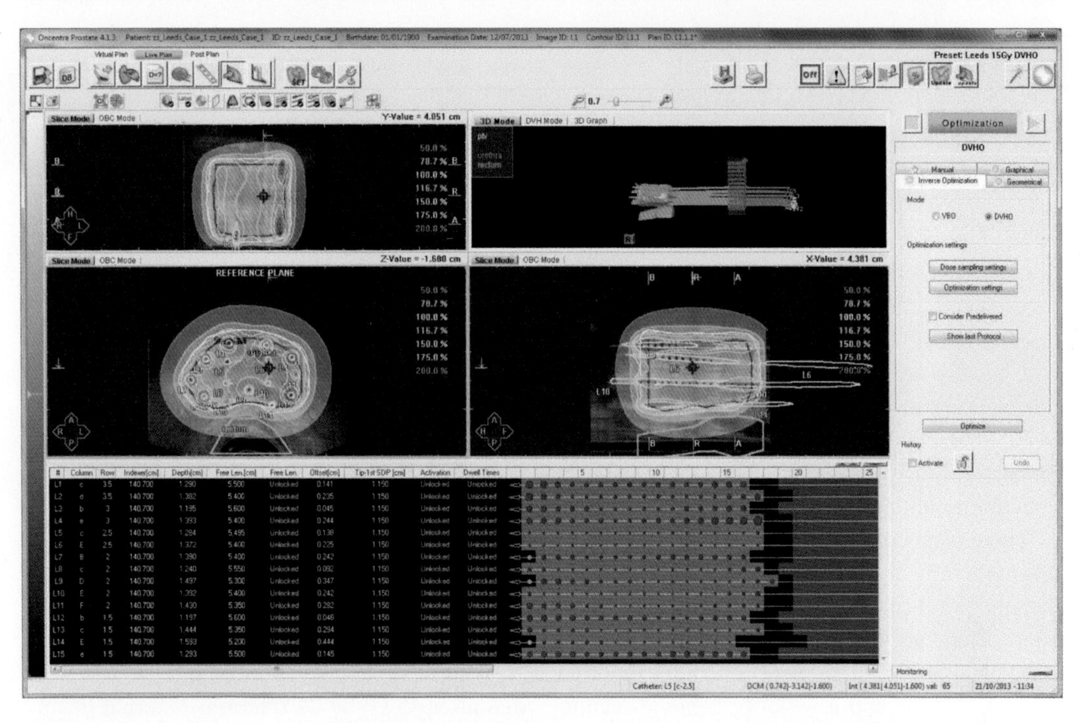

Fig. 6 HDR Treatment planning system generates the optimal radioactive source dwell times and positions to ensure good coverage of the CTV and minimal dose to the urethra and rectum

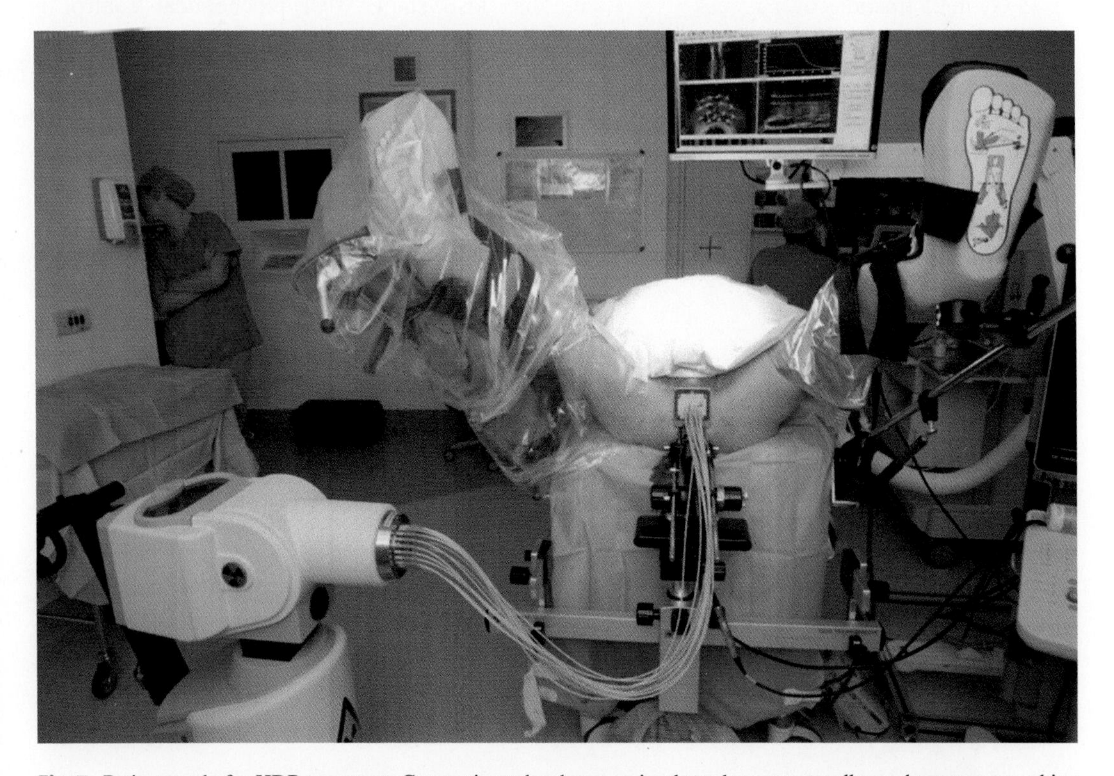

Fig. 7 Patient ready for HDR treatment. Connecting tubes between implanted prostate needles and treatment machine are in place. All staff will leave treatment room during treatment delivery and patient will be monitored remotely

7 HDR Brachytherapy Indications

7.1 HDR Brachytherapy Boost with External Beam

HDR brachytherapy combined with external beam radiotherapy is a treatment option for patients with intermediate and high risk localized disease, but in addition also an option for those with locally advanced and pelvic node positive prostate cancer. The exclusion criteria are similar to LDR brachytherapy apart from the ability to implant glands up to 60 cm^3 and treat patients with higher initial IPS scores (Table 3).

There is no consensus regarding the timing of brachytherapy in relation to external beam radiotherapy and it can be delivered before, during or after. There are also a wide range of external beam volumes and treatment schedules reported in the literature, and it is not possible to recommend one specific prescription. Published schedules include the following:

- 45 Gy in 25 fractions over 5 weeks
- 46 Gy in 23 fractions over 4.5 weeks
- 35.7 Gy in 13 fractions over 2.5 weeks
- 37.5 Gy in 15 fractions over 3 weeks

HDR brachytherapy planning aim doses, defined as a minimum peripheral dose, which have been prescribed with these schedules include:

- 15 Gy in 3 fractions
- 11–22 Gy in 2 fractions
- 12–15 Gy in 1 fraction

It is not possible to make a firm recommendation on planning aim dose; the randomized trial providing level 1 evidence used 17 Gy in 2 fractions (after 35.7 Gy in 13 fractions external beam) [1]. The need for fractionation and repeated treatments has been a logistical disadvantage for HDR brachytherapy but increasingly, a single dose of 15 Gy is gaining acceptance [35, 36].

Table 3 Patient selection criteria for curative high dose rate brachytherapy combined with external beam radiotherapy

Inclusion criteria
Stages T1b-T3b N0-1 M0
Any Gleason score
Any presenting PSA
Exclusion criteria
Limited overall life expectancy
TURP within 3–6 months
Maximal urinary flow rate (Qmax) < 10 ml/s
IPSS > 20
Gland size >60 ml (may be downsized with neo-adjuvant androgen deprivation)
Pubic arch interference
Lithotomy position or anaesthesia not possible
Rectal fistula or previous abdomino-perineal resection (APR)

There is evidence from a large cohort study that after 45 Gy in 25 fractions external beam a dose response exists up to 22 Gy in 2 fractions [33]. An analysis of the dose prescribed and volume treated in patients in a randomized trial has also shown that biochemical control is higher in with a higher delivered dose and volume covered [34].

7.2 HDR Monotherapy

HDR 'monotherapy' is associated with low acute toxicity and high biochemical control rates in the limited series published to date [37–44].

The schedules (planning aim) used include:

- 54 Gy in 9 fractions
- 44 Gy in 6 fractions
- 34 Gy in 4 fractions
- 36–38 Gy in 4 fractions
- 31.5 Gy in 3 fractions
- 26 Gy in 2 fractions
- 19–21 Gy in 1 fraction

Older series have used multiple fractions of HDR but more recent studies are using one or two fractions. Long- term outcome data are not yet available from these cohorts and it is recommended that this treatment is not undertaken outside clinical trials.

7.3 HDR in Recurrence After Previous Radiation

There is limited experience of HDR brachytherapy for locally recurrent prostate cancer after previous irradiation and this is not recommended outside a formal prospective study. Recurrence should be proven by prostate biopsy and patients staged to exclude metastatic disease. Organ at risk constraints are critical in this setting with a significant risk of toxicity due to bladder neck strictures or fistulation. Published schedules (planning aim) include the following:

- 36 Gy in 6 fractions [45]
- 21 Gy in 3 fractions [46]

8 Results

8.1 Results for HDR Prostate Brachytherapy

Multiple single centre series with mature follow-up demonstrate that HDR boost with external beam results in high rates of biochemical control and low toxicity [32, 47]. Biochemical control rates are on average 95 % for low risk, 91 % for intermediate risk and 82 % for high risk disease. Spratt et al. in a single institutional series compared outcomes of contemporaneously treated intermediate risk patients and found that those treated with brachytherapy boost (either LDR or HDR) had improved biochemical disease-free survival and distant metastases-free survival when compared to those treated with dose escalated intensity modulated radiotherapy (IMRT) to a total dose of 86.4 Gy [48]. At a median follow-up of 5.3 years biochemical disease-free survival was 92 % versus 81 %, and distant metastases-free survival 97 % versus 93 % in the brachytherapy boost patients versus IMRT alone patients respectively.

A randomized trial of external beam radiotherapy compared to external beam radiotherapy and HDR brachytherapy boost has been reported [1]. A total of 218 patients with intermediate and high risk prostate cancer were randomized to external beam alone to a dose of 55 Gy in 20 fractions, or external beam to a dose of 35.75 Gy in 13 fractions, followed by HDR brachytherapy to a dose of 17 Gy in two fractions over 24 h. In comparison with external beam alone, the combination showed a significant improvement with 5-, 7- and 10-year estimates of biochemical control at 75, 66 and 46 % for combination treatment compared to 61, 48 and 39 % for external beam alone. No differences in overall survival were noted at a median follow-up time of 85 months. The relatively low total radiation dose in the control arm has been criticized. An on-going trial of the National Cancer Institute of Canada (Clinical Trials. Gov identifier NCT01982786) randomizes patients with intermediate risk disease to either an HDR boost of 15 Gy combined with 37.5 Gy external beam radiotherapy or dose escalated external beam radiotherapy (either 78 Gy in 39 fractions or 60 Gy in 20 fractions) and will provide data on whether dose escalation using HDR boost results in improved disease-free survival when compared to modern dose-escalated radiotherapy.

A systematic review of non-randomized trials has suggested that outcomes with external beam radiotherapy plus HDR brachytherapy are superior to external beam alone or external beam with permanent seed boost [49].

Single centre studies of HDR monotherapy have demonstrated promising results.

Results from the group at California Endocurietherapy, UCLA show 6 and 10-year biochemical control rates of 98 and 97 % in a cohort of 448 low and intermediate risk patients treated over a 13 year period with a median dose of 43.5 Gy in 6 fractions [40]. No significant late rectal toxicity occurred and late (Grade 3+)

urinary toxicity occurred in <5 % after a median follow-up of 6.5 years. Yoshioka et al. reported 93 % and 79 % 5-year biochemical control rates for intermediate and high risk patients respectively using a 7- and 9-fraction protocol [38]. Treatment schedules using fewer fractions are also being investigated and have been shown to have acceptable toxicity [37, 43]. Results on biochemical control rates are awaited and monotherapy remains investigational.

9 HDR Brachytherapy Morbidity

9.1 Urinary Morbidity

Urinary symptoms are common in the 2–3 weeks following HDR brachytherapy but have usually resolved by 6 weeks post-implantation. Dysuria may last for a few days following treatment but is less severe than that associated with LDR brachytherapy. Obstructive symptoms can be relieved with the use of alpha-blockers.

Martinez et al. showed a significantly lower rate of acute dysuria (39 % versus 60 %), frequency/urgency (58 % versus 90 %) and acute rectal pain (6.5 % versus 17 %) with HDR monotherapy compared with LDR monotherapy using palladium-103 seeds [50]. Although late grade 3 toxicity was rare with either technique, there was a significantly increased rate of chronic urinary toxicity with LDR, and a comparable rate of late urethral stricture (3 % versus 1.5 %). Urethral dose seems to be predictive of late urinary symptoms and urinary morbidity can probably be decreased with careful technique to minimize the dose to the urethra [51].

The reported rate of late grade 3 urinary toxicity after HDR boost and external beam radiotherapy is around 5 % (range 2–20 %), with the rate of urethral stricture between 0 and 7 % [52].

9.2 Bowel Morbidity

HDR brachytherapy results in low rectal morbidity. In patients undergoing HDR and external beam radiotherapy, bowel symptoms are generally due to the external beam radiotherapy component. Fewer acute gastrointestinal side effects were noted in the randomized trial comparing external beam alone with external beam and HDR brachytherapy [1], although there was no long term differences. Late rectal toxicity is rarely seen with HDR monotherapy.

9.3 Sexual Dysfunction

Erectile dysfunction is reported in 10–47 % of cases. Patients treated with neo-adjuvant and adjuvant hormone manipulation will experience higher rates of erectile dysfunction.

Conclusions

Prostate brachytherapy is a well-established curative treatment option for men with non-metastatic prostate cancer.

LDR monotherapy for low and selected intermediate risk prostate cancer results in durable prostate cancer progression-free survival. Long term sexual dysfunction, bowel symptom and urinary incontinence rates are lower than that seen with the alternative treatment options.

In intermediate and high risk prostate cancer the use of brachytherapy boost, either HDR or LDR, in addition to external beam radiotherapy improves progression-free survival. Additional long term toxicity has been found and there is a need to demonstrate that refinements in brachytherapy techniques can deliver improved patient outcomes both in terms of cancer control rates and toxicity.

References

1. Hoskin PJ, Rojas AM, Bownes PJ, et al. Randomised trial of external beam radiotherapy alone or combined with high-dose rate brachytherapy boost for localised prostate cancer. Radiother Oncol. 2012;103(2):217–22.
2. Morris W, et al. LDR brachytherapy is superior to 78 Gy of EBRT for unfavourable risk prostate cancer: the results of a randomized trial. Radiother Oncol. 2015;115:S239.

3. Holm HH, Juul N, Pedersen JF, et al. Transperineal125 iodine seed implantation in prostatic cancer guided by transrectal ultrasonography. J Urol. 1983;130:283–6.
4. Blasko JC, Radge H, Schumacher D. Transperineal percutaneous iodine-125 implantation for prostatic carcinoma using transrectal ultrasound and template guidance. Endocurie/Hypertherm Oncol. 1987;3:131–9.
5. Nag S, et al. Intraoperative planning and evaluation of permanent prostate brachytherapy: report of the American Brachytherapy Society. IJROBP. 2001;51(5):1422–30.
6. Ash D, Flynn A, Batterman J, et al. ESTRA/EAU Urological Brachytherapy Group; EORTC Radiotherapy Group. ESTRO/EAU/EORTC recommendations on permanent seed implantation for localized prostate cancer. Radiother Oncol. 2000;57(3):315–21.
7. Salembier C, Lavagnini P, Nickers P, et al. GEC ESTRO PROBATE Group. Tumour and target volumes in permanent prostate brachytherapy: a supplement to the ESTRO/EAU/EORTC recommendations on prostate brachytherapy. Radiother Oncol. 2007;83(1):3–10.
8. Department of veterans affairs office of inspector general health inspection: review of brachytherapy treatment of prostate cancer, Philadelphia, Pennsylvania and Other VA Medical Centers Report No. 09-02815-143. Washington, DC: VA Office of Inspector General. 2010.
9. Davis BJ, Horwitz EM, Lee W, et al. American Brachytherapy Society consensus guidelines for transrectal ultra-sound guided permanent prostate brachytherapy. Brachytherapy. 2012;11(1):6–19.
10. The Royal College of Radiologists. Quality assurance practice guidelines for transperineal LDR permanent seed brachytherapy of prostate cancer. London: The Royal College of Radiologists; 2012.
11. Gelblum DY, Potters L, Ashley R, et al. Urinary morbidity following ultra-sound guided transperineal prostate seed implantation. IJROBP. 1999;45:59–67.
12. Martens C, et al. Relationship of the international prostate symptom score with urinary flow studies and catheterization rates following I-125 prostate brachytherapy. Brachytherapy. 2006;5:9–13.
13. Lee WR. The role of androgen deprivation therapy combined with prostate brachytherapy. Urology. 2002;37:565–9.
14. Sylvester JE, Grimm PD, Wong J, Galbreath RW, Merrick G, Blasko JC. Fifteen-year biochemical relapse-free survival, cause-specific survival, and overall survival following I(125) prostate brachytherapy in clinically localized prostate cancer: Seattle experience. Int J Radiat Oncol Biol Phys. 2011;81(2):376–81.
15. Potters L, Morgenstern C, Calugaru E, et al. 12-year outcomes following permanent prostate brachytherapy in patients with clinically localized prostate cancer. J Urol. 2005;173(5):1562–6.
16. Stone NN, Stone MM, Rosenstein BS, et al. Influence of pretreatment and treatment factors on intermediate to long-term outcome after prostate brachytherapy. J Urol. 2011;185:494–500.
17. Zelefsky MJ, Chou JF, Pei X, et al. Predicting biocehmical control after brachytherapy for clinically localized prostate cancer: the Memorial Sloan-Kettering Cancer Centre experience. Brachytherapy. 2012;11:245–9.
18. Lawton CA, DeSilvio M, Lee WR, et al. Results of a phase II trial of transrectal ultrasound-guided permanent radioactive implantation of the prostate for definitive management of localized adenocarcinoma of the prostate (RTOG 98–05). Int J Radiat Oncol Biol Phys. 2007;67(1):39–47.
19. Henry AM, Al-Qaisieh B, Gould K, et al. Outcomes following iodine-125 monotherapy for localized prostate cancer: the results of Leeds 10-year single-center brachytherapy experience. Int J Radiat Oncol Biol Phys. 2010;76:50–6.
20. Hinnen KA, Battermann JJ, van Roermond JGH, et al. Long term biochemical and survival outcome of 921 patients treated with I-125 permanent prostate brachytherapy. Int J Radiat Oncol Biol Phys. 2010;76:1433–8.
21. Grimm PD, Billiet I, Bostwick D, et al. Comparative analysis of prostate specific antigen free survival outcomes for patients with low, intermediate and high risk prostate cancer treatment by radical therapy. Results from the Prostate Cancer Results Study Group. BJU Int. 2012;109(Suppl1):22–9.
22. Morris WJ, Keyes M, Spadinger I, et al. Population-based 10-year oncologic outcomes after low-dose-rate brachytherapy for low-risk and intermediate-risk prostate cancer. Cancer. 2013;119(8):1537–46.
23. Stock RG, Stone NN. Importance of post-implant dosimetry in permanent brachytherapy. Eur Urol. 2002;41(4):434–9.
24. Rodda SL, Tyldesley S, Morris WJ. Toxicity outcomes in ASCENDE-RT: a multicenter randomized trial of dose-escalation trial for prostate cancer. IJROBP. 2015;93(3):S121.
25. Rodda SL, Duncan G, Hamm J, Morris WJ. Quality of life outcomes: ASCENDE-RT a multicentre randomized trial of radiation therapy for prostate cancer. IJROBP. 2015;93(3):S2.
26. Zelefsky MJ, Shasha D, Branco RD, et al. Prophylactic sildenafil citrate for improvement of erectile function in men treated by radiotherapy for prostate cancer. J Urol. 2014;192(3):868–74.
27. Crook JM, Gomez-Iturriaga A, Wallace K, et al. Comparison of health-related quality of life 5 years after SPIRIT: surgical prostatectomy versus interstitial radiation intervention trial. JCO. 2011;29:362–8.
28. Pardo Y, Guedea F, Aguilo F, et al. Quality of life impacts of primary treatments for localized prostate cancer in patients without hormonal treatment. JCO. 2010;28:4687–96.
29. Chen RC, Clark JA, Talcott JA. Individualizing quality-of-life outcomes reporting: how localized prostate cancer treatments affect patients with different levels of baseline urinary, bowel and sexual function. JCO. 2009;27:3916–22.

30. Ferrer M, et al. Quality of life impact of treatments for localized prostate cancer: cohort study with a 5-year follow-up. Radiother Oncol. 2013;108(2):306–13.
31. Sanda MG, Dunn RL, Michalski J, et al. Quality of life and satisfaction with outcomes among prostate-cancer survivors. New Engl J Med. 2008;358:1250–61.
32. Hoskin PJ, Colombo A, Henry A, et al. GEC/ESTRO recommendations on high dose rate afterloading brachytherapy for localised prostate cancer: an update. Radiother Oncol. 2013;107(3):325–32.
33. Martinez AA, Gonzalez J, Ye H, et al. Dose escalation improves cancer related events at 10 years for intermediate and high risk prostate cancer patients treated with hypofractionated high-dose-rate boost and external beam radiotherapy. IJROBP. 2011;79(2):363–70.
34. Hoskin P, Rojas A, Ostler P, et al. Dosimetric predictors of biochemical control of prostate cancer in patients randomised to EBRT with a boost of HDR. RO. 2014;110:110–3.
35. Morton G, Loblaw DA, Sankreacha A, et al. Single-fraction high dose rate brachytherapy and hypofractionated external beam radiotherapy for men with intermediate risk prostate cancer: an analysis of short and medium term toxicity and quality of life. Int J Radiat Oncol Biol Phys. 2010;77:811–7.
36. Morton G, Loblaw A, Cheung P, Szumacher E, Chahal M, Danjoux C, Chung HT, Deabreu Mamedov A, Zhang L, Sankreacha R, Vigneault E, Springer C. Is single fraction 15 Gy the preferred high dose-rate brachytherapy boost dose for prostate cancer? Radiother Oncol. 2011;100:463–7.
37. Ghilezan M, Martinez A, Gustason G, Krauss D, Antonucci JV, Chen P, et al. High-dose-rate brachytherapy as monotherapy delivered in two fractions within one day for favorable/intermediate-risk prostate cancer: preliminary toxicity data. Int J Radiat Oncol Biol Phys. 2012;83(3):927–32.
38. Yoshioka Y, Konishi K, Sumida I, Takahashi Y, Isohashi F, Ogata T, et al. Monotherapeutic high-dose-rate brachytherapy for prostate cancer: five-year results of an extreme hypofractionation regimen with 54 Gy in nine fractions. Int J Radiat Oncol Biol Phys. 2011;80(2):469–75.
39. Barkati M, Williams SG, Foroudi F, Tai KH, Chander S, van Dyk S, et al. High-dose-rate brachytherapy as a monotherapy for favorable-risk prostate cancer: a Phase II trial. Int J Radiat Oncol Biol Phys. 2012;82(5):1889–96.
40. Hauswald H, Kamrava MR, Fallon JM, et al. High-dose-rate monotherapy for localized prostate cancer: 10 -year results. Int J Radiat Oncol Biol Phys. 2016;94(4):667–74.
41. Prada PJ, Jimenez I, Gonzalez-Suarez H, Fernandez J, Cuervo-Arango C, Mendez L. High-dose-rate interstitial brachytherapy as monotherapy in one fraction and transperineal hyaluronic acid injection into the perirectal fat for the treatment of favorable stage prostate cancer: treatment description and preliminary results. Brachytherapy. 2012;11(2):105–10.
42. Roger CL, Alders AS, Rogers RL, et al. High dose rate brachytherapy as monotherapy for intermediate risk prostate cancer. J Urol 2012;187:109–16.
43. Hoskin P, Rojas A, Ostler P, et al. HDR brachytherapy alone given as two or one fraction to patients for locally advanced prostate cancer: acute toxicity. RO. 2014;110:268–71.
44. Zamboglou N, Tselis N, Baltas D, Buhleier T, Martin T, Milickovic N, et al. High-dose-rate interstitial brachytherapy as monotherapy for clinically localized prostate cancer: treatment evolution and mature results. Int J Radiat Oncol Biol Phys. 2013;85: 672–8.
45. Chen CP, Weinberg V, Shinohara K, et al. Salvage HDR brachytherapy for recurrent prostate cancer after previous definitive radiation therapy: 5-year outcomes. IJROBP. 2013;86:324–9.
46. Tharp M, Hardacre M, Bennett R, et al. Prostate high-dose-rate brachytherapy as salvage treatment of local failure after previous external or permanent seed irradiation for prostate cancer. Brachytherapy. 2008;7:231–6.
47. Morton GC. High-dose-rate brachytherapy boost for prostate cancer: rationale and technique. J Contemp Brachytherapy. 2014;6(3):323–30.
48. Spratt DE, Zumsteg ZS, Ghadjar P, et al. Comparison of high-dose (86.4Gy) IMRT vs. combined brachytherapy plus IMRT for intermediate-risk prostate cancer. BJU Int. 2014;114:360–7.
49. Pieters BR, de Back DZ, Koning CCE, Zwinderman AH. Comparison of three radiotherapy modalities on biochemical control and overall survival for the treatment of prostate cancer: a systematic review. Radiother Oncol. 2009;93(2):168–73.
50. Martinez AA, Demanes J, Vargas C, et al. High-dose-rate prostate brachytherapy: an excellent accelerated-hypofractionated treatment for favorable prostate cancer. Am J Clin Oncol. 2010;33:481–8.
51. Morton GC, Loblaw DA, Chung H, et al. Health-related quality of life after single-fraction high-dose-rate brachytherapy and hypofractionated external beam radiotherapy for prostate cancer. Int J Radiat Oncol Biol Phys. 2011;80:1299–305.
52. Challapalli A, Jones E, Harvey C, Hellawell GO, Mangar SA. High dose rate prostate brachytherapy: an overview of the rationale, experience and emerging applications in the treatment of prostate cancer. Br J Radiol. 2012;85:S18–27.

IMRT, Hypofractionated Radiotherapy and Stereotactic Radiotherapy: Technique, Indications, and Results

Malcolm Mason

1 Introduction

The major technological advance in external beam radiotherapy in the 1990s was the introduction of conformal radiotherapy. For the first time, the high-dose volume was not constrained to be cuboid in shape, because the radiotherapy beam collimators were multi-leaf (instead of single leaf), the radiotherapy beam could be irregular in shape and did not have to be rectangular or square. The high dose volume could thus 'conform' more closely to the shape of the tumour, by tailoring the shape of the beam using multileaf collimators (MLCs); when introduced, this held the promise of reducing the total volume of tissue irradiated, and the randomised trial carried out by the Royal Marsden Hospital confirmed that this was, indeed the case [14]. However, as well as reducing treatment toxicity, conformal radiotherapy also permitted the alternative strategy of dose escalation, which was successfully deployed in a number of randomised trials and is now regarded as standard practice. The current European Association of Urology guidelines recommend a dose of 76–78 Gy in combination with ADT for intermediate-risk and high-risk disease, when given in 'standard' fraction sizes of 1.8–2 Gy per fraction [42].

The main limitation of conformal radiotherapy arises because, although an almost infinite range of irregular high dose volumes can be created, they are in turn constrained by the limitation of such volumes to be convex in topographical terms; a concave surface or component would be encompassed by 'filling in' the dip. In the case of irradiating the prostate, this manifests, for example, as irradiating a greater volume of rectum posteriorly, as shown in Fig. 1 [46].

The consequences of this for prostate cancer are a ceiling on what can be achieved in terms of: (a) dose escalation, (b) reduction in toxicity, (c) irradiation of more complex volumes when desired and (d) more extreme dose-fractionation schedules. These limitations were the major impetus for the development of intensity-modulated radiotherapy (IMRT), which is itself now regarded as a standard of care for external beam radiotherapy. The forerunner to this development was a step change in the paradigm of radiotherapy treatment planning – that of 'inverse planning', in which the starting point was the ideal dose distribution and not the availability and deployment of conventional beam arrangements, multiple beams being placed as needed, as a means of achieving this [41, 52].

M. Mason
Cardiff University, Velindre Hospital, Whitchurch Cardiff CF14 2TL, UK
e-mail: masonmd858@gmail.com

M. Bolla, H. van Poppel (eds.), *Management of Prostate Cancer*,
DOI 10.1007/978-3-319-42769-0_14

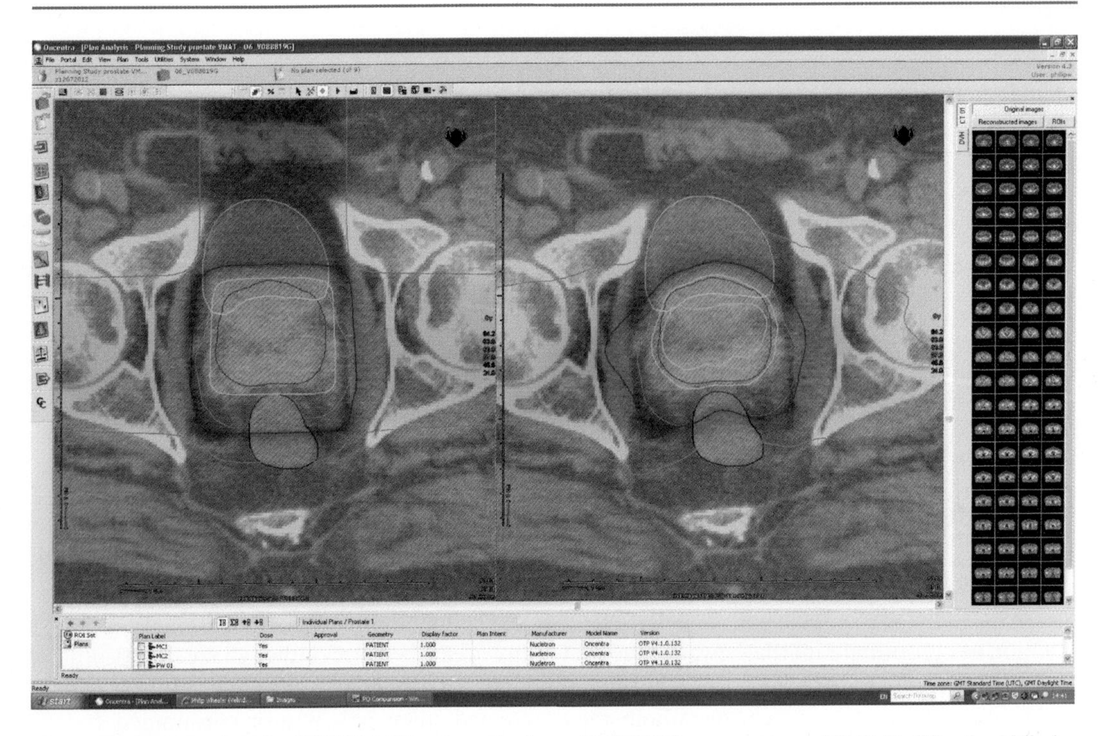

Fig. 1 Dose distributions for IMRT (*right*) and standard, conformal radiotherapy (*left*) to the prostate. Note the improved dose distribution and concave high dose volume with IMRT. Image courtesy of Dr Philip Wheeler, Velindre Cancer Centre, Cardiff, UK

2 Intensity-Modulated Radiotherapy

2.1 Technical Aspects

The main technical difference between conformal radiotherapy and IMRT is that with the former, the multileaf collimators, once set for a particular treatment session, are static; they cannot be moved until after the treatment is complete. With IMRT, the individual collimator leaves move during the period of radiotherapy exposure, and this, finally, allows for the creation of a high dose volume with a concave surface [39]. This advance further allowed the increase in 'conformity' in the treatment of prostate cancer, which was not possible hitherto (see Fig. 1). The practical applications of this new-found ability are considered later, but there are important considerations in relation to the planning process.

For the radiotherapist, just as with conformal radiotherapy, establishment of target volumes such as CTV requires cross-sectional imaging and the definition of the target volume, as well as structures of interest and organs at risk, at each imaging level throughout the proposed treatment volume. It is axiomatic that the treatment planning system must be of a sufficient quality to allow this to be done meticulously and with the greatest possible degree of accuracy. Precise treatment protocols will vary, depending on the proposed dose/schedule/volume, but some consensus guidelines for outlining exist, for example the RTOG guidelines for outlining lymph nodes [37]. Other tissues and organs at risk, which can now be identified with a very high degree of accuracy in prostate radiotherapy include the rectum, the femoral heads, the bladder and the penile bulb. Clinical trials such as CHHIP, which will be discussed later, were also conducted with a very high degree of attention to technical details in the planning protocol [12],[1]

[1] Supplementary appendix describing the CHHIP radiotherapy planning protocol in detail is available at www.thelancet.com.

and these would, in turn, be applicable to routine practice.

The first techniques for IMRT either used a dynamic system, in which the MLCs were in a process of continual movement during the radiation field exposure, or by a sequential, static programme with the MLC positions adjusted for each segment (also called "step-and-shoot") [1, 58]. In both of these instances, the radiation field is static, in the sense that the gantry of the linac remains stationary, and the patient does not change position. Newer variations on static or step-and-shoot IMRT take advantage of the use of rotational arc therapy, or tomotherapy (which, classically, involved the rotation of the linac gantry during a radiation field exposure, sometimes combined with movements of the treatment couch for 'helical' tomotherapy). In the context of IMRT, a commonly used technique is known as VMAT (volumetric modulated arc therapy), which combines the individual, dynamic collimator leaves in standard IMRT with tomotherapy using arc rotation, and this can deliver excellent dose distributions, with all the benefits of IMRT but resulting in an almost infinite variation of complex high dose treatment volumes [54]. A more simple variant of VMAT has also been reported, using sequential tomotherapy, and a comparison of the three techniques (step-and-shoot, serial tomotherapy, and VMAT) with conformal radiotherapy indicated that each IMRT plan was of superior quality, albeit that the conformal radiotherapy used a four-field arrangement which does not allow for the maximum rectal sparing achievable with conventional techniques [54]. A similar system using arc rotation and dynamic IMRT is the RapidArc system [31]. These newer, rotation-therapy based systems do offer the most comprehensive flexibility in terms of defining and shaping an almost limitless range of high dose volumes, but also offer the potential for greater speed of delivery. A major disadvantage of IMRT is the time that it takes to deliver treatment compared with 'conventional' conformal radiotherapy, in these days when machine time is at a premium. As technology evolves, treatment times will continue to fall, but techniques such as VMAT are probably the fastest currently available.

For the physicist, there are several treatment planning systems, and several planning algorithms which can be used. The choice of system will vary from department to department, but consistency in planning, backed up by meticulous quality assurance, is required, especially if non-standard fractionation schedules are employed. As with the outlining, the details of volume and dose constraints may be usefully defined as per protocol, and compliance assured with dose-volume histograms is now routine. A guidance document, which summarises the parameters that the physicist must consider, was published in the early years of IMRT [16]. While the high dose volume can be shaped in a sophisticated manner, and thus reduced in volume, one consequence of the technique is that the volume of normal tissue exposed to a low-dose 'bath' can be higher than it is with conformal radiotherapy. The data on toxicity are discussed later.

Treatment verification is, of course, an important component of high quality treatment delivery, and in modern radiotherapy IMRT is often combined with some form of image-guided radiotherapy (IGRT), in which the prostate/target volume's position is verified by some sort of imaging, before the patient is set up for treatment (or even during treatment). This is now an integral part of the technique; the huge advantage of greater conformity allowed by IMRT is the reduction of treatment margins in the high dose volume. However, it is now well known that the prostate moves, and that this is a potential source of error in treatment set-up [33, 50]. There is no point in treating smaller volumes, whether to reduce toxicity or to increase dose, if prostate movement or other errors result in missing the target. There are, broadly, three approaches to IGRT: orthogonal kilovoltage imaging, cone beam CT imaging, or on-set transabdominal ultrasound based imaging.

For orthogonal imaging, and in some instances for other techniques, fiducial markers can be placed into the prostate; these are often gold seeds, or similar, implanted transperineally

[50]. In an analysis of 453 patients, fiducial markers were found to be reliable, and to detect positional deviations of over 3 mm in over 1/3 of patients, over the entire course of fractionated treatment [50]. The use of fiducial markers was shown to be superior to ultrasound-based treatment verification when these two techniques were compared [47]. Cone-beam CT involves an integrated imaging system which sits on the Linac itself, uses kV irradiation and a large flat panel detector, and is able to produce good resolution images showing soft tissue, and allowing comparison with a treatment plan, under computer control [28]. The potential benefits of IGRT plus IMRT in terms of more accurate localisation, and a reduction in the volume of irradiated tissue, can be modelled, [18], and there is little dispute that these techniques offer, at the very least, theoretical benefits to patients with prostate cancer.

The techniques described thus far address the problem of prostate movement in between treatment fractions, or of inaccuracies in treatment set up. However, emerging techniques such as cine MRI or the Calypso 4D system, might allow for on-line, and real-time correction of positional errors during a treatment exposure [19, 49].

2.2 Indications

The most immediate practical application of IMRT in prostate cancer treatment is well illustrated in Fig. 1, comparing the radiotherapy dose distribution using conformal and Intensity-modulated radiotherapy. The sparing of rectum and other critical normal tissues from the high-dose volume should lead to a reduction in treatment toxicity. However, just as was the case for conformal radiotherapy, it has also been a vehicle for further dose escalation.

However, the potential for IMRT in prostate cancer extends beyond irradiation of the primary tumour. An ongoing uncertainty in the management of this disease by radiotherapy is whether irradiation of pelvic lymph nodes improves outcomes in both N0 and N1 disease. To date, the randomised trials addressing this issue have been negative [6, 36, 45], but the question is still not answered, and recent, though unrandomised data from the UK STAMPEDE trial suggests that there may yet be benefits [29]. One reason for the ongoing uncertainty could be the limited dose that is deliverable to pelvic nodes using conventional or conformal radiotherapy, because of the constraint imposed by the radiation tolerance of small bowel, which is inevitably included in a pelvic radiation field. Could IMRT, by delivering a higher dose to pelvic nodes than was previously possible, yield benefits that could not be demonstrated with lower dose radiotherapy? There are ongoing clinical trials addressing this issue such as the UK PIVOTAL study [22], currently in follow up and awaiting analysis.

3 Results

The programme of dose escalation conducted by the Memorial Sloan-Kettering Hospital has shown that IMRT permits doses in excess of 80Gy to be safely delivered. There must, of course, be some ultimate limit to what is achievable, in terms of dose escalation using IMRT, and it has to be said that, while there is consensus that dose escalation improves biochemical control rates, its impact on overall survival is less clear [8, 13, 23, 35, 60]. It is also unclear just how high a dose is 'enough'; in any event, the potential impact of IMRT in terms of efficacy of eradication of primary tumour, while tangible, must be finite. On the other hand, single institution studies, particularly the MSK's pioneering cohort, do report a reduction in toxicity [59].

For some individual patients, the benefits in terms of reduced toxicity can be expected to be significant, an example being the patient in Fig. 1. However, the degree of benefit will vary from patient to patient, according to their anatomy, and it has to be said that it is hard to prove that every patient benefits from IMRT compared to what they would have achieved with conformal radiotherapy. In some patients, pelvimetry might predict that their anatomy does not lend itself to substantial gains from IMRT [56] This variation, together with the limitations in terms of overall survival, must lie behind some critical and even sceptical assessments of IMRT in the treatment of primary prostate cancer. Two key questions about IMRT are whether it is clinically effective, and whether it is cost effective. That it reduces treatment volumes is generally not in doubt.

A study based on SEER data from nearly 13,000 men receiving IMRT for prostate cancer concluded that it reduced the levels of gastrointestinal toxicity when compared with conformal radiotherapy, but increased the rates of erectile dysfunction [48]. While patients undergoing IMRT were significantly less likely to receive additional anti-cancer treatments, this is probably attributable to their radiotherapy dose escalation and not to IMRT per se. A subgroup of patients in the Dutch dose-escalation study, who were treated with IMRT on the high dose arm have been compared, and lower rates of GI toxicity were seen in the patients treated with IMRT [2].

Two systematic reviews of IMRT in the primary treatment of prostate cancer have been published [7, 26]. Again, advantages to IMRT in terms of biochemical control are probably related to dose escalation, but the overall evidence supported the notion that IMRT improves toxicity, as compared with conformal radiotherapy. Where it is used in association with dose escalation, there is an increase in acute toxicity, as one might expect. A subsequent cost-effectiveness analysis concluded that, in health economic terms, IMRT will be dependent on an improvement in survival if it is to show superiority to conformal radiotherapy; improvements in toxicity did not appear to be enough to win the argument in terms of cost-effectiveness, at least within the parameters of the model used [27]. In some ways, though, this is a sterile argument: IMRT is already used in a variety of tumour indications, and there will, in the future, be costs associated with maintaining a dual infrastructure for both IMRT and conformal therapy. Certainly, the prevalence of IMRT as a technique for the treatment of prostate cancer has rocketed [48].

It is important neither to overestimate nor to underestimate the potential of IMRT, and for now, it justifies its status in treatment guidelines, because it undoubtedly permits a reduction in the volume of tissue treated to high dose. At the same time, a degree of scepticism is warranted [10], and it is noteworthy that the recent patient-reported outcomes reported from the high dose arm of the RTOG 0126 dose escalation study show no differences between IMRT and 3D conformal radiotherapy despite clear evidence that IMRT did reduce treatment volumes [9]. Similarly, cohort data from 9 institutions showed transient but meaningful impacts on quality of life in patients treated with IMRT, and the potential it has to increase acute toxicity, especially urinary toxicity, appears to be consistent, albeit that much of this is associated with dose escalation [21].

A further scenario for the use of IMRT is in postoperative radiotherapy in patients where this is indicated following prior radical prostatectomy. A study from SEER data reports no differences in outcomes (disease control or toxicity) between IMRT and conformal radiotherapy [20], but this study has been criticised because of the unavoidable selection of subjects for the analysis, limiting cases to those with adequate available data [10].

4 Hypofractionation

Prostate cancer is believed to behave like a 'late-reacting' tissue. This is the basis for the recent upsurge of interest in hypofractionation, that is, the use of larger than standard fraction sizes in external beam radiotherapy. The rationale is that tissues which are prone to late (and therefore permanent) radiation damage, such as the spinal cord, are more sensitive to large doses per fraction. If this is true of prostate cancer, then perhaps there will be benefits in altering the schedule for EBRT, from 'standard' fraction sizes of 1.8–2 Gy per fraction, to larger doses, with a concomitant reduction in the total dose (to give an equivalent biological effect).

The evidence for this comes from observational clinical data, and the subsequent insights led by Jack Fowler and colleagues [11, 17]. These data do, indeed suggest that prostate cancer might be best treated by hypofractionation, since it might be regarded as having a low alpha/beta ratio in the region of 1.5 Gy [11], and this is the basis for the BED calculations in the tables in this chapter. The data themselves arose because of disparate clinical practices, which themselves had arisen empirically and based on historical precedent. Thus, while in many parts of the world (Europe, Southern England and the USA), the tradition was to treat with conventional 1.8–2 Gy fraction sizes, other parts of the world (Canada, North of England) used a larger dose per fraction. At that time, typical schedules for the treatment of prostate cancer were 64–66 Gy given in conventional 1.8–2 Gy fractions, or 55 Gy given in 20 fractions of 2.75 Gy per fraction. Clinical outcome data, both in terms of local control, but also normal tissue complications, led to the hypothesis that prostate cancer might be regarded as a late reacting tissue, while the rectum might be regarded as an early reacting tissue, suggesting a possible therapeutic advantage to a Biologically Equivalent Dose (BED) of radiotherapy delivered using hypofractionation.

Before this hypothesis was articulated, and indeed embraced by the clinical community, the clinical trial priorities were to establish whether this disparate practice, at a time before dose escalated radiotherapy was established, was safe, and the trial design was to test the equivalence of these two options. Two randomised trials of this type have been reported; one showed that hypofractionated, conventional dose radiotherapy to be equivalent to standard fractionation, while the other suggested that standard fractionation was superior [40, 55] (Table 1).

The emerging evidence for improved disease control with dose escalation gave new impetus to the study of hypofractionation, taking the total dose beyond what was then standard. From the vantage point of today, it is important to distinguish between two strategies: moderate hypofractionation (which could be regarded as doses per fraction ≤5 Gy), and extreme hypofractionation (which could be regarded as doses per fraction ≥5 Gy). To an extent, the study of extreme hypofractionation can be criticised as being technology led, in that it was partly driven by the development of equipment such as Cyberknife. Of course, the added scientific basis was the potential to deliver an extremely high BED safely, with the added convenience to the patient of having a small number of treatment sessions.

4.1 Technique of Stereotactic Radiotherapy for Extreme Hypofractionation

The principles of stereotactic radiotherapy were well established in neuro-oncology, and briefly comprise: (a) extremely accurate patient positioning (in neuro-oncology this was achieved using a frame that was physically attached to the patient's skull), (b) meticulously accurate radiotherapy planning to define a very small high dose volume and (c) delivery of radiation using a very small 'pencil' beam, and multiple fields to provide adequate coverage of the target.

These principles were modified in the Cyberknife for radiotherapy to the prostate, by creating a free-standing, robotic linear accelerator head that could, if required, deliver a pencil beam of radiation, and was capable of being orientated in any plane of rotation, though still able to do so isocentrically if required. As there is no treatment frame attached to the patient, the machine head must be capable of adjusting rapidly to any changes in patient position. The system is therefore combined with on-board image-guided localisation, with fiducial markers inserted into the prostate (see above).

Today, it is also possible to deliver stereotactic radiotherapy, using the same principles as described above, delivered with a state of the art Linac with full IMRT/IGRT capabilities. This has become a preferred option for some centres, because the equipment can be used in a variety of indications outside of radiotherapy to the prostate gland and indeed outside SBRT.

Table 1 Randomised trials of moderate hypofractionation

Study	Median FU, months	Risk, GS, or NCCN	Technique	Regimen	BED, Gy	n	Outcome	Toxicity
Lukka et al. [15]	68	60 % GS ≤6	3DCRT	52.5 Gy/20 fx	62	466	5 years FFBF 40 % (NS)	Gr ≥3 2 % (NS)
		31 % GS 7	No IGRT					
		9 % GS 8–10		56 Gy/33 fx	66	470	5 years FFBF 43 %	Gr ≥3 1 %
Yeoh et al. [17]	90	n.s.	2D/3DCRT	55 Gy/20 fx	66.8	108	7.5 years FFBF 53 %	Late GU; HR: 1.58 (95 % CI, 1.01–2.47) favouring hypofractionation
			No IGRT				($p<0.05$)	
				64 Gy/32 fx	64	109	7.5 years FFBF 34 %	
Dearnaley et al. [18]	51	n.s.	3D/IMRT	57 Gy/19 fx	73.4	151	n.s.	Gr ≥2 GU 0 % (NS)
			No IGRT					Gr ≥2 GI 1 % (NS)
			3–6 months ADT					
				60 Gy/20 fx	77	153		Gr ≥2 GU 2 %
								Gr ≥2 GI 4 %
				74 Gy/37 fx	74	153		Gr ≥2 GU 2 %
								Gr ≥2 GI 4 %
Kuban et al. [14], Hoffman et al. [19]	60	28 % low	IMRT	72 Gy/30 fx	80.2	102	5 years FFBF 96 % (NS)	5 years Gr ≥2 GU 16 % (NS)
		71 % intermediate	IGRT					5 years Gr ≥2 GI 10 % (NS)
		1 % high	21 % ADT					
				75.6 Gy/42 fx	71.4	101	5 years FFBF 92 %	5 years Gr ≥2 GU 17 %
								5 years Gr ≥2 GI 5 %

(continued)

Table 1 (continued)

Study	Median FU, months	Risk, GS, or NCCN	Technique	Regimen	BED, Gy	*n*	Outcome	Toxicity
Arcangeli et al. [12,13]	70	26 % GS ≤7	3DCRT	62 Gy/20 fx	81.4	83	5 years FFBF 85 %	3 years Gr ≥2 GU 16 % (NS)
		74 % GS >7	No IGRT				($p=0.065$)	3 years Gr ≥2 GI 17 % (NS)
			100 % 9 months ADT				*p ss for GS ≥4+3	
				80 Gy/40 fx	80	85	5 years FFBF 79 %	3 years Gr ≥2 GU 11 %
								3 years Gr ≥2GI 14 %
Pollack et al. [16]	68	34 % GS ≤6	IMRT	70.2 Gy/26 fx	84	151	5 years BCDF 23 % (NS)	5 years Gr ≥2 GU 13 %
		47 % GS 7	IGRT					($p=0.16$)
		19 % GS 8–10						5 years Gr ≥2 GI 9 % (NS)
				78 Gy/36 fx	78	152	5 years BCDF 21 %	5 years Gr ≥2 GU13%
								5 years Gr ≥2 GI 9 %

Reproduced from Koontz et al. [32], with permission

3DCRT three-dimensional conformal radiotherapy, *ADT* androgen-deprivation therapy, *BCDF* biochemical or clinical disease failure, *BED* biologically equivalent dose, calculated to be equivalent in 2 Gy fractions using an α/β of 1.5 Gy; *CI* confidence interval, *FFBF* freedom from biochemical failure, *FU* follow-up, *fx* fractions, *GI* gastrointestinal, *Gr* grade, *GS* Gleason score, *GU* genitourinary, *HR* hazard ratio, *IGRT* image-guided radiation therapy, *IMRT* intensity-modulated radiation therapy, *NCCN* National Comprehensive Cancer Network, *NS* not significant, *n.s.* not stated, *ss* statistically significant

4.2 Indications for Stereotactic Radiotherapy

The role of stereotactic, extreme hypofractionated radiotherapy in the primary, curative treatment of localised prostate cancer is uncertain. To date, there have been no randomised trials, and the status of this technique has to be regarded as 'experimental' in that sense. Nonetheless, it is offered in a number of centres, on the basis of its practical advantages, and based on the results of unrandomised case series (reviewed by [24] and [32]). Patients should be counselled in an open and honest manner about the limited evidence base underpinning this form of treatment, and formal clinical studies should be the only framework within which this treatment is administered.

A second, emerging area which is currently under investigation is in the treatment of oligometastases (usually defined as 3 or less metastatic sites identified after thorough staging investigations) from prostate cancer. This is a relatively uncommon group of patients, and is heterogeneous, in the sense that some present with de novo, advanced, but oligometastatic disease, whereas others develop oligometastases some years after primary treatment. There are two ongoing randomised trials, currently recruiting patients. In the UK, the PACE study is randomising patients with low or intermediate risk localised prostate cancer to stereotactic radiotherapy or conventional radiotherapy, and if laparoscopic surgery is an option, between stereotactic radiotherapy and laparoscopic surgery. In Sweden, the HYPO study is randomising men with intermediate risk, localised disease between IMRT, 78 Gy in 39 fractions, and SBRT, 42.7 Gy in 7 fractions.

4.3 Results of Moderate, Dose-Escalated Hypofractionation for the Treatment of Localised Prostate Cancer

The field of hypofractionation for prostate cancer has been summarised in two recent systematic reviews [32, 57]. These have identified a number of reports from unrandomised case series, and some randomised trials [5, 12, 25, 34, 40, 44, 55]. Subsequent to these reviews, updated results and a new randomised trial report have been published [3, 4, 38, 51, 53], and these are summarised in Table 2 (including the one randomised trial by Vargas et al. using protons and a fraction size of 7.4 Gy RBE). Perhaps disappointingly, none of the trials are powered to report on superiority in terms of efficacy, but many have been non-inferiority trials and powered as such. Understandably, they report in two distinct phases – in the first phase, safety is the main concern, and non-inferiority is absolutely the appropriate endpoint. Often there will be two aspects to safety – acute toxicity, and long-term toxicity (Table 1) – which can usually be inferred from late side effects at 2 years or more. Importantly, the studies vary according to whether toxicity is based on physician-administered scales, such as the RTOG grade, or whether it is from a patient-administered scale such as EPIC. The second phase would be the reporting of efficacy, ideally as overall survival, but more realistically reported as disease-free survival, or biochemical control (Table 1). The reasons are understandable – to yield data on overall survival in localised prostate cancer requires several decades of follow up, and many thousands of patients to power it adequately. The largest trial reporting on disease control is the RTOG 0415 trial, with 1,115 men randomised, all of whom had low risk disease. This was a non-inferiority trial, and at a median follow up of 5.8 years the disease free survival was consistent with the pre-defined criteria for non-inferiority. However, there were more late genitourinary adverse events in patients treated with hypofractionated radiotherapy [38]. The UK CHHIP study has presented disease control outcomes, but at the time of going to press, the peer-reviewed report has not yet been published.

What can be inferred from the results to date is the following:

1. Moderate dose, hypofractionated radiotherapy appears to be safe, in that most studies have not indicated excess levels of toxicity.

Table 2 Randomised trials of hypofractionation published since the systematic reviews

Study	Median FU	Risk, GS, or NCCN	Technique	Regimen	BED Gy	*n*	Outcome	Toxicity
Aluwini et al. [3, 4]	60 months	26 % intermediate 74 % high	IMRT 97 % IGRT 95 %	78 Gy in 29# vs 64.6 Gy in 19#	78 90.4	820	Ns	Late ≥ G3 GI 2.6 % ≥ G3 GU 12.9 % Late ≥ G3 GI 3.3 %, $p=0.55$ ≥ G3 GU 19.0 %, $p=0.021$
Wilkins et al. [53]	50 months	16 % low 73 % intermediate 11 % high	3D/IMRT no IGRT 3–6 months ADT	74 Gy in 37# 60 Gy in 20# 57 Gy in 19#	74 77 73.4	676 686 692	ns	24 months bowel PRO: No bother 66 % 74Gy, 65 % 60 Gy, 65 % 57 Gy Moderate bother 5 % 74Gy, 6 % 60Gy, 5 % 57 Gy Severe bother <1 % all groups
Vargas et al. [51]	18 months	All low risk	Protons All had IGRT	79.2 Gy RBE in 44# 38 Gy RBE in 5#	74.7 98	82	ns	EPIC Bowel score at 24 months 93.28 79.2 Gy, vs 89.24, 38 Gy, $p=0.29$ EPIC urinary 91.31 79.2 Gy, vs 90.92 38 Gy RBE, $p=0.92$
Lee et al. [38]	5.8 years	All low risk	3D/IMRT All IGRT	73.8 Gy in 41# vs 70 Gy in 28#	69.6 80	1115	5 years DFS 85.3 % 73.8 Gy 86.3 Gy 70 Gy	Late GI 14 % ≥ G2 73.8 Gy 22.4 % ≥ G2 70 Gy $p=0.002$ Late GU 22.8 % ≥ G2 73.8 Gy 29.7 % ≥ G2 70 Gy $p=0.06$

Exceptions, however, are the HYPRO study, where non-inferiority in terms of late effects could not be demonstrated, and the RTOG 0415 trial discussed above, and it must be said that the jury is still out [4, 38]. Some authorities have already advocated the adoption of hypofractionation as a standard of care, but perhaps a more prudent policy is that advocated by the European Association of Urology, who state that hypofractionation should be restricted to experienced and expert centres [42]. Certainly, it would seem prudent to continue to collect outcome data, particularly using patient-reported outcome measures, in a 'real-world' setting.

2. Moderate dose, hypofractionated radiotherapy is probably not inferior to standard dose radiotherapy in terms of disease control as determined by disease-specific parameters, including PSA control. This does not, of course, answer the question as to whether hypofractionated radiotherapy might actually be superior, nor does it allow for any assessment regarding its effect on overall survival.

4.4 Results of Extreme Hypofractionation Using Stereotactic Radiotherapy, for Localised Prostate Cancer

To date, there have been no published randomised trials comparing extreme hypofractionation to other schedules. The results of unrandomised case series have been well summarised in the previously referred to reviews [24, 32, 57]. The largest and most mature series of non-randomised patients had been reported by Katz and Kang [30]. In this report, there were 324 low risk and 153 intermediate risk patients treated with Cyberkinife. Following treatment with either 35 or 36.25 Gy delivered in 5 fractions, 7 year biochemical failure rates were 95.6 % and 89.6 % for low and intermediate risk patients, respectively.

With the caveat that the available data are not level one evidence, it appears that this technique is safe, and that disease control rates are good. However, as with any non-randomised data, extreme caution is needed in interpretation. The selection criteria for patients in these studies vary, and in some instances may be difficult to ascertain. In general terms, though, these are fit patients with, predominantly, less than high grade disease, and the same outcomes might not be attainable in a less selected population.

Current guidelines, such as the EAU guidelines, would regard extreme hypofractionation as being experimental, and this reflects the nature of the data, but also that there is a requirement for absolute precision and meticulous attention to detail in the delivery of this form of treatment. It should not be given outside of specialised centres, in the context of a formal clinical trial, and, as a minimum, outcome data in terms of patient-reported toxicity and quality of life, plus oncological outcomes, should be recorded and published.

4.5 Results of Stereotactic Radiotherapy for Oligometastatic Disease

The great hope of radical therapy for oligometastatic disease is that a patient, otherwise harbouring a lethal disease, might be cured. Unfortunately, the available data suggest that this is not commonly achieved [24]. In the largest published series of patients treated with high-dose radiotherapy, using stereotactic techniques, most patients do, unfortunately, progress subsequent to the treatment [43]. However, that does not mean to say that this treatment strategy has no benefits. Indeed, as the 3-year distant progression-free survival was 31 %, it may well be that stereotactic radiotherapy to oligometastases, with or without concomitant radiotherapy to the primary tumour, has an effect on oncological outcomes.

As with extreme hypofractionation, this hypothesis requires testing in a prospective randomised trial, and fortunately, there are two such trials ongoing. The STOMP trial in Europe and the ORIOLE trial in the USA are randomising patients with oligometastatic disease to treatment with SBRT or observation [15].

It will be some time before the outcomes of these trials are known. In the interim, this should be regarded as an experimental approach, best delivered in the context of a trial, and as before, honest counselling of patients must be a prerequisite before this sort of treatment is embarked on.

5 Conclusions: Future Prospects

Randomised trials remain the cornerstone of evidence-based medical practice, and the topics covered here are no exception. IMRT is now firmly established in routine practice, and those centres which are still unable to access it are, in general, moving towards adopting it as a routine for the management of primary prostate cancer. However, IMRT is neither an end in itself, nor can it be utilised without other crucial elements of the treatment process, state-of-the-art treatment planning, verification systems with some form of IGRT. Additionally, other aspects of patient care, such as adequate bowel preparation, though beyond the scope of this Chapter, are vital ingredients of an optimal outcome.

If it is true that a degree of critical evaluation is appropriate for IMRT, it is especially true also of the other two areas covered here – hypofractionation and stereotactic radiotherapy – whether used for extreme hypofractionation in the treatment of localised disease or for oligometastatic disease. In the case of moderate hypofractionation and oligometastatic disease, we have trials which have informed us, or will do so in the future. There are no randomised trials comparing IMRT with conformal radiotherapy for prostate cancer at equivalent doses, and it seems unlikely that any such trials will be performed. The HYPO and PACE trials will be key sources of unprecedented quality data for extreme hypofractionation. These techniques are key components of the blueprint for external beam radiotherapy over the next decade. Let us hope that their place is determined by evidence and not driven by technology.

References

1. Adams EJ, Convery DJ, Cosgrove VP, et al. Clinical implementation of dynamic and step-and-shoot IMRT to treat prostate cancer with high risk of pelvic lymph node involvement. Radiother Oncol. 2004;70:1–10. doi:10.1016/j.radonc.2003.09.004.
2. Al-Mamgani A, Heemsbergen WD, Peeters STH, Lebesque JV. Role of intensity-modulated radiotherapy in reducing toxicity in dose escalation for localized prostate cancer. Int J Radiat Oncol Biol Phys. 2009;73:685–91. doi:10.1016/j.ijrobp.2008.04.063.
3. Aluwini S, Pos F, Schimmel E, et al. Hypofractionated versus conventionally fractionated radiotherapy for patients with prostate cancer (HYPRO): late toxicity results from a randomised, non-inferiority, phase 3 trial. Lancet Oncol. 2016;17:464–74. doi:10.1016/S1470-2045(15)00567-7.
4. Aluwini S, Pos F, Schimmel E, et al. Hypofractionated versus conventionally fractionated radiotherapy for patients with prostate cancer (HYPRO): acute toxicity results from a randomised non-inferiority phase 3 trial. Lancet Oncol. 2015;16:274–83. doi:10.1016/S1470-2045(14)70482-6.
5. Arcangeli G, Saracino B, Gomellini S, et al. A prospective phase III randomized trial of hypofractionation versus conventional fractionation in patients with high-risk prostate cancer. Int J Radiat Oncol Biol Phys. 2010;78:11–8. doi:10.1016/j.ijrobp.2009.07.1691.
6. Asbell SO, Krall JM, Pilepich MV, et al. Elective pelvic irradiation in stage A2, B carcinoma of the prostate: analysis of RTOG 77–06. Int J Radiat Oncol Biol Phys. 1988;15:1307–16.
7. Bauman G, Rumble RB, Chen J, et al. Intensity-modulated radiotherapy in the treatment of prostate cancer. Clin Oncol (R Coll Radiol). 2012;24:461–73. doi:10.1016/j.clon.2012.05.002.
8. Beckendorf V, Guerif S, Le Prisé E, et al. 70 Gy versus 80 Gy in localized prostate cancer: 5-year results of GETUG 06 randomized trial. Int J Radiat Oncol Biol Phys. 2011;80:1056–63. doi:10.1016/j.ijrobp.2010.03.049.
9. Bruner DW, Hunt D, Michalski JM, et al. Preliminary patient-reported outcomes analysis of 3-dimensional radiation therapy versus intensity-modulated radiation therapy on the high-dose arm of the Radiation Therapy Oncology Group (RTOG) 0126 prostate cancer trial. Cancer. 2015;121:2422–30. doi:10.1002/cncr.29362.
10. Cooperberg MR. Expanding utilization of intensity-modulated radiotherapy for prostate cancer: soaring costs, dubious benefits: comment on "Comparative effectiveness of intensity-modulated radiotherapy and conventional conformal radiotherapy in the treatment of prostate cancer after radical prostatectomy". JAMA Intern Med. 2013;173:1143–4. doi:10.1001/jamainternmed.2013.6755.
11. Dasu A, Toma-Dasu I. Prostate alpha/beta revisited – an analysis of clinical results from 14 168 patients. Acta Oncol. 2012;51:963–74. doi:10.3109/0284186X.2012.719635.
12. Dearnaley D, Syndikus I, Sumo G, et al. Conventional versus hypofractionated high-dose intensity-modulated radiotherapy for prostate cancer: preliminary safety results from the CHHiP randomised controlled trial. Lancet Oncol. 2012;13:43–54. doi:10.1016/S1470-2045(11)70293-5.
13. Dearnaley DP, Jovic G, Syndikus I, et al. Escalated-dose versus control-dose conformal radiotherapy for prostate cancer: long-term results from the MRC RT01 randomised controlled trial. Lancet Oncol. 2014;15:464–73. doi:10.1016/S1470-2045(14)70040-3.

14. Dearnaley DP, Khoo VS, Norman AR, et al. Comparison of radiation side-effects of conformal and conventional radiotherapy in prostate cancer: a randomised trial. Lancet. 1999;353:267–72. doi:10.1016/S0140-6736(98)05180-0.
15. Decaestecker K, De Meerleer G, Ameye F, et al. Surveillance or metastasis-directed therapy for OligoMetastatic prostate cancer recurrence (STOMP): study protocol for a randomized phase II trial. BMC Cancer. 2014;14:671. doi:10.1186/1471-2407-14-671.
16. Ezzell GA, Galvin JM, Low D, et al. Guidance document on delivery, treatment planning, and clinical implementation of IMRT: report of the IMRT subcommittee of the AAPM radiation therapy committee. Med Phys. 2003;30:2089–115. doi:10.1118/1.1591194.
17. Fowler JF, Toma-Dasu I, Dasu A. Is the α/β ratio for prostate tumours really low and does it vary with the level of risk at diagnosis? Anticancer Res. 2013;33:1009–11.
18. Ghilezan M, Yan D, Liang J, et al. Online image-guided intensity-modulated radiotherapy for prostate cancer: how much improvement can we expect? A theoretical assessment of clinical benefits and potential dose escalation by improving precision and accuracy of radiation delivery. Int J Radiat Oncol Biol Phys. 2004;60:1602–10. doi:10.1016/j.ijrobp.2004.07.709.
19. Ghilezan MJ, Jaffray DA, Siewerdsen JH, et al. Prostate gland motion assessed with cine-magnetic resonance imaging (cine-MRI). Int J Radiat Oncol Biol Phys. 2005;62:406–17. doi:10.1016/j.ijrobp.2003.10.017.
20. Goldin GH, Sheets NC, Meyer A-M, et al. Comparative effectiveness of intensity-modulated radiotherapy and conventional conformal radiotherapy in the treatment of prostate cancer after radical prostatectomy. JAMA Intern Med. 2013;173:1136–43. doi:10.1001/jamainternmed.2013.1020.
21. Gray PJ, Paly JJ, Yeap BY, et al. Patient-reported outcomes after 3-dimensional conformal, intensity-modulated, or proton beam radiotherapy for localized prostate cancer. Cancer. 2013;119:1729–35. doi:10.1002/cncr.27956.
22. Harris V, South C, Cruickshank C, Dearnaley D. 1299 poster a national phase III trial of pelvic lymph node (LN) IMRT in prostate cancer (pivotal): a comparison of LN outlining methods. Radiother Oncol. 2011;99:S486–7. doi:10.1016/S0167-8140(11)71421-9.
23. Heemsbergen WD, Al-Mamgani A, Slot A, et al. Long-term results of the Dutch randomized prostate cancer trial: impact of dose-escalation on local, biochemical, clinical failure, and survival. Radiother Oncol. 2014;110:104–9. doi:10.1016/j.radonc.2013.09.026.
24. Henderson DR, Tree AC, van As NJ. Stereotactic body radiotherapy for prostate cancer. Clin Oncol (R Coll Radiol). 2015;27:270–9. doi:10.1016/j.clon.2015.01.011.
25. Hoffman KE, Voong KR, Pugh TJ, et al. Risk of late toxicity in men receiving dose-escalated hypofractionated intensity modulated prostate radiation therapy: results from a randomized trial. Int J Radiat Oncol Biol Phys. 2014;88:1074–84. doi:10.1016/j.ijrobp.2014.01.015.
26. Hummel S, Simpson EL, Hemingway P, et al. Intensity-modulated radiotherapy for the treatment of prostate cancer: a systematic review and economic evaluation. Health Technol Assess. 2010;14:1–108. doi:10.3310/hta14470, iii–iv.
27. Hummel SR, Stevenson MD, Simpson EL, Staffurth J. A model of the cost-effectiveness of intensity-modulated radiotherapy in comparison with three-dimensional conformal radiotherapy for the treatment of localised prostate cancer. Clin Oncol (R Coll Radiol). 2012;24:e159–67. doi:10.1016/j.clon.2012.09.003.
28. Jaffray DA, Siewerdsen JH, Wong JW, Martinez AA. Flat-panel cone-beam computed tomography for image-guided radiation therapy. Int J Radiat Oncol Biol Phys. 2002;53:1337–49.
29. James ND, Spears MR, Clarke NW, et al. Failure-free survival and radiotherapy in patients with newly diagnosed nonmetastatic prostate cancer. JAMA Oncol. 2016;2:1–10. doi:10.1001/jamaoncol.2015.4350.
30. Katz AJ, Kang J. Stereotactic body radiotherapy as treatment for organ confined low- and intermediate-risk prostate carcinoma, a 7-year study. Front Oncol 2014;4:240. doi:10.3389/fonc.2014.00240.
31. Kjær-Kristoffersen F, Ohlhues L, Medin J, Korreman S. RapidArc volumetric modulated therapy planning for prostate cancer patients. Acta Oncol. 2009;48:227–32. doi:10.1080/02841860802266748.
32. Koontz BF, Bossi A, Cozzarini C, et al. A systematic review of hypofractionation for primary management of prostate cancer. Eur Urol. 2015;68:683–91. doi:10.1016/j.eururo.2014.08.009.
33. Kotte ANTJ, Hofman P, Lagendijk JJW, et al. Intrafraction motion of the prostate during external-beam radiation therapy: analysis of 427 patients with implanted fiducial markers. Int J Radiat Oncol Biol Phys. 2007;69:419–25. doi:10.1016/j.ijrobp.2007.03.029.
34. Kuban DA, Nogueras-Gonzalez GM, Hamblin L, et al. Preliminary report of a randomized dose escalation trial for prostate cancer using hypofractionation. Int J Radiat Oncol Biol Phys. 2010;78:S58–9. doi:10.1016/j.ijrobp.2010.07.170.
35. Kuban DA, Tucker SL, Dong L, et al. Long-term results of the M. D. Anderson randomized dose-escalation trial for prostate cancer. Int J Radiat Oncol Biol Phys. 2008;70:67–74. doi:10.1016/j.ijrobp.2007.06.054.
36. Lawton CA, DeSilvio M, Roach M, et al. An update of the phase III trial comparing whole pelvic to prostate only radiotherapy and neoadjuvant to adjuvant total androgen suppression: updated analysis of RTOG 94–13, with emphasis on unexpected hormone/radiation interactions. Int J Radiat Oncol

Biol Phys. 2007;69:646–55. doi:10.1016/j.ijrobp.2007.04.003.
37. Lawton CAF, Michalski J, El-Naqa I, et al. RTOG GU radiation oncology specialists reach consensus on pelvic lymph node volumes for high-risk prostate cancer. Int J Radiat Oncol Biol Phys. 2009;74:383–7. doi:10.1016/j.ijrobp.2008.08.002.
38. Lee WR, Dignam JJ, Amin MB, et al. Randomized phase III noninferiority study comparing two radiotherapy fractionation schedules in patients with low-risk prostate cancer. J Clin Oncol. 2016. doi:10.1200/JCO.2016.67.0448.
39. Ling CC, Burman C, Chui CS, et al. Conformal radiation treatment of prostate cancer using inversely-planned intensity-modulated photon beams produced with dynamic multileaf collimation. Int J Radiat Oncol Biol Phys. 1996;35:721–30.
40. Lukka H, Hayter C, Julian JA, et al. Randomized trial comparing two fractionation schedules for patients with localized prostate cancer. J Clin Oncol. 2005;23:6132–8. doi:10.1200/JCO.2005.06.153.
41. Mohan R, Wang X, Jackson A, et al. The potential and limitations of the inverse radiotherapy technique. Radiother Oncol. 1994;32:232–48.
42. Mottet N, Bellmunt J, Briers E, et al. members of the EAU – ESTRO – SIOG prostate cancer guidelines panel. EAU – ESTRO – SIOG guidelines on prostate cancer. Edn. Presented at the EAU Annual congress Munich. ISBN 978-90-79754-98-4. Arnhem: EAU Guidelines Office; 2016.
43. Ost P, Jereczek-Fossa BA, As NV, et al. Progression-free survival following stereotactic body radiotherapy for oligometastatic prostate cancer treatment-naive recurrence: a multi-institutional analysis. Eur Urol. 2016;69:9–12. doi:10.1016/j.eururo.2015.07.004.
44. Pollack A, Walker G, Horwitz EM, et al. Randomized trial of hypofractionated external-beam radiotherapy for prostate cancer. J Clin Oncol. 2013;31:3860–8. doi:10.1200/JCO.2013.51.1972.
45. Pommier P, Chabaud S, Lagrange J-L, et al. Is there a role for pelvic irradiation in localized prostate adenocarcinoma? Preliminary results of GETUG-01. J Clin Oncol. 2007;25:5366–73. doi:10.1200/JCO.2006.10.5171.
46. Sale C, Moloney P. Dose comparisons for conformal, IMRT and VMAT prostate plans. J Med Imaging Radiat Oncol. 2011;55:611–21. doi:10.1111/j.1754-9485.2011.02310.x.
47. Scarbrough TJ, Golden NM, Ting JY, et al. Comparison of ultrasound and implanted seed marker prostate localization methods: implications for image-guided radiotherapy. Int J Radiat Oncol Biol Phys. 2006;65:378–87. doi:10.1016/j.ijrobp.2006.01.008.
48. Sheets N, Goldin GH, Meyer AM, et al. Comparative long-term morbidity of intensity modulated vs. conformal radiation therapy (RT) for prostate cancer: a SEER-Medicare analysis. Int J Radiat Oncol Biol Phys. 2011;81:S43. doi:10.1016/j.ijrobp.2011.06.087.
49. Silva C, Mateus D, Eiras M, Vieira S. Calypso® 4D localization system: a review. J Radiother Pract. 2014;13:473–83. doi:10.1017/S1460396914000223.
50. van der Heide UA, Kotte ANTJ, Dehnad H, et al. Analysis of fiducial marker-based position verification in the external beam radiotherapy of patients with prostate cancer. Radiother Oncol. 2007;82:38–45. doi:10.1016/j.radonc.2006.11.002.
51. Vargas CE, Hartsell WF, Dunn M, et al. Hypofractionated versus standard fractionated proton-beam therapy for low-risk prostate cancer: interim results of a randomized trial PCG GU 002. Am J Clin Oncol. 2015; 1. doi: 10.1097/COC.0000000000000241.
52. Webb S. Optimisation of conformal radiotherapy dose distribution by simulated annealing. Phys Med Biol. 1989;34:1349–70. doi:10.1088/0031-9155/34/10/002.
53. Wilkins A, Mossop H, Syndikus I, et al. Hypofractionated radiotherapy versus conventionally fractionated radiotherapy for patients with intermediate-risk localised prostate cancer: 2-year patient-reported outcomes of the randomised, non-inferiority, phase 3 CHHiP trial. Lancet Oncol. 2015;16:1605–16. doi:10.1016/S1470-2045(15)00280-6.
54. Wolff D, Stieler F, Welzel G, et al. Volumetric modulated arc therapy (VMAT) vs. serial tomotherapy, step-and-shoot IMRT and 3D-conformal RT for treatment of prostate cancer. Radiother Oncol. 2009;93:226–33. doi:10.1016/j.radonc.2009.08.011.
55. Yeoh EE, Botten RJ, Butters J, et al. Hypofractionated versus conventionally fractionated radiotherapy for prostate carcinoma: final results of phase III randomized trial. Int J Radiat Oncol Biol Phys. 2011;81:1271–8. doi:10.1016/j.ijrobp.2010.07.1984.
56. Yirmibeşoğlu Erkal E, Karabey S, Karabey A, et al. Defining the "Hostile Pelvis" for intensity modulated radiation therapy: the impact of anatomic variations in pelvic dimensions on dose delivered to target volumes and organs at risk in patients with high-risk prostate cancer treated with whole pelvic radiation therapy. Int J Radiat Oncol Biol Phys. 2015;92:894–903. doi:10.1016/j.ijrobp.2015.03.014.
57. Zaorsky NG, Ohri N, Showalter TN, et al. Systematic review of hypofractionated radiation therapy for prostate cancer. Cancer Treat Rev. 2013;39:728–36. doi:10.1016/j.ctrv.2013.01.008.
58. Zelefsky MJ, Fuks Z, Happersett L, et al. Clinical experience with intensity modulated radiation therapy (IMRT) in prostate cancer. Radiother Oncol. 2000;55:241–9.
59. Zelefsky MJ, Levin EJ, Hunt M, et al. Incidence of late rectal and urinary toxicities after three-dimensional conformal radiotherapy and intensity-modulated radiotherapy for localized prostate cancer. Int J Radiat Oncol Biol Phys. 2008;70:1124–9. doi:10.1016/j.ijrobp.2007.11.044.
60. Zietman AL, Bae K, Slater JD, et al. Randomized trial comparing conventional-dose with high-dose conformal radiation therapy in early-stage adenocarcinoma of the prostate: long-term results from proton radiation oncology group/american college of radiology 95–09. J Clin Oncol. 2010;28:1106–11. doi:10.1200/JCO.2009.25.8475.

Combination of Androgen Deprivation Therapy and Radiation Therapy for Locally Advanced and Localized Prostate Cancer

Michel Bolla, Camille Verry, and Carole Iriart

1 Introduction

To improve the overall survival of high-risk prostate cancer (PCa) the combination of a local-regional external beam radiotherapy (EBRT) with androgen deprivation therapy (ADT) is imperative, both to potentiate the radiation effect and eventually eradicate microscopic sub-clinical distant metastases. High-risk PCa include men with locally advanced (T3-4 N0-X M0, cN1-pN1 M0-X) or localized PCa (T1-2 N0-X M0) with a Gleason score 8–10 and/or a baseline PSA >20 ng/mL. Since the discovery of hormone dependence of PCa by Huggins and Hodges [28], surgical castration or estrogens have become the cornerstone of treatment in advanced PCa. During the 1980s, conventional hormonal manipulations were replaced by the agonists of the luteinizing hormone-releasing hormone (LHRH) which had the same efficacy with the possibility of reversibility [51] and less side effects. The combination of EBRT and ADT was tried out because of the poor results of definitive EBRT. It has been shown that this combined approach : (1) reduces DNA repair further to DNA damage induced by irradiation [23], (2) improves oxygenation [46], (3) inhibits repopulation during irradiation, (4) decreases both the amount of prostate gland and prostate cancerous tissue, (5) decreases the occurrence of distant metastases, and (6) improves the effectiveness of EBRT by an additive or supra-additive effect [32, 34, 72].

Randomized phase III trials have promoted the combination of long-term adjuvant ADT (≥2 years) as a standard of care for locally advanced PCa. Dose-escalated intensity-modulated radiotherapy (IMRT), with or without image-guided radiotherapy (IGRT), has become the gold standard as it is associated with less toxicity compared to three-dimensional conformal (3D-CRT) techniques by sparing normal tissues (Chap. 13); however, whatever the technique and their degree of sophistication, quality assurance plays a major role in the planning and delivery of EBRT. Since the role of surgery in high-risk PCa is discussed in Chap. 8, we would like to consider the randomized controlled phase III trials devoted to this combined approach for high-risk and intermediate-risk PCa, the new options of EBRT and/or ADT, to conclude with the side effects and quality of life related to ADT.

M. Bolla (✉) • C. Verry • C. Iriart
Clinique Universitaire de Cancérologie-Radiothérapie, Centre Hospitalier Universitaire Grenoble Alpes, Grenoble Alpes Université, BP 217 38043 Grenoble cedex 9, France
e-mail: MBolla@chu-grenoble.fr; CVerry@chu-grenoble.fr; CIriart@chu-grenoble.fr

M. Bolla, H. van Poppel (eds.), *Management of Prostate Cancer*,
DOI 10.1007/978-3-319-42769-0_15

2 Randomized Phase III Trials of Use and Duration of Androgen Deprivation Therapy in Combination with External Beam Radiotherapy (Table 1)

2.1 Locally Advanced Prostate Cancer

The most powerful conclusion from these trials comes from EORTC trial 22863, which is the basis for the combination of EBRT and ADT as standard practice. Radiotherapy is an essential part in management of high-risk PCa and three randomized phase III trials have clearly shown that combined EBRT plus ADT improves overall survival. Androgen deprivation therapy starts either at the onset of EBRT, or 2–3 months before, which may induce size reduction of the prostate and improve lower urinary tract symptoms, but the concomitant component remains crucial to potentiate EBRT. The 2015 current European Association of Urology guidelines recommend a dose of 76–78 Gy in combination with long-term ADT (2–3 years) for high-risk disease, when given in standard fraction sizes of 1.8–2 Gy per fraction [48].

2.1.1 Long Term Androgen Deprivation Therapy

EORTC Trial 22863

This trial was the first to display a significant gain in overall survival in favour of the combined approach [3, 4]. It recruited 415 men classified as T1-2 N0 M0 histological grade 3 WHO or T3-4 N0 M0 to compare EBRT with concomitant and adjuvant ADT to EBRT alone with a deferred ADT in case of relapse: 82 % of patients were T3, 10 % were T4 and 89 %, N0. With a four-field box technique the whole pelvis received 50 Gy followed by a boost to the prostate to a total dose of 70 Gy. Cyproterone acetate was given orally (50 mg three times daily for 1 month) beginning 1 week before the start of EBRT to avoid a flare phenomenon while a monthly subcutaneous injection of Zoladex® was done during 3 years starting the first day of EBRT. At a 9.1-year follow-up, long-term ADT increased 10-year overall survival 58.1 % vs. 39.8 % ($p=0.0004$) and lowered 10-year mortality 10.3 % vs. 30.4 ($p<0.001$); no difference in cardiovascular mortality was noted between treatments groups. These data were confirmed in real life, since after the first publication of this trial, prolonged ADT with EBRT became a standard policy in British Columbia; later on a retrospective analysis was done to evaluate whether population-based survival improved and it was shown that patients with T3–T4 PCa submitted to a long-term ADT had an improved 8-year overall survival ($p=0.0002$) [67].

RTOG Trial 85–31

Nine hundred and seventy seven men with stages T3-4 M0 with or without lymph-node involvement or classified as pT3 after radical prostatectomy were included. Adjuvant monthly administration of Zoladex® was started during the last week of EBRT and continued indefinitely or until signs relapse (arm 1) or started at relapse (arm 2). Fifteen percent of the patients have undergone radical prostatectomy in arm 1 and 14 % in arm 2 and, 29 % and 26 % had lymph-node involvement, respectively. The pelvis received 44–46 Gy followed by a boost to the prostate to a total dose of 65–70 Gy [40]. At a 7.6-year median follow-up the 10-year overall survival was 49 % (arm 1) vs. 39 % (arm 2) ($p<0.002$) [53].

Casodex Early PCa Trialists Group

Three randomized double-blind placebo-controlled trials accruing 1370 patients with T1-4, any N M0 PCa treated by EBRT were merged. A non-steroidal anti-androgen, bicalutamide (Casodex®) was used as an alternative to castration. Casodex® was given orally (150 mg/day) after EBRT during 2 years (trial 23), 5 years (trial 24) or until progression (trial 25). At a median follow-up of 5.3 years bicalutamide significantly reduced the risk of disease progression ($p=0.003$) in patients with locally advanced PCa ($n=305$) [68].

Table 1 Phase III studies addressing use and duration of androgen deprivation therapy in combination with external beam radiotherapy

Study	Year of publication	TNM 2002	Number of patients	Androgen deprivation therapy	External irradiation	Effect on overall survival (OS)
Androgen deprivation + external irradiation versus radiotherapy alone						
EORTC 22863	2010	T1-2 poorly differentiated M0 or T3-4 N0-1 M0	415	LHRHa for 3 years	70 Gy RT	10-year OS: benefit for combined treatment (HR = 0.60, 95 % CI :0.45–0.80, p = 0.0004)
RTOG 85-31	2005	T3 or N1M0	977	Orchiectomy or lifelong LHRHa	65–70 Gy RT	10-year OS: benefit for combined treatment (p = 0.002) seems mostly caused by patients with Gleason score 7–10
Granfors	2006	T3N0-1 M0	91	Orchiectomy	65 Gy RT	Benefit (p = 0.02), mainly caused by lymph node positive tumours
D'Amico	2008	T2N0M0 (localized unfavourable risk)	206	LHRHa + flutamide. 6 months	70 Gy 3D-CRT	8-year OS: significant benefit (HR = 0.55, 95 % CI : 0.34–0.90, p = 0.01) for men with no or minimal co-morbidity
RTOG 94–08	2011	T1b-c T2a-b	1579	2 months neo-adjuvant + concomitant	66.6Gy RT	10 year OS: benefit for combined treatment in subset intermediate risk (p = 0.03)
EORTC 22991	2016	T1-T2 N0M0 Inter- or high-risk	818	LHRHa for 6 months	70-74–78 Gy 3D-CRT	Better 5-year disease-free survival for combined treatment. (HR = 0.63; 95 %: 0.48–0.84, p = 0.001)
TROG 96-01	2011	T2b-T4N0M0	802	LHRHa + flutamide 3 or 6 months before + concomitant	66 Gy 3D-CRT	10-year 0S: no difference. benefit in PCa specific survival (p = 0.04)
RTOG 94-13	2007	T1c-T4N0-1M0	1292	2 months neo-adjuvant + concomitant versus 4 months adjuvant	Whole pelvic RT vs. prostate only 70.2 Gy	No difference in neo-adjuvant + concomitant versus adjuvant ADT groups (interaction suspected)
RTOG 86-10	2008	T2-4N0-1M0	456	LHRHa + flutamide 2 months before + concomitant	65–70 Gy	10-year OS: no difference (p = 0.12)
Short versus long-term androgen deprivation						
RTOG 92-02	2008	T2c-4N0-1 M0	1554	LHRHa 2 years adjuvant after 4 months neo-adjuvant	65–70 Gy RT	10 year OS: benefit in subset with Gleason 8–10 for long-term treatment (p = 0.006)
EORTC 22961	2009	T1c-T2abN1M0 T2c-4N0-1M0	970	LHRHa 6 months versus 3 years	70 Gy 3D-CRT	Better 5-year OS with 3-year treatment (p = 0.008)

(continued)

Table 1 (continued)

Study	Year of publication	TNM 2002	Number of patients	Androgen deprivation therapy	External irradiation	Effect on overall survival (OS)
Androgen deprivation + radiotherapy versus androgen deprivation alone						
SPCGF-7/ SFUO-3	2016	T1b-T2 Grade 2–3 T3N0M0	880	LHRHa 3 months + continuous flutamide	70 Gy RT versus no RT	Lower 10-year PCa mortality for combined treatment ($p=0.0006$)
NCIC CTG PR.3 MRC PRO7/ SWOG	2015	T3-4 N0M0	1205	Continuous LHRHa	60–65 Gy RT versus no RT	10-year OS: benefit for combined treatment (HR = 0.70, 95 % CI 0.57–0.85, $p<0.001$)
French study (Mottet)	2012	T3-4N0M0	273	LHRHa for 3 years	70 Gy 3D-RT versus no RT	Better 5-year progression-free survival for combined treatment ($p<0.001$)

RTOG Trial 92–02

This trial has accrued 1554 patients classified T2c-4 N0 to investigate the value of a long term adjuvant ADT. Androgen deprivation therapy was begun 2 months before the onset of EBRT and continued until it was completed; all patients received flutamide (250 mg three times a day) with Zoladex® (3.6 mg subcutaneously monthly). Patients were randomly assigned to no further treatment or 24 additional months of Zoladex®. The pelvis received 44–46 Gy followed by a boost to the prostate to a total dose of 65–70 Gy. The 10-year results showed no benefit in overall survival ($p=0.35$), but in a subset analysis the overall survival benefit was limited to patients with long term ADT and Gleason score 8–10 ($p=0.006$) [27].

EORTC Equivalence Trial 22961

This trial randomly assigned 970 patients –T1c to T2a-b, pathological nodal stage N1 or N2 or T2c to T4 clinical nodal stages N0 to N2- who received 3D-CRT plus 6-month ADT: 483 patients received no further treatment and 487 patients 2.5 years more of LHRH agonist, triptoreline, Decapeptyl® 11.25 mg. At a median follow-up of 6.4 years, the 5-year overall survival was 84.8 % for long term ADT and 81 % for short term ADT with an estimated hazard ratio of 1.42 ($p=0.008$). The 5-year clinical progression-free survival was 80.5 % for long term ADT and 68.7 % for short term ADT ($p<0.0001$) [5].

36 Months Versus 18 Months of Complete Androgen Deprivation Therapy

This study included 630 N0-X M0 patients with high-risk localized PCa (75.4 %) or locally advanced PCa (24.6 %) who were randomly allocated to 18 months (320 patients) or 36 months (310 patients) ADT. Androgen deprivation therapy consisted of a LHRH agonist plus 1 month of anti-androgen (bicalutamide 50 mg per day) started 4 months before 3D-CRT delivering 44 Gy to the pelvic lymph nodes and 70 Gy to the prostate. With a 77-month median follow-up, 10-year overall survival was 63.6 % (36-month arm) versus 63.2 % (18-month arm) ($p=0.42$), and 10-year disease specific survival was the same for both groups [49]. This trial was not an equivalence trial, which would have required more patients and more poor events. A longer follow-up is needed, but 18-month ADT duration combined with dose-escalated IMRT might be helpful for high-risk localized PCa patients unsuitable for long term ADT, due to co-morbidities.

SPCG-7/SFUO-3 Trial

This study comprised 875 patients T1b-T2, G2-G3 or T3 any WHO histological grade (78 %) with baseline PSA <70 ng/ml; patients were randomly allocated to ADT alone with 3 months of continuous androgen blockade followed by continuous flutamide treatment ($n=439$ patients), or to the same ADT combined with EBRT ($n=436$ patients) [71]. With a median observation time of 12 years the 15-year PCa specific mortality rates were 34 % and 17 % in the ADT arm and ADT + EBRT arm, respectively, ($p<0.001$), 10 (15)-year overall mortality was 35.3 (56.7 %) and 26.4 % (43.4 %) ($p=0.0006$) [22].

MRC PR3/PR07 Trial

This study included 1205 patients with T3-4 ($n=1057$) or T2, PSA >40 ng/ml ($n=119$), or T2, PSA >20 ng and Gleason >8 ($n=25$) and N0-X M0 PCa who were randomized to lifelong ADT (bilateral orchidectomy or LHRH agonist) with or without EBRT (65–70 Gy to prostate ±45 Gy to the pelvic lymph nodes). With a median follow-up time of 8 years, 10-year overall survival was improved in the patients allocated to ADT + EBRT, 55 % vs. 49 % ($p<0.001$) [44].

French Study

The trial comprised 273 patients with locally advanced PCa T3-4 or pT3 pN0 M0 who were randomly assigned to lifelong ADT by LHRH agonist (leuproreline) with or without EBRT (48 ± 2Gy to the whole pelvis followed by a boost to the prostate to a total dose of 70 Gy). With a median follow-up period of 67 months, there was a significant improvement of the 5-year disease-free survival in favour of the combined approach ($p<0.001$) without improvement of overall survival: 71.4 % vs. 71.5 % [47].

2.1.2 Short Term Androgen Deprivation Therapy

RTOG Trial 86–10

This trial investigated the impact of combined ADT prior (2 months) and during EBRT with respect to EBRT alone: 471 patients with bulky tumours (T2-4) with or without regional lymph node involvement were included: 7 % had a positive nodal status in the combined treatment arm versus 9 % in the EBRT alone arm. Thirty percent of patients had a T2 tumour, and 70 % were classified as T3-4. Androgen deprivation therapy consisted of oral flutamide (250 mg three times a day) and a subcutaneous injection of Zoladex®3.6 mg every 4 weeks. The pelvis received 45 Gy and the prostate 65–70 Gy. At 10 years there was a significant difference in disease specific mortality 23 % vs. 36 % ($p=0.01$) but no difference in overall survival [58].

Trans-Tasman Radiation Oncology Group 96.01 Trial

This 3-arm study included 818 patients classified as T2b-4 N0 M0 who were randomly assigned to EBRT alone (66 Gy) or 3-month ADT starting 2 months before radiotherapy or 6-month ADT starting 5 months before radiotherapy; ADT consisted of goserelin and flutamide [14]. After a median follow-up of 10.6 years, 6-month ADT with EBRT decreased cancer specific mortality ($p=0.0008$), and all-cause mortality ($p=0.0008$) compared with RT alone [15].

RTOG Trial 94–13

This four arm trial comprised 1323 patients T1c-4 N0 M0 PSA <100 ng with an estimated risk of lymph-node involvement >15 %. Complete ADT consisted of flutamide 250 mg per os t.i.d. with a LHRH agonist. The first randomization was between 2-month neo-adjuvant and concurrent ADT during EBRT versus 4-month adjuvant ADT after EBRT; the second randomization was between whole pelvis EBRT versus prostate only EBRT. An improvement of the progression-free survival was observed in favour of the whole pelvis EBRT, without any difference between the two ADT modalities [39].

2.2 Intermediate- and High-Risk Localized Prostate Cancer

The Boston Group Trial

This trial comprised 206 men with localized but unfavourable-risk PCa who were randomized to receive 3D-CRT alone (70 Gy) or with 6-month complete ADT. For patients without moderate or severe co-morbidity, the combined approach resulted in an increased 8-year overall survival ($p = 0.01$) [11].

RTOG Trial 94–08

One thousand nine hundred seventy-nine men with intermediate- and high-risk stage T1b-c, T2a-b PCa were randomly assigned to 2-month complete ADT before conventional EBRT and 2-month during or to EBRT alone (46.8 Gy to the lymph nodes and 66.6 Gy to the prostate). The combined approach improved the 10-year overall survival of intermediate-risk patients only ($p = 0.03$) [31].

RTOG Trial 9910

One thousand five hundred seventy-nine men with intermediate PCa were randomly assigned to 8 weeks of complete ADT followed by EBRT (2D- or 3D-CRT) with an additional 8 weeks of concurrent complete ADT (16 weeks total) or to 28 weeks of complete ADT followed by EBRT with an additional 8 weeks of ADT (36 weeks total). The pelvis was to receive 46.8 Gy followed by a boost to the prostate to a total dose of 70.2 Gy. For the 8- and 28-week assignments, the 10-year overall survival rates were, respectively, 66 % and 67 % ($p = 0.62$): extending ADT duration from 8 to 28 weeks before EBRT did not improve outcomes [54].

EORTC Trial 22991

Height 119 patients staged cT1b-c with PSA ≥10 ng/ml or Gleason ≥7 or cT2a (UICC TNM 1997) N0 M0 with PSA ≤50 ng/ml were randomized to receive EBRT alone or EBRT+ 6-month concomitant and adjuvant ADT, the first 3-month depot LHRH-agonist started on day 1. Centres opted for one dose (70, 74 or 78 Gy). 74.8 % of patients were at intermediate risk and 24.8 % at high risk. At 7.2 years median follow-up, EBRT + ADT significantly improved biochemical disease-free survival (HR = 0.53, CI: 0.42–0.67, $p < 0.001$) as well as clinical progression-free survival (HR = 0.63, CI: 0.48–0.84, $p = 0.001$). Results are homogeneous across EBRT doses. In all subgroups EBRT + ADT significantly improved biochemical disease-free survival ($p < 0.00001$) and clinical progression-free survival ($p < 0.01$). Overall survival data are not mature [8].

3 Dose Escalation Combined to Androgen Deprivation Therapy

A meta-analysis of 7 randomized controlled trials accruing 2812 patients, from several risk groups with sometimes the use of ADT, showed a significant reduction in the incidence of biochemical failure in those patients treated with dose-escalated radiotherapy ($p < 0.0001$) [70]. A non-randomized well conducted propensity matched retrospective analysis of the US National Cancer Data Base comprising 42.481 patients has displayed a benefit on overall survival for intermediate ($p < 0.001$) and high-risk patients ($p < 0.001$) treated with dose-escalated EBRT (>75.6 Gy to 90 Gy) [33]. Based on the data of the literature, the current European Association of Urology guidelines recommend a dose of 76–78 Gy in combination with ADT for intermediate-risk and high-risk disease, when given in 'standard' fraction sizes of 1.8–2 Gy per fraction (Mottet et al. 2015). Dose escalation alone may be proposed to patients who are reticent to combined short-term ADT due to co-morbidities or because they want to preserve their sexual health, provided the prostate dose delivered by image-guided IMRT is around 80 Gy.

GETUG 14 Trial

This study comprised 377 patients with intermediate-risk PCa; lymphadenectomy was mandatory when the risk of node involvement was >10 %. Patients were randomly assigned to high dose EBRT (prostate 80Gy; seminal vesicles 46 Gy) either alone or in combination with 4-month complete ADT (flutamide + Decapeptyl ® starting 2 months before EBRT). With 37 months median follow-up, the 3-year biochemical or clinical control probabilities were 86% and 92% in the EBRT arm and complete ADT-RT arm, respectively, ($p=0.09$) and the 3-year biochemical control probabilities 91% and 97% ($p=0.04$) [17].

RTOG Trial 94–06

This phase I/II study investigated dose escalation 3D-CRT to treat 583 men with T1-3 PCa to establish the maximally tolerated dose: 207 men initiated ADT between 2 and 3 months before EBRT, and completed ADT no longer than 3 months after EBRT. The addition of ADT to escalated dose from 73.8 to 84.3 Gy did not significantly improve biochemical or clinical disease-free survival [69].

GICOR Trial

This study was conducted to determine the impact on biochemical control and survival of ADT combined with dose-escalated 3D-CRT: 181 low-risk patients were treated with EBRT alone; 75 intermediate-risk patients were allocated to receive 4- to 6-month ADT before and during EBRT and 160-high risk patients received neo-adjuvant and adjuvant ADT 2 years after EBRT. With a stratification for treatment groups, the 5-year biochemical disease-free survival for high-risk patients with neo-adjuvant and adjuvant ADT was 63% for dose <72 Gy vs. 84% for dose ≥ 72 Gy ($p=0.003$) [73].

DART01/05 GICORC

This study investigated whether long-term ADT was superior to short-term ADT when combined with high-dose EBRT; 355 men with intermediate- and high-risk PCa, were randomly assigned to receive either 4-month ADT before and during 3D-CRT (76–82 Gy) or the same treatment followed by 24-month ADT. After a median follow-up of 63 months, 5-year overall survival was better among patients receiving long-term ADT: 95% vs. 86% ($p=0.009$) with no increase in late radiation toxicity [74].

4 Pelvic Lymph-Node Irradiation Combined with Androgen Deprivation Therapy

In high-risk N0 M0 patients the randomized trials addressing the issue of prophylactic pelvic nodal irradiation (46–50 Gy) have failed to show a benefit [1, 39, 55], but the question is still not answered. One reason for the ongoing uncertainty could be the limited dose that is deliverable to pelvic nodes using conventional or conformal radiotherapy, because of the constraint imposed by the radiation tolerance of small bowel included in a pelvic radiation field, another one the insufficient power of these trials. Although there is no level 1 evidence for prophylactic whole pelvic irradiation, this modality could be recommended for high-risk patients managed with a combined approach since pelvic lymph-node irradiation was achieved for EORTC and RTOG trials which have shown a significant improvement in overall survival. The individual risk of finding positive lymph-node can be estimated using nomograms, bearing in mind that a risk of nodal metastases over 5% is an indication to perform pelvic lymph-node EBRT. The pelvic lymph-node target volume must cover what is harvested during the extended pelvic lymph-node dissection i.e. the nodes overlying the external iliac artery and vein, the nodes within the obturator fossa located cranially and caudally to the obturator nerve, and the nodes medial and lateral to the internal iliac artery; with IMRT, pre-sacral nodes can be included easily.

Clinical or pathological node-positive (N+) patients do not always develop a systemic disease and data shown below suggest that the combination of whole pelvic irradiation plus immediate long term ADT may be beneficial (level of evidence 2b, grade B) [48].

RTOG Trial 85–31

A subset analysis was devoted to 173 patients with biopsy proven pN1 lymph nodes: 98 of them received EBRT plus long-life ADT. With a median follow-up of 6.5 years there was a significant difference in overall survival ($p=0.03$) in favour of the combined arm [38]. These results echo those of the Gransfors' study, prematurely closed [24].

Homogeneous Matched Patients Cohorts
Seven hundred and three consecutive pT2-4 pN+ M0 patients who underwent radical prostatectomy plus pelvic lymph-node dissection were reviewed; of these patients, 171 who received a combination of ADT and EBRT and 532 who received adjuvant ADT alone were selected for a matching process for age, pT stage, Gleason score, number of nodes removed, margin status, duration of follow-up; patients treated with adjuvant EBRT plus ADT had a better overall survival compared with patients with ADT alone ($p<0.001$) [9].

US National Cancer Data Base
A non-randomized matched retrospective analysis comprised 3540 patients: 32.2% of the patients were treated with ADT alone and 51.4% with ADT+EBRT. Using propensity score matching in approximately 600 patients with clinically node-positive patients, the 5-year survival was 72.4% for patients treated with the combined approach vs. 49.4% for those treated with ADT alone ($p<0.001$) [43].

STAMPEDE Trial
This trial has recruited high-risk hormone-naïve men with newly diagnosed PCa starting first-line long-term ADT; a cohort of men with N0M0 and N+M0 disease was included, treated with or without EBRT. These non randomized data have shown that failure-free survival outcomes favoured significantly planned use of EBRT for patients of the N0M0 and N+M0 sub-cohorts [30].

5 Neo-adjuvant or Adjuvant Chemotherapy

Taxanes are radiosensitizer agents, which block the cell cycle during the G2/M-phase, inhibit the anti-apoptotic effect of *bcl-2*, and induce apoptosis [61]. Docetaxel has been shown to produce a cytotoxic effect during the S-phase, known to be radioresistant [26]. Phase III randomized trials in patients with castration resistant PCa have shown a significant improvement of overall survival in favour of docetaxel-containing regimens compared with the reference treatment [52, 66]. Phase II trials have shown the feasibility of concomitant [37] or concomitant and adjuvant docetaxel [6] with EBRT. Preliminary results of neo-adjuvant or adjuvant chemotherapy combined with EBRT and ADT are promising but chemotherapy does not yet have a role in men with locally advanced PCa.

GETUG 12 Trial
This study investigated the role of neo-adjuvant chemotherapy with docetaxel on relapse-free survival based on a cohort of 413 high-risk patients with at least one risk factor (i.e., stage T3-4, Gleason score ≥8, PSA ≥20 ng/ml, pathological node-positive). All patients underwent a staging pelvic lymph node dissection and were randomly assigned to either goserelin 10.8 mg every 3 months for 3 years and 4 cycles of docetaxel 70 mg/m^2 q3w plus estramustine 10 mg/kg/d d1-5 (arm 1) or goserelin alone (arm 2). EBRT was administered at 3 months in 358 patients (87%). Toxicity included grade 3–4 neutropenia (27%) with neutropenic fever in 2% but no toxicity-related death and no secondary leukaemia [20]. At a median follow-up time of 8.8 years, docetaxel-based chemotherapy improves relapse-free survival in patients with high-risk PCa ($p=0.017$), but longer follow-up is needed to assess the impact on overall survival [21].

RTOG Trial 0521
This trial comprised 563 high-risk patients with stage ≥T2, Gleason 8, PSA <20 ng, or any stages with either Gleason ≥9 and PSA <150 ng or Gleason 7–8 and PSA ≥20–150 ng. The 6-year disease-free survival was improved from 55 to 65% ($p=0.04$), but the predefined statistical criteria to obtain an improvement in 4-years OS from 86 to 93% (HR: 0.49) was not met and a longer follow-up is needed [59].

6 New Compounds for Androgen Deprivation Therapy

Before the development of new drugs targeting the androgen axis, maximal surgical or chemical castration combined with anti-androgen was used in advanced PCa [41] and a meta-analysis of 27 randomized trials has shown an improvement of the 5-year survival by about 2 or 3%, with a range of uncertainty between 0 and 5% [45]. Despite surgical or medical castration, PCa cells continue to have sufficient levels of androgen from the adrenal glands or intra-tumoral synthesis to drive tumour growth. In castration resistant PCa, the intracellular androgen level is increased, compared to androgen sensitive cells, and an over-expression of the androgen receptor has been observed. A better understanding of androgen receptor signaling and mechanism underlying resurgent androgen receptor activity have induced major breakthroughs in the development of novel androgen-ablative and androgen receptor antagonist strategies to more effectively inhibit receptor activity [36].

Luteinizing-Hormone-Releasing Hormone Antagonists
LHRH antagonists immediately bind to LHRH receptors, leading to a rapid decrease in LH, FSH and testosterone levels without any flare and therefore without need of anti-androgen to prevent the initial testosterone surge (Chap. 22). The third generation GnRH antagonist degarelix is being used in advanced PCa; compared to leuprolide, degarelix is followed by a more rapid suppression of testosterone and PSA [35]. Its definitive superiority over LHRH analogues remains to be proven by ongoing randomized phase III trials.

Androgen Synthesis Inhibitors
Abiraterone acetate is a potent and selective inhibitor of CYP 17 enzyme which is required for androgen biosynthesis in the testes, adrenal glands and prostate tissue. The combination of abiraterone acetate plus prednisone has been shown to improve overall survival in patients with castration resistant PCa previously treated with docetaxel ($p < 0.001$) [13] or chemotherapy naïve ($p < 0.01$) [57]. Abiraterone acetate is investigated in randomized phase III trials combined with LHRH agonist and EBRT for high-risk PCa.

Androgen Receptors Antagonists
Enzalutamide is a novel androgen receptor antagonist that binds the androgen receptor with a eight times higher affinity than bicalutamide; it has no agonist effects and it prevents both androgen receptor translocation and DNA binding. Enzalutamide significantly prolonged median overall survival of patients with castration resistant PCa previously treated by chemotherapy ($p < 0.001$) [60] and significantly decreased the risk of radiographic progression and death in men with metastattic PCa [2]. Enzalutamide is also investigated with LHRH combined with EBRT for high-risk PCa.

7 Side Effects and Health Related Quality of Life

Androgen deprivation therapy with LHRH agonists may adversely affect quality of life with hot flushes, fatigue, weight gain, loss of libido and erectile dysfunction, insulin resistance, lower bone mineral density with an increase risk of bone fracture, increased cardiovascular events, metabolic syndrome, anaemia and impact on cognitive function [50]. These side effects assessed by a self-administered questionnaire are in relation with the prevalent co-morbidities of the patients and the duration of the treatment [56]. The long-term results of the D'Amico trial with a median follow-up duration of 16 years suggest that the risk of cardiac mortality is increased in patients with moderate or severe co-morbidity treated with short-term (<6 months) LHRH agonists [12]; they also suggest that a 6-month duration is long enough to provoke harmful cardiac effects, [10]. These results are controversial since retrospective analyses of the EORTC and RTOG have shown that long-term ADT did not increase the cumulative incidence estimates of cardiovascular mortality as compared with short term or no ADT [5–7, 18, 19]. Weight is associated with prostate cancer mortality in men undergoing combined treatment, and prevalent diabetes is associated with greater all-cause and non PCa mortality [63]. Many studies demonstrated that long-term ADT was associated with an increased risk of fractures: among men surviving at least 5 years 19.4 % of those who received ADT had a fracture versus 12.6 % of those not receiving this treatment ($p < 0.001$) [62]. Prevention of bone mineral loss through lifestyle modification is recommended, as well as the use of bisphosphonates in case of osteoporosis [65, 15]. After radiotherapy and 6 months of androgen blockade, fatigue, hot flushes and sexual problems increased significantly ($p < 0.001$) [5]; continuing 2.5 years more ADT, induced insomnia ($p = 0{,}006$) and hot flushes ($p < 0{,}001$) and less sexual interest and activity ($p < 0{,}001$) but the overall quality of life did not differ significantly between the two groups ($p = 0{,}37$) [5]. The adverse events encountered with long-term administration of bicalutamide (150 mg per day) are mild to moderate: breast pain (74.8 %), gynaecomastia (66.6 %), diarrhoea (15.4 %), asthenia (13.4 %), impotence (12.7 %), hot flushes (9.8 %).

These potential side-effects have to be discussed with the patients to evaluate the risk-benefit ratio -taking into account age, WHO performance status, co-morbidities, sexual health, lifestyle, tobacco usage and body mass index- to enable them to mitigate adverse effects by stopping smoking, reducing their weight, improving diet and increasing physical exercise. To reduce the risk of adverse effects, other parameters should be assessed- glycaemia, hyperlipidaemia, use of blood pressure medication or oral anti-coagulation, control of bone mineral density- so that co-morbidity treatments are adjusted appropriately by general practitioners, endocrinologists and cardiologists.

Table 2 Guidelines regarding the combination of androgen deprivation therapy with external irradiation

Risk	IMRT	Androgen deprivation therapy
Localized PCa *Low risk* T1c-2a, Gleason ≤6, PSA ≤10 ng/ml	+	
Intermediate risk T2b, or 10 <PSA ≤20 ng/mL or Gleason =7	+	4–6 months[a]
High risk T2c, PSA >20 ng/mL or Gleason >7	+	2–3 years
Locally advanced PCa T3-4 N0 M0	+	2–3 years

[a]For patients unsuitable for ADT consider IMRT at escalated dose or a combination of IMRT and brachytherapy

Conclusions

Within the frame of a radiotherapy management, long-term ADT (≥2 years) with LHRH agonists combined with external irradiation is a gold standard for patients with locally advanced PCa (level 1a of evidence, grade A, Table 2); in patients with high-risk localized PCa, EBRT with a total dose of 76–78 Gy in combination with long-term ADT should be offered (level 1b of evidence, grade A). For intermediate-risk localized PCa, a combined approach with a short-term (4–6 month) ADT should be recommended (level 1b grade A) [48]. Patients have to be informed of the potential morbidity of ADT and a close cooperation is needed with general practitioners and specialists to prevent as much as possible harmful side effects. Dose-escalated image-guided IMRT may offer the opportunity to treat intermediate-risk localized PCa without ADT. New systemic therapies have prolonged the life of men with metastatic castration-resistant prostate cancer and are evaluated in high-risk PCa, combined with EBRT, to reach a complete androgen deprivation and increase clinical disease survival. The best way to tailor and personalize the treatment of the patient is to present his medical chart to a tumour board to benefit from a multidisciplinary approach based on guidelines [25]. Randomized phase III trials require a long period of observation before enabling the evaluation of overall survival, reason why intermediate clinical endpoints are assessed as surrogate to shorten the delay to reach the meaningful endpoints [29]. Ongoing translational research based on DNA-based and RNA-based signatures aims at measuring genomic instability and tumour hypoxia in order to help us to individualize the intensification of treatment in case of high levels of hypoxia and high percentages of tumour genome alteration [42]. To conclude, prostate cancer is a heterogeneous disease and its prognostic landscape is progressively changing: It is likely that one day, oncogenic signatures will give physicians the opportunity to offer the right ADT duration to the right patients at the right time.

References

1. Asbell SO, Krall JM, Pilepich MV, et al. Elective pelvic irradiation in stage A2, B carcinoma of the prostate: analysis of RTOG 77–06. Int J Radiat Oncol Biol Phys. 1988;15:1307–16.
2. Beer TM, Armstrong AJ, Rathkopf DE, et al. Enzalutamide in metastatic prostate cancer before chemotherapy. N Engl J Med. 2014;371:424–33.
3. Bolla M, Gonzalez D, Warde P, et al. Improved survival in patients with locally advanced prostate cancer treated with radiotherapy and goserilin. N Engl J Med. 1997;337:295–300.
4. Bolla M, Collette L, Blank L, et al. Long-term results with immediate androgen suppression and external irradiation in patients with locally advanced prostate cancer (an EORTC study): a phase III randomised trial. Lancet. 2002;360:103–6.
5. Bolla M, de Reijke TM, Van Tienhoven G, et al. Duration of androgen suppression in the treatment of prostate cancer. N Engl J Med. 2009;360: 2516–27.
6. Bolla M, Hannoun-Levi JM, Ferrero JM, et al. Concurrent and adjuvant docetaxel with three-dimensional conformal radiation therapy plus androgen deprivation for high-risk prostate cancer: preliminary results of a multicentre phase II trial. Radiother Oncol. 2010;97:312–7.
7. Bolla M, van Tienhoven G, Warde P, et al. External irradiation with or without long-term androgen suppression for prostate cancer with high metastatic risk: 10-year results of an EORTC randomized study. Lancet Oncol. 2010;11:1066–73.
8. Bolla M, Maingon P, Carrie C, et al. Short term androgen suppression and radiation dose escalation for intermediate and high-rsk localized prostate cancer: results of EORTC trial 22991. J Clin Oncol. 2016;34(15):1748–56. http://jco.ascopubs.org/cgi/doi/10.1200/JCO.2015.64.8055.
9. Briganti A, Karnes RJ, Da Pozzo LP, et al. Combination of adjuvant hormonal and radiation therapy significantly prolongs survival of patients with pT2-4 pN+ prostate cancer: results of a matched analysis. Eur Urol. 2011;59:832–40.
10. D'Amico AV, Denham JW, Crook J, et al. Influence of androgen suppression therapy for prostate cancer on the frequency and timing of fatal myocardial infarctions. J Clin Oncol. 2007;25:2420–5.
11. D'Amico AV, Chen MH, Renshaw AA, Loffredo M, Kantoff PW. Androgen suppression and radiation vs radiation alone for prostate cancer: a randomized trial. JAMA. 2008;299:289–95.
12. D'Amico AV, Chen MH, Renshaw AA, Loffredo M, Kantoff PW. Long-term follow-up of a randomized trial of radiation with or without androgen deprivation therapy for localized prostate cancer. JAMA. 2015;314:1291–3.
13. De Bono JS, Logothetis CJ, Molina A, et al. Abiraterone and increased survival in metastattic prostate cancer. N Engl J Med. 2011;364:1995–2005.
14. Denham JW, Steigler A, Lamb DS, et al. Short-term androgen deprivation and radiotherapy for locally advanced prostate cancer: results from the Trans-Tasman Radiation Oncology Group 96.01 randomised controlled trial. Lancet Oncol. 2005;6:841–50.
15. Denham JW, Steigler A, Lamb DS, et al. Short term neoadjuvant androgen deprivation and radiotherapy for locally advanced prostate cancer: 10-year data from the TROG 96.01 randomised trial. Lancet Oncol. 2011;12(5):451–9.
16. Diamond TH, Higano CS, Smith MR, Guise TA, Singer FR. Osteoporosis in men with prostate carcinoma receiving androgen-deprivation therapy: recommendations for diagnosis and therapies. Cancer. 2004;100:892–9.
17. Dubray BM, Beckendorf V, Guerif S, et al. Does short-term androgen depletion add to high-dose radiotherapy (80 Gy) in localized intermediate-risk prostate cancer? Intermediate analysis of GETUG 14 randomized trial (EU-20503/NCT00104741). J Clin Oncol. 2011;29:(suppl; abstr 4521).
18. Efstathiou JA, Bae K, Shipley WU, et al. Cardiovascular mortality and duration of androgen deprivation for locally advanced prostate cancer: analysis of RTOG 92–02. Eur Urol. 2008;54:816–23.

19. Efstathiou JA, Bae K, Shipley WU, et al. Cardiovascular mortality after androgen deprivation therapy for locally advanced prostate cancer: RTOG 85–31. J Clin Oncol. 2009;27:92–9.
20. Fizazi K, Lesaunier F, Delva R, et al. Docetaxel-estramustine in high-risk localized prostate cancer: first results of the French Genitourinary Tumor Group phase III trial (GETUG12). J Clin Oncol. 2011;29:(suppl; abstr 4513).
21. Fizazi K, Lesaunier F, Delva R, et al. Androgen deprivation therapy plus docetaxel and estramustine versus androgen deprivation therapy alone for high-risk localised prostate cancer (GETUG 12): a phase 3 randomzed trial. Lancet Oncol. 2015;16:787–94.
22. Fossa SD, et al. Ten-and 15-year prostate cancer-specific mortality in patients with non metastatic locally advanced or aggressive intermediate prostate cancer, randomized to lifelong endocrine treatment alone or combined with radiotherapy; final results of the Scandinavian Prostate Cancer Group-7. Eur Urol. 2016;70(4):684–91. http://dx.doi.org/10.1016/j.euro.2016.03.021.
23. Goodwin JF, Schiewer MJ, Dean JL, et al. A hormone-DNA repair circuit governs the response to genotoxic insult. Cancer Discov. 2013;3:1254–71.
24. Granfors T, Modig H, Damber JE, Tomic R. Combined orchiectomy and external radiotherapy versus radiotherapy alone for nonmetastatic prostate cancer with or without pelvic lymph node involvement: a prospective randomized study. J Urol. 1998;159:2030–4.
25. Heidenreich A, Bastian PJ, Bellmunt J, et al. EAU guidelines on prostate cancer. Part 1: screening, diagnosis, and localized treatment with curative intent. Update 2013. Eur Urol. 2014;65:124–37.
26. Hennequin C, Giocanti N, Favaudon V. S-phase specificity of cell killing by docetaxel (Taxotere) in synchronised HeLa cells. Br J Cancer. 1995;71:1194–8.
27. Horwitz EM, Bae K, Hanks GE, et al. Ten-year follow-up of radiation therapy oncology group protocol 92–02: a phase III trial of the duration of elective androgen deprivation in locally advanced prostate cancer. J Clin Oncol. 2008;26:2497–504.
28. Huggins C, Stevens RE, Hodges CV. Studies on prostatic cancer. The effects of castration on advanced carcinoma of the prostate gland. Arch Surg. 1941;43:209–43.
29. ICECap Working Group. The development of intermediate clinical endpoints in cancer of the prostate (ICECaP). J Natl Cancer Inst. 2015;107:1–8.
30. James ND, Spears MR, Clarke NW, et al. Failure-free survival and radiotherapy in patients with newly diagnosed nonmetastatic prostate cancer. JAMA Oncol. 2015;2(3):348–57. doi:10.1001/jamaoncol.2015.4350 1–10.
31. Jones CU, Hunt D, McGowan DG, et al. Radiotherapy and short-term androgen deprivation for localized prostate cancer. N Engl J Med. 2011;365:107–18.
32. Joon DL, Hasegawa M, Sikes C, et al. Supraadditive apoptotic response of R3327-G rat prostate tumors to androgen ablation and radiation. Int J Radiat Oncol Biol Phys. 1997;38:1071–7.
33. Kalbasi A. Dose escalated irradiation and overall survival in men with non metastatic prostate cancer. JAMA Oncol. 2015;1:897–906.
34. Kaminski JM, Hanlon AL, Joon DL, Meistrich M, Hachem P, Pollack A. Effect of sequencing of androgen deprivation and radiotherapy on prostate cancer growth. Int J Radiat Oncol Biol Phys. 2003;57:24–8.
35. Klotz L, Boccon-Gibod L, Shore ND, et al. The efficacy and safety of degarelix: a 12-month, comparative, randomized, open-label, parallel-group phase III study in patients with prosytate cancer. BJU Int. 2008;102:1531–8.
36. Knudsen KE, Scher HI. Starving the addiction: new opportunities for durable suppression of AR signaling in prostate cancer. Clin Cancer Res. 2009;15:4792–8.
37. Kumar P, Perrotti M, Weiss R, et al. Phase I trial of weekly docetaxel with concurrent three-dimensional conformal radiation therapy in the treatment of unfavorable localized adenocarcinoma of the prostate. J Clin Oncol. 2004;22:1909–15.
38. Lawton CA, Winter K, Byhardt R, et al. Androgen suppression plus radiation versus radiation alone for patients with D1/pathologic node-positive adenocarcinoma of the prostate : updated results based on a national prospective randomized trial, Radiation Therapy Oncology Group 85–31. Int J Radiat Oncol Biol Phys. 2005;23:800–7.
39. Lawton CA, DeSivio M, Roach 3rd M, et al. An update of the phase III trial comparing whole pelvis to prostate only radiotherapy and neoadjuvant to adjuvant total androgen suppression.: update analysis of RTOG 94–13, with emphasis on unexpected hormone/radiation interactions. Int J Radiat Oncol Biol Phys. 2007;69:646–55.
40. Lawton CA, Winter K, Murray K, et al. Updated results of the phase III Radiation Therapy Oncology Group (RTOG) trial 85–31 evaluating the potential benefit of androgen suppression following standard radiation therapy for unfavorable prognosis carcinoma of the prostate. Int J Radiat Oncol Biol Phys. 2001;49:937–9.
41. Labrie F, Belanger A, Simard J, Labrie C, Dupont A. Combination therapy for prostate cancer. Endocrine and biologic basis of its choice as new standard first-line therapy. Cancer. 1993;71:1059–67.
42. Lalonde E, Ishkanian AS, Sykes J, et al. Tumour genomic and microenvironmental heterogeneity for integrated prediction of 5-year biochemical recurrence of prostate cancer: a retrospective cohort study. Lancet Oncol. 2014;15:1521–32.
43. Lin CC, Gray PJ, Jemal A, Efstathiou JA. Androgen deprivation with or withoiut radiation therapy for

clinically node-positive prostate cancer. J Natl Cancer Inst. 2015;107:1–10.
44. Mason M. Final report of the Intergroup Randomized Study of Ciombined Androgen deprivationtherapy plus radiotherapy versus androgen deprivation therapy alone in locally advanced prostate cancer. J Clin Oncol. 2015;33:2143–9.
45. Prostate Cancer Trialists' Collaborative Group. Maximum androgen blockade in advanced prostate cancer: an overview of the randomised trials. Lancet. 2000;355:1491–8.
46. Milosevic M, Chung P, Parker C, et al. Androgen withdrawal in patients reduces prostate cancer hypoxia: implications for disease progression and radition response. Cancer Res. 2007;67:6022–5.
47. Mottet N, Peneau M, Mazeron J-J, Molinie V, Richaud P. Addition of radiotherapy to long term androgen deprivation in locally advanced prostate cancer: an open randomised phase 3 trial. Eur Urol. 2012;62:213–9.
48. Mottet N, Bellmunt J, Briers E, et al. members of the EAU – ESTRO – SIOG Prostate Cancer Guidelines Panel. EAU – ESTRO – SIOG guidelines on prostate cancer. Edn. Presented at the EAU Annual Congress Munich 2016. EAU Guidelines Office, Arnhem; 2016. ISBN 978-90-79754-98-4. https://uroweb.org/guideline/prostate-cancer/.
49. Nabid A, Carrier N, Martin AG, et al. High-risk prostate cancer treated with pelvic radiotherapy and 36 months versus 18 months of androgen blockade. Results of a phase III randomized study. J Clin Oncol. 2013;31:(suppl 6; abstr 3).
50. Nguyen PL, Alibhai SMH, Basaria S, et al. Adverse effects of androgen deprivation therapy and strategies to mitigate them. Eur Urol. 2015;67:825–36.
51. Parmar H, Philipps RH, Lightman SL, Edwards L, Allen L, Schally AV. Randomised controlled study of orchidectomy vs long-acting D-Trp-6-LHRH microcapsules in advanced prostatic carcinoma. Lancet. 1985;2:1201–5.
52. Petrylak DP, Tangen CM, Hussain MH, et al. Docetaxel and estramustine compared with mitoxantrone and prednisone for advanced refractory prostate cancer. N Engl J Med. 2004;351:1513–20.
53. Pilepich MV, Winter K, Lawton CA, et al. Androgen suppression adjuvant to definitive radiotherapy in prostate carcinoma – long-term results of phase III RTOG 85–31. Int J Radiat Oncol Biol Phys. 2005;61:1285–90.
54. Pisansky TM, Hunt D, Gomella LG, et al. Duration of androgen suppression before radiotherapy for localized prostate cancer: Radiation Therapy Oncology Group randomized clinical trial 9910. J Clin Oncol. 2015;33:332–9.
55. Pommier P, Chabaud S, Lagrange JL, et al. Is there a role for pelvic irradiation in localized prostate adenocarcinoma? Preliminary results of GETUG-01. J Clin Oncol. 2007;25:5366–73.
56. Potosky AL, Knopf K, Clegg LX, et al. Quality-of-life outcomes after primary androgen deprivation therapy: results from the Prostate Cancer Outcomes Study. J Clin Oncol. 2001;19:3750–7.
57. Ryan CJ, Smith MR, de Bono JS, et al. Abiraterone in metastatic prostate cancer without previous chemotherapy. N Engl J Med. 2013;368:138–48.
58. Roach 3rd M, Bae K, Speight J, et al. Short-term neoadjuvant androgen deprivation therapy and external-beam radiotherapy for locally advanced prostate cancer: long-term results of RTOG 86–10. J Clin Oncol. 2008;26:585–91.
59. Sandler HM, et al. J Clin Oncol. 2015;33:(15S).
60. Scher HI, Fizazi K, Saad F, et al. Increased survival with enzalutamide in proste cancer after chemotherapy. N Engl J Med. 2012;367:1187–97.
61. Schiff PB, Fant J, Horwitz SB. Promotion of microtubule assembly in vitro by taxol. Nature. 1979;277:665–7.
62. Shahinian VB, Kuo YF, Freeman JL, Goodwin JS. Risk of fracture after androgen deprivation for prostate cancer. N Engl J Med. 2007;352:154–64.
63. Smith MR, Bae K, Efstathiou JA, et al. Diabetes and mortality in men with locally advanced prostate cancer. J Clin Oncol. 2008;26:4333–9.
64. Smith MR, Lee H, McGovern F, et al. Metabolic changes during gonadotrophin-releasing hormone agonist therapy for prostate cancer. Differences from the classic metabolic syndrome. Cancer. 2008;112:2188–94.
65. Smith MR, Egerdie B, Hernandez Toriz N, et al. Denosumab in men receiving androgen-deprivation therapy for prostate cancer. N Engl J Med. 2009;361:745–55.
66. Tannock IF, de Wit R, Berry WR, et al. Docetaxel plus prednisone or mitoxantrone plus prednisone for advanced prostate cancer. N Engl J Med. 2004;351:1502–12.
67. Tran E, Paquette M, PicklesT et al. Population-based validation of a policy change to use long-term androgen deprivation therapy for cT3-4 prostate cancer: impact of the EORTC22863 and RTOG 85-31 and 92-02 trials. Radioth Oncol, 2013;107(3):366–71.
68. Tyrell CJ, Payne H, See WA, et al. Bicalutamide ('Casodex') 150 mg as adjuvant to radiotherapy in patients with localised or locally advanced prostate cancer:results from the randomised early prostate cancer programme. Radiat Oncol. 2005;76:4–10.
69. Valicenti RK, Kwounghwa B, Michalski J, et al. Does hormone therapy reduce disease recurrence in prostate cancer patienst receiving dose-escalated radiation therapy? An analysis of Radiation Therapy Oncology Group 94–06. Int J Radiat Oncol Biol Phys. 2011;79:1323–2912.

70. Viani GA, Stefano EJ, Afonso SL. Higher-than-conventional radiation doses in localized prostate cancer treatment: a meta-analysis of randomized, controlled trials. Int J Radiat Oncol Biol Phys. 2009;74(5):1405–18.
71. Widmark A, Klepp O, Solberg A, et al. Endocrine treatment, with or without radiotherapy, in locally advanced prostate cancer (SPCG-7/SFUO-3): an open randomised phase III trial. Lancet. 2009;373:301–30.
72. Zietman AL, Prince EA, Nakfoor BM, Park JJ. Androgen deprivation and radiation therapy: sequencing studies using the Shionogi in vivo tumor system. Int J Radiat Oncol Biol Phys. 1997;38:1067–70.
73. Zapatero A, Valcarcel F, Calvo FA, et al. Risk-adapted androgen deprivation and escalated three-dimensional conformal radiotherapy for prostate cancer: does radiation dose influence outcome of patients treated with adjuvant androgen deprivation? A GICOR study. J Clin Oncol. 2005;23:6561–8.
74. Zapatero A, Guerrero A, Maldonado X, et al. High-dose radiotherapy with short-term or long term androgen deprivation in localized prostate cancer (DART01/05 GICOR): a randomized, controlled, phase 3 trial. Lancet Oncol. 2015;16:320–7.

Postoperative Irradiation: Immediate or Early Delayed?

Dirk Bottke, Detlef Bartkowiak, and Thomas Wiegel

1 Introduction

For patients with localized prostate cancer, radical prostatectomy (RP) and external-beam radiation therapy (RT) enable a 10-year overall survival of 83 % and 89 %, respectively [46]. Following RP, serum prostate-specific antigen (PSA) should become undetectable within 4–6 weeks, as half-life is approximately 2–3 days [89]. Persistent PSA levels indicate residual prostatic tissue, either malignant or benign (e.g. benign prostatic hyperplasia).

A PSA increase of ≥0.2 ng/ml is a common definition of progression of disease following RP [38, 105]. Vital tumor tissue has been found in biopsies form the urethrovesical anastomosis in 35–55 % of all patients with rising PSA after RP without clinical correlates suggestive of recurrent tumor [80]. In these cases, PSA levels predate clinically evident disease and do correlate well with disease progression.

After RP, approximately 15–25 % of the patients experience recurrence [90]. Numerous models are available to predict the probability of relapse [28, 79, 99]. With adverse risk factors such as high baseline levels of PSA, extraprostatic extension, positive surgical margins (R1), and Gleason score ≥8, the 10-year biochemical recurrence rate may grow to 75 % [16, 38, 107]. However, biochemical recurrence is a common event even in patients with favorable prognostic factors. The rate of biochemical progression after 7 years for patients with organ confined tumors (pT2) and positive surgical margins is about 25 % [93].

The optimal management of patients with clinical and pathologic features of increased risk for developing a biochemical recurrence remains controversial. Two treatment approaches for the postoperative management of these patients are adjuvant radiation therapy (ART) in men with an undetectable PSA or observation followed by early salvage radiation therapy (SRT) in men with persisting or rising PSA after initial postoperative undetectable values.

The purpose of this chapter is to review the rationale, results, and possible side effects for the different treatment approaches ART and SRT.

D. Bottke (✉)
Department of Radiotherapy and Radiation Oncology, MVZ (Medical Service Center) Klinikum Esslingen GmbH, Hirschlandstraße 97, 73730 Esslingen, Germany
e-mail: d.bottke@klinikum-esslingen.de

D. Bartkowiak • T. Wiegel
Department of Radiation Oncology and Radiotherapy, University Hospital Ulm, Albert-Einstein-Allee 23, 89081 Ulm, Germany
e-mail: detlef.bartkowiak@uniklinik-ulm.de; thomas.wiegel@uniklinik-ulm.de

M. Bolla, H. van Poppel (eds.), *Management of Prostate Cancer*,
DOI 10.1007/978-3-319-42769-0_16

2 Adjuvant Radiation Therapy

2.1 Randomized Clinical Trials

Three randomized prospective trials (SWOG 8794, EORTC 22911, and ARO 96–02) demonstrated an approximately 20 % absolute benefit for biochemical progression-free survival (bNED) after adjuvant radiation therapy compared with a "wait-and-see" policy, mostly for pT3 cN0 or pN0 tumors (Table 1). The greatest benefit (30 % bNED after 5 years) has been demonstrated in patients with pT3 tumors and positive margins [11, 96, 102, 108]. In the meantime, 10-year follow-up data of the EORTC trial and the ARO trial were reported and confirmed these results [12, 106].

In the prospective study of the South Western Oncology Group (SWOG), overall survival was improved from 13.5 years without to 15.2 years with adjuvant radiation therapy [97].

Notably, central pathological review on the EORTC-trial showed that only surgical margin status had an effect on the outcome, such that the treatment benefit in patients with negative margins did not remain significant. The hazard ratio in the group with negative surgical margins was 0.87 ($p=0.601$), compared to 0.38 ($p<0.0001$) in the group with positive surgical margins according to the review pathology. Excluding the patients with a PSA of >0.2 ng/ml after prostatectomy, the hazard ratio for postoperative irradiation was 1.11 ($p=0.740$) and 0.29 ($p<0.0001$) for the patients with negative and positive margins, respectively [102]. This benefit was also seen in the real adjuvant situation, when the PSA was undetectable before the start of radiation therapy [106, 108]. In the trial of the German Cancer Society 159 patients were randomized into the observation and 148 into the ART arm (60 Gy in 30 fractions over 6 weeks). After a median follow-up of nearly 10 years, there was a significant benefit from ART for bNED: 56 % vs. 35 % ($p<0.0001$). In the subgroup of pT3 R1 tumors, this benefit increased from 21 to 30 % [106].

The three randomized studies have used different definitions of biochemical progression: SWOG: PSA >0.4 ng/ml, EORTC: PSA >0.2 ng/ml, ARO: PSA >0.05 ng/ml. Consequently, biochemical recurrences (as an increase of the PSA out of the undetectable range) were detected earlier in the EORTC and the ARO study. This led to apparently worse results in bNED of the ARO study after 5 years, but long term results are quite similar between the three trials (Table 1).

In the ARO study, a pathology review was performed on 85 % of RP specimens of patients to investigate the influence of pathology review on the analysis. There was fair concordance between pathology review and local pathologists for seminal vesicle invasion (pT3c: 91 %; $k=0.76$), surgical margin status (84 %; $k=0.65$), and for extraprostatic extension (pT3a/b: 75 %; $k=0.74$). Agreement was much less for Gleason score (47 %; $k=0.42$), whereby the review pathology resulted in a shift to Gleason score 7. In contrast to the analysis of progression-free survival with local pathology, the multivariate analysis including review pathology revealed positive surgical margins and Gleason score >6 as significant prognostic factors [14].

It is well known that the location, the extent, and the number of positive surgical margins after radical prostatectomy are predictors of biochemical progression after radical prostatectomy. The investigators of the Cleveland Clinic/Ohio found in their retrospective series of 7160 patients treated with radical prostatectomy 1540 patients with positive margins. The 7-year progression-free probability was 60 % in those patients, resulting in a hazard ratio for biochemical recurrence of 2.3 compared with negative margins. There was also an increased risk of biochemical recurrence in patients with multiple vs. solitary positive surgical margins (HR 1.4) and extensive vs. focal positive surgical margins (adjusted HR 1.3) [93]. From the data of the randomized trials mentioned above, these patients with positive margins and pT3-tumors do stand to profit mostly from ART.

In the EORTC trial, when the data of patients with pT2 tumors and positive surgical margins were analyzed, there was a significant benefit of 10-year biochemical progression-free survival rate in the irradiated group (71.4 % versus 46.8 %

Table 1 Overview of randomized trials for adjuvant radiation therapy after radical prostatectomy

Reference	*n*	Inclusion criteria	Randomization	Definition of biochemical recurrence PSA	Median follow-up	Biochemical progression free survival	Overall survival
SWOG 8794 Thompson et al. [96, 97]	431	pT3 cN0 ± involved SM	60-64 Gy ($n = 214$) versus "wait and see" ($n = 211$)	>0.4 ng/ml	152 months	10 years: 53 % vs. 30 % ($p < 0.05$)	10 years: 74 % vs. 66 % $p = 0.023$
EORTC 22911 Bolla et al. [11, 12]	1005	pT3 cN0 ± involved SM pT2 + involved SM	60 Gy ($n = 502$) versus "wait and see" ($n = 503$)	>0.2 ng/ml	127 months	10 years: 60 % vs. 41 % ($p < 0.0001$)	10 years: 77 % vs 81 % $P = 0.20$
ARO 96–02 Wiegel et al. [106, 108]	388	pT3 pN0 ± involved SM PSA post RP undetectable	60 Gy ($n = 148$) versus "wait and see" ($n = 159$)	>0.05 ng/ml(+ confirmation)	112 months	10 years: 56 % vs. 35 % ($p < 0.0001$)	n.a.

n.s. not significant, *PSA* prostate-specific antigen, *SM* surgical margins

in the wait-and-see group) [12]. However, these data come from a subgroup analysis and biochemical progression-free survival was not the primary endpoint of this study. The possible benefit of radiotherapy must be weighed out carefully in consideration of potential late effects as erectile dysfunction (ED).

2.2 Definition of Clinical Target Volume (CTV)

In the EORTC and SWOG trials, radiation was based on 2D treatment planning, where the prostatic fossa was targeted by using large treatment portals. Obviously, precise definition of target volumes was not essential, which is in great contrast to modern radiation treatment techniques such as IMRT. Compared to 2D based planning, IMRT provides significant normal tissue sparing, but also demands exact definition of target volume.

Consideration of the local failure patterns in the post-RP setting is essential for optimal definition of CTV. The most common sites of local relapse proven by biopsy are the vesicourethral anastomosis (VUA) (66 %), followed by the bladder neck (16 %) and retrotrigone area (13 %) [27]. Recently, endorectal magnetic resonance imaging (MRI) was used to detect local relapse patterns following RP in order to further define the optimal CTV [56]. Based on the results of this study, the authors recommended a cylindrical-shaped CTV centered 5 mm posterior and 3 mm inferior to the VUA, concordant also with the previously mentioned pathologic studies.

To address any uncertainties in the definition of CTV, the Radiation Therapy Oncology Group (RTOG) [53], the EORTC Radiation Oncology Group [73] and other cooperative groups [84, 111] have created consensus guidelines for delineation of target volumes for postprostatectomy patients. In the RTOG recommendations, the CTV extends superiorly from the level of the caudal vas deferens remnant (or 3–4 cm superior to the pubic symphysis, whichever is higher) and inferiorly 8–12 mm inferior to VUA. The VUA is defined as the retropubic region that can be visualized one slice below the most inferior urine-containing image of the bladder. Below the superior border of the pubic symphysis, the anterior border is at the posterior aspect of the pubis and extends posteriorly to the rectum. At this level, the lateral border extends to the levator ani muscles. Above the pubic symphysis, the anterior border should encompass the posterior 1–2 cm of the bladder wall and should extend posteriorly to the mesorectal fascia.

2.3 Use of Image-Guidance to Improve Postprostatectomy Prostatic Fossa Localization

In recent years, several innovative methods have been developed to improve localization of the prostatic fossa and minimize daily internal set-up error. Techniques currently utilized in most practices include daily portal imaging with implanted gold fiducial markers [77], daily cone beam or kilovoltage imaging [59], and the use of electromagnetic transponders [21]. Such image-guidance techniques allow for a minimal (7–10 mm) expansion from a CTV to a planning target volume, thereby providing further normal tissue sparing by minimizing RT dose to the rectum and bladder [83].

2.4 Adjuvant RT of Pelvic Lymph Nodes?

The three randomized trials included only patients with cN0 or pN0-disease. The effect of adjuvant RT in node-positive prostate cancer has not yet been prospectively assessed. A retrospective study by Da Pozzo et al. reported a significant positive impact of RT in combination with hormonal therapy (HT) in patients with nodal metastases treated with RP and pelvic lymph node dissection [31]. However, this study was limited by a potential patient selection bias mainly due to its retrospective and unmatched design. In fact, patients treated with adjuvant RT were those affected by more aggressive disease. Therefore, no effect of adjuvant RT on cancer-specific survival was demonstrated on univariate survival analyses. There was significant gain in predictive accuracy when adjuvant RT was included in multivariable models predicting biochemical recurrence-free and cancer-specific survival (gain: 3.3 % and 3 %, respectively; all $p<0.001$).

In a large retrospective series, Briganti et al. assessed the effect of adjuvant RT in node-positive prostate cancer including two homogeneous matched patient cohorts exposed to either adjuvant RT plus HT or adjuvant HT alone after surgery. In this series from Milan and Jacksonville, a total of 703 patients were assessed at a median follow-up of 95 months. Patients were matched for age at surgery, pathologic T stage and Gleason score, number of nodes removed, surgical margin status, and length of follow-up. The overall survival advantage was 19 % in favor of adjuvant radiation therapy plus hormonal treatment compared with hormonal treatment alone. Similarly, higher survival rates associated with the combination of HT plus RT were found when patients were stratified according to the extent of nodal invasion (namely ≤ 2 versus >2 positive nodes; all $p\leq 0.006$) [15].

In 2014 the same working group has published an analysis of 1107 patients with node-positive prostate cancer. After surgery with elective lymph node dissection, the men received either adjuvant HT alone (intended but not confirmed lifelong, $n=721$) or HT plus ART (66.6–70.2 Gy to the prostate bed and 45–50.4 Gy to the pelvic lymph nodes, $n=386$). The median follow-up was 7.1 years. Based on the pathologic T stage, Gleason score, number of positive lymph nodes, and surgical margin status, five risk groups were defined. In the intermediate-risk group, there was an overall survival advantage from combined therapy of 6 % and 18 %, after 5 and 8 years, respectively. In the high-risk group, the figures were 6 % and 20 %, respectively, in favor of ART plus HT compared with HT alone. In multivariate analysis, two groups had a significant benefit from additional ART, namely: (1) patients with ≤ 2 positive lymph node, Gleason score 7–10, pT3b/pT4 stage, or positive surgical margins; and (2) patients with 3–4 positive lymph nodes irrespective of other features [1]. Because of the retrospective nature of this series with no standardized definition of target volumes, radiation dose, and duration of HT, these results should be interpreted with caution. However, they provide support for this treatment in selected cases, but should be validated in prospective clinical trials.

2.5 Additional Use of Hormone Therapy to ART

It is now clearly established that the standard nonoperative management for patients with locally advanced prostate adenocarcinoma includes long-term hormone therapy. Two cooperative group trials, RTOG 96–02 and EORTC 22961, have demonstrated an overall survival advantage if these patients, and specifically those with additional high-risk factors like Gleason score 8–10, are treated for 2–3 years with hormone therapy [10, 41]. It remains unknown whether men with high risk, node-negative prostate adenocarcinoma initially treated with RP and pelvic lymph node dissection benefit from additional adjuvant hormone therapy. The primary rationale for the use of hormone therapy post-RP is to: (1) improve local control by eradicating disease in a hypoxic scar that may be radioresistant; (2) address micrometastatic disease which may have spread to the lymph nodes or distant sites; and (3) alter PSA kinetics in patients who will eventually relapse [37, 44, 74].

Previous studies have indicated a potential benefit from combination therapy for men at high risk of recurrence. A secondary analysis of Radiation Therapy Oncology Group (RTOG) 85–31, a phase III trial comparing standard external beam RT plus immediate ADT versus RT alone for patients with nonbulky prostate cancer, found improved biochemical control in patients who received combination therapy as compared to men treated with RT alone [29]. With a median follow-up of 5 years, the progression-free survival for men treated with combination therapy was estimated to be 65 % as compared to 42 % for men treated with RT alone ($p=0.002$). Similar results were seen in a retrospective study performed at Stanford University [48].

Two further randomized trials into HT-RT combination therapy, RTOG-P-0011 and EORTC 22043, closed prematurely because of poor recruitment.

The ongoing RADICALS trial will address the question of duration of hormone therapy combined with ART [68].

3 Salvage Radiation Therapy

Salvage radiation therapy (SRT) should be considered for men presenting with persistent PSA after prostatectomy or showing an increase of PSA levels after initial postoperative undetectable values [5, 9, 18, 20, 70, 85, 92, 93, 104].

It remains uncertain whether a PSA increase after RP indicates isolated local disease, distant metastatic progression, or both [80]. Therefore, the best treatment for recurrent prostate cancer in patients with increasing or persisting PSA without clinical evidence of disease still remains controversial. On the other hand, only RT can offer the chance of cure to patients with truly localized malignant disease after RP.

There are indicators for a higher likelihood of local recurrence, e.g. slow PSA rise (PSA doubling time ≥12 months), more than 1 year between RP and the detection of PSA in the serum, Gleason score <7, and negative surgical margins [72]. On the other hand, there are also indicators suggesting metastatic disease such as short PSA doubling time (<12 months) or Gleason score at RP from 8 to 10 [70, 104]. Some authors tried to define combinations of risk factors. For example, patients with a PSA <1 ng/ml before RT, and pre-RP Gleason score <7, and a long PSA doubling time after progression have a high risk of local disease [92]. A predictive model for the outcome of RT for PSA progression after RP has been proposed and validated [58, 91]. Assuming a local nature of the underlying disease, SRT of the prostatic bed has widely been used to treat patients in the absence of biopsy-proven local recurrence. An established standard is conformal radiotherapy to the prostatic fossa with a dose of about 66 Gy, aiming to irradiate the presumed local recurrence and hence to reduce the risk of a "second wave of metastasis" leading to clinical progression of disease [26, 38, 105]. In the light of the well-known problems in detecting local recurrence in the prostatic bed, radiotherapy to the prostatic fossa is one of the rare therapies in which most radiation oncologists irradiate without a histologic proof of tumor recurrence.

3.1 Role of Investigations in Case of Persisting/Rising PSA

Once biochemical failure has been diagnosed, it is essential to distinguish between local recurrence and systemic metastases in order to plan the best therapeutic approach. For this reason, there is a strong need for imaging techniques which may be able to recognize small lesions and to identify their nature (persistent or recurrent neoplastic tissue, healthy residual glandular tissue, and granulation tissue or fibrosis). These techniques should be able to detect residual or recurrent disease when the PSA serum level is very low (less than 1 ng/ml) in order to deliver the more relevant therapeutic option as early as possible.

Currently, transrectal ultrasound (TRUS) has neither good sensitivity nor good specificity in detecting early recurrent cancer [51]. Scattoni et al. showed that TRUS-guided biopsy to detect local relapse after RP has a limited sensitivity (25–54 %) when the PSA serum value is less than 1 ng/ml [76]. TRUS-guided biopsy of the post-prostatectomy fossa is not recommended by EAU-guidelines in patients with PSA serum level less than 1 ng/ml [38].

Over the last few years, technological innovations have allowed the development of superimposed imaging, which links anatomic, functional, and biological information together. Magnetic resonance imaging (MRI) and positron emission computed tomography (PET/CT) have proven to be useful tools in the early diagnosis of prostate cancer recurrence.

The advantages of MRI over TRUS are its superior soft-tissue resolution and its ability to cover the entire postprostatectomy fossa and reveal recurrences that are located beyond the region routinely imaged on ultrasound. The combination of an external and an endorectal coil improves the ability to detect local recurrence of prostate cancer [42]. The anatomic detail and wide coverage of the pelvis by MRI facilitates its increasing use in directing salvage radiation therapy when a recurrence is demonstrated [56]. Additionally, as pelvic lymphadenopathy and osseous metastases are routinely evaluated with MRI, the most common early metastatic sites of prostate cancer are covered by this method.

The reported sensitivity and the specificity of MRI for depicting local recurrences by experienced investigators in 82 patients who underwent prostatectomy were 87 % and 78 %, respectively. PSA levels at MR imaging in patients with clinically proved recurrences ranged from undetectable to 10 ng/ml (mean, 2.18 ng/ml) [78].

Panebianco et al. found that a combined technique of proton magnetic resonance spectroscopic imaging (1H-MRSI) and dynamic contrast-enhanced magnetic resonance imaging (DCE-MRI) at 3 Tesla was a valid tool to detect locoregional relapse. It was more accurate than Cholin-PET/CT in the identification of small lesions in 84 men with low biochemical progression after RP (PSA serum values ranging from 0.2 to 2 ng/ml) [67].

Various targets have been addressed by molecular imaging to improve the detection of recurrent prostate cancer. For PET imaging, mainly ^{11}C- and ^{18}F-labeled choline derivates have been used in the past [39, 49]. However, especially in patients with PSA values below 3 ng/ml, the detection rate is only 40–60 % [7, 23, 49]. Recently, molecular probes have been developed to target for example the gastrin-releasing peptide receptor or the prostate-specific membrane antigen (PSMA), [94, 110]. PSMA is a membrane-bound enzyme with significantly elevated expression in prostate cancer cells in comparison to benign prostatic tissue [86]. A newly developed compound (coupling ^{68}Ga via the chelator HBED-CC to the extracellular PSMA ligand Glu-NH-CO-NH-Lys) demonstrated a high specificity for PSMA expressing tumor cells as well as high and specific uptake in a mouse model [32]. A first preliminary study in prostate cancer patients revealed a higher image contrast and detection rate with ^{68}Ga-PSMA- than with ^{18}F-choline-PET/CT [3]. Afshar-Oromieh et al. performed a retrospective analysis in 319 patients with different primary treatment including 226 patients with recurrent prostate cancer after radical prostatectomy. In 82.8 % of the patients at least one lesion indicative of prostate cancer was detected. A lesion-based analysis of sensitivity, specificity, negative predictive value, and positive predictive value revealed values of 76.6 %, 100 %, 91.4 %, and 100 %, respectively. Of 116 patients available for follow-up, 50 received local therapy after ^{68}Ga-PSMA PET/CT [2]. Eiber et al. investigated the detection rate of ^{68}Ga-PSMA PET/CT in 248 patients with biochemical recurrence after radical prostatectomy. Median PSA level was 1.99 ng/ml. The detection rates were 96.8 %, 93.0 %, 72.7 %, and 57.9 % for PSA levels of ≥2, 1 to <2, 0.5 to <1, and 0.2 to <0.5 ng/ml, respectively. With higher Gleason score (≤7 versus ≥8), detection efficacy was significantly increased ($p=0.019$) [33]. ^{68}Ga-PSMA ligand PET/CT shows substantially higher detection efficacy than reported for other tracers. Most importantly, it reveals a high number of positive findings in the clinically important range of low PSA values (<0.5 ng/ml). However, case numbers in that PSA range are very low in all reports [2, 19, 33, 40].

3.2 Results of Salvage Radiotherapy/ Prognostic Factors

So far, there are no published data available from randomized trials on SRT after RP and the question of whether or not SRT can improve survival is not answered, yet. Numerous retrospective studies focus on biochemical recurrence and there is clear evidence for an advantage from early SRT for that endpoint. However, the definition of "early" varies throughout the literature. European guidelines recommend SRT at a PSA <0.5 ng/ml, AUA/ASTRO suggest a threshold at 0.2 ng/ml, and even lower values (down to 0.05 ng/ml) have been proposed [38, 55, 98]).

Stevenson et al. reported the results of a multi-institutional cohort of 1540 patients. These patients received SRT with a median dose of 66 Gy. Median follow-up was 53 months. A six-years biochemical progression-free survival-rate of 48 % (95 % CI, 40–56 %) could be achieved when the PSA was <0.5 ng/ml compared with only 18 %, when the preradiation therapy PSA was >1.5 ng/ml. In the whole series, the 6-year progression-free survival-rate was 32 % (95 % CI, 28–35 %) [91]. The authors identified several prognostic factors that were associated with a poor response to RT including Gleason score of 8–10, pre-SRT PSA >2 ng/ml, negative surgical margins, postoperative PSA doubling time <10 months and seminal vesicle invasion. Patients without these adverse features had a 6 year progression-free survival of 69 %. Also, some subsets of patients with Gleason score 8–10 would benefit from salvage radiation therapy if the pretreatment PSA was <2.0 ng/ml, surgical margins were positive and PSA doubling time was >10 months [91].

Briganti et al. reported on a multi-institutional cohort of 472 node-negative patients who experienced biochemical recurrence after RP. All patients received SRT at a PSA <0.5 ng/ml. In univariate analysis, pT-stage, Gleason score and margin status were significant predictors of progression. In multivariable Cox regression, also the pre-SRT PSA was a significant predictor (all parameters with $p<0.04$). The study aimed to develop a nomogram predictive for biochemical progression. Therefore, the pre-SRT PSA was a continuous variable with no discrete value to differentiate low versus high risk. Positive margins were a high-risk factor in that data set [17].

Lohm et al. reported the results of 151 patients receiving SRT at a PSA <0.2 ng/ml. After a median follow-up of 82 months, a biochemical progression was diagnosed in 83 patients (55 %). Multivariate analysis confirmed the impact of pre-SRT PSA level, Gleason score, and PSADT on biochemical progression-free survival and tumor stage on overall survival. The margin status was no significant risk factor at all [52]. Also, in a cohort of 409 men who had SRT at higher PSA levels (range 0.3–1.7 ng/ml), surgical margins did not reach significance ($p=0.2$) in the regression model for biochemical failure [43].

Trock et al. conducted a retrospective analysis of a cohort of 675 patients undergoing RP from 1982 to 2004. Median follow-up was 9 years since RP and 6 years since SRT. They show a benefit for prostate cancer-specific survival after SRT (with or without additional hormone treatment) compared with sole androgen deprivation. Particularly, there was an advantage for patients who achieved a post-SRT PSA <0.2 ng/ml (the undetectable range in that study) and for men with a short PSA doubling time (<6 months) at recurrence. However, other established prognostic features such as pT stage or Gleason score failed statistical significance for overall survival [101].

Chang et al. determined the PSA of 164 prostatectomy patients 4 months after the administration of SRT for recurrent prostate cancer. The median follow-up was 53.4 months. If at that time the PSA was ≥0.2 ng/ml or was incompletely reduced (≥45 % of the pre-SRT PSA), then the 5-year rates of clinical recurrence were significantly increased [24].

Jackson et al. identified men with a detectable nadir (0.1–0.2 ng/ml) within 6 months after SRT as a high-risk group regarding biochemical failure, distant metastases, prostate cancer-specific death, and overall mortality. A total of 448 patients (15 % seminal vesicle invasion, 50 % extracapsular extension, 46 % positive margins, 2 % positive lymph nodes) had been followed up for median 64 months. Clinical/pathological risk factors again failed statistical significance in Cox regression analysis when the post-SRT nadir was included [43]. A lower pre-SRT PSA was significantly related with achieving an undetectable post-SRT nadir. The median pre-SRT level was 0.5 ng/ml in responders and 0.7 ng/ml in nonresponders and a PSA maximum of 18 ng/ml. In multivariable analysis, the pre-SRT PSA was a significant parameter for biochemical recurrence ($p=0.005$), metastasis ($p=0.05$) and borderline significant even for OS ($p=0.07$). In a retrospective analysis of 306 patients, the application of SRT at a PSA <0.2 ng/ml correlated significantly with achieving a post-SRT PSA nadir <0.1 ng/ml and with improved freedom from progression (median follow-up 7.2 years). The post-SRT nadir <0.1 ng/ml correlated significantly with less recurrence and with better overall survival [5].

There is now strong evidence that achieving a post-SRT PSA nadir <0.1 ng/ml enables a better overall survival in long-term follow-up. The association of the pre-SRT PSA with post-SRT nadir indicates indirectly that selected patients may have a significant survival benefit from SRT. Moreover, patients whose post-SRT PSA declines to the undetectable range may not need additional hormonal treatment before secondary progress. As a hypothesis, this requires confirmation/validation in the framework of prospective clinical trial (Table 2).

3.3 Total Dose of Salvage Radiotherapy

With reference to the three randomized studies, a dose of 60–64 Gy for adjuvant RT is consensus in the guidelines [38, 105]. The situation is less clear for salvage RT. To avoid radiation toxicity, most SRT studies do not exceed 70 Gy. In the guidelines, total doses of "at least 66 Gy" are recommended [38, 105]. However, some recently published series demonstrated a better outcome with higher total doses [9, 47, 85]. Bernard et al. investigated 364 men with salvage radiation therapy after radical prostatectomy after a median follow-up of 6.0 years. They defined three dose groups (low, <64.8 Gy; moderate, 64.8–66.6 Gy; high, >66.6 Gy). In multivariate analysis, they found that compared with the high dose level, there was a decreased bNED for patients treated with the low dose level (HR 0.60) [9]. This was similar to the results published by Siegmann et al. from the group in Berlin and Ulm. In their retrospective series including 301 patients, 234 received 66.6 Gy while 67 patients with a PSA decrease during salvage radiation therapy were selected and irradiated up to 70.2 Gy. In the multivariate analysis the total dose was a significant predictor of reduced risk of biochemical progression ($p = 0.017$) [85].

The need for a higher irradiation dose remains uncertain; nevertheless it seems justified especially in patients with histologically confirmed local recurrence after radical prostatectomy.

The SAKK 09/10 trial randomized 344 patients without evidence of residual disease between 2011 and 2014 to receive SRT at 70 Gy ($n = 175$) or 64 Gy ($n = 169$). In 44 % of the patients, the RT was applied using a 3D-conformal approach and in 56 % of the patients using an IMRT technique. The primary endpoint was freedom from biochemical failure. The trial was closed for accrual after it met its accrual goal of 350 patients.

A first analysis of the trial reported acute toxicity rates and early quality of life. There was no significant difference in acute genitourinary and gastrointestinal toxicity rates between both arms. Generally, changes in health related quality of life were minor; however, there was a relevant worsening of urinary symptoms in the 70 Gy arm. There was no significant difference in acute toxicity associated with RT technique [35]. The first randomized prospective data regarding freedom from biochemical recurrence and late toxicity are awaited in 2017.

3.4 RT of Pelvic Lymph Nodes?

An important, but unsolved question is the value of an additional whole pelvic irradiation compared with prostate bed irradiation alone. Spioto from the Stanford University reported on 160 patients who underwent adjuvant or salvage radiation therapy, out of which 87 had short course total androgen suppression. A total of 114 patients were considered at high risk of lymph node involvement although cN0 (Gleason score >8, preoperative PSA level >20 ng/ml, seminal vesicle involvement); 72 underwent whole pelvic radiation therapy and 42 underwent prostate bed radiation therapy. The median follow up was >5 years. Limited- to high-risk patients, there was a superior bNED of whole pelvic radiation therapy compared with prostate bed radiation

Table 2 Results for salvage radiotherapy after biochemical recurrence from selected studies

Investigator	Patients (n)	Median PSA (ng/ml)	Median dose (Gy)	bNED
Anscher et al. [4]	89	1.4	66	50 % at 4 years
Bartkowiak et al. [5]	306	0.298	66.6	68 % at 7 years (pre-SRT PSA <0.2 ng/ml) 40 % at 7 years (pre-SRT PSA ≥0.2 ng/ml)
Bernard et al. [9]	364	0.6	64.8	61 % at 5 years
Briganti et al. [18]	390	0.22	66	82 % at 5 years
Buskirk et al. [20]	368	0.7	64.8	35 % at 8 years
Lohm et al. [52]	151	0.34	66.6	40 % at 7 years
Neuhof et al. [61]	171	1.1	60–66	35 % at 5 years
Ost et al. [66]	136	0.8	76	56 % at 5 years
Pazona et al. [70]	307	0.8	64	40 % at 5 years; 25 % at 10 years
Pisansky et al. [72]	166	0.9	64	46 % at 5 years
Siegmann et al. [85]	301	0.28	66.6 vs. 70.2	65 % at 2 years (66.6 Gy) 88 % at 2 years (70.2 Gy)
Stephenson et al. [92]	501	0.72	64.8	45 % at 6 years
Stephenson et al. [91]	1540	1.1	64.8	32 % at 6 years
Ward et al. [104]	211	0.6	64	34 % at 10 years
Wiegel et al. [109]	162	0.33	66.6	54 % at 3.5 years
Wiegel et al. [107]	74	0.6	66	63 % at 10 years (clinical relapse-free)

therapy (5-year rate 47 % vs. 21 %, $p<0.05$) [88]. While these data have to be confirmed in a prospective trial, whole pelvic radiation therapy combined with modern delivery techniques like IMRT can be offered as a promising option for high-risk patients [38, 105].

3.5 Additional Use of Hormone Therapy to SRT

Interesting retrospective data have been reported from the Mayo Clinic and from the University of Michigan [25, 87]. They raise the question of the efficacy of an additional androgen deprivation during and after SRT. Choo and coworkers reported on a prospective pilot study with 75 patients treated with SRT + 2-year androgen deprivation. With a median follow-up from SRT of 6.5 years, all patients achieved an initially complete PSA response (<0.2 ng/ml). Relapse-free survival rate at 7 years was 78 % of the whole population [25]. A group of the University of Michigan treated all together 630 men for salvage indications after RP. In this group, 66 % had high-risk factors. The mean RT dose was 68 Gy and 24 % of all patients received concurrent androgen deprivation. The median ADT duration for these patients was 11 months. With a median follow-up of 3 years, the concurrent androgen deprivation was shown to be a significant independent predictor of progression-free survival in the high-risk group ($p<0.05$) [87]. Therefore, it seems attractive to treat high-risk patients with SRT and an additional androgen deprivation. The optimal duration of this androgen deprivation therapy remains uncertain.

RTOG 96–01 is a randomized, multicenter phase III trial, designed to compare anti-androgen therapy (bicalutamide monotherapy 150 mg/d) plus SRT ($n=384$) with a placebo plus SRT alone ($n=377$) in men with pT3/pT2 R1 N0 M0 prostate cancer who have an elevated PSA after surgery. The primary end-point is overall survival. The results presented at the 2015 Annual Meeting of the American Society for Radiation

Oncology (ASTRO) reveal that the addition of anti-androgen therapy to SRT reduces prostate cancer death and the development of metastatic prostate cancer without increasing radiation toxicity. With a median follow-up of 12.6 years, the actuarial overall survival at 10 years was 82 % for the RT plus HT arm and 78 % for the RT plus placebo arm ($p=0.036$). The 12-year incidence of prostate cancer-related deaths was 2.3 % for the RT plus HT arm, compared with 7.5 % for the RT plus placebo arm. Late bladder and bowel toxicity were low and similar in both groups, whereas 70 % of men in the RT plus HT arm reported swelling of the breasts, compared with 11 % in the RT plus placebo arm [82].

The subgroup analysis on overall survival and time to metastatic prostate cancer presented at the 2016 Genitourinary Cancers Symposium indicates that patients most likely to benefit have Gleason score 7 or 8–10, pre-SRT PSA value of 0.7–4 ng/ml, and positive surgical margins RP [81].

Carrie et al. presented at the 2015 ASCO Annual Meeting the first results of the GETUG-AFU 16. The phase III randomized trial assessed the efficacy of RT alone versus RT+HT on progression-free survival for patients with biochemical recurrence after RP. From 2006 to 2010, 743 patients were randomized to RT alone (66 Gy on prostate bed±pelvic irradiation according to pN status and risk of initial node involvement) or RT+goserelin, for 6 months. With a median follow-up of 63.1 months, 216 cases of progression were noted (138 in RT versus 78 in RT+HT). The intent to treat analysis showed an improved 5-year PFS of 62.1 % versus 79.6 % for RT and RT+HT, respectively ($p<0.0001$). The 5-year overall survival was 94.8 % for RT versus 96.2 % for RT+HT ($p=0.18$). Acute toxicities occurred more frequently in RT+HT arm (89 % versus 79 %). No difference was found in grade 3 acute toxicities and late toxicities [22].

So far, the current data of both studies are published in abstract form only. Until final publication there is no reason to give an additional hormone therapy to all patients. Until now, the recommended type of hormone therapy is also unclear Nevertheless, experience shows that bicalutamide is usually better tolerated than LHRH agonists like Goserelin.

RTOG 0534 is investigating the benefit of short-term ADT as well as pelvic nodal irradiation in the SRT setting. In this trial, patients will be randomized to one of three treatment arms: (1) prostatic fossa irradiation alone; (2) prostatic fossa+whole pelvic irradiation alone; or (3) prostatic fossa+whole pelvic irradiation with short-term ADT. The primary endpoints of this study are to determine: (1) whether the addition of short-term androgen deprivation therapy to prostatic fossa irradiation improves freedom from progression for 5 years over that of prostatic fossa irradiation therapy alone; and (2) whether short-term ADT and whole pelvic RT improve freedom from progression over that of short-term ADT and prostatic fossa irradiation alone for men treated with SRT. The target of accrual for this trial was 1764 patients and, to date, the study is closed to accrual.

4 Radiation Therapy Techniques

Traditionally, a 4-field technique has been used. The conventional treatment volumes were typically very generous, being approximately 10×10 cm in the anterior-posterior fields with the inferior border at the ischial tuberosities. The lateral fields extended from the anterior aspect of the pubic symphysis and split the rectum posteriorly.

After the introduction of modern 3D CRT techniques, a major controversy about the target volumes of postoperative radiation therapy started. Critical evaluation of target volume delineation by different authors and participation of experienced radiation oncologist showed that variations up to 65 % maybe present even in cases of adjuvant or salvage radiation restricted to the prostatic fossa [54].

In 3D CRT, the target volume should include the bladder neck (pulled into the prostate bed), the periprostatic tissue and surgical clips, and the seminal vesicle bed (including any seminal vesicle remnants if present) if initially involved or as a confirmed site of recurrence. Some anatomic landmarks are useful in maximizing/optimizing coverage of the surgical bed: Inferiorly, the vesical–urethral anastomosis should be included. This anastomosis is the most frequent area of positive prostate bed biopsies. By placing the inferior field edge at the top of the bulb of the penis (best seen on magnetic resonance imaging) and adding a margin for uncertainties, there should be adequate coverage. Laterally, the field should extend to about the medial aspect of each obturator internus muscle. Although the rectum is a landmark posteriorly, the relative position of the rectum appears to shift after the prostate is removed as well as during radiation therapy [34, 60]. For this reason, a generous margin from CTV to PTV posteriorly is recommended, such as setting an 8-mm margin with image guidance [69]. The superior margin is more subjective. The former prostate can extend above the pubic symphysis, but it is recommended that the anterior part of the bladder be avoided at this level because this is the least likely area for extracapsular extension and involved margins. Treatment of the seminal vesicle bed, lying behind the bladder, is advised for pT3b tumors. If vascular clips were used at prostatectomy, they are likely to be seen in this region. The level of the posterior-superior clinical target volume is somewhat subjective and should be guided by the extent of disease at the prostate base and by whether or not the seminal vesicles were involved.

The recommendations of the RTOG [53] and of the EORTC [73] are very helpful in delineation of the target volume for irradiation of the prostatic fossa. However, the definition of the target volumes remains difficult. Recently, a study assessed the interobserver agreement of prostate bed delineation after radical prostatectomy as proposed by the EORTC guidelines. Six observers delineated the prostate bed (PB) and the original seminal vesicle position (SV) of ten patients. Contours were then compared for agreement between observers. The mean volume of 100 % agreement was only 5.0 (±3.3) ml for the PB and 0.9 (±1.5) ml for the SV, whereas the mean union of all contours (±1 SD) was 41.1 (±11.8) ml and 25.3 (±13.4) ml, respectively. The overall standard deviation of the outer margins of the PB ranged from 4.6 to 7.0 mm [64].

Furthermore, Croke et al. showed that none of the guidelines adequately covered the prostate bed and/or gross tumor based on preoperative MRI in a nonselect group of 20 patients. On average, 38 % of the prostate volume and 41 % of gross tumor volume on preoperative MRI were not included in the CTV. This suggests that improved target delineation could potentially improve outcomes [30].

Wang et al. recently evaluated regions of local recurrence after RP in relation to whether these would have been covered using the RTOG guidelines. They reported that the RTOG CTV contours did not appear adequate posterolaterally near the rectum/mesorectal fascia and inferiorly at the posterior urogenital diaphragm. Use of the CTV MRI should improve coverage of such regions [103].

Given the potential for late toxicity after postoperative radiation therapy, the use of IMRT is appealing [6]. As with 3D CRT, a generous definition of the prostate bed target volume and adequate margins to account for target motion (especially due to the variation in rectal and bladder filling) and setup uncertainties are critical. The theoretical advantages of IMRT over conventional 3D CRT are its geometrically steep dose falloff and improved conformity with irregularly shaped targets (e.g., the superior-posterior aspect of the postoperative field). A greater sparing of the superior-anterior part of the bladder, the posterior part of the rectum, and the penile bulb can be achieved using IMRT, despite using the same target volume definition [71]. The comparison of a 5-field IMRT and a rotational IMRT (for example "Rapid Arc") technique is displayed in Fig. 1.

For optimization of the margins needed for delivery of IMRT, IGRT remains a helpful tool. Ost and co-workers from Gent University demonstrated a significant reduction of acute toxicity using patient positioning with cone beam CT [63]. Sandhu et al. from the University of California used IGRT in patients undergoing postprostatectomy irradiation. Prostate bed localization was done using image guidance

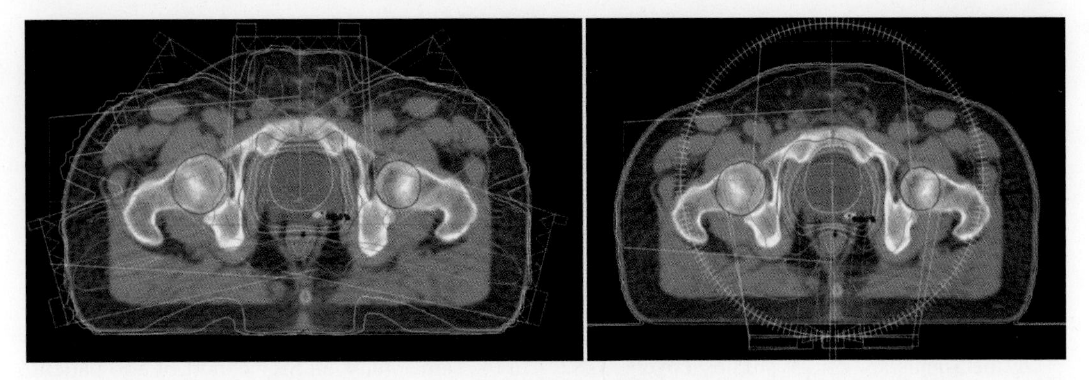

Fig. 1 5-field-IMRT treatment plan (*left*) compared with rotational IMRT (*right*) for prostatic bed irradiation

based on surgical clips, relative to the reference isocenter on the digitally reconstructed radiographs made during radiation therapy planning. They assumed that surgical clips are a useful surrogate for the prostate bed and therefore measured daily shifts of the position of the surgical clips in 3 dimensions. With an average (standard deviation) prostate bed motion in anterior-posterior, superior-inferior, and left-right directions of 2.7 mm (2.1), 2.4 mm (2.1), and 1.0 mm (1.7), respectively, the majority of the patients experienced only grade 1 side effects. The authors recommended daily IGRT for accurate target localization [75]. However the most efficient approach for IGRT during the 6–8 weeks of irradiation remains controversial [50, 77].

5 Side Effects and Toxicity of ART/SRT

The three randomized clinical trials discussed above included prospective collection of data on gastrointestinal and genitourinary toxicity in the two cohorts (ART vs. observation). However, in the EORTC and SWOG trials, radiation was based on 2D treatment planning which did not enable normal tissue sparing to nowadays state-of-the-art. The toxicity data of both studies are therefore no longer relevant.

In contrast, modern 3D based radiation treatment techniques such as IMRT allow for minimization of dose to the rectum and bladder.

A total of 217 patients from the SWOG therapeutic trial patients were eligible and registered to a health-related quality of life (HRQL) study. Patients completed the SWOG Quality of Life Questionnaire at baseline, 6 weeks, 6 months, and annually for 5 years. Patients receiving adjuvant RT reported worse bowel function (through approximately 2 years) and worse urinary function. There were no statistically significant differences for ED. Global HRQL was initially worse for the ART arm but improved over time and was better at the end of the period than the global HRQL reported for RP alone [57].

Unlike the SWOG trial, the EORTC trial did not assess total urinary incontinence; however, in an interim analysis there was no significant difference concerning urinary incontinence between the two treatment arms [11].

In the German study, which utilized 3D-based radiation treatment planning, the incidence of late grade 3 or higher adverse events was only 0.3 % [106]. One patient in the observation arm developed a urethral stricture, compared to two patients in the ART arm. Urinary incontinence was not assessed in this trial.

A low rate of side effects is of particular importance for a therapy without histologic confirmation. The side effects of SRT have so far been reported to be tolerable. Although in general, side effects tend to be underreported in retrospective analyses, a proportion of <3 % severe late side effects seems to be a realistic estimate. Higher rates of 10 % genitourinary grade 3 complications, namely anastomotic strictures and bladder neck contractures requiring dilatation, reported in a series of 115 patients from the Memorial Sloan-Kettering Cancer Center, need to be interpreted with caution [45]. It may be difficult to differentiate side effects of RT from preexisting disabilities and sequelae of RP. At least equivalent rates of severe genitourinary complications following RP alone have been reported in a SEER data base analysis of 11,522 patients published by the same institution [8].

A meta-analysis of 25 studies covers 3282 patients who received 60–72 (median 65) Gy, largely with older albeit 3D-planned techniques. Model calculations predict the 5 % incidence in both organ systems at 68–69 Gy [62].

In a German cohort of 306 patients, there were too few events to test for a dose–response relationship. However, with the majority of our patients receiving 66.6 Gy, a total rate of 1.3 % grade 3 complications compares favorably with previous studies on conventional 3D-SRT [5].

Goenka et al. reported on 285 patients receiving post-RP SRT. The highest doses were 70–72 Gy in conventional 3D technique ($n = 40$) or IMRT ($n = 165$). Five-year actuarial rates for grade ≥2 GI and GU toxicity were 5.2 % and 17 %, respectively [36]. Ost et al. applied salvage IMRT with 70–79 (median 76) Gy to 136 post-RP patients. Their respective figures were 8 % (GI) and 22 % (GU) [66]. Both studies report with 60 months median follow-up. A longer observation and additional studies may be necessary to judge conclusively on the potential side effects of dose escalation with IMRT. Nevertheless, compared to ART with 60–64 Gy, the rate of side effects of SRT with ≥70 Gy appears to be higher.

6 Adjuvant *Versus* Salvage Radiation Therapy

While prospective randomized trials are underway to compare SRT and ART, several retrospective analyses into that question have been conducted. In a first report, 75 patients receiving ART at a median dose of 60 Gy were compared with 71 patients who had SRT at 70 Gy. Although 49 % of the SRT patients and only 3 % of the ART patients received adjuvant HT, the 5-year post-RT bNED rate was 66 versus 88 % in favor of ART ($p < 0.0008$) [95].

In a case–control analysis, 361 ART patients were compared with 722 non-ART patients, who were selected to match the cases by age, pre-RP PSA, tumor stage, Gleason score, and surgical margin status. While 10-year bNED after ART was significantly improved over non-ART (63 vs. 45 %), there was no difference in overall survival. In the same study, an SRT cohort of 856 patients who were treated after biochemical relapse (median PSA: 0.8 ng/ml) was followed up over a median of 5.9 years. A total of 63 % of the SRT patients achieved an undetectable PSA after SRT and the hazard ratio for local recurrence after SRT was 0.13. However, similar to ART, no improved overall survival could be shown after SRT [13].

A straight retrospective comparison with salvage (76 Gy) and adjuvant (74 Gy) IMRT patients ($n = 89$ in both arms) who were matched for personal and tumor characteristics resulted in a significant bNED advantage from ART calculated either from the time of RP or from the end of RT (90 vs. 65 % 3 years post-RT and 91 vs. 84 % post-RP). However, the pre-RT PSA was a key parameter for that difference: a subcohort ($n = 38$) receiving early SRT (at PSA <0.5 ng/ml) had a 3-year post-RT bNED rate of 86 %, quite different from the delayed SRT group, who had 46 % bNED, but very similar to ART patients. Therefore, while overall Kaplan–Meier rates of bNED calculated in either mode suggested a benefit from ART, it was concluded that ART and early SRT did not yield significantly different results. This study included tumor stages from pT2 to pT4 and approximately 30 % of the patients had received HT [65].

Recently, Trabulsi and colleagues studied a group of patients undergoing adjuvant radiation therapy with a matched control group undergoing salvage radiation therapy after biochemical failure. Using a multi-institutional database of 2299 patients, 449 patients with pT3–4N0 disease were eligible, including 211 patients receiving adjuvant radiation therapy and 238 patients receiving salvage radiation therapy. Adjuvant radiation therapy significantly reduced the risk of long-term biochemical progression after radical prostatectomy compared with salvage radiation therapy (5-years freedom from biochemical failure (FFBF) was 73 % after adjuvant radiation therapy compared with 50 % after salvage radiation therapy; $p=0.007$). Gleason score ≥8 was a significant predictor of FFBF [100].

The largest retrospective case-matching study to evaluate ART versus early SRT only included pT3 N0 R0/R1 patients. HT was excluded. A total of 390 out of 500 observation-plus-early-SRT patients (median pre-SRT PSA was 0.2 ng/ml) were propensity matched with 390 ART patients. At 2 and 5 years after surgery, bNED rates were 91 and 78 %, respectively, for ART versus 93 and 82 %, respectively, for SRT. Subgroup analyses, too, yielded no significant differences for the two approaches. The study suggests that timely administration of SRT is comparable to ART in improving BCR-free survival in the majority of pT3pN0 PCa patients [18].

When comparing ART with SRT, it must be kept in mind that a considerable number of ART patients would be relapse-free even without RT. The proportion is likely to be the same as in the observation arms of the three randomized studies which was approximately 35 % after 10 years.

Currently, four prospective randomized trials are investigating the therapeutic benefit of early SRT with or without androgen-deprivation therapy compared with adjuvant RT: *Radiotherapy and Androgen Deprivation in Combination After Local Surgery* (RADICALS), *Radiotherapy Adjuvant Versus Early Salvage* (RAVES), GETUG-17, and EORTC 22043–30031. The results of these prospective studies will certainly contribute to guiding clinical practice in terms of indication and timing of postoperative RT.

Conclusions

Adjuvant radiation therapy (ART) provides improved biochemical relapse-free survival, and, possibly, overall survival for patients with a high-risk of recurrence after prostatectomy, when compared to observation. ART seems clearly indicated for patients with combined risk factors like pT3 and positive margins or positive margins and Gleason score 7–10.

It remains unknown whether early salvage radiation therapy (SRT) initiated after a PSA failure is equivalent to ART. At the present time, there are no published randomized trials to compare ART versus SRT. To this end, the results of the ongoing randomized clinical trials RADICALS, RAVES, GETUG-17 and EORTC 22043–30041 that compare ART and SRT directly are still awaited. When SRT is indicated, it should be initiated as early as possible (with PSA <0.5 ng/ml). In this situation SRT is the only curative therapy option.

The role of AD after adjuvant or salvage RT needs further investigation. But in two trials (RTOG 96–01 and GETUG-AFU 16) the addition of HT during and after RT significantly improved survival. Patients who most likely benefit have Gleason score ≥7, pre-SRT PSA to a maximum of 4.0 ng/ml and positive surgical margins. Up to now, the recommended type of hormone therapy and the optimum duration in this situation is unknown.

Modern radiation therapy techniques like IMRT should be used, ideally with image guidance. Serious side effects are apparently low, thus confirming the suitability of this therapeutic approach.

References

1. Abdollah F, Karnes RJ, Suardi N, et al. Impact of adjuvant radiotherapy on survival of patients with node-positive prostate cancer. J Clin Oncol. 2014;32:3939–47.
2. Afshar-Oromieh A, Avtzi E, Giesel FL. The diagnostic value of PET/CT imaging with the (68) Ga-labelled PSMA ligand HBED-CC in the diagnosis of recurrent prostate cancer. Eur J Nucl Med Mol Imaging. 2015;42:197–209.
3. Afshar-Oromieh A, Zechmann CM, Malcher A, et al. Comparison of PET imaging with a (68) Ga-labelled PSMA ligand and (18)F-choline-based PET/CT for the diagnosis of recurrent prostate cancer. Eur J Nucl Med Mol Imaging. 2014;41:11–20.

4. Anscher MS, Clough R, Dodge R. Radiotherapy for a rising prostate-specific antigen after radical prostatectomy: the first 10 years. Int J Radiat Oncol Biol Phys. 2000;48:369–75.
5. Bartkowiak D, Bottke D, Thamm R, et al. The PSA-response to salvage radiotherapy after radical prostatectomy correlates with freedom from progression and overall survival. Radiother Oncol. 2016;118:131–5.
6. Bastasch MD, Teh BS, Mai WY, et al. Post-nerve-sparing prostatectomy, dose-escalated intensity-modulated radiotherapy: effect on erectile function. Int J Radiat Oncol Biol Phys. 2002;54:101–6.
7. Beer AJ, Eiber M, Souvatzoglou M, et al. Radionuclide and hybrid imaging of recurrent prostate cancer. Lancet Oncol. 2011;12:181–91.
8. Begg CB, Riedel ER, Bach PB, et al. Variations in morbidity after radical prostatectomy. N Engl J Med. 2002;346:1138–44.
9. Bernard Jr JR, Buskirk SJ, Heckman MG, et al. Salvage radiotherapy for rising prostate-specific antigen levels after radical prostatectomy for prostate cancer: dose–response analysis. Int J Radiat Oncol Biol Phys. 2010;76:735–40.
10. Bolla M, De Reijke TM, Van Tienhoven G, et al. Duration of androgen suppression in the treatment of prostate cancer. N Engl J Med. 2009;360:2516–27.
11. Bolla M, Van Poppel H, Collette L, et al. Postoperative radiotherapy after radical prostatectomy: a randomised controlled trial (EORTC trial 22911). Lancet. 2005;366:572–8.
12. Bolla M, van Poppel H, Tombal B. Postoperative radiotherapy after radical prostatectomy for high-risk prostate cancer: long-term results of a randomised controlled trial (EORTC trial 22911). Lancet. 2012;380:2018–27.
13. Boorjian SA, Karnes RJ, Crispen PL, et al. Radiation therapy after radical prostatectomy: impact on metastasis and survival. J Urol. 2009;182:2708–14.
14. Bottke D, Golz R, Störkel S, et al. Phase 3 study of adjuvant radiotherapy versus wait and see in pT3 prostate cancer: impact of pathology review on analysis. Eur Urol. 2013;64:193–8.
15. Briganti A, Karnes RJ, Da Pozzo LF, et al. Combination of adjuvante hormonal and radiation therapy significantly prolongs survival of patients with pT2-4 pN+ prostate cancer: results of a matched analysis. Eur Urol. 2011;59:832–40.
16. Briganti A, Karnes RJ, Gandaglia G, et al. Natural history of surgically treated high-risk prostate cancer. Urol Oncol. 2015;33:163.e7-13.
17. Briganti A, Karnes RJ, Joniau S. Prediction of outcome following early salvage radiotherapy among patients with biochemical recurrence after radical prostatectomy. Eur Urol. 2014;66:479–86.
18. Briganti A, Wiegel T, Joniau S, et al. Early salvage radiation therapy does not compromise cancer control in patients with pT3N0 prostate cancer after radical prostatectomy: results of a match-controlled multi-institutional analysis. Eur Urol. 2012;62:472–87.
19. Budäus L, Leyh-Bannurah SR, Salomon G, Michl U, Heinzer H, Huland H, Graefen M, Steuber T, Rosenbaum C. Initial experience of (68)Ga-PSMA PET/CT imaging in high-risk prostate cancer patients prior to radical prostatectomy. Eur Urol. 2016;69:393–6.
20. Buskirk SJ, Pisansky TM, Schild SE, et al. Salvage radiotherapy for isolated prostate specific antigen increase after radical prostatectomy: evaluation of prognostic factors and creation of a prognostic scoring system. J Urol. 2006;176:985–90.
21. Canter D, Greenberg RE, Horwitz EM, et al. Implantation of electromagnetic transponders following radical prostatectomy for delivery of IMRT. Can J Urol. 2010;17:5365–9.
22. Carrie C, Hasbini A, De Laroche G, et al. Interest of short hormonotherapy (HT) associated with radiotherapy (RT) as salvage treatment for biological relapse (BR) after radical prostatectomy (RP): results of the GETUG-AFU 16 phase III randomized trial. J Clin Oncol Meet Abst. 2015;33(Suppl):5006.
23. Castellucci P, Picchio M. ^{11}C-choline PET/CT and PSA kinetics. Eur J Nucl Med Mol Imaging. 2013;40 Suppl 1:S36–40.
24. Chang JH, Park W, Park JS, et al. Significance of early prostate-specific antigen values after salvage radiotherapy in recurrent prostate cancer patients treated with surgery. Int J Urol. 2015;22:82–7.
25. Choo R, Danjoux C, Gardner S, et al. Efficacy of salvage radiotherapy plus 2-year androgen suppression for postradical prostatectomy patients with PSA relapse. Int J Radiat Oncol Biol Phys. 2009;75:983–9.
26. Coen JJ, Zietman AL, Thakral H, et al. Radical radiation for localized prostate cancer: local persistence of disease results in a late wave of metastases. J Clin Oncol. 2002;20:3199–205.
27. Connolly JA, Shinohara K, Presti Jr JC, et al. Local recurrence after radical prostatectomy: characteristics in size, location, and relationship to prostate-specific antigen and surgical margins. Urology. 1996;47:225–31.
28. Cooperberg MR, Davicioni E, Crisan A, et al. Combined value of validated clinical and genomic risk stratification tools for predicting prostate cancer mortality in a high-risk prostatectomy cohort. Eur Urol. 2015;67:326–33.
29. Corn BW, Winter K, Pilepich MV. Does androgen suppression enhance the efficacy of postoperative irradiation? A secondary analysis of RTOG 85-31. Radiation Therapy Oncology Group. Urology. 1999;54:495–502.
30. Croke J, Malone S, Roustan Delatour N, et al. Postoperative radiotherapy in prostate cancer: the case of the missing target. Int J Radiat Oncol Biol Phys. 2012;83:1160–8.

31. Da Pozzo LF, Cozzarini C, Briganti A, et al. Long-term follow-up of patients with prostate cancer and nodal metastases treated by pelvic lymphadenectomy and radical prostatectomy: the positive impact of adjuvant radiotherapy. Eur Urol. 2009;55:1003–11.
32. Eder M, Schäfer M, Bauder-Wüst U, et al. ^{68}Ga-complex lipophilicity and the targeting property of a urea-based PSMA inhibitor for PET imaging. Bioconjug Chem. 2012;23:688–97.
33. Eiber M, Maurer T, Souvatzoglou M. Evaluation of hybrid ^{68}Ga-PSMA ligand PET/CT in 248 patients with biochemical recurrence after radical prostatectomy. J Nucl Med. 2015;56:668–74.
34. Fiorino C, Foppiano F, Franzone P, et al. Rectal and bladder motion during conformal radiotherapy after radical prostatectomy. Radiother Oncol. 2005;74:187–95.
35. Ghadjar P, Hayoz S, Bernhard J, et al. Acute toxicity and quality of life after dose-intensified salvage radiation therapy for biochemically recurrent prostate cancer after prostatectomy: first results of the randomized trial SAKK 09/10. J Clin Oncol. 2015;33:4158–66.
36. Goenka A, Magsanoc JM, Pei X, et al. Improved toxicity profile following high-dose postprostatectomy salvage radiation therapy with intensity-modulated radiation therapy. Eur Urol. 2011;60:1142–8.
37. Hanlon AL, Horwitz EM, Hanks GE, et al. Short-term androgen deprivation and PSA doubling time: their association and relationship to disease progression after radiation therapy for prostate cancer. Int J Radiat Oncol Biol Phys. 2004;58:43–52.
38. Heidenreich A, Bastian PJ, Bellmunt J, et al. EAU guidelines on prostate cancer. Part II: treatment of advanced, relapsing, and castration-resistant prostate cancer. Eur Urol. 2014;65:467–79.
39. Heinisch M, Dirisamer A, Loidl W, et al. Positron emission tomography/computed tomography with F-18-fluorocholine for restaging of prostate cancer patients: meaningful at PSA <5 ng/ml? Mol Imaging Biol. 2006;8:43–8.
40. Herlemann A, Wenter V, Kretschmer A, Thierfelder KM, Bartenstein P, Faber C, Gildehaus FJ, Stief CG, Gratzke C, Fendler WP. 68Ga-PSMA positron emission tomography/computed tomography provides accurate staging of lymph node regions prior to lymph node dissection in patients with prostate cancer. Eur Urol. 2016;pii: S0302-2838(16)00009-9.
41. Horwitz EM, Bae K, Hanks GE, et al. Ten-year follow-up of radiation therapy oncology group protocol 92–02: a phase III trial of the duration of elective androgen deprivation in locally advanced prostate cancer. J Clin Oncol. 2008;26:2497–504.
42. Huch Boni RA, Meyenberger C, Pok Lundquist J, et al. Value of endorectal coil versus body coil MRI for diagnosis of recurrent pelvic malignancies. Abdom Imaging. 1996;21:345–52.
43. Jackson WC, Johnson SB, Foster B, et al. Combining prostate-specific antigen nadir and time to nadir allows for early identification of patients at highest risk for development of metastasis and death following salvage radiation therapy. Pract Radiat Oncol. 2014;4:99–107.
44. Kaminski JM, Hanlon AL, Joon DL, et al. Effect of sequencing of androgen deprivation and radiotherapy on prostate cancer growth. Int J Radiat Oncol Biol Phys. 2003;57:24–8.
45. Katz MS, Zelefsky MJ, Venkatraman ES, et al. Predictors of biochemical outcome with salvage conformal radiotherapy after radical prostatectomy for prostate cancer. J Clin Oncol. 2003;21:483–9.
46. Kibel AS, Ciezki JP, Klein EA, et al. Survival among men with clinically localized prostate cancer treated with radical prostatectomy or radiation therapy in the prostate specific antigen era. J Urol. 2012;187:1259–65.
47. King CR, Kapp DS. Radiotherapy after prostatectomy: is the evidence for dose escalation out there? Int J Radiat Oncol Biol Phys. 2008;71:346–50.
48. King CR, Presti Jr JC, Gill H, et al. Radiotherapy after radical prostatectomy: does transient androgen suppression improve outcomes? Int J Radiat Oncol Biol Phys. 2004;59:341–7.
49. Krause BJ, Souvatzoglou M, Tuncel M, et al. The detection rate of [11C]choline-PET/CT depends on the serum PSA-value in patients with biochemical recurrence of prostate cancer. Eur J Nucl Med Mol Imaging. 2008;35:18–23.
50. Kupelian PA, Langen KM, Willoughby TR, et al. Daily variations in the position of the prostate bed in patients with prostate cancer receiving postoperative external beam radiation therapy. Int J Radiat Oncol Biol Phys. 2006;66:593–6.
51. Leventis AK, Shariat SF, Slawin KM. Local recurrence after radical prostatectomy: correlation of US features with prostatic fossa biopsy findings. Radiology. 2001;219:432–9.
52. Lohm G, Lütcke J, Jamil B, et al. Salvage radiotherapy in patients with prostate cancer and biochemical relapse after radical prostatectomy: long-term follow-up of a single-center survey. Strahlenther Onkol. 2014;190:727–31.
53. Michalski JM, Lawton C, El Naqa I, et al. Development of RTOG consensus guidelines for the definition of the clinical target volume for postoperative conformal radiation therapy for prostate cancer. Int J Radiat Oncol Biol Phys. 2010;76:361–8.
54. Michalski JM, Roach 3rd M, Merrick G, et al. ACR appropriateness criteria on external beam radiation therapy treatment planning for clinically localized prostate cancer expert panel on radiation oncology – prostate. Int J Radiat Oncol Biol Phys. 2009;74:667–72.
55. Mir MC, Li J, Klink JC, et al. Optimal definition of biochemical recurrence after radical prostatectomy depends on pathologic risk factors: identifying

candidates for early salvage therapy. Eur Urol. 2014;66:204–10.
56. Miralbell R, Vees H, Lozano J, et al. Endorectal MRI assessment of local relapse after surgery for prostate cancer: a model to define treatment field guidelines for adjuvant radiotherapy in patients at high risk for local failure. Int J Radiat Oncol Biol Phys. 2007;67:356–61.
57. Moinpour CM, Hayden KA, Unger JM, et al. Health-related quality of life results in pathologic stage C prostate cancer from a Southwest Oncology Group trial comparing radical prostatectomy alone with radical prostatectomy plus radiation therapy. J Clin Oncol. 2008;26:112–20.
58. Moreira DM, Jayachandran J, Presti Jr JC, et al. Validation of a nomogram to predict disease progression following salvage radiotherapy after radical prostatectomy: results from the SEARCH database. BJU Int. 2009;104:1452–6.
59. Nath SK, Sandhu AP, Rose BS, et al. Toxicity analysis of postoperative image-guided intensity-modulated radiotherapy for prostate cancer. Int J Radiat Oncol Biol Phys. 2010;78:435–41.
60. Naya Y, Okihara K, Evans RB, et al. Efficacy of prostatic fossa biopsy in detecting local recurrence after radical prostatectomy. Urology. 2005;66:350–5.
61. Neuhof D, Hentschel T, Bischof M, et al. Long-term results and predictive factors of three-dimensional conformal salvage radiotherapy for biochemical relapse after prostatectomy. Int J Radiat Oncol Biol Phys. 2007;67:1411–7.
62. Ohri N, Dicker AP, Trabulsi EJ, et al. Can early implementation of salvage radiotherapy for prostate cancer improve the therapeutic ratio? A systematic review and regression meta-analysis with radiobiological modelling. Eur J Cancer. 2012;48:837–44.
63. Ost P, De Gersem W, De Potter B, et al. A comparison of the acute toxicity profile between two-dimensional and three-dimensional image-guided radiotherapy for postoperative prostate cancer. Clin Oncol (R Coll Radiol). 2011;23:344–9.
64. Ost P, De Meerleer G, Vercauteren T, et al. Delineation of the postprostatectomy prostate bed using computed tomography: interobserver variability following the EORTC delineation guidelines. Int J Radiat Oncol Biol Phys. 2011;81:e143–9.
65. Ost P, De Troyer B, Fonteyne V, et al. A matched control analysis of adjuvant and salvage high-dose postoperative intensity-modulated radiotherapy for prostate cancer. Int J Radiat Oncol Biol Phys. 2011;80:1316–22.
66. Ost P, Lumen N, Goessaert AS, et al. High-dose salvage intensity-modulated radiotherapy with or without androgen deprivation after radical prostatectomy for rising or persisting prostate-specific antigen: 5-year results. Eur Urol. 2011;60:842–9.
67. Panebianco V, Sciarra A, Lisi D, et al. Prostate cancer: 1HMRS-DCEMR at 3T versus [(18)F]choline PET/CT in the detection of local prostate cancer recurrence in men with biochemical progression after radical retropubic prostatectomy. Eur J Radiol. 2012;81:700–8.
68. Parker C, Sydes MR, Catton C, et al. Radiotherapy and androgen deprivation in combination after local surgery (RADICALS): a new Medical Research Council/National Cancer Institute of Canada phase III trial of adjuvant treatment after radical prostatectomy. BJU Int. 2007;99:1376–9.
69. Paskalev K, Feigenberg S, Jacob R, et al. Target localization for post-prostatectomy patients using CT and ultrasound image guidance. J Appl Clin Med Phys. 2005;6:40–9.
70. Pazona JF, Han M, Hawkins SA, et al. Salvage radiation therapy for prostate specific antigen progression following radical prostatectomy: 10-year outcome estimates. J Urol. 2005;174(4 Pt 1):1282–6.
71. Pinkawa M, Siluschek J, Gagel B, et al. Postoperative radiotherapy for prostate cancer: evaluation of target motion and treatment techniques (intensity-modulated versus conformal radiotherapy). Strahlenther Onkol. 2007;183:23–9.
72. Pisansky TM, Kozelsky TF, Myers RP, et al. Radiotherapy for isolated serum prostate specific antigen elevation after prostatectomy for prostate cancer. J Urol. 2000;163:845–50.
73. Poortmans P, Bossi A, Vandeputte K, et al. Guidelines for target volume definition in post-operative radiotherapy for prostate cancer, on behalf of the EORTC Radiation Oncology Group. Radiother Oncol. 2007;84:121–7.
74. Rossi Jr CJ, Joe Hsu IC, Abdel-Wahab M, et al. ACR appropriateness criteria postradical prostatectomy irradiation in prostate cancer. Am J Clin Oncol. 2011;34:92–8.
75. Sandhu A, Sethi R, Rice R, et al. Prostate bed localization with image-guided approach using on-board imaging: reporting acute toxicity and implications for radiation therapy planning following prostatectomy. Radiother Oncol. 2008;88:20–5.
76. Scattoni V, Montorsi F, Picchio M, et al. Diagnosis of local recurrence after radical prostatectomy. BJU Int. 2004;93:680–8.
77. Schiffner DC, Gottschalk AR, Lometti M, et al. Daily electronic portal imaging of implanted gold seed fiducials in patients undergoing radiotherapy after radical prostatectomy. Int J Radiat Oncol Biol Phys. 2007;67:610–9.
78. Sella T, Schwartz LH, Swindle PW, et al. Suspected local recurrence after radical prostatectomy: endorectal coil MR imaging. Radiology. 2004;231:379–85.
79. Shariat SF, Karakiewicz PI, Roehrborn CG, et al. An updated catalog of prostate cancer predictive tools. Cancer. 2008;113:3075–99.
80. Shekarriz B, Upadhyay J, Wood Jr DP, et al. Vesicourethral anastomosis biopsy after radical prostatectomy: predictive value of prostate-specific

antigen and pathologic stage. Urology. 1999;54:1044–8.
81. Shipley WU, Pugh SL, Lukka HR, et al. NRG Oncology/RTOG 9601, a phase III trial in prostate cancer patients: anti-androgen therapy (AAT) with bicalutamide during and after salvage radiation therapy following radical prostatectomy and an elevated PSA. J Clin Oncol. 2016;34:(suppl 2S; abstr 3).
82. Shipley WU, Seiferheld W, Lukka H, et al. Report of NRG oncology/RTOG 9601, a phase III trial in prostate cancer: anti-androgen therapy (AAT) with bicalutamide during and after radiation therapy (RT) in patients following radical prostatectomy (RP) with pT2-3pN0 disease and an elevated PSA. ASTRO meeting: Abstract LBA5; 2015.
83. Showalter TN, Nawaz AO, Xiao Y, et al. A cone beam CT-based study for clinical target definition using pelvic anatomy during postprostatectomy radiotherapy. Int J Radiat Oncol Biol Phys. 2008;70:431–6.
84. Sidhom MA, Kneebone AB, Lehman M, et al. Post-prostatectomy radiation therapy: consensus guidelines of the Australian and New Zealand Radiation Oncology Genito-Urinary Group. Radiother Oncol. 2008;88:10–9.
85. Siegmann A, Bottke D, Faehndrich J, et al. Dose escalation for patients with decreasing PSA during radiotherapy for elevated PSA after radical prostatectomy improves biochemical progression-free survival: results of a retrospective study. Strahlenther Onkol. 2011;187:467–72.
86. Silver DA, Pellicer I, Fair WR, et al. Prostate-specific membrane antigen expression in normal and malignant human tissues. Clin Cancer Res. 1997;3:81–5.
87. Soto DE, Passarelli MN, Daignault S, et al. Concurrent androgen deprivation therapy during salvage prostate radiotherapy improves treatment outcomes in high-risk patients. Int J Radiat Oncol Biol Phys. 2011;82:1227–32.
88. Spiotto MT, Hancock SL, King CR. Radiotherapy after prostatectomy: improved biochemical relapse-free survival with whole pelvic compared with prostate bed only for high-risk patients. Int J Radiat Oncol Biol Phys. 2007;69:54–61.
89. Stamey TA, Yang N, Hay AR, et al. Prostate-specific antigen as a serum marker for adenocarcinoma of the prostate. N Engl J Med. 1987;317:909–16.
90. Stephenson AJ, Bolla M, Briganti A, et al. Postoperative radiation therapy for pathologically advanced prostate cancer after radical prostatectomy. Eur Urol. 2012;61:443–51.
91. Stephenson AJ, Scardino PT, Kattan MW, et al. Predicting the outcome of salvage radiation therapy for recurrent prostate cancer after radical prostatectomy. J Clin Oncol. 2007;25:2035–41.
92. Stephenson AJ, Shariat SF, Zelefsky MJ, et al. Salvage radiotherapy for recurrent prostate cancer after radical prostatectomy. JAMA. 2004;291:1325–32.
93. Stephenson AJ, Wood DP, Kattan MW, et al. Location, extent and number of positive surgical margins do not improve accuracy of predicting prostate cancer recurrence after radical prostatectomy. J Urol. 2009;182:1357–63.
94. Sweat SD, Pacelli A, Murphy GP, et al. Prostate-specific membrane antigen expression is greatest in prostate adenocarcinoma and lymph node metastases. Urology. 1998;52:637–40.
95. Taylor N, Kelly JF, Kuban DA, et al. Adjuvant and salvage radiotherapy after radical prostatectomy for prostate cancer. Int J Radiat Oncol Biol Phys. 2003;56:755–63.
96. Thompson Jr IM, Tangen CM, Paradelo J, et al. Adjuvant radiotherapy for pathologically advanced prostate cancer: a randomized clinical trial. JAMA. 2006;296:2329–35.
97. Thompson IM, Tangen CM, Paradelo J, et al. Adjuvant radiotherapy for pathological T3N0M0 prostate cancer significantly reduces risk of metastases and improves survival: long-term followup of a randomized clinical trial. J Urol. 2009;181:956–62.
98. Thompson IM, Valicenti RK, Albertsen P, et al. Adjuvant and salvage radiotherapy after prostatectomy: AUA/ASTRO guideline. J Urol. 2013;190:441–9.
99. Tilki D, Mandel P, Schlomm T, et al. External validation of the CAPRA-S score to predict biochemical recurrence, metastasis and mortality after radical prostatectomy in a European cohort. J Urol. 2015;193:1970–5.
100. Trabulsi EJ, Valicenti RK, Hanlon AL, et al. A multi-institutional matched-control analysis of adjuvant and salvage postoperative radiation therapy for pT3-4N0 prostate cancer. Urology. 2008;72:1298–302; discussion 1302–1294.
101. Trock BJ, Han M, Freedland SJ, et al. Prostate cancer-specific survival following salvage radiotherapy vs observation in men with biochemical recurrence after radical prostatectomy. JAMA. 2008;299:2760–9.
102. Van der Kwast TH, Bolla M, van Poppel H, et al. Identification of patients with prostate cancer who benefit from immediate postoperative radiotherapy: EORTC 22911. J Clin Oncol. 2007;25:4178–86.
103. Wang J, Kudchadker R, Choi S, et al. Local recurrence map to guide target volume delineation after radical prostatectomy. Pract Radiat Oncol. 2014;4:e239–46.
104. Ward JF, Zincke H, Bergstralh EJ, et al. Prostate specific antigen doubling time subsequent to radical prostatectomy as a prognosticator of outcome following salvage radiotherapy. J Urol. 2004;172(6 Pt 1):2244–8.
105. Wenz F, Martin T, Böhmer D, et al. The German S3 guideline prostate cancer: aspects for the radiation oncologist. Strahlenther Onkol. 2010;186:531–4.
106. Wiegel T, Bartkowiak D, Bottke D. Adjuvant radiotherapy versus wait-and-see after radical

prostatectomy: 10-year follow-up of the ARO 96-02/AUO AP 09/95 trial. Eur Urol. 2014;66:243–50.

107. Wiegel T, Bartkowiak D, Bottke D. Prostate-specific antigen persistence after radical prostatectomy as a predictive factor of clinical relapse-free survival and overall survival: 10-year data of the ARO 96–02 trial. Int J Radiat Oncol Biol Phys. 2015;91:288–94.
108. Wiegel T, Bottke D, Steiner U, et al. Phase III postoperative adjuvant radiotherapy after radical prostatectomy compared with radical prostatectomy alone in pT3 prostate cancer with postoperative undetectable prostate-specific antigen: ARO 96-02/AUO AP 09/95. J Clin Oncol. 2009;27:2924–30.
109. Wiegel T, Lohm G, Bottke D, et al. Achieving an undetectable PSA after radiotherapy for biochemical progression after radical prostatectomy is an independent predictor of biochemical outcome – results of a retrospective study. Int J Radiat Oncol Biol Phys. 2009;73:1009–16.
110. Wieser G, Mansi R, Grosu AL, et al. Positron emission tomography (PET) imaging of prostate cancer with a gastrin releasing peptide receptor antagonist-from mice to men. Theranostics. 2014;4:412–9.
111. Wiltshire KL, Brock KK, Haider MA, et al. Anatomic boundaries of the clinical target volume (prostate bed) after radical prostatectomy. Int J Radiat Oncol Biol Phys. 2007;69:1090–9.

High-Intensity Focused Ultrasound (HIFU) for Prostate Cancer

Albert Gelet, Sebastien Crouzet, Olivier Rouviere, and Jean-Yves Chapelon

1 Introduction

The incidence of prostate cancer is increasing worldwide. In Europe, the mortality rate declined from 15 per 100,000 in 1995–12.5 per 100,000 in 2006 [1]. This decline of mortality can be attributed to two factors: firstly, since the use of screening with prostate-specific antigen, 70% of these newly diagnosed prostate cancers are organ confined and therefore suitable for a local, curative therapy; secondly, better control of the disease was secured from a wider adoption of radical prostatectomies and the use of combined androgen deprivation and radiotherapy for patients with locally advanced disease. But the morbidity associated with the radical treatment of both surgery and radiotherapy are significant, suggesting that radical surgery and/or radiation therapy should only be offered to men who are likely to survive more than 10 years. However, the PIVOT trial, started during the PSA era, failed to demonstrate a significant survival advantage in the radical surgery group compared to the observation group [2]. The review of Steyerberg et al. [3] suggests that 49% of men undergoing radical prostatectomy have pathological features in the RP specimen consistent with an insignificant cancer (organ confined cancer <0.5 ml, no Gleason grade 4 or 5 component). Albertsten et al. reported the impact of comorbidity on survival among men with localized prostate cancer. The results suggest that relatively few men diagnosed with moderately differentiated localized prostate cancer older than

A. Gelet, MD (✉)
Department of Urology, Edouard Herriot Hospital, Lyon, France

Therapeutic Ultrasound Research Laboratory, Inserm U1032, Lyon F-69003, France

Université de Lyon, Lyon F-69003, France

Urology and Transplantation Department, Edouard Herriot Hospital, 5 place d'Arsonval, 69437 Lyon Cedex 03, France
e-mail: albert.gelet@chu-lyon.fr

S. Crouzet
Department of Urology, Edouard Herriot Hospital, Lyon, France

Therapeutic Ultrasound Research Laboratory, Inserm U1032, Lyon F-69003, France

Université de Lyon, Lyon F-69003, France

O. Rouviere
Therapeutic Ultrasound Research Laboratory, Inserm U1032, Lyon F-69003, France

Université de Lyon, Lyon F-69003, France

Department of Radiology, Edouard Herriot Hospital, Lyon, France

J.-Y. Chapelon
Therapeutic Ultrasound Research Laboratory, Inserm U1032, Lyon F-69003, France

Université de Lyon, Lyon F-69003, France

M. Bolla, H. van Poppel (eds.), *Management of Prostate Cancer*,
DOI 10.1007/978-3-319-42769-0_17

65 years will die as a result of prostate cancer within 10 years of diagnosis [4]. Most men with either no comorbidity or only one will survive at least 10 years, whereas men with two or more comorbidities have a high risk of dying as a result of a competing medical hazard within this time frame. Thus the quest continues for a reliable alternative to open surgery or radiation therapy and one whose chief objective is to find a procedure as minimally invasive as possible.

Klotz et al. published in 2015 the long term results of a large series of patients treated with active surveillance (watchful-waiting protocol with selective delayed intervention) [5]. Focal therapy is an alternative to active surveillance of low-risk prostate cancer with the aim of achieving local control of the cancer, without the associated morbidity of radical therapies. HIFU is also a very promising technology for focal therapy of prostate cancer.

2 Principles

The first description of HIFU was made in 1942 and the ability to destroy tissue was established in 1944 [6]. HIFU is a nonionizing and nonsurgical physical therapy that produces biological effects by thermal and mechanical means. Heating tissue denatures proteins and leads to cell death, regardless of whether they are normal or abnormal, whereas mechanical effects disrupt cells by the collapse of microbubbles generated by cavitation. In most applications, spherically shaped power transducers are used to focus the ultrasound energy onto a target point deep within the body. This results in thermal tissue coagulation necrosis, cavitation, and heat shock. Each sonication heats only a small focal target, creating an elementary lesion with extreme precision and accuracy (Fig. 1a). Subsequently, multiple sonications, side-by-side and layer after layer, are necessary to create a volume of lesions covering a larger volume of tissue targeted for ablation (Fig. 1b). The main sonication parameters are acoustic intensity, duration of exposure, on/off duty cycle, the distance between two elementary lesions, and the displacement path when multiple lesions are made [7].

3 HIFU in Prostate Cancers Models and First Clinical Trials

In 1992, Chapelon et al. established the ultrasound parameters required to induce irreversible tissue lesions in animals. With the experimental adenocarcinoma of a prostate implanted in rats (R 3327 AT2 Dunning tumor), they demonstrated that HIFU could be used to ablate the tumor and cure cancer without causing metastasis [8]. In 1993, Gelet et al. established that it was possible to induce irreversible coagulation necrosis lesions in dog prostates using transrectal route without damaging the rectal wall [9]. The first in human studies were started in 1993 and included men with benign prostate hypertrophy [10, 11]. Beerlage et al. completed a phase one study of HIFU before prostatectomy demonstrating HIFU being able to deposit a large amount of energy into the tissue, resulting in its destruction through cellular disruption and coagulative necrosis [12]. The results of phase two pilot study were published in 1996 and the preliminary results of the first 50 patients in 1999 [13, 14].

4 Prostate Modern Imaging: A Critical Key for Improving HIFU Ablation Outcome

Imaging is beginning to play a critical role in the management of prostate cancer patients [15]. This role is likely to increase as both imaging and HIFU treatment becomes more precise and evolves towards focal ablation of selected cancer foci. In theory, imaging is useful in four different domains: patient selection, treatment planning, assessment of HIFU ablation, and detection of local recurrences.

4.1 Patient Selection and Treatment Planning: The Need for a Better Prostate Cancer Mapping

The first step of patient selection is to rule out the presence of lymph node and distant metastases.

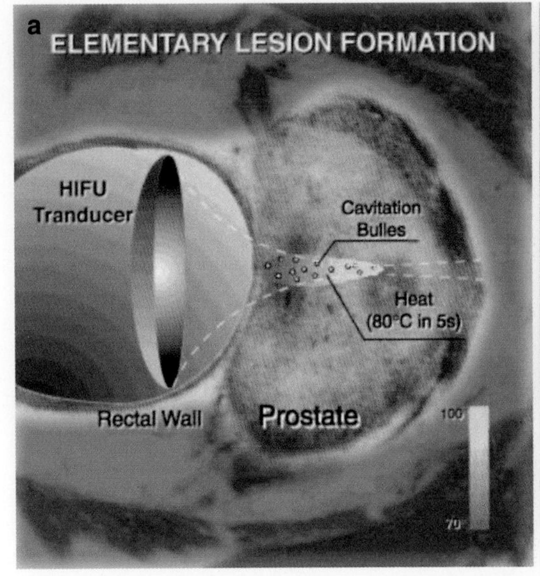

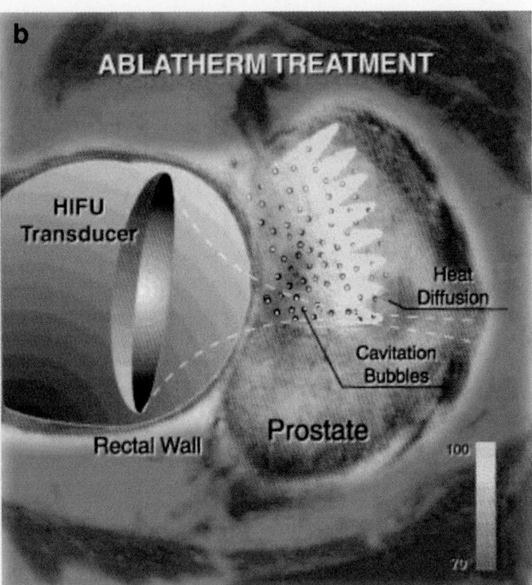

Fig. 1 To treat the prostate, the HIFU transducer is previously covered with a balloon filled with coupling liquid. Then it is inserted into the patient's rectum and positioned close to the rectum wall in such a way that the base of the lesion will stop close to the prostate capsula (**a**). This precise positioning prevents any rectal wall damage. Prostate treatment is performed by the repetition and juxtaposition of several elementary lesions. The sum of these elementary lesions creates a continuous volume where tissue is entire destroyed (**b**)

This step may be optional in low-risk patients, but it is critical in other populations such as the patients with a local recurrence after radiation therapy. The risk of metastases can be assessed by combining clinical and biological data such as the digital rectal examination and biopsy findings, the PSA value, the PSA doubling time or, in case of recurrence, the characteristics of the initial tumor and the delay of the biochemical recurrence. Several nomograms have been shown to predict the onset of metastases and may be useful for clinical decision-making [16]. As detailed in chapters 7 and 8, new MR-based and isotopic techniques can also help in detecting clinically occult metastases.

Once the risk of metastases has been reasonably ruled out, the second step consists of obtaining a precise mapping of the position of cancer foci within the prostate. This is critical for focal ablation candidates, but even in case of whole-gland treatments it helps identify areas where complete tissue destruction is critical. Chapter 7 detailed the progress made in prostate cancer detection and localization, particularly since the advent of multiparametric MRI (mpMRI). MpMRI has a high sensitivity for detecting aggressive cancers [17–19]. At our institution, in 2008 we started a database collecting precise correlation between MR images and prostatectomy specimens. Patients were imaged either at 1.5 T ($n=71$) or 3 T ($n=104$). Images were reviewed by two independent radiologists and compared to histological findings. On a series of 175 consecutive patients, the detection rates for tumors of <0.5 cc, 0.5–2 cc, and >2 cc were 21–29 %, 43–54 %, and 67–75 % for Gleason ≤6 cancers; 63 %, 82–88 %, and 97 % for Gleason 7 cancers; and 80 %, 93 %, and 100 % for Gleason ≥8 cancers, respectively (Fig. 2). Results were not significantly influenced by the field strength [17].

These results underline a limitation of mpMRI: a substantial part of Gleason 6 tumors may be undetected. Another limitation lies in the evaluation of the tumor volume. Accurate assessment of tumor volume is critical for focal ablation. There is a consensus that mpMRI underestimates the histological tumor volume [20–22]. However, some authors found that the volume underestimation was more marked in case of Gleason ≥7 cancers or in case of lesions with a Likert score of 4–5 [19], while others found the opposite [21].

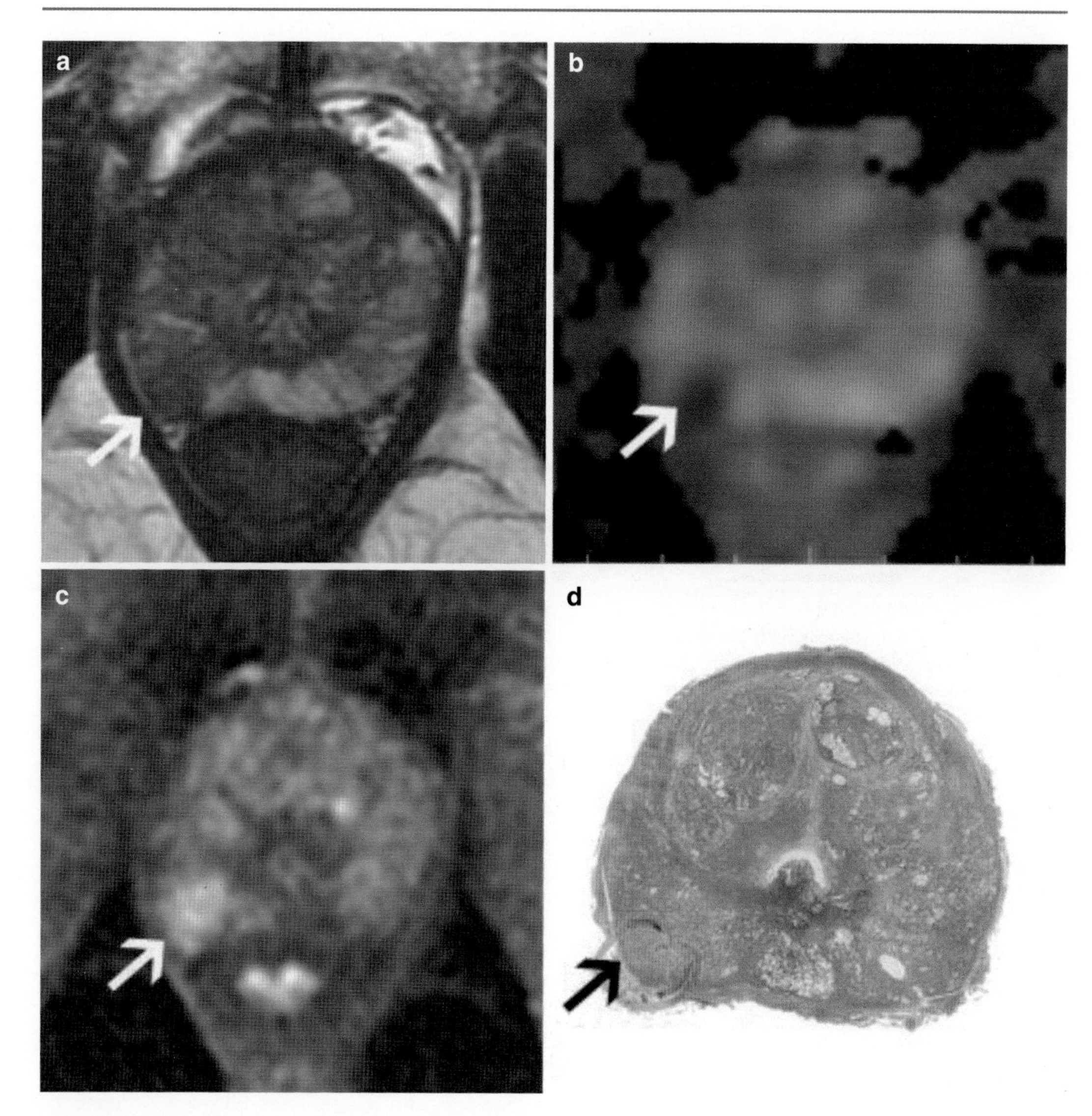

Fig. 2 Multiparametric axial MR images (**a**): T2-weighted image; (**b**): apparent diffusion coefficient (ADC) map computed from diffusion-weighted images (b values: 0 and 2000 s/mm^2); (**c**): dynamic contrast-enhanced image and axial section of the prostatectomy specimen obtained in a 66 year-old patient with a Gleason 8 prostate cancer of the right mid-gland and base at biopsy. MRI images showed a highly suspicious lesion located in the posterolateral part of the peripheral zone of the right midgland, with hyposignal on T2-weighted image (**a**, *arrow*), decreased ADC values (**b**, *arrow*), and early and intense enhancement (**c**, *arrow*). The analysis of the prostatectomy specimen (**d**, *arrow*) was confirmative and showed in that area a Gleason 8 cancer. The rest of the gland did not contain cancer

Thus, further research is needed to better evaluate the safety margin that needs to be used around lesions seen on mpMRI in case of focal ablation.

It is of note that mpMRI seems much more accurate in delineating intraprostatic local recurrences after radiotherapy. Several independent groups reported a strong agreement between mpMRI and biopsy findings in patients with rising PSA after radiotherapy, at the patient, lobe, and even sextant level [23–25]. The contrast between recurrent cancer and post-radiation fibrosis seems high, both on diffusion-weighted imaging and on dynamic contrast-enhanced imaging (Fig. 3). As a result, mpMRI interpretation is easier and interreader agreement is good, even with junior readers

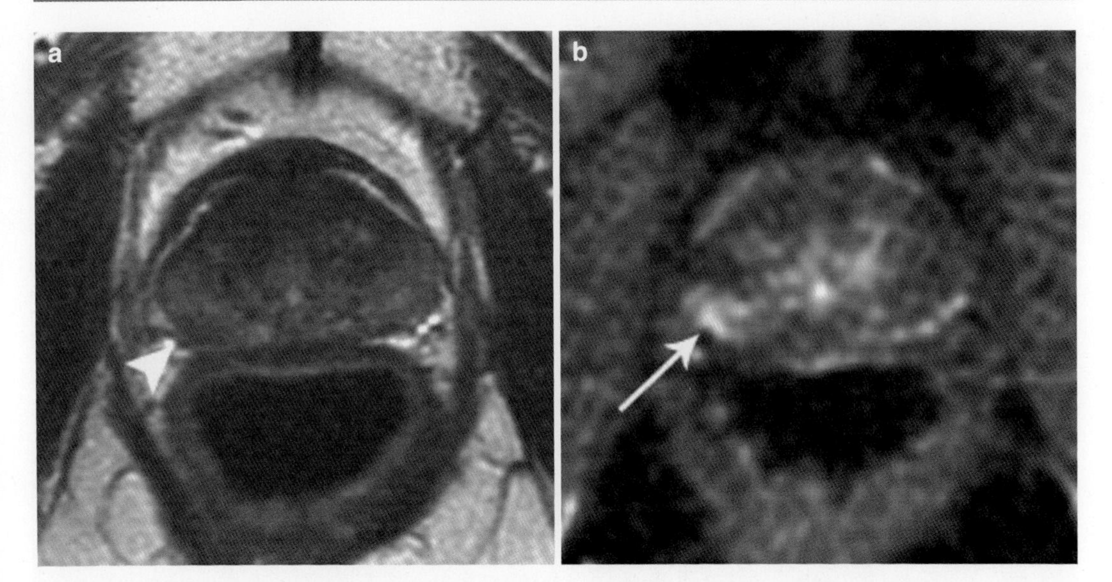

Fig. 3 Multiparametric MR images (**a**): T2-weighted image; (**b**): dynamic contrast-enhanced image) obtained in a 69-year-old patient with history of radiation therapy for prostate cancer 10 years before. The nadir of the PSA level after radiation therapy was 0.8 ng/ml. The PSA level had slowly increased to 3.21 ng/ml at the time of MRI. MR images showed a suspicious lesion of the right midgland, with mild hyposignal on T2-weighted imaging (**a**, *arrowhead*) and marked enhancement on dynamic imaging (**b**, *arrow*). Biopsy showed Gleason 6 recurrent cancer in the right midgland

[25]. In the postradiation setting, mpMRI also provides prognostic information; in a series of 46 patients with postradiotherapy local recurrences treated with HIFU at our institution, the position of the recurrence anterior to the urethra (as determined by DCE MRI) was shown to be an independent negative predictive factor along with the pre-HIFU PSA value [26].

4.2 Postoperative Evaluation of the Ablated Area

Ideally, imaging could show the prostate volume destroyed at the end of the HIFU ablation session so that in case of unsatisfactory results, a new HIFU ablation could be immediately performed. Unfortunately, transrectal ultrasound, used to guide HIFU treatment, cannot accurately show the ablated area [27].

Gadolinium-enhanced (nondynamic) MRI clearly reveals the treated volume as a devascularized zone (corresponding to the central core of the coagulation necrosis) surrounded by a peripheral rim of enhancement (corresponding to edema), but MRI cannot be obtained in the operating room [28, 29].

We have recently shown that contrast-enhanced ultrasound (CEUS), using Sonovue™ as contrast agent, can show the ablated volume immediately at the end of the treatment with an excellent correlation with MR and biopsy findings. All prostate sectors showing no enhancement at CEUS at the end of HIFU ablation can be considered entirely destroyed. In contrast, prostate sectors showing any degree of enhancement can be considered containing living (benign or malignant) tissue [30] (Fig. 4). These results should allow immediate re-treatment of the parts of the gland showing residual enhancement and that are within the range of the transducer.

4.3 Detection of Post-HIFU Local Recurrences

After HIFU ablation, residual prostate is composed of scarring fibrosis and benign prostate hyperplastic (BPH) tissue that has not been destroyed because of its anterior location.

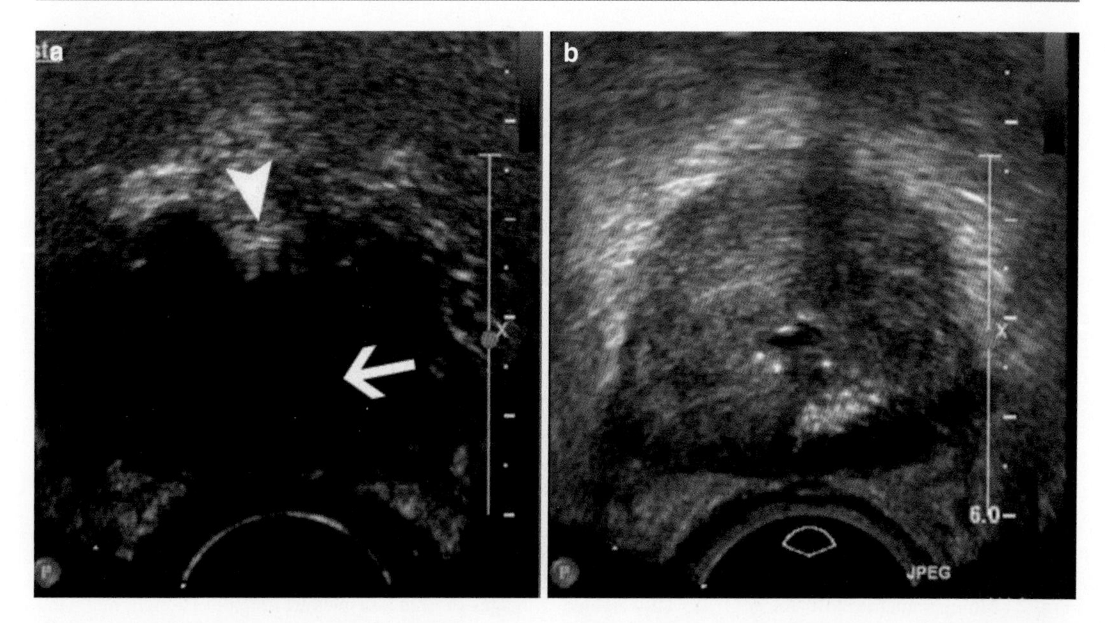

Fig. 4 Contrast-enhanced ultrasound (CEUS) axial image (**a**) with corresponding low mechanical index gray-scale image (dual mode; **b**), obtained after HIFU ablation of a local recurrence of prostate cancer after radiation therapy in a 68-year-old patient. CEUS image showed the nearly complete devascularization of the gland (*large arrow*), with a small strip of anterior and median residual parenchyma that still enhanced (*arrowhead*). Note that tissue destruction is not visible on the gray-scale image

Because local recurrences (or residual cancers) can be treated with a second session of HIFU ablation or by radiation therapy [31], it is important to detect them early. The precise location of these recurrences can also help in selecting an appropriate salvage treatment (e.g., anterior recurrences may be better treated by radiation therapy).

Even if color Doppler can sensitize TRUS [32], US-based techniques are not accurate enough to detect local recurrences early and guide biopsy.

MRI, and particularly DCE MRI, seems to provide early detection and accurate localization of recurrent cancers that enhance earlier and more than post-HIFU fibrosis [33, 34] (Fig. 5). However, DCE MRI lacks specificity. It is indeed difficult to distinguish recurrent cancer from residual BPH tissue. In a retrospective study of 65 patients with biochemical recurrence after HIFU ablation performed at our institution, neither the enhancement pattern nor the apparent diffusion coefficient (ADC) was able to significantly distinguish BPH nodules from recurrent cancers, even if the latter had, on average, higher wash-in rates, lower wash-out rates, and lower ADCs (unpublished results).

Thus, to date, all patients with rising PSA after HIFU ablation should undergo prostate MRI, and all areas with early and intense enhancement should be biopsied to distinguish cancers from BPH residual tissue.

4.4 Towards an Increased Integration of Imaging and Therapy

Imaging is so essential for patient selection, treatment planning and guidance, assessment of tissue destruction, and detection of local recurrences that it is likely that imaging and therapy will become increasingly intertwined in the future.

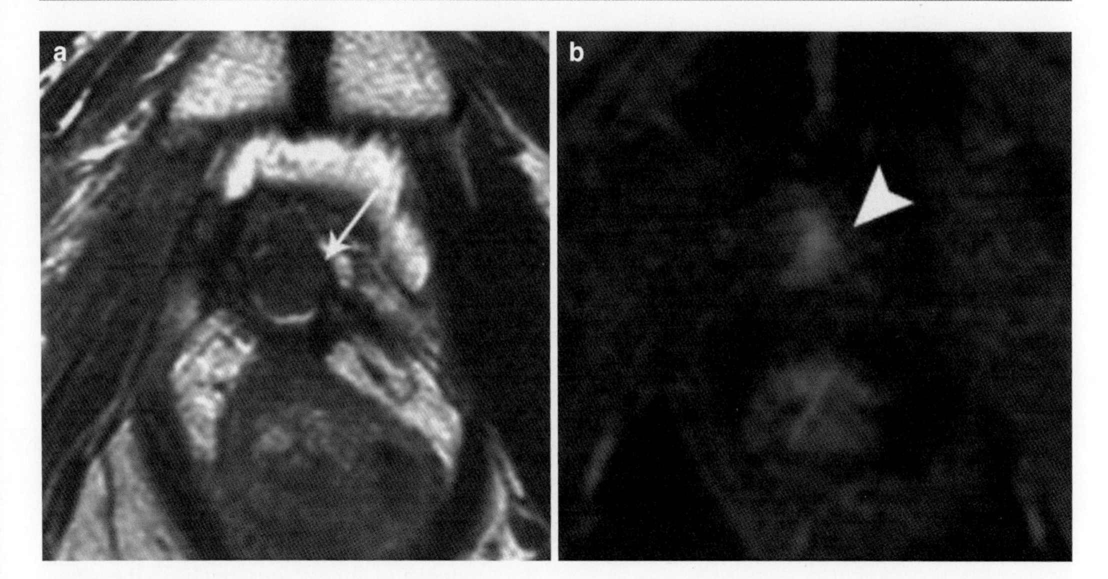

Fig. 5 Multiparametric MR images (**a**): T2-weighted image; (**b**): dynamic contrast-enhanced image) obtained in a 76-year-old patient with history of HIFU ablation for prostate cancer 5 years before. The nadir of the PSA level after HIFU ablation was 0.03 ng/ml. The PSA level had slowly increased to 1.47 ng/ml at the time of MRI. MR images showed an atrophic residual prostate (approximately 4 cc; **a**, *arrow*) with a marked enhancement of its anterior and central part (**b**, *arrowhead*). Targeted biopsy showed recurrent Gleason 6 cancer in this area

Two possible technological strategies can be foreseen.

The first one is the development of prostate cancer HIFU ablation under MR guidance. This approach would directly benefit of MR cancer detection/location capabilities. It can also provide real-time temperature monitoring during treatment [35]. The volume of tissue ablated could be immediately assessed by contrast-enhanced MRI and re-treatment would be easily possible in case of incomplete tissue destruction. This MR-guided integrated approach is probably the ideal solution, but will be expensive and will necessitate dedicated scanners.

Another approach, much less expensive, will consist in keeping the traditional US guidance, but after taking into account preoperative MR cancer mapping by using US/MR fusion software. The assessment of the ablated volume at the end of the treatment will be obtained using CEUS, and thus immediate re-treatment will be possible.

It is too soon to know which approach will prevail in the future.

5 HIFU Devices and Techniques

Three commercially available devices are currently used for the treatment of prostate cancer: Sonablate® (Focus surgery Inc., Indianapolis IN, USA), Ablatherm®, and Focal One® (EDAP-TMS SA, Vaulx en Velin, France).

The Sonablate uses a single transducer (4 MHz) for both imaging and treatment (Fig. 6). Several probes are available with many focal lengths (from 25 to 45 mm). The size of elementary lesion is 10 mm in length and 2 mm in diameter. The Sonablate procedure is conducted in a dorsal position with a patient lying on a regular operating table. Sonablate uses a single treatment protocol in which the power has to be adapted manually by the operator. The treatment is usually made in three consecutive coronal layers, starting from the anterior part of the prostate and moving to the posterior part, with at least one probe switch during the procedure [36]. The probe chosen depends on the prostate size, with

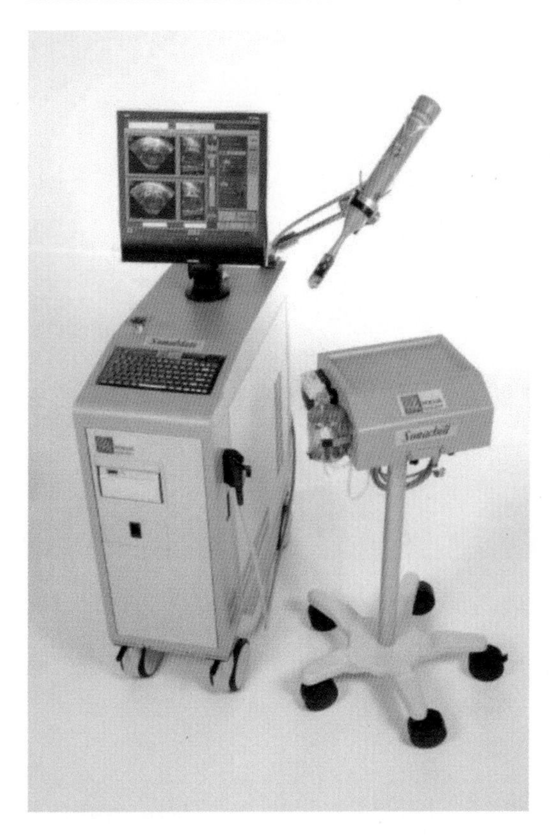

Fig. 6 Sonablate 500

larger glands requiring longer focal length probes.

The Ablatherm has both the imaging (7.5 MHz) and therapeutic (3 MHz) transducers included in a unique endorectal probe focused at 40 mm (Fig. 7a, b). Ablatherm requires a specific bed with a patient on a lateral position. Lateral position treatment allows gas bubbles produced through the heating of the prostate tissue to rise with gravity to a position lateral to the prostate, which will reduce the risk of acoustic interference with the HIFU waves. The Ablatherm includes three treatment protocols with specifically designed treatment parameters depending on the clinical use (standard, HIFU re-treatment, and radiation failure). The size of the HFU induced lesion can be precisely controlled by adjusting the power and the duration of the ultrasound pulse. The size of the elementary lesion may vary from 19 to 26 mm in length (1.7 mm in diameter). HIFU efficacy was mathematically modeled [37]. This allows the calculation of the optimal acoustic intensity necessary to achieve an irreversible necrosis lesion in several clinical situations, particularly for an irradiated prostate. The Ablatherm integrated imaging offers a real-time ultrasonic monitoring of the treatment. The HIFU probe is robotically adjusted with a permanent control of the distance between the transducer and the rectal wall. By repeating the shots and moving the transducer a precise volume can be treated, defined by the operator (planning phase). The treatment is made in transversal layers. The prostate is usually divided into four to six volume boundaries and treated from the apex to the base, slice by slice, by an entirely computer-driven probe. The risk of urethrorectal fistula has been reduced to almost zero thanks to the refinement of the acoustic parameters and many safety features (control of the distance transducer/rectal wall, cooling system, patient motion detector). The standard treatment parameters used 100 % of the acoustic power with a 6-s pulse of energy to create each discrete HIFU lesion with a 4-s delay between each shots. For HIFU re-treatment, the shot duration was reduced to 5 s with the acoustic power of 100 % and a 4-s delay between each shot. Starting in March 2002, specific postradiation treatment parameters were adopted (5-s pulse, 5-s waiting period, 90 % of the acoustic power). These were developed because of the decreased vascularity of the previously irradiated tissue. The goal was to optimize the thermal dose delivered within the gland while minimizing the damage probability to the surrounding tissues, and particularly the rectal wall, caused by the conductive heat transfer. Finally, postbrachytherapy parameters have been developed with 85 % of the acoustic powers with 4-s of energy and 5-s waiting period. In contemporary series, the incidence of urethrorectal fistula was reported between 0 and 0.6 % for primary procedures.

Focal One is a new device specifically designed for focal therapy of prostate cancer, combining the necessary tools to visualize, target, treat, and validate the focal treatment (Fig. 8a). MR images are imported through the hospital's network or USB drive. The operator defines the contours of the prostate and the

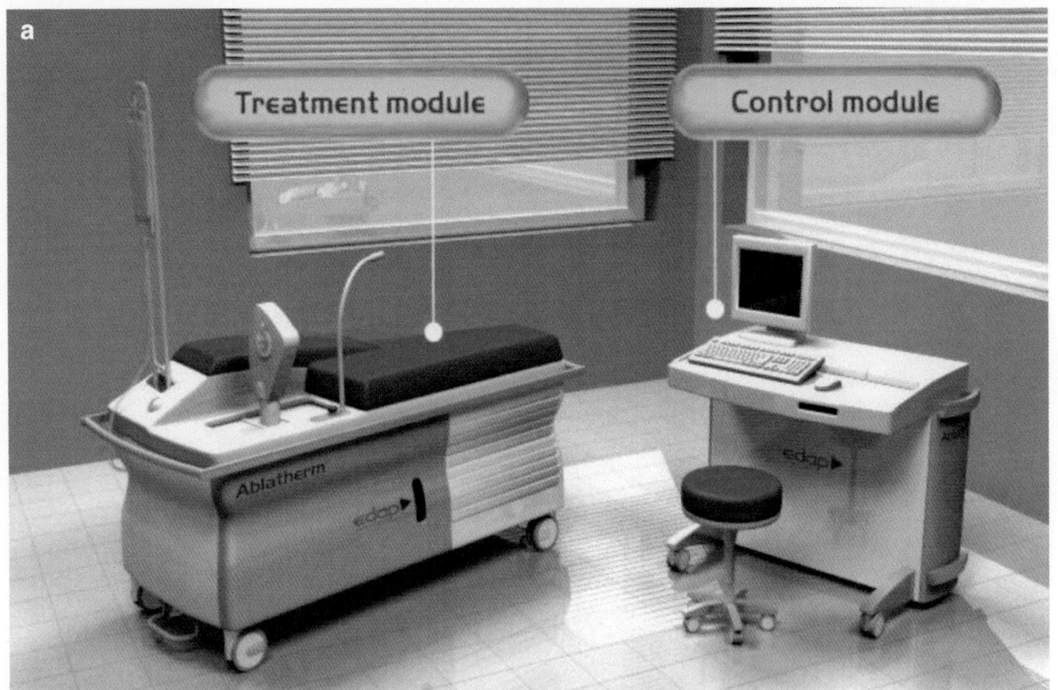

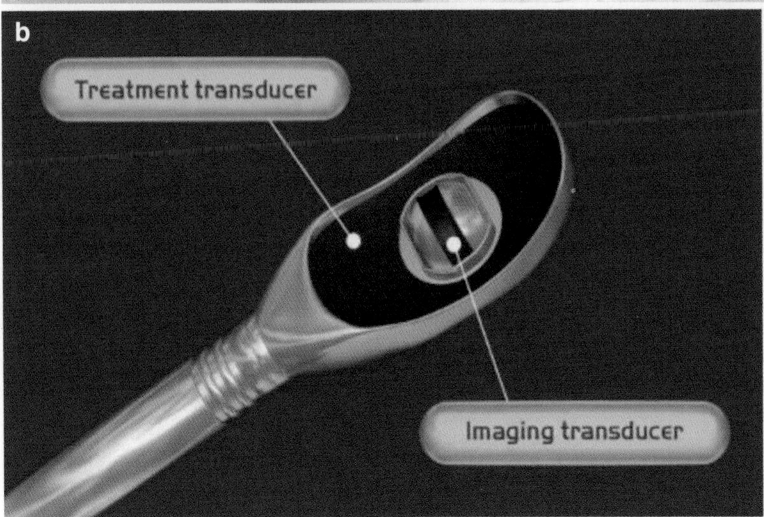

Fig. 7 Ablatherm integrated imaging (device and probe)

regions of interests that have been confirmed as prostate tumors. The same contouring of the prostate is performed on the live ultrasound volume acquired by the transrectal probe. The software proceeds to an "elastic fusion": the live ultrasound volume is considered as the reference volume and the MR volume is smoothly deformed so the 3D contour of the prostate on the MR volume matches perfectly the contours of the prostate on the ultrasound volume. The same 3D elastic transformation is applied to the ROIs initially indicated on the MR image so they appear at the adequate position on the live ultrasound image, guiding the planning process (Fig. 9).

Focal One is equipped with a new generation of HIFU probe able to electronically vary the focal point along the acoustic axis using a HIFU multielement transducer (Fig. 8b). The

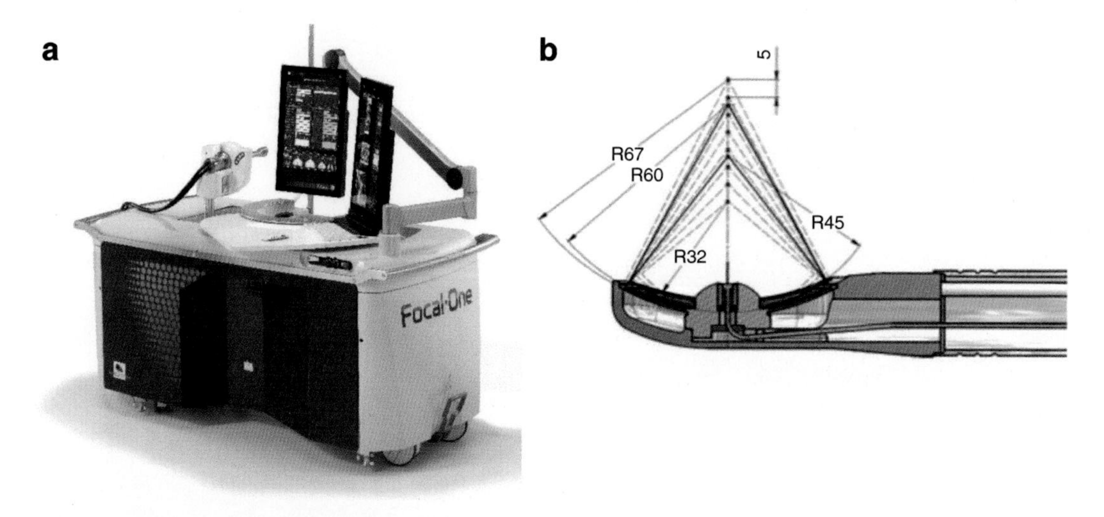

Fig. 8 (**a, b**) Focal one (device and phase array transducer)

Dynamic Focusing transducer is made of 16 isocentric rings that allowed an electronic displacement of the focal point to a maximum of 8 different points 32–67 mm from the transducer. The Dynamic Focusing treatment consists in stacking several unitary HIFU lesions (Fig. 9a–c). The unitary HIFU lesion height is 5 mm and stacking two to eight unitary lesions leads to necrotic lesion of 10–40 mm height. The shooting process is 1 s fire at foci and no OFF between different foci. Compare to Fixed Focusing treatment the Dynamic Focusing allow the treatment of bigger prostates with maximum lesion height of 40 mm instead of 26 mm. The wide range of lesion heights (10–40 mm) allows to a better contouring of the prostate. The HIFU treatment of prostate cancer should be faster due to the shooting process with no time OFF between firings. The last advantages of Dynamic Focusing HIFU treatment could be a more homogeneous necrotic zone due to a better energy distribution. During the HIFU energy delivery process, the operator sees a live ultrasound image of what is being treated and, if necessary, can readjust the treatment planning. At the end of the treatment process, a contrast-enhanced ultrasound volume is acquired showing the devascularized areas. This CEUS volume can be fused with the treatment planning as well as the initial MR image showing immediate concordance between targeted and treated areas.

MRgFUS Devices: Magnetic resonance guided focused ultrasound surgery (MRgFUS) was recently presented as a method for ablation with focused ultrasound under magnetic resonance imaging guidance. This approach has the advantage of improved targeting and real-time temperature monitoring. To date, two different approaches have been used for MRgFUS of the prostate: one with a transrectal probe compatible with the ExAblate ® system (InSightec, Haifa, Israel) under a 1.5 T GE MRI, and another with an MRI-compatible ultrasound applicator to deliver controlled thermal therapy to the regions of the prostate gland via a transurethral approach (Profound Medical Inc., Toronto, Canada). The potential of both technologies is currently being demonstrated in Phase I clinical trials, but only a few studies have been conducted in therapy of PCa with human patients [38, 39].

6 HIFU Contraindications

All HIFU devices are size limited and it is not yet possible to treat a prostate gland greater than 60 cc. In order to reduce the size of the prostate, and in particular the distance between the rectal

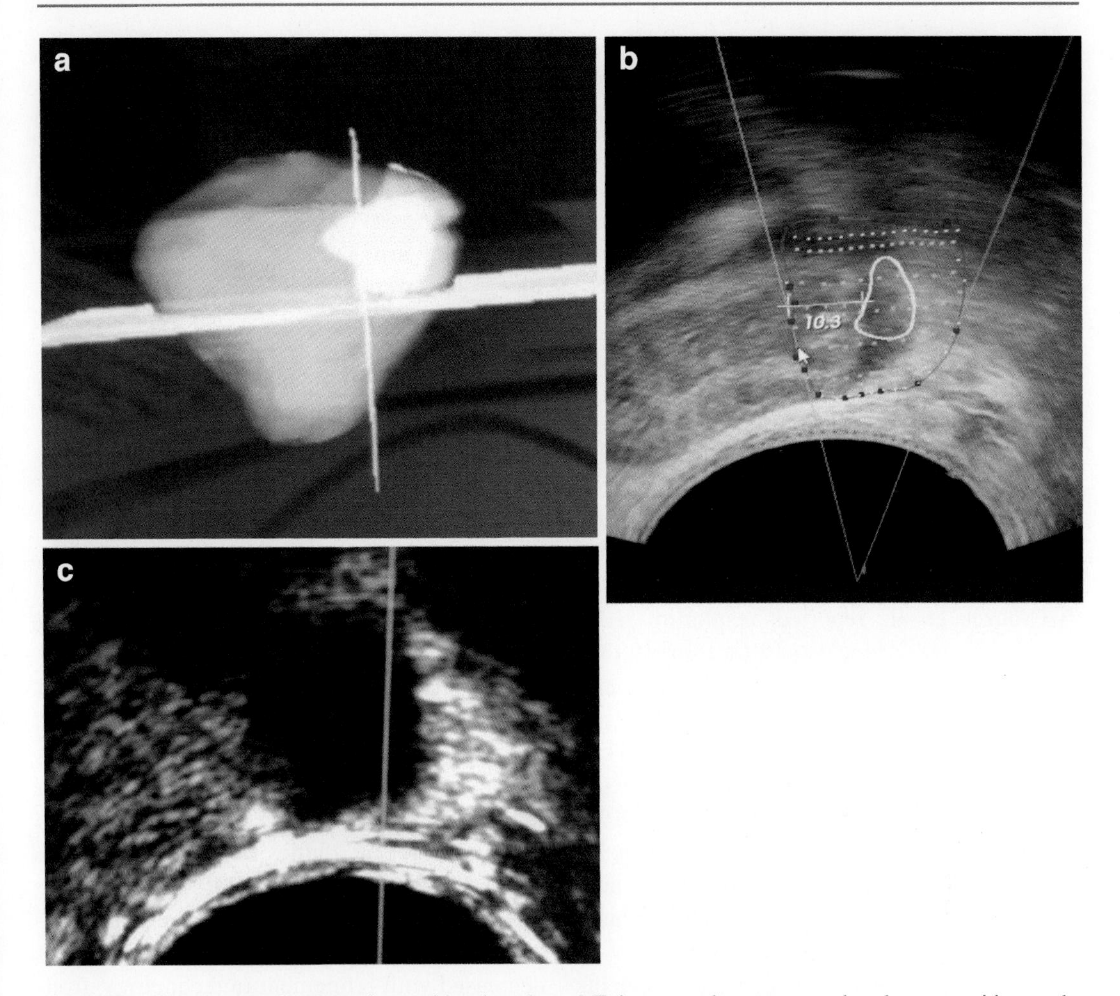

Fig. 9 The live ultrasound volume is considered as the reference volume and the MR volume is smoothly deformed so the 3D contour of the prostate on the MR volume matches perfectly the contours of the prostate on the ultrasound volume (**a**) The same 3D elastic transformation is applied to the ROIs initially indicated on the MR image so they appear at the adequate position on the live ultrasound image, guiding the planning process (**b**). At the end of the treatment process, a contrast-enhanced ultrasound volume is acquired showing the devascularized areas (**c**)

wall and the prostate's anterior, a TURP could be carried out at the time of HIFU or 2 months before the session. TURP dramatically reduces the catheter duration after the HIFU [40–44] and also reduces the risk of bladder outlet obstruction, which is one of the main side effects observed after HIFU.

The HIFU contraindications included a rectal wall thickness >6 mm (Ablatherm device) or >10 mm (Focal One device), a rectal stenosis, chronic inflammatory disease of the intestines, or intense prostate calcifications not removed by the TURP.

7 HIFU as Primary Care Treatment

The usual recommendations on the choice of HIFU for prostate cancer as a primary treatment concern patients with localized prostate cancer (clinical stage T1–T2, NX/0 MX/0) for whom radical prostatectomies are not an option for one the following reasons: age >70 year old, life expectancy ≤10 years, major comorbidities which preclude surgery, or the simple refusal on the part of the patient to undergo one [45, 46]. Among publications on HIFU as a primary therapy for prostate cancer, 18 studies report a series of at least 50 patients [47–64], while the five most recent studies report a series of at least 500 patients [65–69]. In most cases, the PSA nadir was reached 3–4 months after the HIFU treatment. Many studies have demonstrated that the PSA nadir was a significant predictor of HIFU failure. Patients with a PSA nadir over 0.5 ng/ml must be carefully monitored [56, 62]. A PSA nadir >0.2 ng/ml after HIFU has been associated with a four times greater risk of treatment failure (as defined by cancer on biopsy after HIFU) [65].

Articles published from three European urology departments confirmed the long-term efficacy (mean follow-up 76–97 months) of HIFU treatment with Ablatherm device [65–67].

Crouzet et al. reported results of 1002 patients treated for localized PCa from 1997 to 2009 [65]. At 10 years, the PCa-specific survival rates (PCSSR) and metastasis-free survival rates (MFSR) were 97 % and 94 %, respectively. Salvage therapies included external beam radiation therapy (EBRT) (13.8 %), EBRT+ androgen deprivation (ADT) (9.7 %), and ADT alone (12.1 %). Thuroff et al. published outcomes of 709 patients with primary localized prostate cancer [66]. Mean follow-up was 5.3 years (1.3–14 years). Cancer specific survival was 99 %, metastasis-free survival was 95 %, and 10-year salvage treatment-free rates were 98 % in low-risk, 72 % in intermediate-risk, and 68 % in high-risk patients respectively. The HIFU re-treatment rate has been 15 % since 2005. Ganzer et al. reported results of a prospective study on 538 consecutive patients who underwent primary HIFU for clinically localized PCa [67]. The mean follow-up was 8.1 years. Metastatic disease was reported in 0.4, 5.7, and 15.4 % of low-, intermediate-, and high-risk patients, respectively. The salvage treatment rate was 18 %. PCa-specific death was registered in 18 (3.3 %) patients.

Two recent articles confirm the efficacy of whole-gland HIFU treatment (median follow-up 46–78 months) with Sonablate device. Uchida et al. included 918 patients treated with Sonablate™ devices during 1999–2012 and followed-up for >2 years [68]. The 10-year overall and cancer-specific survival rates were 89.6 % and 97.4 %, respectively. The 5-year biochemical disease-free survival rates in the SB200/500, SB500 version 4, and SB500 tissue change monitor groups were 48.3 %, 62.3 %, and 82.0 %, respectively ($p<0.0001$). Dickinson et al. reported medium-term outcomes in 569 men receiving primary whole-gland HIFU [69]. Of the 569, 163 (29 %) required a total of 185 redo-HIFU procedures. Median follow-up was 46 months. Failure-free survival at 5 years after first HIFU was 70 %; it was 87 %, 63 %, and 58 % for low-, intermediate-, and high-risk groups, respectively.

Complication rates are low with sloughing occurring in 0.3–8.6 %. Urethrorectal fistula occurs in 0.23–0.7 % in the large studies treated with Ablatherm device [65–67]. Erectile dysfunction (ED) occurs in 35–45 % of previous potent patients and bladder outlet obstruction in 24–28 % [66, 67]. Incontinence rates reported in recent studies were: 4–5.5 % grade I and 1.5–3.1 % grade II/III [66, 67]. In the largest study published [65], severe incontinence and bladder outlet obstruction (BOO) decreased with refinement in technology, from 5.7 % and 10.2 % to 3.1 % and 5.9 %, respectively.

In a study from a prospective database, Shoji et al. included 326 patients who filled out self-administered questionnaires on urinary function, QOL, and sexual assessment [70]. Maximum flow rate and residual urine volume were significantly impaired at 6 months ($P=0.010$) after HIFU, even if they returned to baseline values at 12 or 24 months after HIFU. At 6, 12, and 24 months after HIFU, 52 %, 63 %, and 78 %, respectively, of the patients who hadn't received neoadjuvant hormonal therapy were potent.

In a prospective study, Li et al. compared the IIEF score, penile color Doppler ultrasound, penile length, and circumference on patients treated for prostate cancer with HIFU or cryoablation [71]. At 36 months, cryoablation patients experienced a lower erectile function recovery rate compared to HIFU patients (cryoablation = 46.8 %; HIFU = 65.5 %; $P = 0.021$).

Finally, the oncologic outcomes achieved in large HIFU studies are remarkably consistent across series.

8 HIFU Re-treatment

In case of incomplete treatment or treatment failure, HIFU does not result in a therapeutic impasse. Unlike radiation, there is no dose limitation and no limited number of sessions. In large series, the re-treatment rate is estimated to be between 15 % and 42 % [65–67]. The morbidity related to repeat HIFU treatment for localized prostate cancer has been studied on 223 patients with a re-treatment rate of 22 %. While urinary infection, bladder outlet obstruction and chronic pelvic pain did not significantly differ after one or more sessions, a significant increase was observed for urinary incontinence and impotence in the group which required retreatment [72].

9 Salvage EBRT After HIFU Failure

In a retrospective study, Pasticier et al. presented results of salvage radiation after HIFU [73]. A total of 100 patients were included with a median follow-up of 33 months. Mean doses of radiation were 71.9 ± 2.38Gys. The mean delay between HIFU and ERBT was 14.9 ± 11.8 months. Mean PSA before salvage ERBT was 2.1 ± 1.8 ng/ml and the nadir PSA after ERBT was 0.28 ± 0.76 ng/ml with 17.4 ± 10.8 months to reach nadir. The incontinence rate was the same before and 1 year after salvage ERBT. The progression-free survival rate was 76.6 % at 5 years, and was 93, 70, and 57.5 % for low-, intermediate-, and high-risk group respectively. The predicting factors of failure were the PSA nadir after salvage ERBT and the time to reach this nadir. Recently, Munoz et al. reported the outcomes of 24 patients treated by salvage EBRT after HIFU [74]. The median follow-up was 40.3 months. The 3-years biochemical disease-free rate (bDFS) was 77.8 % (Phoenix definition). Patients achieving nadir PSA ≤ 0.35 ng/ml had a significantly higher bDFS (87.7 % at 3-years).

SRT provides satisfactory oncologic control after HIFU failure with little (or mild) additional toxicity.

10 Salvage Surgery After HIFU Failure

Salvage surgery is feasible after HIFU but with a higher morbidity than after primary surgery. Lawrentschuk et al. reported the results in 15 men with a rising PSA and biopsy-verified prostate cancer after HIFU treatment [75]. Perioperative morbidity was limited to one transfusion in a patient with a rectal injury. Pathological extensive periprostatic fibrosis was found in all patients. Postoperative PSA value was undetectable in 14 patients (93.3 %). Six of ten patients experienced no postoperative incontinence at 12 months, but with uniformly poor erectile function.

Kane reported short term results of 13 men with locally recurrent prostate cancer after HIFU undergoing salvage radical laparoscopic surgery [76]. There was no perioperative mortality and no conversion to open surgery was necessary. None of the patients received any transfusion. On histopathologic evaluation, eight patients had extracapsular extension (pT3a). Positive surgical margins (PSMs) were detected in two patients in the pT3a group. Four patients showed mild incontinence and used two pads per day. None of the patients were potent.

This study confirms that salvage surgery is feasible for men in whom whole-gland HIFU ablation has failed but has a higher morbidity rate than primary surgery. Salvage surgery after whole-gland HIFU is feasible but difficult to perform due to fibrotic reaction.

11 Salvage HIFU After EBRT or Brachytherapy

11.1 EBRT Failure

The rate of positive biopsy after external beam radiotherapy (ERBT) for prostate cancer in the literature is between 25 and 32 % [77, 78].

There appears to be a role for salvage HIFU therapy with curative intents for patients with a locally proven recurrence after external-beam radiation therapy and no metastasis that are usually treated with androgen deprivation [79]. Crouzet et al. examined the outcomes of salvage HIFU in 290 consecutive patients with biopsy-confirmed locally radiorecurrent PCa, without evidence of metastasis [80]. Progression was defined using Phoenix biochemical failure criteria or androgen deprivation (AD) introduction. Local cancer control with negative biopsy results was obtained in 169 patients out of 208 who underwent post-HIFU biopsies (81 %). The median PSA nadir was 0.14 ng/ml. The cancer-specific and metastasis-free survival rates at 7 years were 80 % and 79.6 % respectively. The PFSR was significantly influenced by three factors: the pre-HIFU PSA level, the Gleason score and a previous AD treatment. With the use of dedicated acoustic parameters, the rate of severe side effects decreased significantly from standard parameters: rectourethral fistula (0.4 %), grade II/III incontinence (19.5 %), and bladder outlet obstruction (14 %). Rouvière et al. demonstrated [81] that the MRI localization of cancer recurrence anterior to the urethra is an independent significant predictor of salvage HIFU failure after EBRT. Therefore, MRI may be useful for patient selection before post-EBRT salvage HIFU ablation. Similar outcomes were reported by Berge et al. [82].

Two articles reported outcome of salvage HIFU performed with the Sonablate, the biochemical survival rate was 71 % at 9 months and 52 % at 5 years [83, 84].

Nevertheless, the risk–benefit ratio of salvage HIFU compares favorably with those of the other available techniques and with less morbidity and similar oncological outcomes. In this context, HIFU appears to be an effective curative treatment option for local recurrence after radiation failure.

11.2 Salvage High-Intensity Focused Ultrasound for Patients with Recurrent Prostate Cancer After Brachytherapy

Sylvester et al. reported 15-year biochemical relapse-free survival rate and cause-specific survival following I^{125} prostate brachytherapy in 215 patients: 15-year BRFS for the entire cohort was 80.4 % and the cancer specific survival rate was 84 % [85]. There was no significant difference between the low- and intermediate-risk group. Salvage surgery is a challenging procedure after brachytherapy [86]. Forty-seven patients treated with salvage HIFU for biopsy-proven recurrence after brachytherapy are under evaluation in an ongoing clinical trial in Lyon (unpublished data); 38 patients underwent 1 HIFU session and 9 underwent 2 HIFU sessions. The mean follow-up is 28 months. The mean PSA before HIFU was 4.97 ± 2.9 ng/ml and the median nadir PSA is 0.35 ng/ml. The overall survival rate is 89 %. Cancer specific, metastases-free, and the additional treatment-free survival rates were 94 %, 87 %, and 50 %, respectively. For the first patients, we used post-EBRT treatment parameters. Because of the high rates of side effects, new treatment parameters for brachytherapy failure were developed with a decrease in the acoustic dose according to the intense prostate fibrosis. Main complications were urethrorectal fistula in two patients (4 %) and pubic osteitis in one patient (2 %). Incontinence grade 2/3 and bladder neck stenosis occurred in 17 % and 8.5 % of the cases, respectively. Yutkin reported the outcomes of 19 patients with locally recurrent prostate cancer after brachytherapy treated with whole-gland HIFU [87]. Thirteen men had grade 3a or 3b complications by the Clavien system; there were no grade 4 or 5 complications. The most common postoperative complication was dysuria, which was self-limited. Three men developed rectourethral fistulae. The overall continence rate was 68.4 %. At a mean follow-up of 51.6 months, all men were alive. The overall biochemical recurrence-free survival rate was 73.3 % using the Astro-Phoenix criteria.

The oncologic outcomes of salvage HIFU after brachytherapy is similar to the outcomes achieved with salvage HIFU after EBRT, but the risk of rectal injury seems higher.

12 Focal Therapy

HIFU focal therapy is another pathway that must be explored when considering the accuracy and reliability for PCa mapping techniques. HIFU would be particularly suitable for such a therapy since it is clear that HIFU results and toxicity are relative to treated prostate volume.

12.1 Focal Therapy as Primary Care Treatment

Active surveillance has been adopted as an option for men who have a low-risk prostate cancer. The advantages of active surveillance must be weighed against the very real possibility of missing the "window" to cure some cancers because of delayed treatment. In the Canadian trial, overall, 30 % of patients have been reclassified as higher risk and have been offered definitive therapy [88]. Of 117 patients treated radically, the PSA failure rate was 50 %, which was 13 % of the total cohort. Focal therapy is emerging as an alternative to active surveillance in the management of low-intermediate risk, selected patients. In patient candidates for active surveillance, the risk of extracapsular extension was found to range from 7 to 19 % and seminal vesicle invasion ranged from 2 to 9 %, depending on the inclusion of patients with Gleason 7 disease [89]. Mouraviev et al. identified unilateral cancers in 19.2 % of 1184 radical prostatectomy specimens [90]. This study suggests, without taking into account cancer significance, that almost a fifth of the patients who are candidates for radical surgery could be amenable to hemiablation using thermal therapy targeting one lobe of prostate. The literature showed a direct correlation between the Gleason score and the outcomes after radical surgery [91]. Stamey et al. demonstrated that tumor volume was associated with biochemical relapse: recurrence occurs in only 14 % of men with a tumor volume of less than 2.0 ml [92]. Focal therapy must be used only in carefully selected patients (Gleason 6 or Gleason 7 3+4, small solitary cancer foci) included in prospective trials. As discussed above, mp-MRI may be useful in the evaluation of patients considering active surveillance or focal therapy [93]. The concept of a index tumor does, however, potentially allow for the use of focal therapy on patients with bilateral tumors. Some evidence exists which shows the largest tumor (the index lesion) is the main driver of progression, outcome, and prognosis; small secondary cancers might be clinically irrelevant [94, 95]. HIFU might be one of the best techniques for focal therapy because it is performed under real time control using ultrasound or MRI. An immediate control of the boundaries of the necrosis area is possible using contrast agents (either with ultrasound and MRI). HIFU procedures can also be repeated if necessary. Finally, salvage standard curative therapies are feasible after HIFU (EBRT, surgery or cryoablation).

In 2008, Muto et al. reported the outcomes of 29 patients treated with Sonablate™ device [96]. In selected patients whose cancer was confined to only one lobe by multiregional biopsies, the total peripheral zone and a half portion of the transitional zone were ablated. The PSA level decreased from 5.36 ± 5.89 ng/ml to 1.52 ± 0.92 at 36 months. Twenty-eight patients underwent control biopsies 6 months after the procedure: a residual cancer foci was found in three patients (10.7 %). Seventeen patients underwent control biopsies 12 months after the procedure: a residual cancer foci was found in four patients (23.5 %). No significant change was found on

IPSS score and maximal flow rate before and 12 months after the procedure.

The first study (20 patients) of prostate hemiablation with HIFU was published in 2011 [97]. Inclusion criteria were men with low-moderate risk (Gleason = 7, PSA = 15 μg/ml), unilateral PCa on TRUS biopsy underwent MRI and 5 mm-spaced trans-perineal template biopsies to localize disease. Of the men, 25 % had low-risk and 75 % intermediate-risk cancer. The mean PSA pre-HIFU was 7.3 ng/ml. Mean PSA decreased to 1.5 ng/ml ± 1.3 at 12 months. A total of 89 % of the patients had no histological evidence of any cancer. Two patients (11.1 %) had positive protocol biopsy at 6 months with residual 1 mm Gleason 3 + 3: one elected for retreatment and the other active surveillance. An erection sufficient for penetrative sex occurred in 95 % of the patients and 95 % of patients were pad free after focal HIFU.

Ahmed et al. reported in 2015, the outcomes of 56 patients with multifocal localized prostate cancer treated with HIFU focal ablation targeted to the index lesion [98]. The mean age was 63.9 years and median prostate-specific antigen (PSA) was 7.4 ng/ml. There were 7 (12.5 %) low-risk, 47 (83.9 %) intermediate-risk, and 2 (3.6 %) high-risk cancers. The median PSA nadir was 2.4 ng/ml. At 12 months, 42/52 (80.8 %) patients had histological absence of clinically significant cancer (Gleason <7, <2 positive cores, and no cancer core length > 3 mm regardless of grade) and 85.7 % (48/56) had no measurable prostate cancer (biopsy and/or mpMRI). Two (3.6 %) patients had clinically significant disease in untreated areas not detected at baseline. Pad-free and leak-free plus pad-free continence was preserved in 92.3% and 92.0% of patients, respectively. Erections sufficient for intercourse were preserved in 76.9 % of patients.

The French Urological Association (AFU) has started a multi-institutional study to evaluate hemiablation with HIFU as a primary treatment for patients >50 years, T1C or T2A, PSA < 10 ng/ml, Gleason 6 or 7 (3 + 4), in no more than one lobe after MRI, random, and targeted biopsies. To be included, the tumor must be >6 mm from apex and >5 mm from the midline. Only one prostatic lobe is treated. The primary outcome was the absence of clinically significant cancer (CSC) on control biopsy (Gleason <7, <2 positive cores, and no cancer core length >3 mm regardless of grade). Secondary outcomes were the presence of any cancer on biopsy, biochemical response, or radical treatment-free survival (RTFS). A total of 111 patients were treated (mean age 64.8 ± 6.2 years; mean PSA 6.2 ± 2.6 ng/ml; 74 % Gleason ≤6; 26 % Gleason 7). On control biopsy, 12 patients (11.9 %) had a CSC (5 ipsilateral; 7 contralateral). Secondary treatments were technically uneventful and the radical treatment-free survival rate at 2 years was 89 %. The mean PSA decrease at 2 years was 62.8 %. The rate of adverse events was 12.6 % Clavien III. At 12 months, urinary and erectile functions were preserved in 97.2 and 78.4 % of patients. No significant decrease in QOL score was observed at 12 months. Similar results were reported by Cordeiro Feijoo et al. [99].

Van Velthoven published the first long term results of a prospective clinical trial of HIFU hemiablation for clinically localized prostate cancer [100]. Hemiablation HIFU was primarily performed in 50 selected patients with biopsy-proven clinically localized unilateral, low-intermediate risk prostate cancer in complete concordance with the prostate cancer lesions identified by magnetic resonance. The median follow-up was 39.5 months. The mean nadir PSA value was 1.6 ng/ml, which represents 72 % reduction compared with initial PSA pretreatment value ($P < 0.001$). Biochemical recurrence, according to Phoenix definition, occurred in 28 % of patients, respectively. The 5-year actuarial metastases-free survival, cancer-specific survival, and overall survival rates were 93, 100, and 87 %, respectively. Out of the eight patients undergoing biopsy, six patients had a positive biopsy for cancer occurring in the untreated contralateral ($n = 3$) or treated ipsilateral lobe ($n = 1$) or bilaterally ($n = 2$). A Clavien-Dindo grade 3b complication occurred in two patients. Complete continence (no pads) and erection sufficient for intercourse were documented in 94 or 80 % of patients, respectively.

After hemiablation HIFU, the rate of clinically significant disease was low and associated with low morbidity and preservation of quality of life. This treatment strategy does not preclude future definitive therapies.

New devices (i.e., Focal One) will make HIFU an even more effective treatment option for focal therapy. Preliminary results compare favorably with those of hemiablation studies [101].

12.2 Focal Therapy as Salvage Treatment (Focal Salvage HIFU)

Early identification of a local relapse after radiation therapy failure is feasible using MRI and targeted biopsies performed soon after the biochemical failure (Phoenix criteria). Focal Salvage HIFU is a new therapeutic option. The aim of focal salvage HIFU (FSH) is to destroy the recurrent cancer with a minimal risk of severe side effects.

The study of Ahmed et al. demonstrated that, focal therapy with HIFU can achieve a local control of the disease with minimal morbidity in patients with unilateral relapse after EBRT [102]. Baco and Gelet reported outcomes of 48 men with unilateral radio-recurrent prostate cancer prospectively enrolled in two European centers and treated with hemisalvage HIFU [103]. After HSH, the mean PSA nadir was 0.69 ng/mL at a median follow-up of 16.3 months. Disease progression occurred in 16 patients. Of these, four had local recurrence in the untreated lobe and four bilaterally, six developed metastases, and two had rising PSA levels without local recurrence or radiological confirmed metastasis. Progression-free survival rates at 12, 18, and 24 months were 83, 64, and 52 %. Severe incontinence occurred in 4 of the 48 patients (8 %), 8 (17 %) required one pad a day, and 36/48 (75 %) were pad-free. The mean IPSS and erectile function (IIEF-5) scores decreased from a mean of 7.01–8.6 and from 11.2 to 7.0, respectively.

13 Androgen Deprivation and Chemotherapy Associated with HIFU for High-Risk Prostate Cancer

13.1 Androgen Deprivation

Promising preliminary results on HIFU and hormonal deprivation in patients with locally advanced disease and/or high-risk PCa have been published [61]. At 12 months after the procedure, 28 patients (93 %) were continent. Seven of the 30 men (23 %) had a positive prostate biopsy. At the 1-year follow-up, only three of the 30 patients with high-risk prostate cancer had a PSA level of >0.3 ng/m. Long term outcome was unknown.

13.2 Chemotherapy

Experimental studies have demonstrated the potential of chemotherapy associated with HIFU. In a rat model, Paparel et al. evaluated the therapeutic effect of HIFU combined with Docetaxel on AT2 Dunning adenocarcinoma [104, 105]. They showed a synergistic inhibitory effect of the HIFU + Docetaxel association.

In an ethical committee approved study, 27 high-risk patients (Gleason ≥ 4 + 3 and/or PSA >15 ng/ml and/or >2/3 of positive biopsy) underwent HIFU associated with Docetaxel. Chemotherapy was delivered 30 min before the HIFU treatment. The protocol included a dose escalation starting at 30 mg/ml. Fifteen patients received 30 mg/m^2 of Docetaxel with no adverse effects, two patients received 50 mg/m2 with 1 febrile neutropenia and 1 transient alopecia grade 1 and the next seven patients received 40 ml/m2 without adverse effects. A PSA nadir ≤0.30 ng was achieved in 15 patients (55.5 %). At 7 years, the cancer-specific survival rate and the metastasis-free survival rate were estimated at 90 % (CI:47–98) and 77 % (CI:48–91), respectively. An additional therapy was used in 13 cases: salvage EBRT alone in five patients, salvage EBRT + AD in two patients, and palliative

AD was started in six patients. At 5 years, the progression-free survival rate was 48 % (95 %CI: 27–66). Randomized studies with long term follow-up are required to evaluate the potential role of chemotherapy associated with HIFU in high-risk patients.

Conclusion

The outcomes achieved for primary care patients seem close to those obtained by standard definitive therapies. HIFU does not represent a therapeutic impasse: EBRT is a safe salvage option after HIFU failure and salvage surgery is possible in young and motivated patients. On the other hand, HIFU has a considerable potential for local recurrence after radiation failure. Recently, some early experiences on focal therapy suggest that HIFU provides an excellent opportunity to achieved local control of the disease in low-intermediate risk prostate cancer and in early identified local relapse after EBRT.

References

1. Bosetti C, Bertuccio P, Chatenoud L, Negri E, La Vecchia C, Levi F. Trends in mortality from urologic cancers in Europe, 1970–2008. Eur Urol. 2011;60(1):1–15.
2. Wilt TJ, Brawer MK, Jones KM, Barry MJ, Aronson WJ, Fox S, et al. Radical prostatectomy versus observation for localized prostate cancer. N Engl J Med. 2012;367(3):203–13.
3. Steyerberg EW, Roobol MJ, Kattan MW, van der Kwast TH, de Koning HJ, Schröder FH. Prediction of indolent prostate cancer: validation and updating of a prognostic nomogram. J Urol. 2007;177(1):107–12.
4. Albertsen PC, Moore DF, Shih W, Lin Y, Li H, Lu-Yao GL. Impact of comorbidity on survival among men with localized prostate cancer. J Clin Oncol. 2011;29(10):1335–41.
5. Klotz L, Vesprini D, Sethukavalan P, Jethava V, Zhang L, Jain S, Yamamoto T, Mamedov A, Loblaw A. Long-term follow-up of a large active surveillance cohort of patients with prostate cancer. J Clin Oncol. 2015;33(3):272–7.
6. Lynn JG, Putnam TJ. Histology of cerebral lesions produced by focused ultrasound. Am J Pathol. 1944;20(3):637–49.
7. Chapelon JY, Ribault M, Birer A, Vernier F, Souchon R, Gelet A. Treatment of localised prostate cancer with transrectal high intensity focused ultrasound. Eur J Ultrasound. 1999;9:31–8.
8. Chapelon JY, Margonari J, Vernier F, Gorry F, Ecochard R, Gelet A. In vivo effects of high-intensity ultrasound on prostatic adenocarcinoma Dunning R3327. Cancer Res. 1992;52(22):6353–7.
9. Gelet A, Chapelon JY, Margonari J, Theillere Y, Gorry F, Cathignol D, et al. Prostatic tissue destruction by high-intensity focused ultrasound: experimentation on canine prostate. J Endourol. 1993;7(3):249–53.
10. Gelet A, Chapelon JY, Margonari J, Theillere Y, Gorry F, Souchon R, et al. High-intensity focused ultrasound experimentation on human benign prostatic hypertrophy. Eur Urol. 1993;23 Suppl 1:44–7.
11. Madersbacher S, Kratzik C, Szabo N, Susani M, Vingers L, Marberger M. Tissue ablation in benign prostatic hyperplasia with high-intensity focused ultrasound. Eur Urol. 1993;23 Suppl 1:39–43.
12. Beerlage HP, van Leenders GJ, Oosterhof GO, Witjes JA, Ruijter ET, van de Kaa CA, et al. High-intensity focused ultrasound (HIFU) followed after one to two weeks by radical retropubic prostatectomy: results of a prospective study. Prostate. 1999;39(1):41–6.
13. Gelet A, Chapelon JY, Bouvier R, Souchon R, Pangaud C, Abdelrahim AF, et al. Treatment of prostate cancer with transrectal focused ultrasound: early clinical experience. Eur Urol. 1996;29(2):174–83.
14. Gelet A, Chapelon JY, Bouvier R, Pangaud C, Lasne Y. Local control of prostate cancer by transrectal high intensity focused ultrasound therapy: preliminary results. J Urol. 1999;161(1):156–62.
15. Rouviere O, Gelet A, Crouzet S, Chapelon JY. Prostate focused ultrasound focal therapy – imaging for the future. Nat Rev. 2012;9(12):721–7.
16. Sartor O, Eisenberger M, Kattan MW, Tombal B, Lecouvet F. Unmet needs in the prediction and detection of metastases in prostate cancer. Oncologist. 2013;18(5):549–57.
17. Bratan F, Niaf E, Melodelima C, et al. Influence of imaging and histological factors on prostate cancer detection and localisation on multiparametric MRI: a prospective study. Eur Radiol. 2013;23(7):2019–29.
18. Turkbey B, Mani H, Shah V, et al. Multiparametric 3T prostate magnetic resonance imaging to detect cancer: histopathological correlation using prostatectomy specimens processed in customized magnetic resonance imaging based molds. J Urol. 2011;186(5):1818–24.
19. Turkbey B, Pinto PA, Mani H, et al. Prostate cancer: value of multiparametric MR imaging at 3 T for detection – histopathologic correlation. Radiology. 2010;255(1):89–99.
20. Le Nobin J, Orczyk C, Deng FM, et al. Prostate tumour volumes: evaluation of the agreement between magnetic resonance imaging and histology

using novel co-registration software. BJU Int. 2014;114(6b):E105–12.
21. Bratan F, Melodelima C, Souchon R, et al. How accurate is multiparametric MR imaging in evaluation of prostate cancer volume? Radiology. 2015;275(1):144–54.
22. Cornud F, Khoury G, Bouazza N, et al. Tumor target volume for focal therapy of prostate cancer-does multiparametric magnetic resonance imaging allow for a reliable estimation? J Urol. 2014;191(5):1272–9.
23. Donati OF, Jung SI, Vargas HA, et al. Multiparametric prostate MR imaging with T2-weighted, diffusion-weighted, and dynamic contrast-enhanced sequences: are all pulse sequences necessary to detect locally recurrent prostate cancer after radiation therapy? Radiology. 2013;268(2):440–50.
24. Abd-Alazeez M, Ramachandran N, Dikaios N, et al. Multiparametric MRI for detection of radiorecurrent prostate cancer: added value of apparent diffusion coefficient maps and dynamic contrast-enhanced images. Prostate Cancer Prostatic Dis. 2015;18(2):128–36.
25. Alonzo F, Melodelima C, Bratan F, et al. Detection of locally radio-recurrent prostate cancer at multiparametric MRI: can dynamic contrast-enhanced imaging be omitted? Diagn Interv Imaging. 2016;97(4):433–41.
26. Rouviere O, Sbihi L, Gelet A, Chapelon JY. Salvage high-intensity focused ultrasound ablation for prostate cancer local recurrence after external-beam radiation therapy: prognostic value of prostate MRI. Clin Radiol. 2013;68(7):661–7.
27. Rouviere O, Souchon R, Salomir R, Gelet A, Chapelon JY, Lyonnet D. Transrectal high-intensity focused ultrasound ablation of prostate cancer: effective treatment requiring accurate imaging. Eur J Radiol. 2007;63(3):317–27.
28. Rouviere O, Lyonnet D, Raudrant A, et al. MRI appearance of prostate following transrectal HIFU ablation of localized cancer. Eur Urol. 2001;40(3):265–74.
29. Kirkham AP, Emberton M, Hoh IM, Illing RO, Freeman AA, Allen C. MR imaging of prostate after treatment with high-intensity focused ultrasound. Radiology. 2008;246(3):833–44.
30. Rouvière O, Glas L, Girouin N, et al. Transrectal HIFU ablation of prostate cancer: assessment of tissue destruction with contrast-enhanced ultrasound. Radiology. 2011;259(2):583–91.
31. Pasticier G, Chapet O, Badet L, et al. Salvage radiotherapy after high-intensity focused ultrasound for localized prostate cancer: early clinical results. Urology. 2008;72(6):1305–9.
32. Rouviere O, Mege-Lechevallier F, Chapelon JY, et al. Evaluation of color Doppler in guiding prostate biopsy after HIFU ablation. Eur Urol. 2006;50(3):490–7.
33. Ben Cheikh A, Girouin N, Ryon-Taponnier P, et al. MR detection of local prostate cancer recurrence after transrectal high-intensity focused US treatment: preliminary results. J Radiol. 2008;89(5 Pt 1):571–7.
34. Rouviere O, Girouin N, Glas L, et al. Prostate cancer transrectal HIFU ablation: detection of local recurrences using T2-weighted and dynamic contrast-enhanced MRI. Eur Radiol. 2010;20(1):48–55.
35. Salomir R, Delemazure AS, Palussiere J, Rouviere O, Cotton F, Chapelon JY. Image-based control of the magnetic resonance imaging-guided focused ultrasound thermotherapy. Top Magn Reson Imaging. 2006;17(3):139–51.
36. Uchida T, Ohkusa H, Nagata Y, Hyodo T, Satoh T, Irie A. Treatment of localized prostate cancer using high-intensity focused ultrasound. BJU Int. 2006;97(1):56–61.
37. Chavrier F, Chapelon JY, Gelet A, Cathignol D. Modeling of high-intensity focused ultrasound-induced lesions in the presence of cavitation bubbles. J Acoust Soc Am. 2000;108(1):432–40.
38. Chopra R, Colquhoun A, Burtnyk M, N'djin WA, Kobelevskiy I, Boyes A, Siddiqui L, Foster H, Sugar L, Haider MA, Bronskill M, Klotz L. MR imaging-controlled transurethral ultrasound therapy for conformal treatment of prostate tissue: initial feasibility in humans. Radiology. 2012;265:303–13.
39. Zini C, Hipp E, Thomas S, Napoli A, Catalano C, Oto A. Ultrasound- and MR-guided focused ultrasound surgery for prostate cancer. World J Radiol. 2012;4:247 52.
40. Vallancien G, Prapotnich D, Cathelineau X, Baumert H, Rozet F. Transrectal focused ultrasound combined with transurethral resection of the prostate for the treatment of localized prostate cancer: feasibility study. J Urol. 2004;171(6 Pt 1):2265–7.
41. Chaussy C, Thuroff S. The status of high-intensity focused ultrasound in the treatment of localized prostate cancer and the impact of a combined resection. Curr Urol Rep. 2003;4(3):248–52.
42. Thuroff S, Chaussy C. High-intensity focused ultrasound: complications and adverse events. Mol Urol. 2000;4(3):183–7;discussion 9.
43. Netsch C, Pfeiffer D, Gross AJ. Development of bladder outlet obstruction after a single treatment of prostate cancer with high-intensity focused ultrasound: experience with 226 patients. J Endourol. 2010;24(9):1399–403.
44. Sumitomo M, Asakuma J, Sato A, Ito K, Nagakura K, Asano T. Transurethral resection of the prostate immediately after high-intensity focused ultrasound treatment for prostate cancer. Int J Urol. 2010;17(11):924–30.
45. Rebillard X, Davin JL, Soulie M. Treatment by HIFU of prostate cancer: survey of literature and treatment indications. Prog Urol. 2003;13(6):1428–56. Epub 2004/03/06. Traitement par HIFU du cancer de la prostate: revue de la litterature et indications de traitement.
46. Rebillard X, Soulié M, Chartier-Kastler, et al. High-intensity focused ultrasound in prostate cancer; a

systematic literature review of the French Association of Urology. BJU Int. 2008;101(10):1205–13.
47. Lee HM, Hong JH, Choi HY. High-intensity focused ultrasound therapy for clinically localized prostate cancer. Prostate Cancer Prostatic Dis. 2006;9(4):439–43.
48. Poissonnier L, Chapelon JY, Rouviere O, Curiel L, Bouvier R, Martin X, et al. Control of prostate cancer by transrectal HIFU in 227 patients. Eur Urol. 2007;51(2):381–7.
49. Uchidaa T, Nakanoa M, Shojia S, Omataa T, Haranoa Y, Nagataa Y, Usuib Y, Terachib T, et al. Ten year biochemical disease free survival after high intensity focused ultrasound (HIFU) for localised prostate cancer: comparison with three different generation devices. J Urol. 2009;181(4):228.
50. Ahmed HU, Zacharakis E, Dudderidge T, Armitage JN, Scott R, Calleary J, et al. High-intensity-focused ultrasound in the treatment of primary prostate cancer: the first UK series. Br J Cancer. 2009;101(1):19–26.
51. Blana A, Brown SCW, Chaussy C, Conti GN, Eastham JA, Ganzer R, et al. Primary prostate HIFU without pretreatment hormone therapy: biochemical survival of 468 patients tracked with the @-registry. J Urol. 2009;181(4):227.
52. Mearini L, D'Urso L, Collura D, Zucchi A, Costantini E, Formiconi A, et al. Visually directed transrectal high intensity focused ultrasound for the treatment of prostate cancer: a preliminary report on the Italian experience. J Urol. 2009;181(1):105–11; discussion 11–2.
53. Blana A, Murat FJ, Walter B, Thuroff S, Wieland WF, Chaussy C, et al. First analysis of the long-term results with transrectal HIFU in patients with localised prostate cancer. Eur Urol. 2008;53(6):1194–201. Epub 2007/11/13.
54. Misrai V, Roupret M, Chartier-Kastler E, Comperat E, Renard-Penna R, Haertig A, et al. Oncologic control provided by HIFU therapy as single treatment in men with clinically localized prostate cancer. World J Urol. 2008;26(5):481–5.
55. Blana A, Rogenhofer S, Ganzer R, Lunz JC, Schostak M, Wieland WF, et al. Eight years' experience with high-intensity focused ultrasonography for treatment of localized prostate cancer. Urology. 2008;72(6):1329–33; discussion 33–4.
56. Ganzer R, Rogenhofer S, Walter B, Lunz JC, Schostak M, Wieland WF, et al. PSA nadir is a significant predictor of treatment failure after high-intensity focussed ultrasound (HIFU) treatment of localised prostate cancer. Eur Urol. 2008;53(3):547–53.
57. Uchida T, Ohkusa H, Yamashita H, Shoji S, Nagata Y, Hyodo T, et al. Five years experience of transrectal high-intensity focused ultrasound using the Sonablate device in the treatment of localized prostate cancer. Int J Urol. 2006;13(3):228–33.
58. Thuroff S, Chaussy C, Vallancien G, Wieland W, Kiel HJ, Le Duc A, et al. High-intensity focused ultrasound and localized prostate cancer: efficacy results from the European multicentric study. J Endourol. 2003;17(8):673–7.
59. Chaussy C, Thuroff S. Results and side effects of high-intensity focused ultrasound in localized prostate cancer. J Endourol. 2001;15(4):437–40; discussion 47–8.
60. Gelet A, Chapelon JY, Bouvier R, Rouviere O, Lasne Y, Lyonnet D, et al. Transrectal high-intensity focused ultrasound: minimally invasive therapy of localized prostate cancer. J Endourol. 2000;14(6):519–28.
61. Ficarra V, Antoniolli SZ, Novara G, Parisi A, Fracalanza S, Martignoni G, et al. Short-term outcome after high-intensity focused ultrasound in the treatment of patients with high-risk prostate cancer. BJU Int. 2006;98(6):1193–8.
62. Uchida T, Illing RO, Cathcart PJ, Emberton M. To what extent does the prostate-specific antigen nadir predict subsequent treatment failure after transrectal high-intensity focused ultrasound therapy for presumed localized adenocarcinoma of the prostate? BJU Int. 2006;98(3):537–9.
63. Chaussy C, Thuroff S, Rebillard X, Gelet A. Technology insight: high-intensity focused ultrasound for urologic cancers. Nat Clin Pract Urol. 2005;2(4):191–8.
64. Crouzet S, Poissonnier L, Murat FJ, Pasticier G, Rouviere O, Mege-Lechevallier F, et al. Outcomes of HIFU for localised prostate cancer using the Ablatherm Integrate Imaging(R) device. Prog Urol. 2011;21(3):191–7.
65. Crouzet S, Chapelon JY, Rouvière O, Mege-Lechevallier F, Colombel M, Tonoli-Catez H, Martin X, Gelet A. Whole-gland ablation of localized prostate cancer with high-intensity focused ultrasound: oncologic outcomes and morbidity in 1002 patients. Eur Urol. 2014;65(5):907–1464.
66. Thüroff S, Chaussy C. Evolution and outcomes of 3 MHz high intensity focused ultrasound therapy for localized prostate cancer during 15 years. J Urol. 2013;190(2):702–10. 65.
67. Ganzer R, Fritsche HM, Brandtner A, Bründl J, Koch D, Wieland WF, Blana A. Fourteen-year oncological and functional outcomes of high-intensity focused ultrasound in localized prostate cancer. BJU Int. 2013;112(3):322–9.
68. Uchida T, Tomonaga T, Kim H, Nakano M, Shoji S, Nagata Y, Terachi T. Improved outcomes with advancements in high intensity focused ultrasound devices for the treatment of localized prostate cancer. J Urol. 2015;193(1):103–10.
69. Dickinson L, Arya M, Afzal N, Cathcart P, Charman SC, Cornaby A, Hindley RG, Lewi H, McCartan N, Moore CM, Nathan S, Ogden C, Persad R, van der Meulen J, Weir S, Emberton M, Ahmed HU. Medium-term outcomes after whole-gland high-intensity

focused ultrasound for the treatment of nonmetastatic prostate cancer from a multicentre registry cohort. Eur Urol. 2016. pii: S0302–2838(16)00244-X. doi:10.1016/j.eururo.2016.02.054. [Epub ahead of print].
70. Shoji S, Nakano M, Nagata Y, Usui Y, Terachi T, Uchida T. Quality of life following high-intensity focused ultrasound for the treatment of localized prostate cancer: a prospective study. Int J Urol. 2010;17(8):715–9.
71. Li LY, Lin Z, Yang M, Gao X, Xia TL, Ding T. Comparison of penile size and erectile function after high-intensity focused ultrasound and targeted cryoablation for localized prostate cancer: a prospective pilot study. J Sex Med. 2010;7(9):3135–42.
72. Blana A, Rogenhofer S, Ganzer R, Wild PJ, Wieland WF, Walter B. Morbidity associated with repeated transrectal high-intensity focused ultrasound treatment of localized prostate cancer. World J Urol. 2006;24(5):585–90; Epub 2006/07/20.
73. Pasticier G, Riviere J, Wallerand H, Robert G, Bernhard JC, Ferriere JM, et al. Salvage radiotherapy (SRT) for local recurrence of prostate adenocarcinoma after primary treatment with high intensity focused ultrasound (HIFU): first series of 100 patients. 2010 ASCO annual meeting. 2010.
74. Munoz F, Guarneri A, Botticella A, Gabriele P, Moretto F, Panaia R, Ruggieri A, D'Urso L, Muto G, Filippi AR, Ragona R, Ricardi U. Salvage external beam radiotherapy for recurrent prostate adenocarcinoma after high-intensity focused ultrasound as primary treatment. Urol Int. 2013;90(3):288–93.
75. Lawrentschuk N, Finelli A, Van der Kwast TH, Ryan P, Bolton DM, Fleshner NE, et al. Salvage radical prostatectomy following primary high intensity focused ultrasound for treatment of prostate cancer. J Urol. 2011;185(3):862–8. Epub 2011/01/18.76 Kane C. Salvage laparoscopic radical prostatectomy following high-intensity focused ultrasound for treatment of prostate cancer.Urol Oncol. 2013 Feb;31(2):273–4.
76. Kane C. Salvage laparoscopic radical prostatectomy following high-intensity focused ultrasound for treatment of prostate cancer. Urol Oncol. 2013;31(2):273–4.
77. Borghede G, Aldenborg F, Wurzinger E, Johansson KA, Hedelin H. Analysis of the local control in lymph-node staged localized prostate cancer treated by external beam radiotherapy, assessed by digital rectal examination, serum prostate-specific antigen and biopsy. Br J Urol. 1997;80(2):247–55.
78. Zelefsky MJ, Fuks Z, Hunt M, Lee HJ, Lombardi D, Ling CC, et al. High dose radiation delivered by intensity modulated conformal radiotherapy improves the outcome of localized prostate cancer. J Urol. 2001;166(3):876–81. Epub 2001/08/08.
79. Murat FJ, Poissonnier L, Rabilloud M, Belot A, Bouvier R, Rouviere O, et al. Mid-term results demonstrate salvage high-intensity focused ultrasound (HIFU) as an effective and acceptably morbid salvage treatment option for locally radiorecurrent prostate cancer. Eur Urol. 2009;55(3):640–7.
80. Sébastien C, Francois-Joseph M, Pascal P, Laura P, Gilles P, Olivier R, Jean-Yves C, Muriel R, Aurélien B, Florence M-L, Hélène T-C, Xavier M, Albert G. Locally recurrent prostate cancer after initial radiation therapy: early salvage high-intensity focused ultrasound improves oncologic outcomes. Radiother Oncol. 2012. doi:10.1016/j.radonc.2012.09.014.
81. Rouvière O, Sbihi L, Gelet A, Chapelon JY. Salvage high-intensity focused ultrasound ablation for prostate cancer local recurrence after external-beam radiation therapy: prognostic value of prostate MRI. Clin Radiol. 2013;68(7):661–7. doi:10.1016/j.crad.2012.12.010.
82. Berge V, Baco E, Karlsen SJ. A prospective study of salvage high-intensity focused ultrasound for locally radiorecurrent prostate cancer: early results. Scand J Urol Nephrol. 2010;44(4):223–7.
83. Zacharakis E, Ahmed HU, Ishaq A, Scott R, Illing R, Freeman A, et al. The feasibility and safety of high-intensity focused ultrasound as salvage therapy for recurrent prostate cancer following external beam radiotherapy. BJU Int. 2008;102(7):786–92.
84. Uchida T, Shoji S, Nakano M, Hongo S, Nitta M, Usui Y, et al. High-intensity focused ultrasound as salvage therapy for patients with recurrent prostate cancer after external beam radiation, brachytherapy or proton therapy. BJU Int. 2010;107(3):378–82.
85. Sylvester JE, Grimm PD, Wong J, Galbreath RW, Merrick G, Blasko JC. Fifteen-year biochemical relapse-free survival, cause-specific survival, and overall survival following I(125) prostate brachytherapy in clinically localized prostate cancer: seattle experience. Int J Radiat Oncol Biol Phys. 2010;81:376–81.
86. Heidenreich A, Richter S, Thuer D, Pfister D. Prognostic parameters, complications, and oncologic and functional outcome of salvage radical prostatectomy for locally recurrent prostate cancer after 21st-century radiotherapy. Eur Urol. 2010;57(3):437–43.
87. Yutkin V, Ahmed HU, Donaldson I, McCartan N, Siddiqui K, Emberton M, Chin JL. Salvage high-intensity focused ultrasound for patients with recurrent prostate cancer after brachytherapy. Urology. 2014;84(5):1157–62.
88. Klotz L, Zhang L, Lam A, Nam R, Mamedov A, Loblaw A. Clinical results of long-term follow-up of a large, active surveillance cohort with localized prostate cancer. J Clin Oncol. 2010;28(1):126–31.
89. Conti SL, Dall'era M, Fradet V, Cowan JE, Simko J, Carroll PR. Pathological outcomes of candidates for active surveillance of prostate cancer. J Urol. 2009;181(4):1628–33; discussion 33–4.
90. Mouraviev V, Mayes JM, Sun L, Madden JF, Moul JW, Polascik TJ. Prostate cancer laterality as a

rationale of focal ablative therapy for the treatment of clinically localized prostate cancer. Cancer. 2007;110(4):906–10.
91. Blute ML, Bergstralh EJ, Iocca A, Scherer B, Zincke H. Use of Gleason score, prostate specific antigen, seminal vesicle and margin status to predict biochemical failure after radical prostatectomy. J Urol. 2001;165(1):119–25.
92. Stamey TA, McNeal JE, Yemoto CM, Sigal BM, Johnstone IM. Biological determinants of cancer progression in men with prostate cancer. JAMA. 1999;281(15):1395–400.
93. Mullins JK, Bonekamp D, Landis P, Begum H, Partin AW, Epstein JI, Carter HB, Macura KJ. Multiparametric magnetic resonance imaging findings in men with low-risk prostate cancer followed using active surveillance. BJU Int. 2013;111(7):1037–45.
94. Wise AM, Stamey TA, McNeal JE, Clayton JL. Morphologic and clinical significance of multifocal prostate cancers in radical prostatectomy specimens. Urology. 2002;60(2):264–9.
95. Noguchi M, Stamey TA, McNeal JE, Nolley R. Prognostic factors for multifocal prostate cancer in radical prostatectomy specimens: lack of significance of secondary cancers. J Urol. 2003;170(2 Pt 1):459–63.
96. Muto S, Yoshii T, Saito K, Kamiyama Y, Ide H, Horie S. Focal therapy with high-intensity-focused ultrasound in the treatment of localized prostate cancer. Jpn J Clin Oncol. 2008;38(3):192–9. Epub 2008/02/19.
97. Ahmed HU, Freeman A, Kirkham A, Sahu M, Scott R, Allen C, et al. Focal therapy for localized prostate cancer: a phase I/II trial. J Urol. 2011;185(4):1246–54.
98. Ahmed HU, Dickinson L, Charman S, Weir S, McCartan N, Hindley RG, Freeman A, Kirkham AP, Sahu M, Scott R, Allen C, Van der Meulen J, Emberton M. Focal ablation targeted to the index lesion in multifocal localised prostate cancer: a prospective development study. Eur Urol. 2015;68(6):927–36.
99. Feijoo ER, Sivaraman A, Barret E, Sanchez-Salas R, Galiano M, Rozet F, Prapotnich D, Cathala N, Mombet A. Cathelineau X focal high-intensity focused ultrasound targeted hemiablation for unilateral prostate cancer: a prospective evaluation of oncologic and functional outcomes. Eur Urol. 2016;69(2):214–20.
100. Van Velthoven R, Aoun F, Marcelis Q, Albisinni S, Zanaty M, Lemort M, Peltier A, Limani K. A prospective clinical trial of HIFU hemiablation for clinically localized prostate cancer. Prostate Cancer Prostatic Dis. 2016;19(1):79–83.
101. Albert G, Sebastien C, Olivier R, Flavie B, Jean-Yves C. Focal treatment of prostate cancer using focal one device: pilot study results. J Ther Ultrasound. 2015;3(Suppl 1):O54 (30 June 2015).
102. Ahmed HU, Cathcart P, McCartan N, Kirkham A, Allen C, Freeman A, Emberton M. Focal salvage therapy for localized prostate cancer recurrence after external beam radiotherapy: a pilot study. Cancer. 2012;118(17):4148–55.
103. Baco E, Gelet A, Crouzet S, Rud E, Rouvière O, Tonoli-Catez H, Berge V, Chapelon JY, Eggesbø HB. Hemi salvage high-intensity focused ultrasound (HIFU) in unilateral radiorecurrent prostate cancer: a prospective two-centre study. BJU Int. 2014;114(4):532–40.
104. Paparel P, Curiel L, Chesnais S, Ecochard R, Chapelon JY, Gelet A. Synergistic inhibitory effect of high-intensity focused ultrasound combined with chemotherapy on Dunning adenocarcinoma. BJU Int. 2005;95(6):881–5.
105. Paparel P, Chapelon JY, Bissery A, Chesnais S, Curiel L, Gelet A. Influence of the docetaxel administration period (neoadjuvant or concomitant) in relation to HIFU treatment on the growth of Dunning tumors: results of a preliminary study. Prostate Cancer Prostatic Dis. 2008;11(2):181–6.

Prostate Cryotherapy

Kae Jack Tay, Matvey Tsivian,
and Thomas J. Polascik

1 Introduction

Cryosurgery has been applied in oncologic treatments for over 150 years [1], constantly evolving into the modern minimally invasive approach for the treatment of prostate cancer (PCa). Today, modern cryosurgery is an accepted option for both the primary and salvage treatment of localized PCa recognized by the international guidelines [2, 3]. Herein we review cryobiology, treatment indications, procedure details, as well as contemporary results of cryotherapy for PCa.

2 Elements of Cryobiology

The basis of cryogenic injury is local tissue destruction by subtraction of energy and achievement of low temperatures. There are three main mechanisms that can be considered as the principal pathways of cryoinjury, and these consist of cellular damage caused by ice crystal formation, failure of the microcirculation after thawing, and the induction of apoptosis and necrosis [4].

The direct cell injury process can be summarized by two topographically distinct processes: intracellular and extracellular ice formation. Extracellular ice formation subtracts water from the extracellular environment and, aside from its mechanical damage, induces extracellular hypertonicity that in turn draws water from within the cells, dehydrating them and disrupting normal enzymatic processes and membrane properties [5, 6]. Intracellular ice crystal formation occurs secondarily and causes lethal cell disruption. These ice crystals mechanically disrupt and damage vital cell structures such as organelles and the membrane. While the relative contributions of intra- and extracellular ice formations are debatable, it is generally recognized that they are synergistic [7]. During the thawing phase, when frozen tissue temperature rises above −40 °C, smaller ice crystals fuse to form larger structures in a process known as recrystallization, and additional structural damage is inflicted upon cell structures. As thawing proceeds, extracellular ice melts and a hypotonic environment is created driving overloading water shifts into the cells [6].

Extreme temperatures mainly affect the small vessels, damaging the endothelium whereby the vessel cell lining sloughs and impedes blood flow, thereby inducing a typical inflammatory response with permeability of the vessels, distention of vessel walls, thrombosis, ischemia, and necrosis of the supplied tissue [7]. Moreover, during the thawing phase of cryotherapy, reperfusion injury enhances endothelial damage stimulating the inflammatory response with release of oxygen radicals and augmenting tissue damage.

K.J. Tay • M. Tsivian • T.J. Polascik, MD, FACS (✉)
Division of Urology, Department of Surgery, Duke University Medical Center, Durham, NC, USA
e-mail: polas001@mc.duke.edu

M. Bolla, H. van Poppel (eds.), *Management of Prostate Cancer*,
DOI 10.1007/978-3-319-42769-0_18

Lastly, advances in understanding post-thaw molecular events have led to the recognition that postthaw apoptosis may occur after the cryoinjury due to extrinsic, or membrane-modulated, and intrinsic, or mitochondrial-modulated, pathways [8]. The extrinsic pathway appears to involve the activation of caspases 8 and 9, while the intrinsic pathway involves the disruption of normal mitochondrial function by upregulation of Bax, a proapoptotic protein of the Bcl-2 family. It has also been shown that cryoinjury sensitizes cancer, but not normal prostate cells, to pathways of apoptosis suggesting a potential role for combination strategies in PCa cryosurgery to enhance targeted damage to cancerous tissue [9–11].

Alongside local mechanisms of destruction, cryotherapy may provide an additional aspect to cancer control. Since cancerous tissue is not removed by the procedure and cancer-specific antigens are left in situ, these can theoretically be recognized by the immune system and stimulate a cancer-specific immune response towards them. However, there is controversy regarding the nature of such immunologic response with conflicting data reported in the literature. While some studies support an anticancer response after cryoablation, others indicate that immunosuppression or tolerance to these antigens may, in fact, be induced [12–16]. It appears that the nature of the immune response depends on local and systemic factors such as cytokines, antigen-presenting cells, as well as the type of antigen presented that comprise the immune system response [17].

Below temperatures of −40 °C, recognized as the lethal temperature where majority of cell kill occurs, virtually all water is transformed to ice [18, 19]. Reaching temperatures below this threshold has also been shown to ensure effective PCa cell destruction [20]. At the periphery of the ice ball, where temperatures are not as cold, cryoinjury may be reversible (at temperatures −20 to 0 °C) and, rather than harness the full spectrum of lethal effects, only induce apoptosis [21]. Cryoinjury is also time-dependent as cryoinjury progresses with freezing. In general, achieving a nadir temperature of at least −40 °C for "a few minutes" has been thought to reach a lethal dose [22]. It must be noted that the exact dose achieved is confounded by biological variability such as cell-type (neoplastic versus normal), cell-cycle stage, vascular supply (large vessels act as a heat sink), and reflex vasoconstrictive variations which may influence the generation of a uniform cryoablative dose field [4]. These factors must be understood by practitioners in order to apply the lethal effects of cryoinjury judiciously to achieve the desired outcomes.

3 Indications for Cryosurgery

Cryosurgery for PCa is a recognized treatment option; however, there is no agreement to date upon the indications and contraindications for this approach and international guidelines remain cautious in this regard [2, 23].

In the setting of primary cryotherapy for localized PCa, the American Urological Association (AUA) guidelines state that cryosurgery is an option for patients who do not desire or are not good candidates for conventional surgery [2]. On the other hand, the EAU guidelines state that primary cryotherapy, as with all other primary ablative techniques, should only be applied in a trial setting [23].

Doubtlessly, patient and disease characteristics need to be taken into account when considering cryotherapy as an option for prostate cancer. However, the current lack of homogeneous, high-quality data in the literature, specific to low-, intermediate-, and high-risk prostate cancer, has hampered the adoption of clear recommendations from the major guidelines. As long term outcomes of primary cryosurgery become available, we are likely to see a refinement of the guidelines with stronger and more precise recommendations made.

There are several technical contraindications to cryosurgery that apply both in the primary and salvage settings. A history of transurethral resection of the prostate or similar procedures should be considered relative contraindications, as large defects in the prostatic fossa may impair the effectiveness of the urethral warmer, a device that safeguards against mucosal slough, by preventing it from coapting with the urethral wall. Additionally, major rectal pathology may be considered a contraindication, particularly if the procedure cannot be monitored under transrectal ultrasound guidance. Moreover, extensive counseling is needed for potent patients expecting to maintain erectile function, as potency is typically impaired to some degree, similar to other procedures, following whole gland cryoablation. Large prostate glands (>60 cc) may be difficult to treat due to sheer size alone or interference of the pubic arch. The latter obstacle can be overcome with either manual positioning of the probes that is void of transperineal grid constraints or extended lithotomy position of the patient. For larger prostates, gland downsizing using hormonal agents can be utilized prior to intervention.

Cryotherapy in the salvage setting represents an attractive alternative to salvage prostatectomy offering reduced morbidity and technical challenge [24]. Salvage cryosurgery has been used both after external beam radiation and interstitial radiotherapy, along with other failed primary therapies such as cryoablation, high-intensity focused ultrasound, etc. Therefore, patients with local, biopsy proven recurrence of prostate cancer after radiation or other primary therapy with no evidence of metastatic disease represent potential candidates for salvage cryotherapy. Due to a higher chance of seminal vesicle invasion, we recommend considering seminal vesicle biopsies and lymph node sampling in the evaluation of potential high-risk candidates.

Several studies have suggested factors associated with greater success of salvage cryotherapy and these can be summarized as favorable disease characteristics: low PSA nadir after primary treatment, low PSA presalvage cryotherapy (<4 ng/mL), PSA doubling time >16 months, as well as the Gleason grade of the recurrent disease [25–27].

In summary, although cryoablation is a recognized option both in the primary and salvage settings for the treatment of localized prostate cancer, there is difficulty in reaching a consensus on selection criteria and to define ideal candidates for this approach. This is mainly due to the paucity of data in the literature and is likely to resolve in the near future as more studies on cryoablation add their results to the pool of available information. There is agreement that currently cryoablation should be considered as a treatment option for patients that are not willing or are not good candidates for conventional surgery.

4 Cryoablation Procedure

Herein we describe the general steps of the procedure using third generation cryotechnology that utilizes the Joule-Thompson principle of gas expansion and therefore heat delivery and subtraction by means of ultrathin needle-like cryoprobes. Translating the physical principle into practice, as compressed gas is delivered to the tip of the cryoprobe in a closed circuit and allowed to expand through a minute opening (s), gas pressure falls, and it changes its physical properties (internal state). For argon gas, the change of state subtracts energy resulting in reduction of the temperature and freezing. The opposite is true regarding the properties of helium gas that upon expansion releases energy to the environment, thereby generating heat that translates into active thawing. The opposite effects of helium and argon derive from differences in attractive and repulsive forces of the molecules (internal energy) of these gasses. A newer cryotechnology that has been introduced relies on argon gas as the sole cryogen whereby both freezing and thawing phases are achieved by regulating the properties of this gas, since Joule-Thompson coefficients of gasses vary with pressure and temperature. At pressures of 3500 PSI, expansion of argon gas results in temperature drop, and thus freezing. When this gas is allowed to expand under lower pressures (200–500 PSI), when Joule-Thompson coefficient of argon is very low and only negligible cooling takes place, and the gas is used to heat the needle shaft by spreading the heat generated by an electrical heating source embedded in the needle. This technical modification allows for the use of a single gas (argon) for both freezing and thawing during cryoablation.

Several cryoablation platforms are commercially available and these consist of a console for treatment planning and monitoring that receives information from the probes and regulates the freezing/thawing phases. The console is connected to peripherals such as a urethral warming catheter, a transrectal ultrasound mounted on a stepper, cryoprobes, and temperature sensors. Gas tanks (argon with or without helium) are connected to the system. On the console monitor, the live information from the treatment is integrated with ultrasound imaging in real time which allows for precise monitoring of the procedure as well as input from temperature sensors and cryoprobes. For treatment planning, the desired ice coverage can be precisely sculptured by varying the configuration of the probes as well as by using different probes generating different shapes and sizes of ice balls. The probes are positioned in the gland through a transperineal grid template under ultrasonographic guidance to produce a series of overlapping ice balls that cover the entire gland or regions to be treated

Typically, cryoablation is performed as an outpatient procedure under spinal, locoregional, or general anesthesia. With the patient in lithotomy position, cryoprobes are positioned under transrectal ultrasonographic guidance using both sagittal and transverse views. In addition to cryoprobes, temperature sensor probes are placed to allow for precise monitoring of ice ball development. These thermocouples can be positioned in Denonvillier's fascia, the urinary sphincter, and/or the neurovascular bundles to monitor the freezing process and avoid injury to adjacent structures. Once the probes are in place, flexible cystoscopy is used to verify the integrity of the urethra and bladder and to place a super-stiff guidewire for the introduction of the urethral warming catheter placed by Seldinger technique. A double freeze/thaw cycle is performed and monitored by ultrasonography and readings from the temperature probes. At the end of the procedure, the urethral warming device is replaced with a urethral catheter, although some prefer placing a suprapubic cystostomy to ensure adequate bladder drainage in the postoperative period. Acute swelling and inflammatory processes following cryoablation typically resolve within 1–2 weeks. In our experience, most patients are able to void spontaneously by 1 week after treatment.

5 Primary Cryotherapy: Complications

Cryoablation of the prostate is a minimally invasive surgical technique and its morbidity profile has been extensively studied. Table 1 provides a summary of the reported complications. The majority of the postoperative events reported in the literature are self-limiting. Transient penile and scrotal swelling and paresthesia have been reported to occur within 2–3 weeks in up to 10 % of patients, and typically resolve in 2–6 months [31, 42]. Major complications are rare with a reported incidence of rectourethral fistula ranging from 0 to 2.4 %, urethral sloughing occurring in <5 % with the use of urethral warming devices, and incontinence requiring pads being reported in less than 10 % with most cases resolving spontaneously. It remains unclear whether urge or stress incontinence is the predominant type since only one study did distinguish between the types of incontinence: Caso et al. reported that 10.4 % of men had urge incontinence, 2.8 % had stress incontinence, and in 1.9 % it was mixed [39]. Notably, only 4.7 % of men in this study required the use of pads at 1 year. Similarly, episodes of urinary retention have been reported in <5 % of patients following cryoablation [30, 35], albeit the definitions of urinary retention vary and most retention episodes are transitory and resolve within several weeks of surgery. Urethral stricture rates are approximately 2.5 % (compared to 8.4 % with radical prostatectomy) [43].

Incontinence and erectile dysfunction are among the most widely used measures of functional outcomes following treatments for localized PCa. For cryoablation, erectile dysfunction occurs in the majority of patients treated with

Table 1 Complication rates after primary cryoablation of the prostate using third generation technology

Reference	# patients	Complication rates (%) Slough	Perineal pain	Urinary retention	UTI/sepsis	Urethral stricture	Fistula	Incontinence	ED
Bahn [28]	210	NR	NR	3	NR	NR	2.4	9	41
Shinohara [29]	102	NR	3	23	3/3	NR	1	4 (15[a])	86
Han [30]	106	5	2.6	3.3	0	NR	0	3	87
Wake [31]	100	1	NR	20	NR	2	0	8	NR
DiBlasio [32]	78	NR	NR	NR	NR	1	NR	7.7	84.6
Cohen [33]	98	2	NR	NR	NR	NR	0	0	NR
Prepelica [34][b]	65	NR	0	3.1	NR	NR	0	3.1	NR
Hubosky [35]	89	2	6	4	1/0	NR	1	2	NR
Donnelly [36]	117	NR	NR	15.4	NR	NR	NR	32.5	70.9
Chin [37][c]	33	NR	32	NR	NR	NR	NR	7	29
Lian [38]	102	4.9	NR	0	NR	0	0	4	64.1
Caso [39]	106	2.8	3.8	3.8	5.7/0	NR	0	4.7	NR
Rodriguez [40]	108	5.6	11.1	NR	NR	NR	0.9	5.6	98.1
Ward [41]	366	NR	NR	6	NR	NR	1.1	2.6	69.6

UTI urinary tract infection, *ED* erectile dysfunction, *NR* not reported
[a]Including patients who underwent transurethral resection of prostate following cryoablation
[b]High-risk patients
[c]Locally-advanced disease

whole gland ablation although some studies report that many patients did remain potent (Table 1). A recent study using the Surveillance Epidemiology End Results (SEER) database reported on complications of primary cryotherapy derived from Medicare claims [44]; the authors estimate 20.1 % of erectile dysfunction following cryotherapy, along with 9.8 % incontinence.

An accurate assessment of the rates of erectile dysfunction and urinary incontinence is hampered by the varying definitions of these outcome measures and only scattered use of validated instruments to adequately identify these conditions. For future studies it is of paramount importance to use validated tools (e.g. questionnaires) to evaluate both erectile function and continence.

Kimura et al. used validated tools to assess urinary function after cryoablation and found that while urinary function and bother scores dropped immediately following cryoablation, they recovered steadily and persistently in a 12-month period [45]. Notably, men with preoperative moderate to severe urinary symptoms and larger prostate volumes showed *improvement* of urinary symptoms after cryosurgery. Another study reported excellent voiding function outcomes with no apparent change in urinary function scores after primary cryoablation [32]. Malcolm and colleagues reviewed quality of life outcomes comparing brachytherapy, robotic and open radical prostatectomy, and cryotherapy [46]. These authors have shown that cryotherapy as well as brachytherapy were associated with a better health-related quality of life, especially that related to urinary function and bother along with sexual bother as assessed by validated tools. When directly compared to brachytherapy, cryoablation resulted in worse sexual function scores for up to 12 months while urinary scores were similar; however, after 18 and 24 months, cryoablation has shown consistently better urinary domain scores compared to brachytherapy [35].

Kimura and colleagues [47] assessed erectile function outcomes using validated questionnaires and found that 77.4 % of patients had moderate to severe erectile dysfunction following cryoablation and suggested that the use of erectile aids may assist in the recovery of potency to preoperative levels. Similarly, Ellis et al. [48] have suggested that penile rehabilitation strategies (regular use of vacuum devices and oral agents) after cryoablation may increase potency rates. In fact, the authors report steady recovery of erectile function over time with over 50 % of preoperatively potent patients regaining erections sufficient for intercourse over a 4-year follow-up [48]. Despite encouraging reports, more studies are needed to determine the appropriate strategies to enhance both urinary and sexual function in men undergoing cryoablation.

6 Salvage Cryotherapy: Complications

The complication profile of salvage cryotherapy for radiorecurrent prostate cancer appears to be similar to that in the primary setting with higher rates of events (Table 2). Urethral mucosal sloughing remains a rare event using third generation technology and has been reported in <2 % of patients. Specifically, fistula rates appear to be higher, up to 3.4 % as well as incontinence rates that remain in most series under 10 % compared to an incontinence rate of approximately 3 % in primary series. In the few series reporting erectile function outcomes, only a minority of patients regain potency. However, many patients are impotent due to their prior primary treatment. These results favorably compare to conventional salvage radical prostatectomy series [24] suggesting that salvage treatment with cryosurgery may be considered as a relatively low morbidity option, particularly in maintaining urinary continence.

7 Primary Cryotherapy: Oncological Outcomes

Oncological outcomes reported in the literature are summarized in Table 3. The various definitions of biochemical recurrence make it very challenging to adequately compare the different series emphasizing the need for a consensus on the matter. Conventional criteria of biochemical failure adopted for radical prostatectomy are most likely not suitable for cryoablation since a portion of PSA producing tissue is intentionally spared periurethrally due to the use of urethral warming devices and therefore undetectable PSA levels are not always achievable. Similarly, biochemical failure criteria used in radiation oncology are likely not suitable as well since an effective ablation of the entire gland is carried out and most PSA-producing tissue is destroyed. Many of the earlier, and thus longer-running series, have used the ASTRO criteria, and data from the COLD registry now support the use of the Phoenix (nadir PSA + 2) criteria to define biochemical failure [58]. Biochemical disease-free survival (bDFS) has been reported at 5 years in 7 studies showing consistent results of approximately 75 % in general series and 48–60 % in series comprising higher-risk cohorts [32, 36, 40, 41, 54, 56, 57].

To date, only two studies reported 10-year oncological outcomes following primary cryoablation [59, 60]. Both studies are based on early cohorts of patients (1990s) often treated with liquid nitrogen and therefore may not represent accurately the outcomes of third generation technology. Cohen et al. [59] reported on biochemical disease-free survival in 370 men treated with primary cryosurgery before 1999. The authors have found that in low-, intermediate-, and high-risk groups bDFS at 10 years were 80.5, 74.2, and 45.5 %, respectively. Cheetham et al. [60] focused on overall and cancer-specific survival. They report on 25 patients treated between 1994 and 1999 with 10 years of follow-up where only 2 patients died of prostate cancer compared to 8 deaths attributed to other causes.

Table 2 Complication rates after salvage cryoablation using third generation cryotechnology

		Complication rates (%)							
Reference	# patients	Slough	Perineal pain	Urinary retention	UTI/sepsis	Urethral stricture	Fistula	Incontinence	ED
Ng [25]	187	NR	14	21	10	2.1	2	40	NR
Han [49]	29	NR	NR	NR	NR	NR	0	7	NR
Ismail [27]	100	2	4	2	NR	NR	1	13	86
Pisters [50][a]	279	NR	NR	NR	NR	NR	1.2	4.7	69.2
Ghafar [42]	38	0	39.5	0	2.6	NR	0	7.9	NR
Cresswell [51]	20	NR	NR	4	NR	NR	0	4	86
Bahn [52]	59	NR	NR	NR	NR	NR	3.4	8	NR
Kvorning Ternov [53]	30	10	23.3	10	NR	10	3.3	46	NR

UTI urinary tract infection, *ED* erectile dysfunction, *NR* not reported
[a]Series includes a portion of cases treated using second generation technology

Table 3 Oncologic outcomes of primary cryoablation

Reference	# patients	Definition	bDFS 1–2 years	bDFS 3 years	bDFS 5 years	bDFS 7 years	bDFS 8 years
Hubosky [35]	89	ASTRO	94 %	–	–	–	–
		≤0.4	70 %	–	–	–	–
DiBlasio [32]	78	ASTRO	97.9 %	95.7 %	71.1 %	–	–
Prepelica [34][a]	65	ASTRO	83.3 %	–	–	–	–
Cresswell [51]	31	≤0.5	60 %	–	–	–	–
Donnelly [36]	117	Phoenix	–	82.9 %	75 %	–	–
Bahn [28][b]	590	ASTRO	–	–	–	89.5 %	–
Jones [54][b]	1198	ASTRO	–	–	77.1 %	–	–
Lian [38]	102	<0.5	92.2 %	–	–	–	–
Chin [55][c]	62	Phoenix	–	–	–	–	17 %
Guo [56][c]	75	Phoenix	–	–	48 %	–	–
Ward [41][c]	366	Phoenix	–	65 %	52 %	–	–
Rodriguez [40]	108	Phoenix	–	–	75	–	–
Tay [57][d]	300	Phoenix	77.2 %	–	59 %	–	–

bDFS biochemical disease-free survival
[a]High-risk patients
[b]Contains a proportion of patients treated with earlier generation technology
[c]Majority/all clinical T3 disease
[d]Clinically localized, high-grade patients

Oncological outcomes of primary cryoablation are strongly dependent on disease characteristics. Logically, favorable disease characteristics translate to better bDFS rates and this is corroborated with the observed data: Those with clinically low-risk cancer, lower pretreatment PSA, lower prostate volume, lower clinical stage, and Gleason score have better outcomes [28, 35, 61]. Post treatment, Caso et al. [62] have evaluated predictors of biopsy-proven recurrence after primary cryotherapy and found that on multivariate analysis only time of undetectable PSA (TUPSA) was associated with both biochemical and biopsy-proven disease-free survival suggesting that TUPSA may be used as a potential informative tool during follow-up. Additionally, among men with high-grade clinically localized disease, Tay et al. demonstrated a worse prognosis in men failing to achieve a PSA nadir < 0.4 ng/ml [57]. As the experience with primary cryotherapy matures, we are likely to be able to identify additional factors associated with oncologic outcomes and produce predictive models as well as more accurate recommendations on patient selection for this approach.

It is also important to compare cryotherapy to other, well-standardized approaches for the treatment of localized PCa. Two randomized clinical trials comparing cryosurgery to radiation were published yielding conflicting results. Chin et al. [37] found cryoablation to be inferior to external beam radiation in bDFS. However, a similar trial by Donnelly et al. [36] concluded that the two approaches have comparable oncological efficacy. This discrepancy may be due to differences in study designs: Chin et al. included only patients with locally advanced PCa while Donnelly and colleagues excluded bulky disease from their study. While the trial by Donnelly et al. had a greater sample size, the design was noninferiority. Ultimately, both trials suffered from insufficient accrual leading to difficulty in meeting their primary endpoints. Nonetheless, the experience from these two trials suggests that primary cryotherapy may be more suited to treating localized prostate cancer rather than locally advanced disease. This observation is mirrored in the COLD registry report from Ward et al. examining 366 patients with cT3 prostate cancer with a rather low 3- and 5-year estimated bDFS of 65 and 52 % [41]. At 8 year follow-up of their trial, Chin et al. report a 17 % disease free survival with cryotherapy compared to 59 % with external beam radiation [55].

It appears from the available data that the oncological outcomes of primary cryotherapy are acceptable and competitive with other primary treatments for PCa, provided that treatment is used in patients with clinically localized disease. The outcomes in this group may yet improve further with better selection using advanced imaging techniques. Yet, it is paramount to emphasize the need to standardize reporting regarding the definition of biochemical failure, report more biopsy-based outcomes, and to follow up patients for a longer period of time.

8 Salvage Cryotherapy: Oncological Outcomes

The data on oncological outcomes following salvage cryotherapy for radiorecurrent PCa are affected by the same difficulties of the lack of consistency in the definition of biochemical failure and therefore the inability to perform an effective comparison between the published results. The summary of the literature is provided in Table 4.

Despite various definitions of biochemical failure, it is apparent that bDFS at 1 year can be as high as 86 %. Long term data suggest that with a strict definition of PSA ≤ 0.5 ng/mL following salvage cryosurgery, 59 % of patients are disease-free at 7 years [52] and these results are comparable to >55 % bDFS at 5 years from other studies [25, 50]. Recently, Cheetham et al. [60] reported on 10-years data regarding outcomes after salvage cryoablation focusing on overall and cancer-specific survival. In their report, 8 out of 51 patients (15.7 %) who underwent salvage cryotherapy died of PCa over 10 years. Williams et al. [65] reported on 176 men undergoing salvage cryotherapy with long-term follow-up; the authors found that 47 %, 39 %, and 39 % of patients were disease-free at 5, 8, and 10 years, respectively. This study has also evaluated metastasis-free survival, indicating 87 % at 5 and 82 % at 10 years.

Several studies attempted to identify prognostic factors associated with the outcome of salvage cryoablation. A report from the COLD (Cryo On Line Data) registry analyzed 455 patients and found that PSA nadir levels <0.6 ng/mL after salvage cryotherapy were associated with better cancer control outcomes offering 80 % bDFS at 1 year and 67 % bDFS at 3 years, whereas higher PSA nadirs were associated with progressively worsening outcomes [66]. In this study, it was also determined that Gleason scores of the recurrent cancer correlated with the outcome. These findings were confirmed when follow-up was

Table 4 Oncologic outcomes of salvage cryoablation

Reference	# patients	Definition	bDFS 1 year	bDFS 3 years	bDFS 5 years	bDFS 7 years
Ng [25]	187	Nadir+2	–	–	56 %	–
Ghafar [42]	38	Nadir+0.3	86 %	74 %	–	–
Ismail [27]	100	ASTRO	83 %	59 %	–	–
Cresswell [51]	20	≤0.5	66.7 %	–	–	–
Bahn [52][a]	59	≤0.5	–	–	–	59 %
Pisters [50][a]	279	ASTRO	–	–	59 %	–
Williams [63][b]	176	Phoenix	–	–	47 %	39 %
Castro Abreu [64]	25	Phoenix	–	–	86.5 %	–

bDFS biochemical disease-free survival
[a]Includes earlier generation technology
[b]Definition of recurrence was a composite of biochemical, radiological, and histological

extended to 5-years, with a posttreatment PSA nadir <0.4 ng/ml being the most objective predictor of bDFS at 5 years [67]. Another prognosticator is disease burden (the ratio of positive cores to prostate volume) [68]. One study showed that preradiation PSA, Gleason score, as well as presalvage PSA level and postsalvage PSA nadir were associated with biochemical disease-free survival [65]. The authors showed that patients with presalvage Gleason score of ≤6 had a 54 % bDFS at 10 years, underlining the importance of disease characteristics in defining cancer control outcomes.

Spiess and colleagues [69] developed a nomogram that quantifies the risk of biochemical failure after salvage cryotherapy based on initial PSA level, Gleason score, and clinical stage. This tool may be useful to generate realistic expectations with regards to the probability of biochemical failure in candidates for salvage cryoablation. However, further validation is required.

9 Focal Therapy: Maintaining Quality of Life

Technological advances, specifically those that brought cryotherapy to be recognized as an option in the treatment of prostate cancer, have enabled physicians to rethink treatment schemes and potentially move away from whole gland treatments towards a targeted, partial ablation of the gland [70, 71]. The concept of focal therapy relies on a selective, targeted destruction of known cancer while sparing the uninvolved tissue, thereby potentially reducing morbidity and improving quality of life compared to traditional treatment forms. The concept of focal therapy for PCa has gained interest and popularity, especially in the era of growing evidence that overdiagnosis and overtreatment of prostate cancer is becoming a pressing public concern [72].

Advances in imaging of the prostate, namely magnetic resonance and novel ultrasound techniques, are permitting the physician to visualize PCa foci within the prostate and characterize those with a guided, targeted biopsy. The same imaging technology can then potentially be used, in appropriate candidates to guide the targeted ablation of these lesions while leaving intact the remainder of the prostate.

Early results of focal therapy are promising, albeit based on a small number of single institution, small-sized, studies and one community-based registry analysis [73–81]. Despite heterogeneous reporting of complications (Table 5), in general, continence and erectile function outcomes appear to be quite good. The rates of rectourethral fistulae and other similar complications appear to be lower than that reported in whole gland series as well. Biochemical disease-free survival is again subject to varying definitions. In addition, bDFS becomes less reliable as the portion of prostate left untreated increases. The reported bDFS rates range from 71 to 98 %. Correspondingly, as the

Table 5 Complication rates after primary focal cryoablation using third generation technology

		Complication rates (%)							
Reference	# patients	Slough	Perineal pain	Urinary retention	UTI/sepsis	Urethral stricture	Fistula	Incontinence	ED
Ellis [76]	60	NR	NR	NR	NR	NR	0	3.6	29.4
Onik [79]	48	NR	NR	NR	NR	NR	NR	0	10
Ward [81]	1160	NR	NR	1.2	NR	NR	0.1	1.4	41.9
Bahn [73]	73	NR	NR	NR	NR	NR	0	0	26
Hale [77]	26	NR	NR	4	4/0	NR	NR	0	0
Durand [75]	48	NR	NR	15	NR	2	2	0	0
Lian [78]	41	NR	NR	3.4	NR	NR	NR	0	23.1

Table 6 Oncological outcomes after primary focal ablation

Reference	# patients	bDFS Definition	bDFS[a]	Biopsy trigger	Positive biopsy rate (treated zone)	Positive biopsy rate (untreated zone)
Ellis [76]	60	ASTRO	80.4 %	PSA	2.9 %	37.1 %
Onik [79]	48	ASTRO	92 % (1 year)	Mandatory	14.3 %	
Truesdale [80]	77	Phoenix	72.7 %	PSA	13.6 %	36.3 %
Ward [81]	1160	ASTRO	75.7 % (2 year)	NR	26.2 %	
Bahn [73]	73	NR	NR	Mandatory	2.1 %	23 %
Hale [77]	26	Nadir +0.5	88 %	PSA	Only 2 biopsied, both positive	
Barqawi [74]	62	> preoperative PSA	71 %	Mandatory	12.9 %	8.1 %
Durand [75]	48	Phoenix	98 %	Mandatory	13 %	15.2 %
Lian [78]	41	Phoenix	95 %	Mandatory	6.3 %	15.6 %

[a]Absolute unless otherwise stated

volume of prostate left untreated increases, the problem of undergrading and understaging the cancer prior to treatment is magnified, particularly in series where patients are selected using conventional 12-core biopsies. In order to deal with this problem, several studies have mandatory prostate biopsies at a set follow-up interval. The actual biopsy rates in these "mandatory rebiopsy" series are, on average, about 79 %, with a positive biopsy rate of approximately 20 % (Table 6). Li et al., leveraging on the concept of gland preservation, reported on 91 men undergoing salvage focal prostate cryoablation, reporting bDFS of 95.3 % at 1 year, 72.4 % at 3 years, and 46.5 % at 5 years. However, in this series, while potency preservation was superior to whole gland salvage ablation, the rates of rectourethral fistula and incontinence appeared similar [82].

There remains a lack of consensus on the appropriate candidates and selection methods for focal therapy, as well as tools to be used in postablation follow-up. Despite the hurdles, the focal therapy approach is being investigated intensively and international consensus panels are providing guidance. Randomized trials are under way to set stage for the introduction of this intriguing therapeutic option.

References

1. Arnott J. Practical illustrations of the remedial efficacy of a very low or anaesthetic temperature.-I. In Cancer. Lancet. 1850;56(1411):316–8.
2. Babaian RJ, Donnely B, Bahn D, Baust JG, Dineen M, Ellis D, et al. Best practice policy statement on cryosurgery for the treatment of localized prostate

cancer. AUA Clinical Guidelines [Internet]. 2008 2/8/2010. Available from: http://www.auanet.org/content/guidelines-and-quality-care/clinical-guidelines.cfm.
3. Heidenreich A, Bastian PJ, Bellmunt J, Bolla M, Joniau S, van der Kwast T, et al. EAU guidelines on prostate cancer. part 1: screening, diagnosis, and local treatment with curative intent-update 2013. Eur Urol. 2014;65(1):124–37.
4. Baust JG, Gage AA, Bjerklund Johansen TE, Baust JM. Mechanisms of cryoablation: clinical consequences on malignant tumors. Cryobiology. 2014;68(1):1–11.
5. Mazur P. Freezing of living cells: mechanisms and implications. Am J Physiol. 1984;247(3 Pt 1):C125–42.
6. Theodorescu D. Cryotherapy for prostate cancer: what we know, what we need to know. J Urol. 2008;180(2):437–8.
7. Hoffmann NE, Bischof JC. The cryobiology of cryosurgical injury. Urology. 2002;60(2 Suppl 1):40–9.
8. Robilotto AT, Baust JM, Van Buskirk RG, Gage AA, Baust JG. Temperature-dependent activation of differential apoptotic pathways during cryoablation in a human prostate cancer model. Prostate Cancer Prostatic Dis. 2013;16(1):41–9.
9. Clarke DM, Robilotto AT, VanBuskirk RG, Baust JG, Gage AA, Baust JM. Targeted induction of apoptosis via TRAIL and cryoablation: a novel strategy for the treatment of prostate cancer. Prostate Cancer Prostatic Dis. 2007;10(2):175–84.
10. Kimura M, Rabbani Z, Mouraviev V, Tsivian M, Caso J, Satoh T, et al. Role of vitamin D(3) as a sensitizer to cryoablation in a murine prostate cancer model: preliminary in vivo study. Urology. 2010;76(3):764 e14–20.
11. Santucci KL, Snyder KK, Baust JM, Van Buskirk RG, Mouraviev V, Polascik TJ, et al. Use of 1,25alpha dihydroxyvitamin D3 as a cryosensitizing agent in a murine prostate cancer model. Prostate Cancer Prostatic Dis. 2011;14(2):97–104.
12. Ablin RJ. Cryosurgery of the rabbit prostate. Comparison of the immune response of immature and mature bucks. Cryobiology. 1974;11(5):416–22.
13. Urano M, Tanaka C, Sugiyama Y, Miya K, Saji S. Antitumor effects of residual tumor after cryoablation: the combined effect of residual tumor and a protein-bound polysaccharide on multiple liver metastases in a murine model. Cryobiology. 2003;46(3):238–45.
14. Udagawa M, Kudo-Saito C, Hasegawa G, Yano K, Yamamoto A, Yaguchi M, et al. Enhancement of immunologic tumor regression by intratumoral administration of dendritic cells in combination with cryoablative tumor pretreatment and Bacillus Calmette-Guerin cell wall skeleton stimulation. Clin Cancer Res. 2006;12(24):7465–75.
15. Yamashita T, Hayakawa K, Hosokawa M, Kodama T, Inoue N, Tomita K, et al. Enhanced tumor metastases in rats following cryosurgery of primary tumor. Gann. 1982;73(2):222–8.
16. Miya K, Saji S, Morita T, Niwa H, Sakata K. Experimental study on mechanism of absorption of cryonecrotized tumor antigens. Cryobiology. 1987;24(2):135–9.
17. Sabel MS. Cryo-immunology: a review of the literature and proposed mechanisms for stimulatory versus suppressive immune responses. Cryobiology. 2009;58(1):1–11.
18. Gage AA, Baust JG. Cryosurgery for tumors. J Am Coll Surg. 2007;205(2):342–56.
19. Klossner DP, Robilotto AT, Clarke DM, VanBuskirk RG, Baust JM, Gage AA, et al. Cryosurgical technique: assessment of the fundamental variables using human prostate cancer model systems. Cryobiology. 2007;55(3):189–99.
20. Tatsutani K, Rubinsky B, Onik G, Dahiya R. Effect of thermal variables on frozen human primary prostatic adenocarcinoma cells. Urology. 1996;48(3):441–7.
21. Gage AA, Baust JM, Baust JG. Experimental cryosurgery investigations in vivo. Cryobiology. 2009;59(3):229–43.
22. Gage AA, Baust J. Mechanisms of tissue injury in cryosurgery. Cryobiology. 1998;37(3):171–86.
23. Heidenreich A, Bellmunt J, Bolla M, Joniau S, Mason M, Matveev V, et al. EAU guidelines on prostate cancer. Part 1: screening, diagnosis, and treatment of clinically localised disease. Eur Urol. 2011;59(1):61–71.
24. Kimura M, Mouraviev V, Tsivian M, Mayes JM, Satoh T, Polascik TJ. Current salvage methods for recurrent prostate cancer after failure of primary radiotherapy. BJU Int. 2010;105(2):191–201.
25. Ng CK, Moussa M, Downey DB, Chin JL. Salvage cryoablation of the prostate: followup and analysis of predictive factors for outcome. J Urol. 2007;178(4 Pt 1):1253–7; discussion 7.
26. Spiess PE, Lee AK, Leibovici D, Wang X, Do KA, Pisters LL. Presalvage prostate-specific antigen (PSA) and PSA doubling time as predictors of biochemical failure of salvage cryotherapy in patients with locally recurrent prostate cancer after radiotherapy. Cancer. 2006;107(2):275–80.
27. Ismail M, Ahmed S, Kastner C, Davies J. Salvage cryotherapy for recurrent prostate cancer after radiation failure: a prospective case series of the first 100 patients. BJU Int. 2007;100(4):760–4.
28. Bahn DK, Lee F, Badalament R, Kumar A, Greski J, Chernick M. Targeted cryoablation of the prostate: 7-year outcomes in the primary treatment of prostate cancer. Urology. 2002;60(2 Suppl 1):3–11.
29. Shinohara K, Connolly JA, Presti Jr JC, Carroll PR. Cryosurgical treatment of localized prostate cancer (stages T1 to T4): preliminary results. J Urol. 1996;156(1):115–20; discussion 20–1.
30. Han KR, Cohen JK, Miller RJ, Pantuck AJ, Freitas DG, Cuevas CA, et al. Treatment of organ confined prostate cancer with third generation cryosurgery: preliminary multicenter experience. J Urol. 2003;170(4 Pt 1):1126–30.

31. Wake RW, Hollabaugh Jr RS, Bond KH. Cryosurgical ablation of the prostate for localized adenocarcinoma: a preliminary experience. J Urol. 1996;155(5):1663–6.
32. DiBlasio CJ, Derweesh IH, Malcolm JB, Maddox MM, Aleman MA, Wake RW. Contemporary analysis of erectile, voiding, and oncologic outcomes following primary targeted cryoablation of the prostate for clinically localized prostate cancer. Int Braz J Urol. 2008;34(4):443–50.
33. Cohen JK. Cryosurgery of the prostate: techniques and indications. Rev Urol. 2004;6 Suppl 4:S20–6.
34. Prepelica KL, Okeke Z, Murphy A, Katz AE. Cryosurgical ablation of the prostate: high risk patient outcomes. Cancer. 2005;103(8):1625–30.
35. Hubosky SG, Fabrizio MD, Schellhammer PF, Barone BB, Tepera CM, Given RW. Single center experience with third-generation cryosurgery for management of organ-confined prostate cancer: critical evaluation of short-term outcomes, complications, and patient quality of life. J Endourol. 2007;21(12):1521–31.
36. Donnelly BJ, Saliken JC, Brasher PM, Ernst SD, Rewcastle JC, Lau H, et al. A randomized trial of external beam radiotherapy versus cryoablation in patients with localized prostate cancer. Cancer. 2010;116(2):323–30.
37. Chin JL, Ng CK, Touma NJ, Pus NJ, Hardie R, Abdelhady M, et al. Randomized trial comparing cryoablation and external beam radiotherapy for T2C-T3B prostate cancer. Prostate Cancer Prostatic Dis. 2008;11(1):40–5.
38. Lian H, Guo H, Gan W, Li X, Yan X, Wang W, et al. Cryosurgery as primary treatment for localized prostate cancer. Int Urol Nephrol. 2011.
39. Caso JR, Tsivian M, Mouraviev V, Kimura M, Polascik TJ. Complications and postoperative events after cryosurgery for prostate cancer. BJU Int. 2012;109(6):840–5.
40. Rodriguez SA, Arias Funez F, Bueno Bravo C, Rodriguez-Patron Rodriguez R, Sanz Mayayo E, Palacios VH, et al. Cryotherapy for primary treatment of prostate cancer: intermediate term results of a prospective study from a single institution. Prostate Cancer. 2014;2014:571576.
41. Ward JF, DiBlasio CJ, Williams C, Given R, Jones JS. Cryoablation for locally advanced clinical stage T3 prostate cancer: a report from the Cryo-On-Line Database (COLD) Registry. BJU Int. 2014;113(5):714–8.
42. Ghafar MA, Johnson CW, De La Taille A, Benson MC, Bagiella E, Fatal M, et al. Salvage cryotherapy using an argon based system for locally recurrent prostate cancer after radiation therapy: the Columbia experience. J Urol. 2001;166(4):1333–7; discussion 7–8.
43. Elliott SP, Meng MV, Elkin EP, McAninch JW, Duchane J, Carroll PR. Incidence of urethral stricture after primary treatment for prostate cancer: data From CaPSURE. J Urol. 2007;178(2):529–34; discussion 34.
44. Roberts CB, Jang TL, Shao YH, Kabadi S, Moore DF, Lu-Yao GL. Treatment profile and complications associated with cryotherapy for localized prostate cancer: a population-based study. Prostate Cancer Prostatic Dis. 2011.
45. Kimura M, Mouraviev V, Tsivian M, Moreira DM, Mayes JM, Polascik TJ. Analysis of urinary function using validated instruments and uroflowmetry after primary and salvage prostate cryoablation. Urology. 2010;76(5):1258–65.
46. Malcolm JB, Fabrizio MD, Barone BB, Given RW, Lance RS, Lynch DF, et al. Quality of life after open or robotic prostatectomy, cryoablation or brachytherapy for localized prostate cancer. J Urol. 2010;183(5):1822–8.
47. Kimura M, Donatucci CF, Tsivian M, Caso JR, Moreira DM, Mouraviev V, et al. On-demand use of erectile aids in men with preoperative erectile dysfunction treated by whole gland prostate cryoablation. Int J Impot Res. 2011;23(2):49–55.
48. Ellis DS, Manny Jr TB, Rewcastle JC. Cryoablation as primary treatment for localized prostate cancer followed by penile rehabilitation. Urology. 2007;69(2):306–10.
49. Han KR, Belldegrun AS. Third-generation cryosurgery for primary and recurrent prostate cancer. BJU Int. 2004;93(1):14–8.
50. Pisters LL, Rewcastle JC, Donnelly BJ, Lugnani FM, Katz AE, Jones JS. Salvage prostate cryoablation: initial results from the cryo on-line data registry. J Urol. 2008;180(2):559–63; discussion 63–4.
51. Cresswell J, Asterling S, Chaudhary M, Sheikh N, Greene D. Third-generation cryotherapy for prostate cancer in the UK: a prospective study of the early outcomes in primary and recurrent disease. BJU Int. 2006;97(5):969–74.
52. Bahn DK, Lee F, Silverman P, Bahn E, Badalament R, Kumar A, et al. Salvage cryosurgery for recurrent prostate cancer after radiation therapy: a seven-year follow-up. Clin Prostate Cancer. 2003;2(2):111–4.
53. Kvorning Ternov K, Krag Jakobsen A, Bratt O, Ahlgren G. Salvage cryotherapy for local recurrence after radiotherapy for prostate cancer. Scand J Urol. 2015;49(2):115–9.
54. Jones JS, Rewcastle JC, Donnelly BJ, Lugnani FM, Pisters LL, Katz AE. Whole gland primary prostate cryoablation: initial results from the cryo on-line data registry. J Urol. 2008;180(2):554–8.
55. Chin JL, Al-Zahrani AA, Autran-Gomez AM, Williams AK, Bauman G. Extended followup oncologic outcome of randomized trial between cryoablation and external beam therapy for locally advanced prostate cancer (T2c-T3b). J Urol. 2012;188(4):1170–5.
56. Guo Z, Si T, Yang X, Xu Y. Oncological outcomes of cryosurgery as primary treatment in T3 prostate cancer: experience of a single centre. BJU Int. 2015;116(1):79–84.

57. Tay KJ, Polascik TJ, Elshafei A, Cher ML, Given RW, Mouraviev V, et al. Primary cryotherapy for high-grade clinically localized prostate cancer: oncologic and functional outcomes from the COLD registry. J Endourol. 2016;30(1):43–8.
58. Levy DA, Ross AE, ElShafei A, Krishnan N, Hatem A, Jones JS. Definition of biochemical success following primary whole gland prostate cryoablation. J Urol. 2014;192(5):1380–4.
59. Cohen JK, Miller Jr RJ, Ahmed S, Lotz MJ, Baust J. Ten-year biochemical disease control for patients with prostate cancer treated with cryosurgery as primary therapy. Urology. 2008;71(3):515–8.
60. Cheetham P, Truesdale M, Chaudhury S, Wenske S, Hruby GW, Katz A. Long-term cancer-specific and overall survival for men followed more than 10 years after primary and salvage cryoablation of the prostate. J Endourol/Endourol Soc. 2010;24(7):1123–9.
61. Elshafei A, Kovac E, Dhar N, Levy D, Polascik T, Mouraviev V, et al. A pretreatment nomogram for prediction of biochemical failure after primary cryoablation of the prostate. Prostate. 2015;75(13):1447–53.
62. Caso JR, Tsivian M, Mouraviev V, Polascik TJ. Predicting biopsy-proven prostate cancer recurrence following cryosurgery. Urol Oncol. 2010.
63. Williams AK, Martinez CH, Lu C, Ng CK, Pautler SE, Chin JL. Disease-free survival following salvage cryotherapy for biopsy-proven radio-recurrent prostate cancer. Eur Urol. 2011;60(3):405–10.
64. de Castro Abreu AL, Bahn D, Leslie S, Shoji S, Silverman P, Desai MM, et al. Salvage focal and salvage total cryoablation for locally recurrent prostate cancer after primary radiation therapy. BJU Int. 2013;112(3):298–307.
65. Williams AK, Martinez CH, Lu C, Ng CK, Pautler SE, Chin JL. Disease-free survival following salvage cryotherapy for biopsy-proven radio-recurrent prostate cancer. Eur Urol. 2010;60:405.
66. Levy DA, Pisters LL, Jones JS. Prognostic value of initial prostate-specific antigen levels after salvage cryoablation for prostate cancer. BJU Int. 2010;106(7):986–90.
67. Kovac E, Elshafei A, Tay KJ, Mendez MH, Polascik T, Jones JS. 5-Year biochemical progression-free survival following salvage whole-gland prostate cryoablation: defining success with nadir PSA. J Endourol. 2016.
68. Levy DA, Li J, Jones JS. Disease burden predicts for favorable post salvage cryoablation PSA. Urology. 2010;76(5):1157–61.
69. Spiess PE, Katz AE, Chin JL, Bahn D, Cohen JK, Shinohara K, et al. A pretreatment nomogram predicting biochemical failure after salvage cryotherapy for locally recurrent prostate cancer. BJU Int. 2010;106(2):194–8.
70. Polascik TJ, Mouraviev V. Focal therapy for prostate cancer is a reasonable treatment option in properly selected patients. Urology. 2009;74(4):726–30.
71. Polascik TJ, Mayes JM, Mouraviev V. Nerve-sparing focal cryoablation of prostate cancer. Curr Opin Urol. 2009;19(2):182–7.
72. Welch HG, Black WC. Overdiagnosis in cancer. J Natl Cancer Inst. 2010;102(9):605–13.
73. Bahn D, de Castro Abreu AL, Gill IS, Hung AJ, Silverman P, Gross ME, et al. Focal cryotherapy for clinically unilateral, low-intermediate risk prostate cancer in 73 men with a median follow-up of 3.7 years. Eur Urol. 2012;62(1):55–63.
74. Barqawi AB, Stoimenova D, Krughoff K, Eid K, O'Donnell C, Phillips JM, et al. Targeted focal therapy for the management of organ confined prostate cancer. J Urol. 2014;192(3):749–53.
75. Durand M, Barret E, Galiano M, Rozet F, Sanchez-Salas R, Ahallal Y, et al. Focal cryoablation: a treatment option for unilateral low-risk prostate cancer. BJU Int. 2014;113(1):56–64.
76. Ellis DS, Manny Jr TB, Rewcastle JC. Focal cryosurgery followed by penile rehabilitation as primary treatment for localized prostate cancer: initial results. Eur J Cancer Care. 2007;70(6 Suppl):9–15.
77. Hale Z, Miyake M, Palacios DA, Rosser CJ. Focal cryosurgical ablation of the prostate: a single institute's perspective. BMC Urol. 2013;13:2.
78. Lian H, Zhuang J, Yang R, Qu F, Wang W, Lin T, et al. Focal cryoablation for unilateral low-intermediate-risk prostate cancer: 63-month mean follow-up results of 41 patients. Int Urol Nephrol. 2015.
79. Onik G, Vaughan D, Lotenfoe R, Dineen M, Brady J. The "male lumpectomy": focal therapy for prostate cancer using cryoablation results in 48 patients with at least 2-year follow-up. Urol Oncol. 2008;26(5):500–5.
80. Truesdale MD, Cheetham PJ, Hruby GW, Wenske S, Conforto AK, Cooper AB, et al. An evaluation of patient selection criteria on predicting progression-free survival after primary focal unilateral nerve-sparing cryoablation for prostate cancer: recommendations for follow up. Cancer J (Sudbury, Mass). 2010;16(5):544–9.
81. Ward JF, Jones JS. Focal cryotherapy for localized prostate cancer: a report from the national Cryo On-Line Database (COLD) Registry. BJU Int. 2012;109(11):1648–54.
82. Li YH, Elshafei A, Agarwal G, Ruckle H, Powsang J, Jones JS. Salvage focal prostate cryoablation for locally recurrent prostate cancer after radiotherapy: initial results from the cryo on-line data registry. Prostate. 2015;75(1):1–7.

Salvage Prostate Brachytherapy for Postradiation Local Failure

Gilles Créhange, I-Chow Hsu, Albert J Chang, and Mack Roach III

1 Introduction

For a long time, one drawback of both prostate external-beam radiotherapy (EBRT) and brachytherapy was linked to the risk of morbidity associated with any local salvage therapy such as radical prostatectomy. For this reason, some patients may choose primary radical prostatectomy, following which salvage local EBRT still remains a possible curative salvage option, as recommended by many urologists. Life-long androgen deprivation therapy (ADT) was the standard of care for patients with rising PSA levels after primary radiotherapy [1, 2]. However, ADT is associated with a number of toxicities, such as erectile dysfunction, decreased libido, gynecomastia, hot flashes, osteoporosis, and metabolic syndrome. An alternative that has recently emerged is intermittent life-long androgen deprivation, which in theory results in an improvement in quality of life compared to continuous androgen deprivation therapy, though this may not be the case [3–5]. However, all patients are doomed to progress to castrate-resistant prostate cancer and develop metastases, making this treatment palliative only.

2 Natural History of Postradiation Local Failure

In a large prostate cancer registry of 5277 men initially treated with radical prostatectomy or external-beam radiotherapy, patients with recurrent disease were more likely to have bone metastases (15 % vs. 1 %, $p<0.01$), higher prostate cancer-specific mortality (45 % vs. 0 %, $p<0.01$) and overall deaths (19 % vs. 3 %, $p<0.01$) than those without recurrence [1].

Among patients who have salvage therapy, only 7 % die whereas 25 % die if there is no salvage [1, 2]. This observation paves the way for more curative intent salvage therapies. Before the advent of modern functional imaging, such as multiparametric MRI and MR spectroscopy, and salvage therapies, most of these failures were treated with life-long palliative hormones (93.5 %) [1].

There is a strong relationship between failure to eradicate all intraprostatic cancer cells and the

G. Créhange (✉)
Department of Radiation Oncology, Centre Georges François Leclerc, 1 Rue du Professeur Marion, F-21000 Dijon, France
e-mail: gcrehange@cgfl.fr

I.-C. Hsu • A.J. Chang • M. Roach III
Department of Radiation Oncology, Helen Diller Family Comprehensive Cancer Center, University of California San Francisco, 1600 Divisadero Street, 94143 San Francisco, CA, USA
e-mail: IChow.Hsu@ucsf.edu; Albert.Chang@ucsf.edu; MRoach@radonc.ucsf.edu

M. Bolla, H. van Poppel (eds.), *Management of Prostate Cancer*,
DOI 10.1007/978-3-319-42769-0_19

subsequent appearance of metastases [6]. It is hypothesized that this relationship may be explained by two processes: first, the local persistence of cancer cells in the prostate may be a prognostic marker of distant metastases associated with a more aggressive pathobiology; and second, by the reseeding theory [7]. In the first case, any local salvage intervention may be judged unhelpful, while in the latter, the late wave of metastases may be avoided by eradicating potentially shedding cells with a local salvage intervention.

In a cohort of 1427 and 42 patients treated with external-beam radiation therapy (EBRT) and interstitial brachytherapy, respectively, Coen et al. found large differences in distant metastasis-free survival at 10 and 15 years when local control was achieved (77 %, and 72 %, respectively) when compared to patients with locally persistent disease (61 %, and 37 %, respectively). The median time to the appearance of metastasis was longer in patients who failed to achieve local control, 54 months, which is in keeping with a late wave of metastases in the reseeding theory [8].

2.1 Patterns of Local Failure After Prostate EBRT

After EBRT, a positive biopsy can occur in 14–91 % of rebiopsied patients [9]. The association of a positive rebiopsy with higher PSA nadirs and higher PSA at the time of biopsy supports the use of PSA as a surrogate marker of residual prostate cancer. A positive rebiopsy has been associated with both local and distant failure in several series. Crook et al. reported a 30 % positive rebiopsy rate at 30 months [10]. Dugan et al. found that for T3 to T4 tumors, the positive rebiopsy rate 2 years after radiation was 8 % for patients with PSA levels less than 1.0 versus 63 % if the PSA level was greater than 1 at the time of biopsy [11]. In their prostate dose-escalated EBRT program, Zelefsky et al. reported significantly lower rates of positive rebiopsy in patients receiving higher doses: 7 %, 48 %, 45 %, and 57 % after 81 Gy, 75.6 Gy, 70.2 Gy, and 64.8 Gy, respectively [12]. Similar results were observed by Shipley et al. in a randomized trial comparing 75.6 GyE of protons to 67.2 GyE for T3 to T4 tumors: 28 % versus 45 % of positive rebiopsies, respectively [13].

In another randomized trial by Huang et al., 125 patients with prostate biopsy at 2 years after EBRT, among whom 86 patients had pre- and posttreatment sextant biopsies, were analyzed [14]. Compared with the distribution of positive biopsies before EBRT, the authors found that after EBRT persistent prostate tumor cells increased from the base to the apex. These findings suggest that daily image guidance and MRI-based delineation may help to prevent apical failures.

Multiple studies of salvage prostatectomy after failure following external-beam radiotherapy have provided useful information on the sites of recurrence within the prostate. Huang et al. described 70 cancer foci after 46 radical prostatectomies [15]. All the foci were in the peripheral zone: at the apex in 93 % of the patients, at the mid-gland in 93 %, and at the base in 50 % of the patients. Leibovici et al. found that the base, apex, and base + apex were involved in 46 %, 74 % and 46 % of the specimens, respectively, in 50 salvage radical prostatectomies after radiation therapy [16]. Median tumor volume was 1.27 cm^3 (range 0.05 to 12.96). While two thirds of the patients had a single cancer focus at relapse, bilateral involvement was found in three quarters (74 %) and within 5.0 mm of the urethra in another three quarters. These results must warn physicians against focal salvage therapy in patients without a comprehensive workup that includes multiparametric MRI and 3D transperineal biopsy-based mapping.

Of note, they also found that 28 % of patients with local failure on salvage radical prostatectomy after EBRT had microscopic involvement of the seminal vesicles [15].

2.2 Patterns of Local Failures After Prostate Brachytherapy

Based on their cohort of 2223 patients treated with low-dose-rate (LDR) prostate brachytherapy, the group from Vancouver, British Columbia estimated that <2.7 % would have true local failure, indicating that this rate might be lower than that after radical prostatectomy [17].

In another large cohort, 1,562 men with localized prostate cancer were treated with permanent prostate brachytherapy. Among the 508 who underwent rebiopsy 2 years after prostate brachytherapy [18], 44 % percent of those with a positive biopsy at 2 years had negative results on subsequent biopsy, while only 2.2 % of patients with negative 2-year biopsies went on to show positive results. With a median follow-up of 6.7 years (max 14.6 years), only 39 (7.7 %) had a final positive biopsy. Independent predictors of a positive biopsy on multivariate analysis were low-dose prostate brachytherapy and no hormonal therapy. However, in both of these series, the investigators were very experienced and it remains unclear whether this reflects the pattern of failure among community physicians. An early report by Stone and Stock suggests that there is a learning curve and that in the earlier years dosimetry is likely to be problematic [19].

In a study at the University of California San Francisco (UCSF), in a cohort of patients with a positive sextant rebiopsy at biochemical failure after primary prostate brachytherapy with iodine seeds, we found that 75 % of cold areas were located at the apex, 62.5 % at the base, and 54 % at the base + apex. Cold areas were found to correlate with positive posttreatment biopsies [20]. Of note, this sextant mapping of postbrachytherapy failures was similar to that observed in post-EBRT failures [16].

Among patients with biopsy-proven failure, Stone et al. found that 20 % had seminal vesicle involvement [18]. Thus, biopsies of the seminal vesicles should be strongly encouraged in patients with local failure who are referred for local salvage therapy.

3 Imaging in Postradiation Local Failure

While failures after primary EBRT and/or prostate brachytherapy could be due to a more challenging delineation of the base and apex on planning CT or US, other studies have reported that more than 90 % of patients with a proven local failure have recurrences in an area that overlaps the site of the primary index lesion [21–23]. The latter observations may suggest that an inadequate radiation dose was initially delivered to the primary index site, thus leading to local failure. The above has implications not only with regard to reducing the trauma and risk of infection due to posttreatment biopsies by reducing the number of biopsy samples needed, but also with regard to improving the detection and confirmation yield from biopsies, as they can be targeted to the visible lesion on MRI. A more compelling argument in favor of the accurate and sensitive localization of recurrent disease within the prostate is that targets for focal salvage therapy can be identified. Nevertheless, even with multiparametric MRI performed by experienced GU radiologists with a high volume of prostate MRI spanning two decades, the UCSF found that an additional intraprostatic but noncapsular margin of 5 mm around the index lesion should be added in the case of a focal plan so as to include 95 % of the pathological tumor volume as determined on radical prostatectomy [24]. In other words, caution must be paid to ultrafocal salvage brachytherapy because excessively tight volumes could lead to higher rates of failure by geographical misses.

With the introduction of multiparametric MRI, it is now feasible to identify areas of failure within the prostate. In a study by Haider et al., DCE-MRI was compared with T2-weighted MRI in identifying locally recurrent prostate cancer after external-beam radiotherapy [25]. All of the patients had a sextant biopsy in the wake of biochemical relapse. DCE-MRI was significantly better than T2-weighted MRI in terms of sensitivity (72 % vs. 38 %), positive predictive value (46 % vs. 24 %), and negative predictive value (95 % vs. 88 %) (Fig. 1). Specificities were similar for both modalities (85 % vs. 80 %). In another study that correlated spatial recurrence, as identified on endorectal MRI, with whole-mount salvage prostatectomy specimens, there was strong correlation between the two, confirming that MRI can accurately visualize recurrent

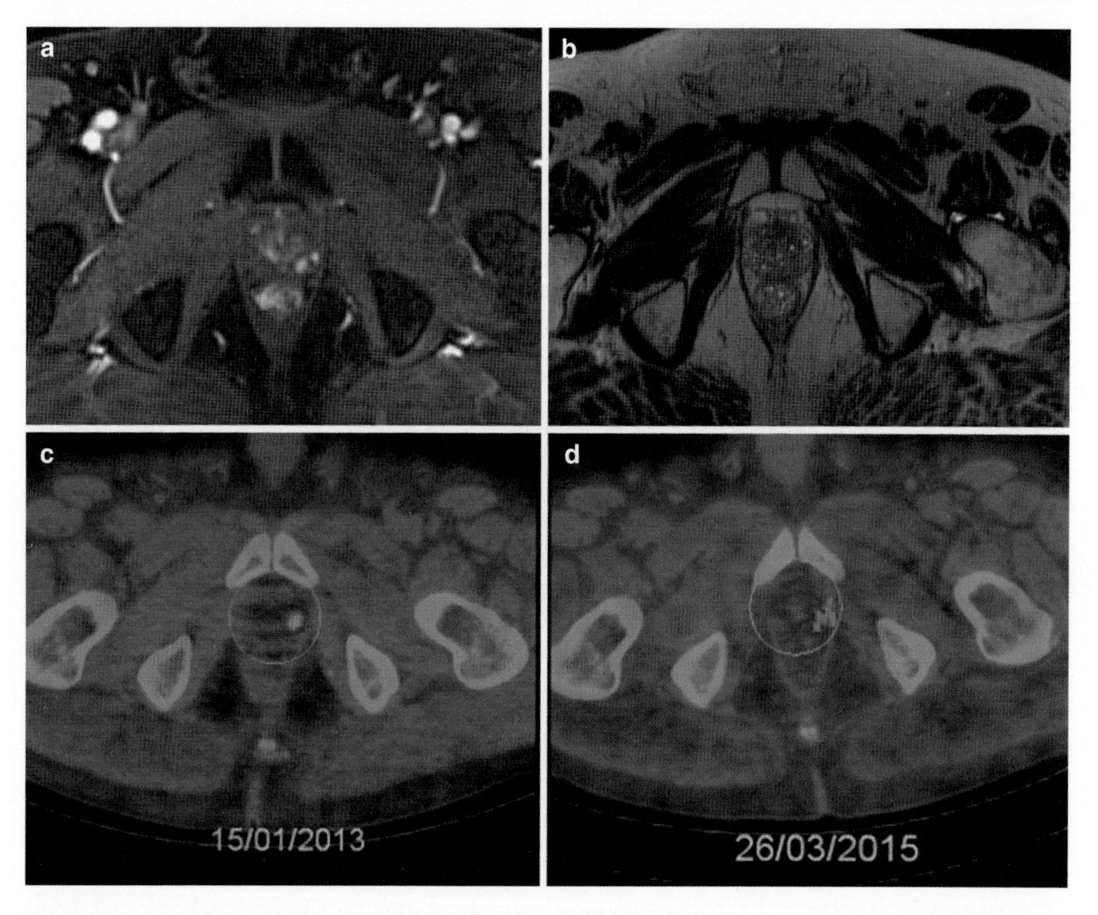

Fig. 1 Post-external-beam radiation therapy local failure of the left lobe assessed on multiparametric MRI and ^{18}F-fluorocholine PET-CT before (**a**) and (**c**) after (**b**) and (**d**) focal salvage LDR brachytherapy with iodine seeds

disease [23]. However, an important limitation is that even previously untreated patients with biopsy-proven disease may have a negative MRI. This point highlights the fact that a previously irradiated prostate with a negative MRI may be more suitable for focal therapy than a previously untreated gland.

In keeping with the MRI studies cited above, Chopra et al. at the Princess Margaret Hospital in Toronto found that most of the patients (95 %) had recurrences at the original site of the index lesion on imaging or in regions with a prostate core length involved on biopsy >40 % while 44 % also experienced recurrences in regions of non-dominant core involvement <40 % and/or regions with a negative biopsy at baseline [22].

Due to the lower accuracy of prostate T-staging only after local radiation therapy, choline PET may guide radiation oncologists in focal optimization of the dose distribution. However, choline PET should not be recommended alone when mapping local failure as multiparametric MRI is superior for focal-only salvage brachytherapy (Fig. 1) [26–28].

4 Salvage Brachytherapy for Postradiation Local Failure

4.1 Selection of Patients for Salvage Brachytherapy

In one of the first published experiences in patients treated with salvage prostate LDR brachytherapy for local relapse, Beyer et al. demonstrated a 5-year actuarial freedom from a second relapse of 53% [29]. A low presalvage PSA value (≤10 ng/mL) and a low pathological grade were found to be associated with better disease-free survival [46].

The group from Mount Sinai Hospital in New York found that the 10-year freedom from biochemical failure and cancer-specific survival rates following salvage prostate brachytherapy were 54% and 96%, respectively [30]. Patients with a presalvage PSA<6 ng/mL had improved biochemical control. Clearly, the wide range of PSA control rates after salvage brachytherapy across different studies primarily reflects differences in patients' characteristics. The selection of patients is critical to ensure that salvage brachytherapy, with its associated risk of complications, is not offered to patients with metastatic disease [31].

In a review of salvage therapies after prostate EBRT including salvage cryotherapy, radical prostatectomy, and brachytherapy, Nguyen et al. suggested more stringent selection criteria for salvage brachytherapy to identify patients who are more likely to have an isolated local relapse [31]. These criteria include at baseline a clinical T1c or T2 tumor, a Gleason score of 6 or less, and a PSA less than 10 ng/mL (i.e. favorable risk group of patients at baseline) as well as a pretreatment PSA velocity <2.0 ng/mL per year at baseline, interval between prior radiotherapy and biochemical failure >3 years, PSA doubling time >12 months, negative bone scan and pelvic imaging studies, and positive rebiopsy.

In a study of 2694 prostate cancer patients who underwent dose-escalated EBRT (75.6–86.4 Gy) with a median follow up of 10 years, the group from the Memorial Sloan Kettering Cancer Center identified 609 with biochemical failure. In these patients, the median time from biochemical failure to the occurrence of distant metastases and to death from prostate cancer was 5.4 years and 10.5 years, respectively. Patients with a Gleason score of 8 or higher, T3b to T4 disease at baseline or a PSA doubling time of less than 3 months and an interval between the end of radiotherapy and biochemical failure of less than 3 years were more likely to develop clinical progression. Patients with distant metastases were more likely to die from their prostate cancer [32]. Patients with two risk factors had a significantly higher incidence of distant metastases and prostate cancer specific mortality following biochemical failure than those with zero or one risk factor. These findings provided opportunities for a more aggressive salvage intervention in selected patients [33]. Peters et al. evaluated prognostic factors in a cohort of 62 men with local failure after radiotherapy with a median follow-up of 6 years after salvage LDR prostate brachytherapy. Among patients with a PSA doubling time >30 months and a disease-free interval >60 months, the biochemical control rates at 3 years with whole-gland salvage LDR brachytherapy were >75%. A PSA doubling time of >24 months and >33 months, respectively, gave a >80% probability of prostate cancer specific and overall survival 8 years after whole-gland salvage I-125-brachytherapy while a PSA doubling time of 12 months was associated with a 50% probability of survival at 8 years [34, 35].

A consensus of experts on this topic found a majority of agreement on the following patient and tumor criteria for selecting patients for salvage brachytherapy: age less than 80 years, life expectancy >5 years, <T3b, GS<8, whatever the Gleason score at relapse, PSA doubling time greater than 6 months, no maximal prostate volume, MR-guided biopsies, evaluation of local and distant disease using choline PET and pelvic MRI, and an interval between primary radiotherapy and salvage brachytherapy over 2 years [36]. Given the inconsistency in evaluating the postradiation Gleason score, some prognostic markers, such as the Ki67 proliferation index and DNA repair kinase (DNA-PKcs), have been shown to correlate with survival outcomes [37–39]. The Ki67 proliferation index with immunostaining was shown to correlate with the pathological Gleason score, and thus in postradiation biopsies, it may help to better identify patients with a clinically more aggressive local relapse. DNA repair kinase DNA-PKcs is another potential driver of cell migration, invasion, and metastasis [39]. Table 1 illustrates the characteristics of patients and the disease that may guide physicians in selecting patients for salvage prostate brachytherapy [40].

4.2 Salvage LDR Prostate Brachytherapy

Salvage brachytherapy has been mostly developed and reported in patients with local recurrence after external-beam radiotherapy. Most studies delivered salvage brachytherapy to the whole gland, rather than parts of the gland, using iodine-125 seeds with doses ranging between 90 Gy and 144 Gy (Table 2) [29, 30, 41–46].

Among the preliminary results of salvage prostate permanent implants with seeds, the first report published in 1999 by Beyer et al. found a 53 % control rate at 5 years in 17 patients treated with this strategy after a primary EBRT of 63 Gy (median dose) [29]. The late genitourinary morbidity was not insignificant, with 24 % incontinent at 5 years. The early series by Grado et al. reported in 49 patients treated with salvage prostate brachytherapy after 66 Gy of primary EBRT that 5-year disease-free survival and disease-specific survival rates were 34 % and 79 %, respectively. Genitourinary morbidities were infrequent as were rectal ulcer and colostomy rates (4 % and 2 %, respectively) [43].

A series of larger reports published since 2007 showed higher biochemical control rates (50–70 % with 3–5 years of follow-up) with lower rates of gastrointestinal or genitourinary toxicity and rare grade 3 or higher toxicity [41, 42, 44, 46–48]. Surprisingly, the only prospective phase II trial with MRI-guided salvage brachytherapy demonstrated a higher than expected rate of gastrointestinal toxicity (8 % of proctitis requiring Argon plasma coagulation and 12 % of fistula) [47]. Twelve of the 25 patients selected (48 %) had undergone primary prostate brachytherapy with seeds.

A few small series have reported the outcomes of salvage LDR prostate brachytherapy after prior prostate LDR brachytherapy, most of which mixed primary EBRT and brachytherapy with seeds [30, 45, 47, 49]. The University of California San Francisco (UCSF) found 71 % of biochemical control rates at 3 years with no grade 3 or higher toxicity using a focal salvage prostate permanent implant with iodine seeds [44]. Lacy et al. reported biochemical control in one half of the patients at 5 years with salvage focal LDR prostate brachytherapy after primary LDR brachytherapy with one rectourethral fistula and one bladder neck contracture only among the 21 patients [50].

In the long term, after salvage prostate LDR brachytherapy, the group from Mount Sinai Hospital in New York found that the 10-year freedom from biochemical failure and cancer-specific

Table 1 Patient selection for salvage brachytherapy for local failure

	Recommended	To be discussed
Primary disease	<cT3 <GS 8–10 PSA < 20 ng/mL	T3a or T3b cN+/pN+ GS ≤ 6 PSA < 10 ng/mL PSA velocity < 2 ng/mL/year
Local failure	Biopsy-proven prostate failure Life expectancy > 10 years <clinical T3 by DRE (if LDR) Interval between the end of primary radiotherapy and/or ADT > 3 years PSA <10 ng/mL PSADT > 6 months GS <7 (on a rebiopsy sample without significant RT effects, otherwise whatever the Gleason score) Negative bone scan and pelvic CT IPSS < 10	Life expectancy > 5 years but comorbidities Negative biopsy of seminal vesicles (if LDR) Choline PET/CT (No mets) Rectoscopy (No severe radiation effects) Cystoscopy (No severe radiation effects) Transperineal 3D biopsy mapping (if focal salvage) Multiparametric MRI (if focal salvage) Urinary flow max > 10–12 ml/s No recent TURP

GS Gleason score, *PSA* prostate specific antigen, *Mets* metastases, *DRE* digital rectal examination, *LDR* low dose rate, *ADT* androgen deprivation therapy, *PET/CT* positron emission tomography/computed tomography, *MRI* magnetic resonance imaging, *IPSS* International Prostate Symptom Score, *TURP* transurethral resection of the prostate

Table 2 Salvage LDR brachytherapy after external beam or prostate brachytherapy local failure: literature reports

References	Type of PBT	Salvage dose prescription	*N*	Primary treatment EBRT/brachy	Primary radiation dose prescription Median (range)	FU (months)	Biochemical control	Late toxicity
Beyer [29] (1999)	LDR Whole gland	88 % I^{125}: 120 Gy 22 % Pd ^{103}: 90 Gy Activity: NR	17	17/0	63.6 Gy (NR)	62	53 % (5-years)	GU: 24 % incontinence GI: 0
Grado [43] (1999)	LDR Whole gland	76 % Pd^{103}: 120 Gy (range 80–180), 24 % I^{125}: 160 Gy (range 80–180) Activity: NR	49	46/3	66.2 Gy (range 20.0–70.2)	64	34 % (5-years)	GU: 4 % hematuria 6 % painful penile dysuria GI: 4 % rectal ulcers 2 % colostomy
Allen [42] (2007)	LDR Whole gland	I^{125}: 109–112.5 Gy Pd^{103}: 90–97 Gy Activity: NR	12	12/0	70 Gy (range, 59.4–70.2)	45	63 % (4-years)	GU: 16 % G2 incontinence 8 % G1 hematuria GI: 0
Nguyen [47] (2007)	LDR Partial gland	I^{125}: 137 Gy Activity: 0.40 mCi/seed	25	13/12	EBRT: (66–70.2) PBT:137 Gy; MRI-guided	47	70 % (4-years)	GI: 8 % Argon for proctitis GU: 8 % 12 % fistula
Aaronson [41] (2009)	LDR Whole gland + SIB	I125: 108 Gy whole gland + 144 Gy focal boost Activity: 13.32 MBq/seed	24	24/0	EBRT 72 Gy (65–80)	30	89.5 % (3-years)	GU: 1 G3 Hematochezia/0 G4 GI: 0 G3/0 G4
Burri [30] (2010)	LDR Whole gland	–97 % Pd ^{103}: 110 Gy Activity: 0.9–1.7 mCi/seed –3 % I^{125}: 135 Gy Activity: 0.4 mCi/seed	37	32/5	EBRT: 67.8 Gy (range, 63.0–75.6 Gy) PBT: 47.5–113.1 Gy	86	54 % (10-years)	GU: 5 % TURP 3 % hematuria 3 % fistula
Moman [45] (2010)	LDR Whole gland	I^{125}: 145 Gy Activity: NR	31	20/11	EBRT: 66 Gy (NR)	73	23 % (5-years)	GU: 19 % G3/0 G4 GI: 6 % G3/0 G4
Rose [56] (2015)	LDR Whole gland	I^{125}: 130–144 Gy Activity: 0.33 mCi	18	18/0	EBRT : 70.5 (range : 66–78 Gy)	31.5	88 %	GU : 1G3+, 3 urethral strictures, urinary catheterization 33 % GI : 44 % G1–2 0G3+

(continued)

Table 2 (continued)

References	Type of PBT	Salvage dose prescription	*N*	Primary treatment EBRT/brachy	Primary radiation dose prescription Median (range)	FU (months)	Biochemical control	Late toxicity
Hsu [44] (2013)	LDR Partial gland	I^{125}: 144 Gy Pd^{103}: 125 Gy	15	0/15	LDR seeds	23	71.4 % (3-years)	No G3+ GI/GU (13 % G1 GI/33 % G2 GU)
Peters M [48] (2014)	LDR Partial gland	I125: ≥144 Gy	20	20/0	EBRT: NR	36	14 bNED (70 %) (3 out of 6 BF with no initial response)	1 G3 GU (stricture)
Sasaki [46] (2014)	LDR Partial gland	I^{125}: 144 Gy Activity: 0.29–0.33 mCi/seed	7	0/7	LDR seeds Median D90 135.9 Gy	27	5/7 bNED (71.5 %)	No G3+ GU/GI
Lacy (2016) [50]	LDR Partial gland	I^{125}: 108–144 Gy	21	0/21	LDR seeds 115–144 Gy	61	52.4 % (5-years)	2 G1 incontinence 1 bladder neck contracture 1 rectourethral fistula 1 leiomyosarcoma

FU follow-up, *NR* not reported, *LDR* low dose rate, *GU* genitourinary, *GI* gastrointestinal, *EBRT* external beam radiotherapy, *PBT* prostate brachytherapy, *bNED* biochemically nonevolutive disease, *BF* biochemical failure, *TURP* transurethral resection of the prostate

survival rates with salvage prostate brachytherapy were 54 % and 96 %, respectively, with only 3 % fistula [30].

Although urinary incontinence appears to be much less frequent after salvage brachytherapy than after salvage radical prostatectomy (41 %) or cryosurgery (36 %), patients who receive salvage brachytherapy face a 17 % risk of grade 3 or 4 genitourinary complications and a fistula risk that ranges from 0 to 11 %. Such treatments must be handled only by teams with expertise in prostate brachytherapy and after the careful selection of patients (see referred paragraph above). In the United States, the prospective multi-institutional phase II study by the Radiation Therapy Oncology Group (RTOG 0526: NCT00450411) of whole-gland iodine-125 seed brachytherapy to a dose of 140 Gy has completed accrual, and the results are expected soon. In France, results from a prospective multicenter single-arm study (CAPRICUR) with whole-gland iodine-125 seeds brachytherapy (90 Gy) with a simultaneous focal MR-guided brachytherapy boost (144 Gy) and rectal spacer are also expected soon (NCT01956058) (Fig. 2).

4.3 Salvage HDR Prostate Brachytherapy

Given the improved outcomes achieved in more recent salvage LDR reports, a growing number of salvage HDR brachytherapy studies have been also published since 2007, but data remains limited as compared with LDR brachytherapy [51–53]. Only a few centers have published their preliminary experience of delivering 22 to 36 Gy in 2–6 fractions over 1 or 2 implants. The group from UCSF has published the largest study with salvage whole-gland HDR prostate brachytherapy using 6 fractions of 6 Gy in 2 separate implants 1 week apart [51]. With a 5-year median follow-up, half of the patients survived without any biochemical relapse and very few toxicities (2 % grade 3 acute and late genitourinary toxicities with no grade 3 or higher acute or late gastrointestinal toxicity). Of note, neoadjuvant or concomitant short-course hormonal therapy was prescribed to 24 out of the 52 patients. Some authors also reported promising results with few toxicities with 2 fractions of 11 Gy in 1 implant with a 6 h interval in between or 13.5 Gy over 2 implants, 1–2 weeks apart (Fig. 3) (Table 3) [52, 54].

4.4 Dose and Techniques

Doses delivered during primary EBRT in series reporting outcomes of salvage brachytherapy were commonly ≤72 Gy [29, 42, 45, 47, 49]. Only a few reports in the dose escalation era have evaluated the feasibility of salvage brachytherapy for isolated local relapses only [52, 53, 55]. Nevertheless, data from salvage focal brachytherapy after a first brachytherapy would suggest its feasibility with no increased risk of harm or toxicity [44, 50]. In this setting, a composite plan which sums the dose distribution from the primary plan and the salvage plan would be ideal to predict late urethral and rectal toxicities, but this remains technically challenging. Given the aforementioned, late toxicity may certainly be related to salvage implant volumes, favoring partial implants, whenever possible. Although a majority of physicians with experience in prostate brachytherapy indicated they would never take the primary dose into account when deciding the retreatment [36], the most important precautions to take into account before salvage brachytherapy are how much additional dose can be given safely and where should the additional dose be delivered to, with more careful attention paid to surrounding tissues than is the case for dose prescription in primary brachytherapy.

Regarding the technique, most physicians consider both HDR and LDR prostate brachytherapy with seeds suitable for salvage brachytherapy. No recommendation is given on the complementary dose that would be required to cure a local relapse but the same dose as the primary brachytherapy is often given [51].

One may hypothesize that if radiotherapy failure is related to a radioresistant relapse, either dose escalation or modifying the dose rate or the dose per fraction may help circumvent resistance to the first treatment.

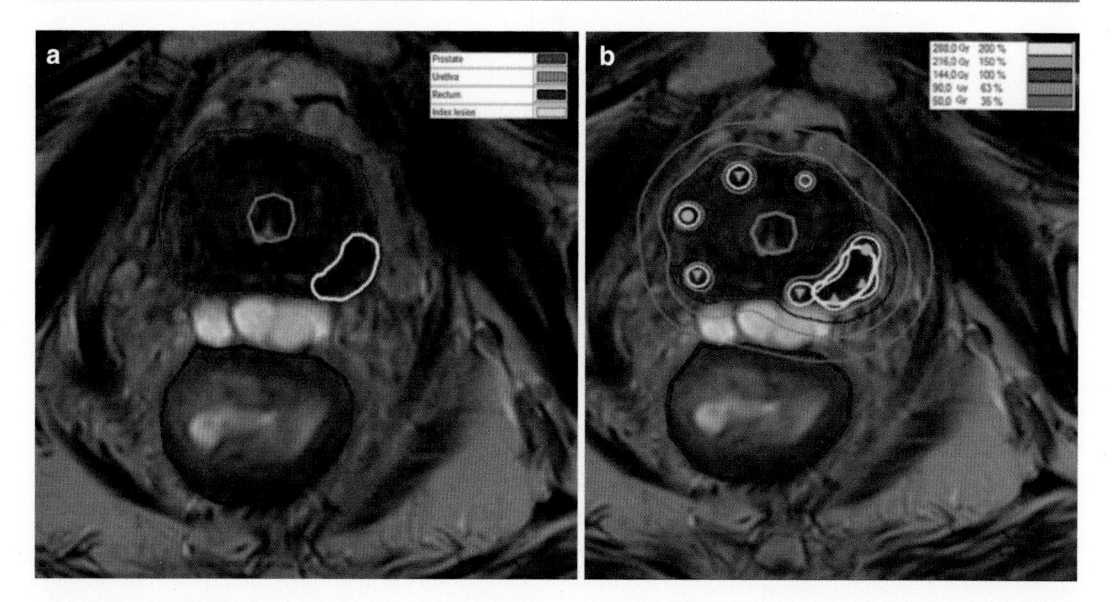

Fig. 2 Salvage whole-gland LDR prostate brachytherapy with iodine seeds with a focal simultaneous integrated boost (SIB) in the CAPRICUR study. (**a**): post-EBRT T2-weighted MRI; (**b**): post-EBRT DCE-MRI, the white arrow shows the left lobe median peripheral zone nodular relapse; (**c**): T2-weighted MRI-based delineation of the prostate (*red*) and the local relapse (*yellow*) with hyaluronic acid gel at the rectum-prostate interface (*white*); (**d**): MRI-based dosimetry of the whole-gland salvage post implant with I^{125} seeds

When Pd^{103} and I^{125} are used for LDR brachytherapy, the doses delivered range between 90–110 Gy and 109–180 Gy, respectively [29, 30, 41, 42, 44–47, 49]. Rose et al. from Vancouver (British Columbia, Canada) found that all five patients with significant toxicities (28 %) after salvage LDR brachytherapy had a higher whole-prostate D90% (median, 151 Gy; range, 135–180 Gy) than did those without late complications (median, 134 Gy; range, 105–165 Gy) [56]. There are no recommendations on the required activity of the seeds but as the prostate shrinks over the years, mostly resulting in small prostate volumes at the time of relapse, a lower than usual activity per seed may be considered.

Concerning protection of previously irradiated healthy organs surrounding the prostate, every effort must be centered on protection of the rectum to avoid any risk of fistula.

The group from Utrecht (the Netherlands) has assessed the relationship between the volume of rectum reirradiated and the likelihood of grade 3 or higher gastrointestinal toxicity in a cohort of 48 patients treated with salvage prostate permanent implant with iodine-125 seeds (D90% = 145 Gy; median primary EBRT radiation dose: 64.4–76 Gy in 28–35 fractions and LDR with I^{125} seeds: 145 Gy) [57]. Fistulas (rectourethral and rectovesical) were defined as either grade 3 or grade 4 when they required elective or emergency surgery, or ICU hospitalization, respectively. Of the 60 patients evaluable for late gastrointestinal toxicity, 20 % had Argon plasma coagulation for radiation proctitis. One patient had a grade 3 rectal ulcer, two patients a grade 3 rectourethral fistula, two patients a grade 3 rectovesical fistula, and one patient a grade 4 rectovesical fistula. No late gastrointestinal toxicity occurred in the subgroup of 28 patients treated with focal salvage brachytherapy. Although patients with focal salvage brachytherapy had a GTV median D90 > 200 Gy, this did not translate into higher rectal D0.1 cc or D1cc or D2cc when compared with whole-gland salvage plans.

Regarding patients treated to the whole gland, intraoperative rectal dose metrics were significantly poorer in patients with late grade 2 or higher gastrointestinal toxicity. The following intraoperative rectal constraints were found to have 100 % sensitivity with maximum specificity

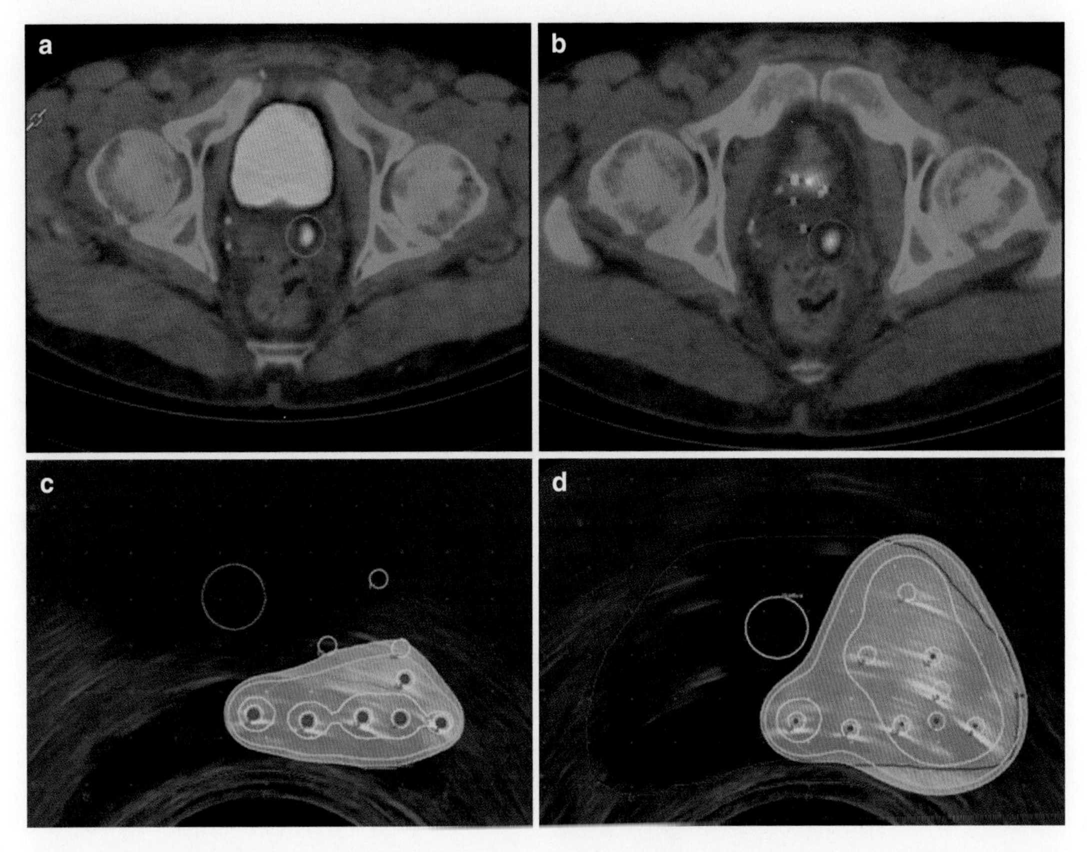

Fig. 3 Salvage focal HDR brachytherapy for a local relapse of base of the left lobe and the left seminal vesicle after a primary whole-gland prostate permanent implant with iodine seeds. Figure shows US-based axial images of a salvage focal HDR (2 fractions of 13.5 Gy) performed in Dijon (C and D), for a patient with a left biopsy-proven seminal vesicle local recurrence diagnosed on ^{18}F-fluorocholine PET-CT (**a**, **b**) with 2 positive cores of the left base of the prostate on 3D mapping transperineal biopsies

in predicting rectal toxicity: D0.1 cc < 160 Gy, D1cc < 120 Gy, D2cc < 100 Gy and V100% < 0.35 cc (compared to D0.1 cc < 200 Gy, D2cc < 145 Gy and V100% < 1 cc in a primary prostate permanent implant according to the American Brachytherapy Society) [58].

Our group in Dijon (Burgundy, France) has assessed the cumulative rectal biological effective dose (BED) by cumulating the first primary dose of escalated EBRT and a salvage prostate permanent implant with iodine seeds [55]. We found that focal salvage allowed a lower rectal BED when compared with whole-gland salvage brachytherapy. Nevertheless, rectal hot spots remain possible even with a focal approach. Only a rectal spacer may significantly decrease hot spots (Fig. 2).

Regarding urinary function, the older the patient, the worst the urinary function. Given this, one might hypothesize that patients treated with salvage brachytherapy are older than patients with primary brachytherapy. Peters et al. found that older patients had a higher rate of grade 3 or higher genitourinary toxicity [59]. Whole-gland salvage brachytherapy provides higher rates of grade 3 or higher genitourinary toxicity while fewer urinary toxicities occur with focal plans [59]. A volume of urethra receiving 100 % of the prescribed dose as determined on US planning the day of the implant higher than 0.4 cc seems to be related to significant rates of genitourinary toxicities, such as urethral strictures and/or urinary retention while the dose to the bulbomembranous urethra

Table 3 Salvage HDR brachytherapy after local failure following external beam or prostate brachytherapy: literature reports

References	Type of PBT	Salvage dose prescription	*N*	Primary treatment EBRT/brachy	Primary radiation dose prescription Median (range)	FU (months)	Biochemical control	Late toxicity
Lee [31] (2007)	HDR Whole gland	36 Gy/6fx	21	21/0	EBRT 72 Gy (63–78)	19	89 % (2-years)	GU: 14%G3/0G4 GI: 0G3+
Jo Y [52] (2012)	HDR Whole gland	22 Gy/2fx	11	1/10	EBRT 36.8 Gy + HDR boost 24 Gy/4fx HDR monotherapy: 37.5 Gy/5fx	29	67 %	GU : 0G3+ GI : 0G3+
Yamada [53] (2014)	HDR Whole gland	32 Gy/4fx	42	42/0	Median dose: 81 Gy (68.4–86.4)	36	68.5 % (5-years)	GU : 1 G3 GI 1G3/0G4
Chen [51] (2013)	HDR Whole gland	36 Gy/6fx	52	42/10	NR	59.6	51 % (5-years)	GU: 2%G3/0G4 GI: 0G3+

FU follow-up, *NR* not reported, *HDR* high dose rate, *GU* genitourinary, *GI* gastrointestinal; *EBRT* external beam radiotherapy, *PBT* prostate brachytherapy

does not. Peters et al. also advised to keep the bladder D2cc below 70 Gy.

With HDR brachytherapy, the UCSF reported good PSA control with low toxicity in their experience using 36 Gy in 6 fractions [51, 60]. Other groups have reported promising results with fewer fractions or implants with a shorter follow-up (32 Gy in 4 fractions or 22 Gy in 2 fractions over 1 implant) [52, 54].

5 Role of Hormones

Short-term and long-term ADT have definitely proved to improve survival outcomes in localized or locally advanced prostate cancer treated with exclusive radiotherapy [61–64].

A randomized trial from Quebec demonstrated lower positive rebiopsy rates in patients treated with neoadjuvant hormone suppression followed by radiation. Thus, neoadjuvant ADT can play a role in improving the local eradication of residual prostate cancer cells with radiation therapy [65].

In the RTOG 9408 phase III trial, a post hoc analysis of 831 patients with postradiation rebiopsy showed that positive postradiation rebiopsy was associated with increased rates of distant metastases and diminished disease-specific survival in patients treated with definitive EBRT and with diminished overall survival in patients with high-grade tumors [66]. The rate of positive rebiopsy in patients treated with short-term ADT combined with external-beam radiotherapy was half that in patients treated with radiation alone (39 % vs. 21 %), suggesting the radiosensitizing effect of hormones and their impact on local control. In the absence of data from salvage radical prostatectomy after ADT and radiation therapy vs. radiation therapy alone, these results may be used to select or counsel patients for additional hormone therapy in the case of local relapse with a higher risk of radioresistance or early distant progression. Nevertheless, one should keep in mind that biological interactions between ADT and LDR/HDR brachytherapy remain less well understood than those between ADT and EBRT.

Some experts claim that even if patients may have been given salvage ADT at the time of biochemical relapse, hormonal therapy should not be given concomitantly or adjuvantly with salvage brachytherapy [36]. Prostate shrinkage observed shortly after neoadjuvant ADT may also increase urethra and rectal doses at the time of the salvage brachytherapy plan.

An intriguing point was raised by colleagues from London, who found in a few patients who underwent salvage prostate brachytherapy for hormone-resistant local failure that sensitivity to hormones may be reversed at the time of failure after salvage brachytherapy, suggesting that if radiation is delivered to hormone-resistant clones, microscopic metastatic disease may recover sensitivity to androgen deprivation therapy [67]. This report suggests that even if some patients may not be definitely cured with salvage brachytherapy, the strategy may postpone the occurrence of castration-resistant prostate cancer.

Conclusions

Salvage brachytherapy for postradiation local failure is rapidly growing worldwide but patients should still be referred to experienced academic centers. In 2015, the National Comprehensive Cancer Network (NCCN) proposed salvage brachytherapy as a validated therapeutic option in patients with isolated local postradiation failure [68]. Although the prognosis of patients treated with a salvage treatment for postradiation local failure is still worse than that after a first biochemical failure, nearly 75 % of patients seem biochemically controlled in the first 3–4 years following salvage brachytherapy with more than half of the patients with no biochemical failure at 10 years with a low risk of late sequelae. Data of prospective phase II studies are expected soon to validate the reproducibility and feasibility of this strategy in experienced hands only. The notion that a patient who had first-line pelvic radiotherapy should not undergo secondary salvage radiation due to the risk of rectal fistulas and diffuse hemorrhagic cystitis has become obsolete.

References

1. Agarwal PK, Sadetsky N, Konety BR, Resnick MI, Carroll PR, Cancer of the Prostate Strategic Urological Research E. Treatment failure after primary and salvage therapy for prostate cancer: likelihood, patterns of care, and outcomes. Cancer. 2008;112(2):307–14.
2. Kimura M, Mouraviev V, Tsivian M, Mayes JM, Satoh T, Polascik TJ. Current salvage methods for recurrent prostate cancer after failure of primary radiotherapy. BJU Int. 2010;105(2):191–201.
3. Crook JM, O'Callaghan CJ, Duncan G, Dearnaley DP, Higano CS, Horwitz EM, et al. Intermittent androgen suppression for rising PSA level after radiotherapy. N Engl J Med. 2012;367(10):895–903.
4. Hussain M, Tangen CM, Berry DL, Higano CS, Crawford ED, Liu G, et al. Intermittent versus continuous androgen deprivation in prostate cancer. N Engl J Med. 2013;368(14):1314–25.
5. Hershman DL, Unger JM, Wright JD, Ramsey S, Till C, Tangen CM, et al. Adverse health events following intermittent and continuous androgen deprivation in patients with metastatic prostate cancer. JAMA Oncol. 2016;2(4):453–61.
6. Fuks Z, Leibel SA, Wallner KE, Begg CB, Fair WR, Anderson LL, et al. The effect of local control on metastatic dissemination in carcinoma of the prostate: long-term results in patients treated with 125I implantation. Int J Radiat Oncol Biol Phys. 1991;21(3):537–47.
7. Zagars GK, von Eschenbach AC, Ayala AG, Schultheiss TE, Sherman NE. The influence of local control on metastatic dissemination of prostate cancer treated by external beam megavoltage radiation therapy. Cancer. 1991;68(11):2370–7.
8. Coen JJ, Zietman AL, Thakral H, Shipley WU. Radical radiation for localized prostate cancer: local persistence of disease results in a late wave of metastases. J Clin Oncol. 2002;20(15):3199–205.
9. Zietman AL, Westgeest JC, Shipley WU. Radiation-based approaches to the management of T3 prostate cancer. Semin Urol Oncol. 1997;15(4):230–8.
10. Crook JM, Perry GA, Robertson S, Esche BA. Routine prostate biopsies following radiotherapy for prostate cancer: results for 226 patients. Urology. 1995;45(4):624–31; discussion 31–2.
11. Dugan TC, Shipley WU, Young RH, Verhey LJ, Althausen AF, Heney NM, et al. Biopsy after external beam radiation therapy for adenocarcinoma of the prostate: correlation with original histological grade and current prostate specific antigen levels. J Urol. 1991;146(5):1313–6.
12. Zelefsky MJ, Leibel SA, Gaudin PB, Kutcher GJ, Fleshner NE, Venkatramen ES, et al. Dose escalation with three-dimensional conformal radiation therapy affects the outcome in prostate cancer. Int J Radiat Oncol Biol Phys. 1998;41(3):491–500.
13. Shipley WU, Verhey LJ, Munzenrider JE, Suit HD, Urie MM, McManus PL, et al. Advanced prostate cancer: the results of a randomized comparative trial of high dose irradiation boosting with conformal protons compared with conventional dose irradiation using photons alone. Int J Radiat Oncol Biol Phys. 1995;32(1):3–12.
14. Huang KT, Stoyanova R, Walker G, Sandler K, Studenski MT, Dogan N, et al. Post-radiotherapy prostate biopsies reveal heightened apex positivity relative to other prostate regions sampled. Radiother Oncol. 2015;115(1):101–6.
15. Huang WC, Kuroiwa K, Serio AM, Bianco Jr FJ, Fine SW, Shayegan B, et al. The anatomical and pathological characteristics of irradiated prostate cancers may influence the oncological efficacy of salvage ablative therapies. J Urol. 2007;177(4):1324–9; quiz 591.
16. Leibovici D, Chiong E, Pisters LL, Guo CC, Ward JF, Andino L, et al. Pathological characteristics of prostate cancer recurrence after radiation therapy: implications for focal salvage therapy. J Urol. 2012;188(1):98–102.
17. Lo AC, Morris WJ, Pickles T, Keyes M, McKenzie M, Tyldesley S. Patterns of recurrence after low-dose-rate prostate brachytherapy: a population-based study of 2223 consecutive low- and intermediate-risk patients. Int J Radiat Oncol Biol Phys. 2015;91(4):745–51.
18. Stone NN, Stock RG, White I, Unger P. Patterns of local failure following prostate brachytherapy. J Urol. 2007;177(5):1759–63; discussion 63–4.
19. Stock RG, Stone NN, Tabert A, Iannuzzi C, DeWyngaert JK. A dose–response study for I-125 prostate implants. Int J Radiat Oncol Biol Phys. 1998;41(1):101–8.
20. Lepinoy A, Cochet A, Cueff A, Cormier L, Martin E, Maingon P, et al. Pattern of occult nodal relapse diagnosed with (18)F-fluoro-choline PET/CT in prostate cancer patients with biochemical failure after prostate-only radiotherapy. Radiother Oncol. 2014;111(1):120–5.
21. Arrayeh E, Westphalen AC, Kurhanewicz J, Roach 3rd M, Jung AJ, Carroll PR, et al. Does local recurrence of prostate cancer after radiation therapy occur at the site of primary tumor? Results of a longitudinal MRI and MRSI study. Int J Radiat Oncol Biol Phys. 2012;82(5):e787–93.
22. Chopra S, Toi A, Taback N, Evans A, Haider MA, Milosevic M, et al. Pathological predictors for site of local recurrence after radiotherapy for prostate cancer. Int J Radiat Oncol Biol Phys. 2012;82(3):e441–8.
23. Pucar D, Hricak H, Shukla-Dave A, Kuroiwa K, Drobnjak M, Eastham J, et al. Clinically significant prostate cancer local recurrence after radiation therapy occurs at the site of primary tumor: magnetic resonance imaging and step-section pathology evidence. Int J Radiat Oncol Biol Phys. 2007;69(1):62–9.
24. Anwar M, Westphalen AC, Jung AJ, Noworolski SM, Simko JP, Kurhanewicz J, et al. Role of endorectal MR imaging and MR spectroscopic imaging in defining treatable intraprostatic tumor foci in prostate cancer: quantitative analysis of imaging contour compared to whole-mount histopathology. Radiother Oncol. 2014;110(2):303–8.

25. Haider MA, Chung P, Sweet J, Toi A, Jhaveri K, Menard C, et al. Dynamic contrast-enhanced magnetic resonance imaging for localization of recurrent prostate cancer after external beam radiotherapy. Int J Radiat Oncol Biol Phys. 2008;70(2):425–30.
26. Testa C, Schiavina R, Lodi R, Salizzoni E, Corti B, Farsad M, et al. Prostate cancer: sextant localization with MR imaging, MR spectroscopy, and 11C-choline PET/CT. Radiology. 2007;244(3):797–806.
27. Van den Bergh L, Koole M, Isebaert S, Joniau S, Deroose CM, Oyen R, et al. Is there an additional value of (1)(1)C-choline PET-CT to T2-weighted MRI images in the localization of intraprostatic tumor nodules? Int J Radiat Oncol Biol Phys. 2012;83(5):1486–92.
28. Chang JH, Lim Joon D, Davis ID, Lee ST, Hiew CY, Esler S, et al. Comparison of [(11)C]choline positron emission tomography with T2- and diffusion-weighted magnetic resonance imaging for delineating malignant intraprostatic lesions. Int J Radiat Oncol Biol Phys. 2015;92(2):438–45.
29. Beyer DC. Permanent brachytherapy as salvage treatment for recurrent prostate cancer. Urology. 1999;54(5):880–3.
30. Burri RJ, Stone NN, Unger P, Stock RG. Long-term outcome and toxicity of salvage brachytherapy for local failure after initial radiotherapy for prostate cancer. Int J Radiat Oncol Biol Phys. 2010;77(5):1338–44.
31. Nguyen PL, D'Amico AV, Lee AK, Suh WW. Patient selection, cancer control, and complications after salvage local therapy for postradiation prostate-specific antigen failure: a systematic review of the literature. Cancer. 2007;110(7):1417–28.
32. Zumsteg ZS, Spratt DE, Romesser PB, Pei X, Zhang Z, Polkinghorn W, et al. The natural history and predictors of outcome following biochemical relapse in the dose escalation era for prostate cancer patients undergoing definitive external beam radiotherapy. Eur Urol. 2015;67(6):1009–16.
33. Roach 3rd M. Natural history after biochemical failure following dose-escalated external beam radiation: an opportunity to improve outcomes? Eur Urol. 2015;67(6):1017–8.
34. Peters M, van der Voort van Zyp JR, Moerland MA, Hoekstra CJ, van de Pol S, Westendorp H, et al. Development and internal validation of a multivariable prediction model for biochemical failure after whole-gland salvage iodine-125 prostate brachytherapy for recurrent prostate cancer. Brachytherapy. 2016.
35. Peters M, van der Voort van Zyp JR, Moerland MA, Hoekstra CJ, van de Pol S, Westendorp H, et al. Multivariable model development and internal validation for prostate cancer specific survival and overall survival after whole-gland salvage Iodine-125 prostate brachytherapy. Radiother Oncol. 2016.
36. Kaljouw E, Pieters BR, Kovacs G, Hoskin PJ. A Delphi consensus study on salvage brachytherapy for prostate cancer relapse after radiotherapy, a Uro-GEC study. Radiother Oncol. 2016;118(1):122–30.
37. Tretiakova MS, Wei W, Boyer HD, Newcomb LF, Hawley S, Auman H, et al. Prognostic value of Ki67 in localized prostate carcinoma: a multi-institutional study of >1000 prostatectomies. Prostate Cancer Prostatic Dis. 2016.
38. Zellweger T, Gunther S, Zlobec I, Savic S, Sauter G, Moch H, et al. Tumour growth fraction measured by immunohistochemical staining of Ki67 is an independent prognostic factor in preoperative prostate biopsies with small-volume or low-grade prostate cancer. Int J Cancer. 2009;124(9):2116–23.
39. Goodwin JF, Kothari V, Drake JM, Zhao S, Dylgjeri E, Dean JL, et al. DNA-PKcs-mediated transcriptional regulation drives prostate cancer progression and metastasis. Cancer Cell. 2015;28(1):97–113.
40. Crehange G, Roach 3rd M, Martin E, Cormier L, Peiffert D, Cochet A, et al. Salvage reirradiation for locoregional failure after radiation therapy for prostate cancer: who, when, where and how? Cancer Radiother. 2014;18(5–6):524–34.
41. Aaronson DS, Yamasaki I, Gottschalk A, Speight J, Hsu IC, Pickett B, et al. Salvage permanent perineal radioactive-seed implantation for treating recurrence of localized prostate adenocarcinoma after external beam radiotherapy. BJU Int. 2009;104(5):600–4.
42. Allen GW, Howard AR, Jarrard DF, Ritter MA. Management of prostate cancer recurrences after radiation therapy-brachytherapy as a salvage option. Cancer. 2007;110(7):1405–16.
43. Grado GL. Benefits of brachytherapy as salvage treatment for radiorecurrent localized prostate cancer. Urology. 1999;54(2):204–7.
44. Hsu CC, Hsu H, Pickett B, Crehange G, Hsu IC, Dea R, et al. Feasibility of MR imaging/MR spectroscopy-planned focal partial salvage permanent prostate implant (PPI) for localized recurrence after initial PPI for prostate cancer. Int J Radiat Oncol Biol Phys. 2013;85(2):370–7.
45. Moman MR, van der Poel HG, Battermann JJ, Moerland MA, van Vulpen M. Treatment outcome and toxicity after salvage 125-I implantation for prostate cancer recurrences after primary 125-I implantation and external beam radiotherapy. Brachytherapy. 2010;9(2):119–25.
46. Sasaki H, Kido M, Miki K, Kuruma H, Takahashi H, Aoki M, et al. Salvage partial brachytherapy for prostate cancer recurrence after primary brachytherapy. Int J Urol. 2014;21(6):572–7.
47. Nguyen PL, Chen MH, D'Amico AV, Tempany CM, Steele GS, Albert M, et al. Magnetic resonance image-guided salvage brachytherapy after radiation in select men who initially presented with favorable-risk prostate cancer: a prospective phase 2 study. Cancer. 2007;110(7):1485–92.
48. Peters M, Maenhout M, van der Voort van Zyp JR, Moerland MA, Moman MR, Steuten LM, et al. Focal salvage iodine-125 brachytherapy for prostate cancer recurrences after primary radiotherapy: a retrospective study regarding toxicity, biochemical outcome and quality of life. Radiother Oncol. 2014;112(1):77–82.

49. Grado GL, Collins JM, Kriegshauser JS, Balch CS, Grado MM, Swanson GP, et al. Salvage brachytherapy for localized prostate cancer after radiotherapy failure. Urology. 1999;53(1):2–10.
50. Lacy JM, Wilson WA, Bole R, Chen L, Meigooni AS, Rowland RG, et al. Salvage brachytherapy for biochemically recurrent prostate cancer following primary brachytherapy. Prostate Cancer. 2016;2016:9561494.
51. Chen CP, Weinberg V, Shinohara K, Roach 3rd M, Nash M, Gottschalk A, et al. Salvage HDR brachytherapy for recurrent prostate cancer after previous definitive radiation therapy: 5-year outcomes. Int J Radiat Oncol Biol Phys. 2013;86(2):324–9.
52. Jo Y, Fujii T, Hara R, Yokoyama T, Miyaji Y, Yoden E, et al. Salvage high-dose-rate brachytherapy for local prostate cancer recurrence after radiotherapy – preliminary results. BJU Int. 2012;109(6):835–9.
53. Yamada Y, Kollmeier MA, Pei X, Kan CC, Cohen GN, Donat SM, et al. A Phase II study of salvage high-dose-rate brachytherapy for the treatment of locally recurrent prostate cancer after definitive external beam radiotherapy. Brachytherapy. 2014;13(2):111–6.
54. Chung HT, Loblaw A, D'Alimonte L, Ravi A, Haider MA, Morton G. Pilot study of focal salvage high-dose rate (HDR) prostate brachytherapy in patients with local recurrence after definitive external-beam radiotherapy (XRT). J Clin Oncol. 2014: ASCO Vol 32, No 4_suppl, 2014: 264.
55. Guimas V, Quivrin M, Bertaut A, Martin E, Maingon P, Mazoyer F, Cormier L, Crehange G. Focal or whole-gland salvage prostate brachytherapy with iodine seeds with or without a rectal spacer for postradiotherapy local failure: how best to spare the rectum? Brachytherapy. 2016;15(4):406–11.
56. Rose JN, Crook JM, Pickles T, Keyes M, Morris WJ. Salvage low-dose-rate permanent seed brachytherapy for locally recurrent prostate cancer: association between dose and late toxicity. Brachytherapy. 2015;14(3):342–9.
57. Peters M, Hoekstra CJ, van der Voort van Zyp JR, Westendorp H, van de Pol SM, Moerland MA, et al. Rectal dose constraints for salvage iodine-125 prostate brachytherapy. Brachytherapy. 2016;15(1):85–93.
58. Davis BJ, Horwitz EM, Lee WR, Crook JM, Stock RG, Merrick GS, et al. American Brachytherapy Society consensus guidelines for transrectal ultrasound-guided permanent prostate brachytherapy. Brachytherapy. 2012;11(1):6–19.
59. Peters M, van der Voort van Zyp J, Hoekstra C, Westendorp H, van de Pol S, Moerland M, et al. Urethral and bladder dosimetry of total and focal salvage Iodine-125 prostate brachytherapy: Late toxicity and dose constraints. Radiother Oncol. 2015;117(2):262–9.
60. Lee B, Shinohara K, Weinberg V, Gottschalk AR, Pouliot J, Roach 3rd M, et al. Feasibility of high-dose-rate brachytherapy salvage for local prostate cancer recurrence after radiotherapy: the University of California-San Francisco experience. Int J Radiat Oncol Biol Phys. 2007;67(4):1106–12.
61. Roach 3rd M, Bae K, Speight J, Wolkov HB, Rubin P, Lee RJ, et al. Short-term neoadjuvant androgen deprivation therapy and external-beam radiotherapy for locally advanced prostate cancer: long-term results of RTOG 8610. J Clin Oncol. 2008;26(4):585–91.
62. Bolla M, Van Tienhoven G, Warde P, Dubois JB, Mirimanoff RO, Storme G, et al. External irradiation with or without long-term androgen suppression for prostate cancer with high metastatic risk: 10-year results of an EORTC randomised study. Lancet Oncol. 2010;11(11):1066–73.
63. D'Amico AV, Chen MH, Renshaw A, Loffredo M, Kantoff PW. Long-term follow-up of a randomized trial of radiation with or without androgen deprivation therapy for localized prostate cancer. JAMA. 2015;314(12):1291–3.
64. Jones CU, Hunt D, McGowan DG, Amin MB, Chetner MP, Bruner DW, et al. Radiotherapy and short-term androgen deprivation for localized prostate cancer. N Engl J Med. 2011;365(2):107–18.
65. Jalloh M, Leapman MS, Cowan JE, Shinohara K, Greene KL, Roach 3rd M, et al. Patterns of local failure following radiation therapy for prostate cancer. J Urol. 2015;194(4):977–82.
66. Krauss DJ, Hu C, Bahary JP, Souhami L, Gore EM, Chafe SM, et al. Importance of local control in early-stage prostate cancer: outcomes of patients with positive post-radiation therapy biopsy results treated in RTOG 9408. Int J Radiat Oncol Biol Phys. 2015;92(4):863–73.
67. Smith D, Plowman PN. Recovery of hormone sensitivity after salvage brachytherapy for hormone refractory localized prostate cancer. Int Braz J Urol. 2010;36(3):283–91.
68. Mohler JL, Armstrong AJ, Bahnson RR, Boston B, Busby JE, D'Amico AV, et al. Prostate cancer, version 3.2012: featured updates to the NCCN guidelines. J Natl Compr Canc Netw. 2012;10(9):1081–7.

Follow-Up After Radical Treatments and Relapse

Friederike Haidl and Axel Heidenreich

1 Introduction

Organ confined and locally advanced prostate cancer can be treated by various surgical or radiooncological methods [1, 2]. In addition, nonsurgical treatment options such as focal MRI-based HIFU treatment and cryosurgery are becoming more popular although these methods are currently not guideline recommended due to small patient numbers and only short-term follow-up [1, 2]. For all local therapies, the type and the frequency of follow-up procedures depends on the local extent of the cancer and the potentially available treatment options.

Following all nonsurgical treatment options, radical salvage prostatectomy might be performed in well selected relapsing patients with a high chance of locally recurrent but organ confined prostate cancer [3]. These patients need a specific and different follow-up from patients who underwent RP for treatment-naive PCA.

Relapse rates of patients who have undergone maximum local therapy including radical prostatectomy and salvage radiation therapy of the prostatic fossa represent another cohort of men who will need an individualized follow-up in order to identify additional potentially available local treatment strategies.

It is the purpose of the current chapter to summarize the follow-up procedures after local radical treatment of PCA based on an individualized, risk-adapted model which depends on tumor biology, patient comorbidities, patient age, and patient wishes.

2 Why to Perform Follow-Up?

Follow-up strategies after local radical prostate cancer therapy aim to reach two goals: [1] early detection of local or systemic relapse which might enable second-line therapy to improve long-term prognosis and [2] early detection of treatment related side effects to allow early intervention and thereby to improve quality of life for the patients. Early detection of both oncological relapse and functional impairment will allow a profound discussion with the patient and his family concerning active treatment or watchful waiting. It remains to be shown, however, that early treatment of micrometastatic disease has a fundamental impact on long-term survival.

F. Haidl • A. Heidenreich (✉)
Department of Urology, Uro-Oncology, Robot-assisted and Specialized Urologic Surgery, University of Cologne, Kerpener Str. 62, 50937 Cologne, Germany
e-mail: axel.heidenreich@uk-koeln.de

M. Bolla, H. van Poppel (eds.), *Management of Prostate Cancer*, DOI 10.1007/978-3-319-42769-0_20

3 Methods of Follow-Up

Follow-up examinations after radical prostatectomy might include digital rectal examination, evaluation of PSA serum levels and imaging studies such as computed tomography of the abdomen and small pelvis, bone scintigraphy or positron emission tomography (PET/CT). It depends on individual tumor characteristics which method or which combination of studies might be best to early detect the presence and the location of relapse [4].

4 Prostate Specific Antigen (PSA) Monitoring

PSA is the most sensitive marker to identify relapsing PCA in patients following RP. It is generally recommended that the first PSA should be obtained about 6 weeks following RP. At this time, PSA should have decreased to non detectable serum levels and any PSA above measurable PSA is an indicator for persisting local prostate cancer elements or micrometastatic lymph node or systemic spread [5, 6].

Recurrent PSA is an indicator of relapsing disease and it usually precedes clinical relapse by months to years depending on the biological aggressiveness of the individual cancer [7, 8].

A single, elevated PSA serum levels should always be confirmed twice at 4-week intervals before therapeutic consequences in terms of second-line therapy are drawn.

Following RP, PSA relapse is defined by two consecutive PSA values ≥ 0.2 ng/ml. The background of this definition is the finding of a retrospective study demonstrating as a subsequent increase in PSA in 49 %, 62 %, and 72 % of patients with PSA levels of 0.2, 0.3, and 0.4 ng/mL, respectively [9].

The use of ultrasensitive PSA assays in daily routine is discussed controversially due to its unclear prognostic value. About two thirds of men with postoperative ultrasensitive PSA levels > 0.05 ng/ml remain free of biochemical disease at 5 years. However, if a continuous PSA rise from < 0.1 ng/ml to > 0.1 ng/ml is observed, treatment failure can be anticipated and early salvage therapy might be initiated [10, 11].

Early salvage treatment might improve oncological outcome especially in men with high probability of local relapse [12].

Time interval between RP and PSA rise and PSA kinetics play an important role in the potential localization of residual disease and on its second-line treatment. Slowly increasing PSA levels most probably indicate local recurrence, whereas rapidly rising PSA serum levels with a doubling time well below 1 year indicate lymph node involvement or systemic disease.

Local failure following RP might be predicted with an 80 % probability by a PSA increase > 3 years after RP, a PSA DT > 11 mos, a Gleason score < 7, and stage ≤ pT3a pN0, pTx R1. Systemic failure following RP might be predicted with > 80 % accuracy by a PSA increase < 1 year after RP, a PSA DT of 4–6 mos, a Gleason score of 8–10, and stage pT3b, pTxpN1. In a cohort of 148 men with rising PSA and a PSA DT < 12 mos following local treatment, the PFS was associated with Gleason grade ($p = 0.006$), PSA at time of treatment ($p < 0.001$) and PSA DT ($p < 0.001$) [13]. The median PFS was 19 mos, with a 3- and 5-year metastasis PFS of 32 % and 16 %, respectively.

5 PSA Relapse After HIFU and Cryotherapy

Following cryosurgery, an objective assessment of PSA outcome is not easy because of the lack of internationally accepted PSA nadir PSA levels defining relapse. With regard to modern cryosurgery techniques, a threshold PSA level of 0.5 ng/ml might be best used to define relapsing disease based on the data of Long et al. [14]. The authors retrospectively evaluated the oncological outcome of 975 PCA patients at three different risk groups. At a mean follow-up of 2 years, the biochemical disease-free survival rates were calculated for PSA nadir levels of 1.0 ng/ml and 0.5 ng/ml, respectively with the following relapse rates at 5 years:

- 76 % and 60 %, respectively, for the low-risk group
- 71 % and 45 %, respectively, for the intermediate-risk group
- 61 % and 36 %, respectively, for the high-risk group

With regard to HIFU, the Stuttgart criteria (> PSA nadir + 1.2 ng/mL) have been proposed to define biochemical relapse [15]. However, these data are only valid for patients who have undergone whole gland HIFU therapy. In patients who have undergone focal therapy, PSA threshold levels which might define relapse are discussed controversially [16].

Once PSA relapse has been identified following HIFU or cryosurgery, local versus systemic recurrence must be differentiated which should be done by multiparametric MRI of the prostate and PSMA- PET/CT (see below).

6 Digital Rectal Examination

Locally recurrent PCA without concomitant PSA rise can be detected in patients with undifferentiated PCA and low PSA serum levels at time of diagnosis. Since the combination of both DRE and PSA represents the most useful combination, it should be performed in every single patient [4].

7 When and How Long to Perform Follow-Up Studies?

The first PSA serum level should be checked 6 weeks postoperatively to exclude PSA persistence. Thereafter, the frequency of follow-up examinations should be tailored according to the individual risk profile [1, 2].

The risk of PSA relapse in low-risk disease is extremely low during the first 20 years of follow-up and it does not exceed 10 %. Therefore, it might be sufficient to use a “relaxed” follow-up strategy with PSA serum levels measured 6 weeks, 3 months, and 6 and 12 months postoperatively followed by 6 months intervals if no relapse was detected.

In the high-risk group, biochemical PFS (BPFS) at 5- and 10-years follow-up ranged between 35–51 % and 24–39 %, respectively, while the CSS at 5-, 10-, and 15-years follow-up was 96 %, 84–88 %, and 66 %, respectively [17–20]. It is obvious that follow-up strategies need to be different depending on the risk profile of the tumor.

In a recent retrospective study including more than 5000 patients after RP, three risk groups with different annual hazard rates of biochemical recurrence could be identified [21]. The low-risk group comprised 23.7 % of the patients with an annual hazard rate of only 0–2.6 % throughout the follow-up period. Therefore, follow-up examinations at 6–2 months might be sufficient. The low-risk group was defined as PSA < 11 ng/ml, clinical stage T1c and pathological Gleason score ≤ 6 plus organ-confined disease and negative surgical margins. The high-risk group comprised 19 % of the total patient cohort and it includes patients with PSA > 22 ng/ml, pathological seminal vesicle invasion or clinical stage T3 disease, or pathological Gleason score 8–10 or positive lymph nodes. Annual hazard rates are as high as 32 throughout follow-up so that these patients need close and continuous follow-up examination at 3 months intervals. The intermediate-risk group comprised 57 % of the patients and the annual hazard rates were between 1.3 and 7.2 throughout the follow-up period.

Similar data have been produced by a recent German multicentric retrospective study comprising 956 patients with pT2 disease and positive surgical margins but without adjuvant treatment [22]. The mean follow-up was 48 months and biochemical recurrence was observed in 25.4 % of patients. In multivariate analysis, Gleason score (GS) of the prostatectomy specimen was the only significant parameter for BCR. Median time to recurrence for GS ≤ 6 was not reached; 5-year BCR-free survival was 82 %; and they were 127 months and 72 % for GS 3 + 4, 56 months and 54 % for GS 4 + 3, and 27 months and 32 % for GS 8–10.

In patients with pT3a PCA and positive surgical margins without adjuvant treatment, biochemical relapsed occurred in 39.7 % of patients after a mean follow-up of 48 months [23]. In multivariate analysis, Gleason score was the only independent prognostic factor ($p<0.001$) for BCR. Five-year BCR-free survival rates were 74 %, 70 %, 38 %, and 51 % with Gleason score 6, 3+4=7a, 4+3=7b, and 8–10, respectively. The mean time to PSA relapse was *not reached in patients with Gleason score 6 and it was 100 months in patients with a Gleason Score 7a indicating that long time intervals can be safely performed during follow-up without negative consequences on oncological outcome. In patients with Gleason score 7b and 8–10, the mean time interval until PSA relapse was in the range of 65 and 43 months, respectively*, indicating that PSA follow-up examinations must be performed more frequently at 3–6 months intervals.

Follow-up strategies also need to take into consideration if RP was performed as monotherapy or if fit was combined with adjuvant radiation therapy in the presence of positive surgical margins or adjuvant androgen deprivation therapy for the management of lymph node metastases or a triple combination of surgery, RT, and ADT in case of a high-risk profile.

8 Imaging Studies During Follow-Up

There is no indication to perform routine imaging studies in patients without PSA relapse and in the absence of symptoms of clinical progression. It must be remembered that PSA failure after RP might precede clinical metastases by up to 7–8 years [10, 11].

The indication for any imaging study should be based on its potential therapeutic consequences. E.g., in patients with oligometastatic disease, local treatment of pelvic lymph node metastases by salvage lymphadenectomy or localized radiation therapy might be an option in order to prolong time to initiation of systemic therapy [24, 25].

If, however, the patient is no candidate for such a localized salvage procedure, imaging studies at low PSA serum levels do not make sense since these will not change the therapeutic strategy. In such a scenario, it might be better to follow the patient with serial measurements and no imaging study until a certain PSA threshold value or until the development of clinical symptoms.

Systemic androgen deprivation therapy can be postponed to PSA levels as high as 5 ng/ml in the presence of prostatectomy Gleason score < 8 and/or a PSA doubling time with no negative impact on survival or metastasis-free survival as compared to early ADT [26]. In patients with Gleason score 8–10 and/or a PSA-DT < 12 months, early ADT is associated with an improved metastasis-free survival.

However, baseline imaging studies should be performed once systemic will be started to be able to evaluate objective remission or progression during treatment.

It is common sense that skeletal scintigraphy and computed tomography of the abdomen/pelvis are not helpful with a positive finding in < 5 % except in patients with PSA serum levels > 20 ng/ml or a PSA velocity > 2 ng/ml/year [27, 28]. Another study demonstrated that the probability of a positive bone scan is less than 5 % if the PSA level is < 7 ng/ml. The sensitivity of an abdominal and pelvic CT scan is in the range of 11–15 % even in patients with a PSA level > 20 ng/ml and a PSA velocity of 1.8 ng/ml/year. Based on these data it becomes evident that we need more sensitive methods to early detect low volume metastases.

Positron-emission tomography has been successfully used in many human cancers for early identification of local, locoregional, or systemic recurrences. In PCA, there are few, even if promising, published data on the clinical efficacy of PET in detecting locoregional recurrences after RP, especially in situations of a PSA value > 1.0 ng/ml [29, 30]. As recently reported by Giovaccini et al. [31], the accuracy of PET correlates with PSA values, PSADT, and other pathological features. Certainly, a PSADT < 3 months can be regarded as a strong predictor of PET positivity.

In patients with biochemical failure after RP, PET/CT detection rates are only 5–24 % when the PSA level is < 1 ng/mL, but rises to 67–100 % when the PSA level is > 5 ng/mL. Similarly, PET/CT sensitivity seems much higher when the PSA velocity is high or the PSA-DT is short. In a recent meta-analysis, Choline PET/CT detection rates were 65 % (95 % CI, 58 %–71 %) when the PSA-DT was < 6 months, and were 71 % (95 % CI, 66 %–76 %) and 77 % (95 % CI, 71 %–82 %) when the PSA velocity was > 1 and > 2 ng/mL/year, respectively [32].

However, even in patients with PSA values > 2 ng/mL and negative imaging studies, 11C-choline PET/CT is positive in only 28 % of patients. Choline PET/CT is generally not recommended for patients with prostate specific antigen (PSA) levels <1–2 ng/ml or for initial staging [29–31].

^{11}C-Choline PET/CT may detect multiple bone metastases in patients showing a single metastasis on bone scan and may be positive for bone metastases in up to 15 % of patients with biochemical failure after RP and negative bone scan [32]. The specificity of ^{11}C-Choline PET-CT is also higher than bone scan with less false positive and indeterminate findings.

The prostate specific membrane antigen (PSMA) is generally overexpressed in prostate cancer (PCA), correlating with the Gleason score [33, 34]. PSMA is therefore considered as a target for radionuclide imaging and therapy [35].

Positron emission tomography/computed tomography (PET/CT) using ^{68}Ga-labeled ligand [^{68}Ga]PSMA-HBED-CC was recently presented as a novel imaging modality for the detection of prostate cancer (PCA) recurrence and/or metastases [36, 37]. Initial studies showed that [^{68}Ga]PSMA-HBED-CC-PET/CT might be able to offer a high rate of lesion detection, even at very low prostate specific antigen (PSA) levels or in staging at initial diagnosis [36, 37].

In a recent study, [^{68}Ga]PSMA-HBED-CC PET/CT was positive in 44 %, 79 %, and 90 % of patients with PSA levels of ≤1, 1–2, or ≥2 ng/ml. Especially at low levels this compares favorably to choline PET/CT, e.g., in a recent large series [29] the lesion detection rates in 1000 patients undergoing choline PET/CT at these same levels were 31 %, 43 %, and 81 %, respectively. In another series of 325 patients, Chondrogiannis et al. [30] reported detection rates of ~28 % and ~35 % for patients with PSA levels of 0.1–0.5 and 0.5–1.5 ng/ml, respectively. Based on the various studies, [^{68}Ga]PSMA-HBED-CC PET/CT is a novel and promising imaging modality for prostate cancer patients which compares favorably to the current de-facto standard of choline PET/CT. [^{68}Ga]PSMA-HBED-CC PET/CT can yield clinically useful diagnostic results even in patients with very low PSA levels as has been also reported by the groups of Verburg et al. [38] and Eiber et al. [39].

In a group of 167 consecutive patients, PET/CT was positive in 44 %, 79 %, and 90 % of patients with PSA levels of ≤1, 1–2, or ≥2 ng/ml, respectively. Patients with high PSA levels showed higher rates of locally recurrent ($p < 0.001$) lesions or bone metastases ($p = 0.03$). Patients with a shorter PSA doubling time (PSAdt) significantly more often showed distant metastases in the paraaortal lymph nodes ($p = 0.028$), bones ($p = 0.014$), and organs ($p = 0.028$). Gleason score was not related to imaging findings except for the frequency of bone metastases ($p = 0.048$). Based on results of biopsies, surgeries or radiation therapy in 29/167 patients sensitivity, specificity, positive and negative predictive value were 100 %, 40 %, 88 % and 100 %, respectively. Eiber et al. reported similar results.

Recently, a direct comparison of the diagnostic value of ^{18}FEC-PET/CT and ^{68}Ga-PSMA-PET/CT was performed in patients with PSA relapse following RP who all underwent pelvic salvage lymphadenectomy [25].

In 30/38 ^{18}FEC and 22/27 ^{68}Ga-PSMA patients ≥1 focus of PCA was identified in postsurgical histology, leading to a per-patient PPV of 78.9 % for ^{18}FEC and 81.5 % for ^{68}Ga-PSMA. In ^{18}FEC and ^{68}Ga-PSMA patients, a total of 378 and 308 lymph nodes and local lesions were removed, respectively. For ^{18}FEC and ^{68}Ga-PSMA, the respective sensitivity (95 % confidence interval) was 71.2 % (64.5–79.6 %) and 86.9 % (75.8–94.2 %), specificity 86.9 % (82.3–90.6 %) and

93.1 % (89.2–95.9 %), PPV 67.3 % (57.7–75.9 %) and 75.7 % (64.0–98.5 %), NPV 88.8 % (84.4–92.3 %) and 96.6 % (93.5–98.5 %) and accuracy 82.5 % (78.3–86.8 %) and 91.9 % (88.7 %–95.1 %). In their series, ^{68}Ga-PSMA PET/CT shows a better performance than the current de-facto PET/CT standard tracer ^{18}FEC with a significantly higher NPV and accuracy. Due to these results, ^{68}Ga-PSMA-PET/CT should be recommended as imaging study of choice even at PSA levels < 1.0 ng/ml.

If ^{68}Ga-PSMA-PET/CT identifies local relapse, its anatomically exact localization is needed before salvage treatment and/or if this localization changes treatment planning. Especially with the introduction of PSMA-PET/CT, the finding of remnants of prostatic tissue or seminal vessels is not quite unusual [40]. These local relapses might be managed by surgical resection or by radiation therapy.

Dynamic contrast-enhanced MRI produces sensitivities and specificities of 84–88 % and 89–100 %, respectively, at mean PSA serum levels of 0.8–1.9 ng/ml [41, 42]. In patients with PSA level < 0.5 ng/mL, the results are controversial in 2 studies. Whereas one found a sensitivity of only 13 % in men with PSA level < 0.3 ng/mL [43], the second series reported a sensitivity of 86 % in patients with PSA level < 0.4 ng/mL [44]. Based on these data, MRI does not represent the primary imaging study of choice in men with biochemical failure and low PSA serum levels.

9 Follow-Up for Treatment-Related Side Effects

Increased life expectancy in PCA makes post-treatment quality of life a key issue. For patients after RP, incontinence and erectile dysfunction are of major concern. In order to counsel the patient adequately, every surgeon should know his/her own results with regard to functional outcome following RP which makes continuous follow-up by standardized questionnaires necessary. Health-related QoL (HRQoL) refers to the impact of disease and treatment on well-being and physical, emotional, and social functioning, including daily functioning. HRQoL is measured using standardized questionnaires, which provide an objective assessment of general and disease-specific domains. It is, however, of utmost importance to define and to assess condition-specific outcomes that matter to patients. Recently, Martin et al. defined a standard set of patient-centered outcomes for men with localized PCA [45]. They suggested to include information about treatment approaches, baseline characteristics of the patients and the cancer, acute complications, survival, and disease control, as well as the patient-reported health status using the standardized EPIC-26 questionnaire [46].

10 Summary

Follow-up strategies after local radical prostate cancer therapy aim to reach two goals: (1) early detection of local or systemic relapse which might enable second-line therapy to improve long-term prognosis and (2) early detection of treatment related side effects to allow early intervention and thereby to improve quality of life for the patients. As described above, PSA monitoring is the cornerstone of follow-up after radical prostatectomy. PSA should be undetectable 6 weeks postoperatively and any PSA rise might be an indicator for relapsing cancer. Imaging studies at PSA levels < 1.0 ng/ml in terms of PSMA-PET/CT scans are only indicated if the results will be associated with therapeutic consequences such as salvage lymphadenectomy. In all other cases, imaging studies such as computed tomography of the abdomen/pelvis or bone scans are only indicated as baseline study prior to initiation of androgen deprivation therapy or in case of new symptoms which might be related to metastases.

Concerning the follow-up of treatment related side effects, erectile dysfunction and incontinence are of major concern to the patient. As pointed out, every center and every surgeon should now his/her own functional and oncological results so that patients need to be followed continuously. As proposed recently, the EPIC-26 questionnaire and the Charlson Comorbidity Score seem to represent the most valid tool for follow-up strategies [45–47].

References

1. Heidenreich A, Bastian PJ, Bellmunt J, Bolla M, Joniau S, van der KT, Mason M, Matveev V, Wiegel T, Zattoni F, Mottet N. EAU guidelines on prostate cancer. Part 1: screening, diagnosis, and local treatment with curative intent-update 2013. Eur Urol. 2014;65:124–37.
2. Parker C, Gillessen S, Heidenreich A, Horwich A, ESMO Guidelines Committee. Cancer of the prostate: ESMO Clinical Practice Guidelines for diagnosis, treatment and follow-up. Ann Oncol. 2015;26 Suppl 5:v69–77.
3. Heidenreich A, Richter S, Thüer D, Pfister D. Prognostic parameters, complications, and oncologic and functional outcome of salvage radical prostatectomy for locally recurrent prostate cancer after 21st-century radiotherapy. Eur Urol. 2010;57(3):437–43.
4. Heidenreich A, Bastian PJ, Bellmunt J, Bolla M, Joniau S, van der KT, Mason M, Matveev V, Wiegel T, Zattoni F, Mottet N. EAU guidelines on prostate cancer. Part II: treatment of advanced, relapsing, and castration-resistant prostate cancer. Eur Urol. 2014;65:467–79.
5. Stamey TA, Kabalin JN, McNeal JE, et al. Prostate specific antigen in the diagnosis and treatment of adenocarcinoma of the prostate. II. Radical prostatectomy treated patients. J Urol. 1989;141:1076–83.
6. Wiegel T, Bartkowiak D, Bottke D, Thamm R, Hinke A, Stöckle M, Rübe C, Semjonow A, Wirth M, Störkel S, Golz R, Engenhart-Cabillic R, Hofmann R, Feldmann HJ, Kälble T, Siegmann A, Hinkelbein W, Steiner U, Miller K. Prostate-specific antigen persistence after radical prostatectomy as a predictive factor of clinical relapse- free survival and overall survival: 10-year data of the ARO 96–02 trial. Int J Radiat Oncol Biol Phys. 2015;91(2):288–94.
7. Horwitz EM, Thames HD, Kuban DA, et al. Definitions of biochemical failure that best predict clinical failure in patients with prostate cancer treated with external beam radiation alone: a multi-institutional pooled analysis. J Urol. 2005;173:797–802.
8. Stephenson AJ, Kattan MW, Eastham JA, et al. Defining biochemical recurrence of prostate cancer after radical prostatectomy: a proposal for a standardized definition. J Clin Oncol. 2006;24:3973–8.
9. Amling CL, Bergstralh EJ, Blute ML, et al. Defining prostate specific antigen progression after radical prostatectomy: what is the most appropriate cut point? J Urol. 2001;165:1146–51.
10. Shen S, Lepor H, Yaffee R, et al. Ultrasensitive serum prostate specific antigen nadir accurately predicts the risk of early relapse after radical prostatectomy. J Urol. 2005;173:777–80.
11. Eisenberg ML, Davies BJ, Cooperberg MR, et al. Prognostic implications of an undetectable ultrasensitive prostate-specific antigen level after radical prostatectomy. Eur Urol. 2010;57:622–9.
12. Siegmann A, Bottke D, Faehndrich J, Brachert M, Lohm G, Miller K, Bartkowiak D, Hinkelbein W, Wiegel T. Salvage radiotherapy after prostatectomy–what is the best time to treat? Radiother Oncol. 2012;103(2):239–43.
13. Slovin SF, Wilton AS, Heller G, Scher HI. Time to detectable metastatic disease in patients with rising prostate-specific antigen values following surgery or radiation therapy. Clin Cancer Res. 2005;11(24 Pt 1):8669–73.
14. Long JP, Bahn D, Lee F, et al. Five-year retrospective, multi-institutional pooled analysis of cancer-related outcomes after cryosurgical ablation of the prostate. Urology. 2001;57:518–23.
15. Blana A, Brown SC, Chaussy C, et al. High-intensity focused ultrasound for prostate cancer: comparative definitions of biochemical failure. BJU Int. 2009;104:1058–62.
16. Feijoo ER, Sivaraman A, Barret E, Sanchez-Salas R, Galiano M, Rozet F, Prapotnich D, Cathala N, Mombet A, Cathelineau X. Focal high-intensity focused ultrasound targeted hemiablation for unilateral prostate cancer: a prospective evaluation of oncologic and functional outcomes. Eur Urol. 2016;69(2):214–20.
17. Donohue JF, Bianco Jr FJ, Kuroiwa K, et al. Poorly differentiated prostate cancer treated with radical prostatectomy: long-term outcome and incidence of pathological downgrading. J Urol. 2006;176:991–5.
18. Bastian PJ, Gonzalgo ML, Aronson WJ, et al. Clinical and pathologic outcome after radical prostatectomy for prostate cancer patients with a preoperative Gleason sum of 8 to 10. Cancer. 2006;107:1265–72.
19. Yossepowitch O, Eggener SE, Serio AM, et al. Secondary therapy, metastatic progression, and cancer-specific mortality in men with clinically high-risk prostate cancer treated with radical prostatectomy. Eur Urol. 2008;53:950–9.
20. Walz J, Joniau S, Chun FK, et al. Pathological results and rates of treatment failure in high-risk prostate cancer patients after radical prostatectomy. BJU Int. 2011;107:765–70.
21. Walz J, Chun FK, Klein EA, Reuther A, Graefen M, Huland H, Karakiewicz PI. Risk-adjusted hazard rates of biochemical recurrence for prostate cancer patients after radical prostatectomy. Eur Urol. 2009;55(2):412–9.
22. Karl A, Buchner A, Tympner C, Kirchner T, Ganswindt U, Belka C, Ganzer R, Burger M, Eder F, Hofstädter F, Schilling D, Sievert K, Stenzl A, Scharpf M, Fend F, Vom Dorp F, Rübben H, Schmid K,

Porres-Knoblauch D, Heidenreich A, Hangarter B, Knüchel-Clarke R, Rogenhofer M, Wullich B, Hartmann A, Comploj E, Pycha A, Hanspeter E, Pehrke D, Sauter G, Graefen M, Stief C, Haese A. The natural course of pT2 prostate cancer with positive surgical margin: predicting biochemical recurrence. World J Urol. 2015;33(7):973–9.
23. Karl A, Buchner A, Tympner C, Kirchner T, Ganswindt U, Belka C, Ganzer R, Wieland W, Eder F, Hofstädter F, Schilling D, Sievert KD, Stenzl A, Scharpf M, Fend F, Vom Dorp F, Rübben H, Kurt Werner S, Porres-Knoblauch D, Heidenreich A, Hangarter B, Knüchel-Clarke R, Rogenhofer M, Wullich B, Hartmann A, Comploj E, Pycha A, Hanspeter E, Pehrke D, Sauter G, Graefen M, Gratzke C, Stief C, Wiegel T, Haese A. Risk and timing of biochemical recurrence in pT3aN0/Nx prostate cancer with positive surgical margin–a multicenter study. Radiother Oncol. 2015;116(1):119–24.
24. Suardi N, Gandaglia G, Gallina A, Di Trapani E, Scattoni V, Vizziello D, Cucchiara V, Bertini R, Colombo R, Picchio M, Giovacchini G, Montorsi F, Briganti A. Long-term outcomes of salvage lymph node dissection for clinically recurrent prostate cancer: results of a single-institution series with a minimum follow-up of 5 years. Eur Urol. 2015;67:299–309.
25. Pfister D, Porres D, Heidenreich A, Heidegger I, Knuechel R, Steib F, Behrendt FF, Verburg FA. Detection of recurrent prostate cancer lesions before salvage lymphadenectomy is more accurate with $_{68}$Ga-PSMA-HBED-CC than with $_{18}$F-Fluoroethylcholine PET/CT. Eur J Nucl Med Mol Imaging. 2016;43(8):1410–7 [Epub ahead of print].
26. Moul JW, Wu H, Sun L, McLeod DG, Amling C, Donahue T, Kusuda L, Sexton W, O'Reilly K, Hernandez J, Chung A, Soderdahl D. Early versus delayed hormonal therapy for prostate specific antigen only recurrence of prostate cancer after radical prostatectomy. J Urol. 2008;179(5 Suppl):S53–9.
27. Kane CJ, Amling CL, Johnstone PAS, Pak N, Lance RS, Thrasher B, Foley JP, Riffenburgh RH, Moul JW. Limited value of bone scintigraphy and computed tomography in assessing biochemical failure after radical prostatectomy. Urology. 2003;61(3):607–11.
28. Gomez P, Manoharan M, Kim SS, Soloway MS. Radionuclide bone scintigraphy in patients with biochemical recurrence after radical prostatectomy: when is it indicated? BJU Int. 2004;94(3):299–302.
29. Cimitan M, Evangelista L, Hodolic M, Mariani G, Baseric T, Bodanza V, Saladini G, Volterrani D, Cervino AR, Gregianin M, Puccini G, Guidoccio F, Fettich J, Borsatti E. Gleason score at diagnosis predicts the rate of detection of 18F-choline PET/CT performed when biochemical evidence indicates recurrence of prostate cancer: experience with 1,000 patients. J Nucl Med. 2015;56:209–15.
30. Chondrogiannis S, Marzola MC, Ferretti A, Grassetto G, Maffione AM, Rampin L, Fanti S, Giammarile F, Rubello D. Is the detection rate of 18F-choline PET/CT influenced by androgen-deprivation therapy? Eur J Nucl Med Mol Imaging. 2014;41:1293–300.
31. Giovacchini G, Picchio M, Parra RG, Briganti A, Gianolli L, Montorsi F, Messa C. Prostate-specific antigen velocity versus prostate-specific antigen doubling time for prediction of 11C choline PET/CT in prostate cancer patients with biochemical failure after radical prostatectomy. Clin Nucl Med. 2012;37(4):325–31.
32. Treglia G, Ceriani L, Sadeghi R, et al. Relationship between prostate-specific antigen kinetics and detection rate of radiolabelled choline PET/CT in restaging prostate cancer patients: a meta-analysis. Clin Chem Lab Med. 2014;52(5):725–32.
33. Schmittgen TD, Teske S, Vessella RL, True LD, Zakrajsek BA. Expression of prostate specific membrane antigen and three alternatively spliced variants of PSMA in prostate cancer patients. Int J Cancer. 2003;107:323–9.
34. Mannweiler S, Amersdorfer P, Trajanoski S, Terrett JA, King D, Mehes G. Heterogeneity of prostate-specific membrane antigen (PSMA) expression in prostate carcinoma with distant metastasis. Pathol Oncol Res. 2009;15:167–72.
35. Hillier SM, Maresca KP, Femia FJ, Marquis JC, Foss CA, Nguyen N, Zimmerman CN, Barrett JA, Eckelman WC, Pomper MG, Joyal JL, Babich JW. Preclinical evaluation of novel glutamate-urea-lysine analogues that target prostate-specific membrane antigen as molecular imaging pharmaceuticals for prostate cancer. Cancer Res. 2009;69:6932–40.
36. Afshar-Oromieh A, Avtzi E, Giesel FL, Holland-Letz T, Linhart HG, Eder M, Eisenhut M, Boxler S, Hadaschik BA, Kratochwil C, Weichert W, Kopka K, Debus J, Haberkorn U. The diagnostic value of PET/CT imaging with the (68)Ga-labelled PSMA ligand HBED-CC in the diagnosis of recurrent prostate cancer. Eur J Nucl Med Mol Imaging. 2015;42:197–209.
37. Afshar-Oromieh A, Malcher A, Eder M, Eisenhut M, Linhart HG, Hadaschik BA, Holland-Letz T, Giesel FL, Kratochwil C, Haufe S, Haberkorn U, Zechmann CM. PET imaging with a [68Ga]gallium-labelled PSMA ligand for the diagnosis of prostate cancer: biodistribution in humans and first evaluation of tumour lesions. Eur J Nucl Med Mol Imaging. 2013;40:486–95.
38. Verburg FA, Pfister D, Heidenreich A, Vogg A, Drude NI, Vöö S, Mottaghy FM, Behrendt FF. Extent of disease in recurrent prostate cancer determined by [(68)Ga]PSMA-HBED-CC PET/CT in relation to PSA levels, PSA doubling time and Gleason score. Eur J Nucl Med Mol Imaging. 2016;43(3):397–403.
39. Eiber M, Maurer T, Souvatzoglou M, Beer AJ, Ruffani A, Haller B, Graner FP, Kubler H, Haberhorn U, Eisenhut M, Wester HJ, Gschwend JE, Schwaiger M. Evaluation of hybrid 68Ga-PSMA ligand PET/CT in 248 patients with biochemical recurrence after radical prostatectomy. J Nucl Med. 2015;56:668–74.

40. Nguyen DP, Giannarini G, Seiler R, Schiller R, Thoeny HC, Thalmann GN, Studer UE. Local recurrence after retropubic radical prostatectomy for prostate cancer does not exclusively occur at the anastomotic site. BJU Int. 2013;112(4):E243–9.
41. Cirillo S, Petracchini M, Scotti L, et al. Endorectal magnetic resonance imaging at 1.5 Tesla to assess local recurrence following radical prostatectomy using T2-weighted and contrast-enhanced imaging. Eur Radiol. 2009;19(3):761–9.
42. Sciarra A, Panebianco V, Salciccia S, et al. Role of dynamic contrast-enhanced magnetic resonance (MR) imaging and proton MR spectroscopic imaging in the detection of local recurrence after radical prostatectomy for prostate cancer. Eur Urol. 2008;54(3):589–600.
43. Liauw SL, Pitroda SP, Eggener SE, et al. Evaluation of the prostate bed for local recurrence after radical prostatectomy using endorectal magnetic resonance imaging. Int J Radiat Oncol Biol Phys. 2013;85(2):378–84.
44. Linder BJ, Kawashima A, Woodrum DA, et al. Early localization of recurrent prostate cancer after prostatectomy by endorectal coil magnetic resonance imaging. Can J Urol. 2014;21(3):7283–9.
45. Martin NE, Massey L, Stowell C, et al. Defining a standard Set of patient-centered outcomes for men with localized prostate cancer. Eur Urol. 2015;67:460–7.
46. Wei JT, Dunn RL, Litwin MS, Sandler HM, Sanda MG. Development and validation of the Expanded Prostate Cancer Index Composite (EPIC) for comprehensive assessment of health-related quality of life in men with prostate cancer. Urology. 2000;56:899–905.
47. Habbous S, Chu KP, Harland LT, et al. Validation of a one-page patient-reported Charlson comorbidity index questionnaire for upper aerodigestive tract cancer patients. Oral Oncol. 2013;49:407–12.

First-Line Hormonal Manipulation: Surgical and Medical Castration with LHRH Agonists and Antagonists, Steroids, and Pure Antiandrogens

Tobias Gramann and Hans-Peter Schmid

1 Introduction to Topic

Over the past years, many different approaches to the treatment of advanced, metastatic carcinoma of the prostate have been introduced, and with impressive speed. Today, endocrine therapy, in the form of androgen deprivation (ADT), as first suggested by Charles Huggins, is still the standard treatment and is always the first step in any systemic therapy for metastatic, hormone-sensitive carcinoma of the prostate [1]. Charles Huggins and Clarence V Hodges were awarded the Nobel Prize for Physiology and Medicine in 1966 for their research in 1941 into the effects of androgens on prostate carcinoma cells [2]. Andrew V Schally developed the LHRH agonists and, together with Roger Guillemin, received the Nobel Prize in 1977 for their research on peptide hormone production in the brain. In 1971, Schally et al. were the first to isolate and elucidate the structure and synthesis of the hypothalamic "luteinizing hormone releasing hormone" (LHRH) [3–5]. Recognizing the importance of the hypothalamic-pituitary-gonadal axis in the growth of prostate carcinoma cells and the elucidation of gonadotropin releasing hormone (GnRH) resulted in the gradual development of hormone therapy for carcinoma of the prostate in the last century. Numerous agonistic and antagonistic therapeutic substances that intervene in the testosterone synthesis feedback loop have been established in clinical practice. Despite decades of clinical use, much controversy still reigns over the best approach to ADT (surgical vs. medical), the best time to start treatment (immediate or delayed), the type of ADT (simple vs. total), and the modality and duration of treatment (intermittent or continuous) [6]. Moreover, the gold standard of ADT alone as first-line therapy may well be modified soon thanks to study findings published in 2015 that so far show – at least for patients with metastatic carcinoma of the prostate – statistically significant and clinically relevant advantages of first-line therapy of ADT combined with chemotherapy rather than ADT alone [7–9]. Curative treatment of metastatic disease is still not yet possible. This applies to both carcinoma of the prostate, which is metastatic at the time of diagnosis, and to recurrences of disease after initial treatment with curative intent (including salvage therapy).

This chapter describes and discusses surgical and medical aspects of first-line ADT, and looks at possible future developments in the light of recent study findings with a combination of ADT and docetaxel-based chemotherapy.

T. Gramann, MD (✉) • H.-P. Schmid, MD
Department of Urology, EBU Certified Training Center, Kantonsspital,
CH-9007 St. Gallen, Switzerland
e-mail: tobias.gramann@kssg.ch

M. Bolla, H. van Poppel (eds.), *Management of Prostate Cancer*,
DOI 10.1007/978-3-319-42769-0_21

2 Fundamental Aspects of Hormone Manipulation in Carcinoma of the Prostate

The growth of the prostate cells is androgen-dependent. Testosterone is converted into the biologically active metabolite dihydrotestosterone (DHT) by the enzyme 5-alpha reductase. DHT binds to the androgen receptor of the prostate cell and in so doing mediates a general proliferation of androgen-dependent tissue. At the same time, it also suppresses programmed cell death (apoptosis). The synthesis of testosterone is controlled by a negative feedback mechanism of the hypothalamic-pituitary-gonadal axis and takes place mainly (about 95 %) in the Leydig cells in the testes and to a small extent (about 5 %) in the adrenal cortex. LHRH is formed in the hypothalamus and triggers the release of the gonadotropin luteinizing hormone (LH) and follicle-stimulating hormone (FSH) in the anterior lobe of the pituitary. LH stimulates androgen synthesis in the Leydig cells of the testes. The adrenal formation of testosterone is also controlled by the pituitary via adrenocorticotropic hormone (ACTH), which mediates the release of corticosteroids and androgens from the reticular zone.

Therapeutic intervention in the androgen-mediated growth of prostate tumor cells can either take the form of reducing the body's own androgen synthesis to the castration level or blocking the androgen receptors in the target organ, or both. The combination of these two approaches achieves the maximum androgen blockade (MAB), also termed complete or total ADT. The castration level of testosterone defined more than 40 years ago used in most studies so far is <50 ng/dl. A lower threshold value of <20 ng/dl that can be determined with modern laboratory methods is closer to the actual testosterone level achieved after castration [1, 10]. The activity of the enzyme 5-alpha reductase can also be limited so that less testosterone is converted into biologically active DHT. Complete inhibition of the 5-alpha reductase isoenzymes is, however, not possible, which means that monotherapy with a 5-alpha reductase inhibitor is not suitable for the treatment of hormone-sensitive, metastatic carcinoma of the prostate. All antiandrogenic approaches have in common the problem that they can cause muscular atrophy and osteoporosis to differing extents. Concomitant vitamin D and calcium, and physical exercise are therefore recommended. The different possibilities for first-line therapy with surgical and medical hormone manipulation are discussed in the next sections.

3 Surgical Androgen Deprivation

Surgical androgen deprivation is achieved by (subcapsular) bilateral orchiectomy. Since the introduction of the LHRH agonists, surgical castration has played an increasingly smaller role in everyday clinical practice, but is definitely not obsolete. Surgery according to Riba consists of enucleation of the hormone-secreting testicular parenchyma via a small scrotal incision leaving the spermatic cord, epididymis, and testicular coat intact. The scrotal cavity is therefore not empty after surgery. The testosterone level falls to the castration level (<50 ng/ml) within 12 h after surgery [1, 6]. Surgical castration is an effective, rapid, safe, and simple form of ADT, which sets a high standard for other (medical) therapy options to achieve [1]. It does not depend on patient compliance and is comparatively cheap. The principal disadvantage of surgical castration is that it is not reversible and does not permit intermittent ADT. Orchiectomy also causes mental stress in some men. In a study by Cassileth et al., most of the men with advanced prostate carcinoma opted for medical castration with goserelin and only about 20 % for surgical castration [11]. In a small study, Bonzani et al. found an advantage in favor of surgical castration for general quality of life [12]. Surgical and medical castration with LHRH analogs appear to be equieffective with regard to tumor control [13, 14]. A study by Sun et al. showed that surgical castration may offer advantages over long-term treatment with LHRH analogs with regard to adverse reactions, and in particular the fracture risk and cardiac complications [14]. This retrospective, nonrandomized study did, however, have some limitations. A further study showed a similar or slightly increased fracture risk with orchiectomy, depending on the number of doses of the LHRH analog [15].

4 Medical Androgen Deprivation

4.1 LHRH Agonists

After Schally et al. isolated hypothalamic LHRH and elucidated its structure and synthesis for the first time in 1971, they went on to develop the endocrine therapy of carcinoma of the prostate based on LHRH agonists throughout the 1980s [5, 16–18]. Thousands of LHRH analogs have been synthesized over the past few decades, but only a few are of importance in urological tumor therapy. The most important agents are triptorelin, leuprorelin, buserelin, and goserelin, which all have receptor affinities and therefore biological activities many times higher than physiological LHRH [5]. They are therefore referred to as superagonists. Long-term administration of LHRH agonists downregulates the pituitary LHRH receptors and decreases LH and FSH concentrations in the blood. As a result of this, the testosterone level drops to the castration level after 3–4 weeks [1, 5]. A transient increase in pituitary hormone secretion occurs in the first few days after the first administration, which in turn leads to an increase in testosterone synthesis. This initial stimulation of testosterone synthesis is referred to as the "flare-up phenomenon," and in patients with metastatic carcinoma of the prostate it can become clinically evident in progressive bone pain and problems with urination, even extending up to compression of the spinal cord with symptoms of hemiplegia [1, 6]. An antiandrogen therefore has to be given for a short period at the beginning of treatment with an LHRH agonist to prevent such symptoms. Recommendations as to the best time to start the antiandrogen – before LHRH administration or at the same time – and the duration of treatment are not consistent. The current EAU Guidelines recommend a 4-week course of antiandrogen started at the same time as the LHRH agonist or 1 week before starting the LHRH agonist in symptomatic patients [1]. Important advantages of medical castration with LHRH analogs over surgical castration are that it is reversible and is well accepted by patients with injections at up to 6-monthly intervals [5]. A depot preparation, histrelin, is even available with a duration of effect of 12 months. The histrelin implant is placed in the nondominant upper arm under local anesthetic and is renewed each year [19]. Adverse reactions of LHRH agonist treatment are possible hypercoagulability, hot flushes, loss of libido, and impotence. Moreover, long-term ADT is associated with osteoporosis and a subsequent increased fracture risk [20, 21]. With regard to tumor control, LHRH analog treatment is as effective as orchiectomy [13].

4.2 LHRH Antagonists

Abarelix, in 2004, and degarelix, in 2008, were the first LHRH antagonists approved for the treatment of advanced carcinoma of the prostate [22]. They also cause androgen deprivation, but with a different mechanism of action from that of the LHRH agonists. The LHRH antagonists directly and competitively block the pituitary LHRH receptors and in this way cause an immediate and significant decrease in FSH and LH concentration, which in turn leads to a decrease in the testosterone level to the castration level [22]. The testosterone concentration drops rapidly and no flare-up phenomenon (testosterone surge) occurs, as with the LHRH agonists [23]. Adjunctive treatment with an antiandrogen at the beginning of treatment is therefore not necessary. The most widely used and best researched antagonist is degarelix [22, 24–26]. It is administered monthly by subcutaneous injection, with a loading dose of 240 mg, followed by 80 mg monthly. Degarelix is as effective at maintaining the decreased testosterone level for 1 year as the LHRH agonist leuprolide [24]. The castration level and a decrease in PSA were achieved more rapidly than with leuprolide. Furthermore, studies indicate that the PSA progression-free survival period with degarelix may be longer than with leuprolide, which may also be accompanied by a delayed occurrence of castration resistance [22]. The adverse reaction profile of the LHRH antagonists is mainly due to the androgen deprivation. Severe systemic allergic reactions may also occur under treatment with abarelix [22, 27]. An increased incidence of local reactions at the injection site has been reported under degarelix, especially after the first injection [24]. Systemic anaphylactic reactions have, however, not been observed under degarelix. It has to be injected monthly, which means that it is less convenient in the clinical setting than the long-acting depot preparations of some LHRH agonists [1]. The LHRH antagonists offer the greatest advantage in patients who need immediate treatment so that the castration level is reached as soon as possible. This may be the case in patients with boney metastases threatening to attack the spinal canal or local complaints due to obstructive carcinoma of the prostate. Studies indicate that a better response in laboratory terms is achieved under degarelix than under leuprolide in patients with a high baseline PSA value of >20 ng/ml [28]. Switching to an LHRH agonist as treatment progresses is possible. The tolerance and effects on the testosterone concentration of an oral LHRH antagonist (relugolix) have been tested in a recent Phase I study [29]. It appears that oral administration may be an option in the future.

4.3 Antiandrogens

Antiandrogens competitively block the peripheral androgen receptors and thereby inhibit the effects of circulating testosterone [1, 30]. Steroidal and nonsteroidal forms are available, depending on their chemical structure. Cyproterone acetate (CPA), megestrol acetate, and medroxyprogesterone acetate are steroidal antiandrogens. Flutamide, nilutamide, and bicalutamide are nonsteroidal antiandrogens.

4.3.1 Steroidal Antiandrogens

In addition to the above-mentioned inhibitory effects of the antiandrogens on the peripheral androgen receptor, the steroidal antiandrogens also have inhibitory effects on gonadotropin secretion due to their progesterone-like active components [30]. The decreased release of LH also results in a decrease in testosterone concentration under continuous therapy with steroidal antiandrogens. The first widely used antiandrogen was CPA, a synthetic derivative of hydroxyprogesterone [30]. It was associated with a similar incidence of decreased libido and erectile dysfunction as castration [30, 31]. Data comparing CPA as monotherapy and castration with regard to tumor control and survival are limited, and partially contradictory [30, 32–34]. Furthermore, no dose-finding studies have been conducted for CPA monotherapy, so that the effective dose is not known [1]. No significant differences for general or tumor-specific survival were seen in a study comparing CPA and flutamide monotherapy in metastatic carcinoma of the prostate. The results, however, are only of limited validity as the patient numbers were so small [32]. Because of its central antigonadotropic effect, CPA can be used to alleviate hot flushes under ADT.

4.3.2 Nonsteroidal Antiandrogens

The nonsteroidal antiandrogens act exclusively on the androgen receptor and have no direct gonadotropic effect [6]. They are therefore referred to as pure antiandrogens. The competitive blockade of the androgen receptors inhibits the effects of the peripheral androgens. An increase in LH secretion under monotherapy with a nonsteroidal antiandrogen brings about a paradoxical increase in testosterone synthesis [30, 31]. Libido and potency may be preserved.

Nilutamide is not approved for monotherapy of carcinoma of the prostate [1]. No studies comparing the efficacy of nilutamide monotherapy and castration have been performed. Adverse reactions such as visual disturbances, alcohol intolerance, interstitial pneumonitis, and hepatotoxicity appear to outweigh the benefits of treatment [1, 6].

As monotherapy, flutamide, which has been in use for many years, had similar efficacy to surgical castration and exerted a maximum androgen blockade (MAB) in two comparative studies

[30, 35]. Its active metabolite has a short half-life and it is therefore given in a three-times-daily regimen. Due to the absence of dose-finding studies, the most effective dosage is not known. Adverse reactions that are relatively frequent are diarrhea and potentially severe hepatotoxicity.

The recommended standard dose of bicalutamide as monotherapy is 150 mg/day. At this dosage, it achieved a similar PSA response to castration [36]. To avoid the flare-up phenomenon at the start of treatment with an LHRH agonist, short-term adjunctive treatment with an antiandrogen is recommended (Table 1). For this indication, the bicalutamide dosage is 50 mg/day.

For a discussion of monotherapy with nonsteroidal antiandrogens, and their side effects and treatment, see the section "Monotherapy with antiandrogens" in this chapter.

4.4 Estrogens

Estrogens bring about an inhibition of testicular testosterone synthesis. In the past, diethylstilbestrol was used to treat advanced carcinoma of the prostate as an alternative to orchiectomy. Studies showed similar efficacy with both [37]. The considerable incidence of thromboembolic and cardiovascular adverse reactions has resulted, however, in only very restricted use of estrogens at present. The incidence of these adverse reactions was not able to be reduced, or at least only partially, by either parenteral estrogen administration (polyestradiol phosphate) to avoid the hepatic first-pass metabolism, or the prophylactic administration of anticoagulants with low-dose diethylstilbestrol [38, 39]. Estrogens are not recommended as first-line therapy.

Table 1 "Flare-up" prevention

Use of Antiandrogens	Recommendation
"Flare-up" prevention	In M1 patients treated with an LHRH agonist offer short-term administration of antiandrogens to reduce the risk of the "flare-up" phenomenon Start antiandrogens used for "flare-up" prevention on the same day as an LHRH analogue is started or for up to 7 days before the first LHRH analogue injection in symptomatic patients Treat for 4 weeks

Recommendations of EAU-guidelines for hormonal treatment of metastatic carcinoma of the prostate [1]

5 Therapeutic Strategies

5.1 Simple Versus Maximum Androgen Blockade

The combination of medical or surgical castration with the administration of an antiandrogen is referred to as maximum, complete, or total androgen blockade. Via the adjunctive administration of an antiandrogen, this approach combines the deprivation of testicular testosterone synthesis with an additional blockade of adrenally synthesized androgens. It was suggested that this would improve the response to therapy in metastatic carcinoma of the prostate [6]. In 1982, a good response to a combination of an LHRH agonist and a pure androgen was reported. Such a combination was not established at the time, and this was followed by numerous studies comparing MAB with medical or surgical castration as monotherapy [40]. Even today, the findings are still contradictory [1, 41]. Some studies showed a statistically significant survival advantage of MAB over castration alone. The NCI Intergroup Study INT-0036 compared daily subcutaneous injections of leuprolide with and without flutamide and showed an improvement in overall survival of 7 months in favor of MAB [42, 43]. The results of this study are, however, not uncontroversial. In the absence of flare-up prophylaxis and because of possible suboptimal compliance with the then daily injection regimen, there was, for example, some discussion as to whether an initial flare-up and even possibly a second flare-up might have had a negative influence on the outcome in the LHRH monotherapy group [41]. Since no flare-up phenomenon occurs after orchiectomy, one criticism was that a comparison of MAB for androgen deprivation alone should ideally be made with orchiectomy, to provide a reliable basis for the efficacy of MAB. Exactly this was investigated in the NCI Intergroup Study INT-0105 with a comparison of orchiectomy plus flutamide as MAB with orchiectomy plus placebo [44]. Although a small survival advantage of just under 4 months was found in favor of the MAB in this study, the difference was not statistically significant. Results of the EORTC 30853 Study were published several times in the 1990s [45–47]. During long-term follow-up, a statistically significant overall survival advantage over orchiectomy was shown for goserelin plus flutamide (MAB). However, a large meta-analysis comprising 27 studies did not show any statistically significant advantage for overall survival with MAB [48, 49]. Only for the two antiandrogens flutamide and nilutamide given as part of MAB was it possible to show a statistically significant survival advantage of just less than 3 % – with questionable clinical relevance, however. Indeed, in a critical review on the suitability of Phase III studies for the evaluation of MAB vs. castration, the authors state that the statistically significant survival advantage for flutamide is no longer present if the studies that did not include prophylaxis with an antiandrogen against flare-up at the start of LHRH agonist treatment are excluded [41]. Investigations into quality of life under MAB showed that it was associated with more adverse reactions and poorer quality of life than castration alone [50]. Treatment costs are also higher for MAB than for monotherapy. MAB is not generally recommended in the current guidelines for the treatment of metastatic carcinoma of the prostate. The potential benefit of MAB should be weighed up against the associated side effects [1].

5.2 Immediate Versus Delayed Therapy

It is generally agreed that ADT should be started immediately in patients with symptomatic metastatic carcinoma of the prostate (M1) [1]. The current EAU Guidelines also recommend, regardless of symptoms, that treatment should be started immediately in patients with metastatic carcinoma of the prostate to delay tumor-related complications; the possibility of a delayed start of treatment should, however, also be discussed with the patient [1]. Reference is also made to the ASCO Guidelines, which give no clear recommendation either for or against immediate androgen deprivation and attribute this to the contradictory present state of knowledge [51]. Also controversial is the ideal time to begin androgen deprivation in patients with locally advanced, nonmetastatic carcinoma of the prostate who do not qualify for curative treatment and for patients with histologically confirmed lymph node metastases following radical prostatectomy.

The first "Veterans Administration Cooperative Urological Research Group" (VACURG) Study showed no survival advantage for immediate orchiectomy versus placebo in locally advanced or metastatic carcinoma of the prostate after 9 years. This study was, however, underpowered with regard to sample size and, like other earlier studies with similar aims, was carried out in the pre-PSA era [37, 52]. A Cochrane Review comprising 4 studies was only able to demonstrate a small, statistically significant survival advantage for an immediate start of treatment compared to a delayed start of ADT after 10 years' follow-up [53]. Tumor-specific survival showed no significant difference. Also, the SAKK 08/88 Study did not show a statistically significant difference between an immediate and delayed start of ADT, either for overall survival or tumor-specific survival [54]. The first interim analysis of a study by the "Medical Research Council" showed a statistically significant advantage in favor of early ADT for overall survival, but this was not maintained during the remainder of the study, as shown by a later analysis with a longer follow-up period [54, 55]. In patients with locally advanced nonmetastatic carcinoma of the prostate, the EORTC 30891 Study showed a moderate, statistically significant advantage in favor of an immediate start of ADT, also in the final evaluation after a 12-year follow-up [56]. Tumor-specific and symptom-free survival did not differ statistically significantly between the two study arms after 7.8 years of follow-up [52]. The evaluation also showed that patients with a baseline PSA value of >50 ng/ml had a higher risk of dying of carcinoma of the prostate than those with a baseline value of <8 ng/ml [57]. For baseline PSA values in the range of 8–50 ng/ml, a time to doubling of the PSA value (PSAdt) of <12 months was associated with a markedly increased risk of dying of carcinoma of the prostate. The authors concluded that above all patients with PSA values of >50 ng/ml and/or a PSAdt <12 months could benefit from immediate ADT.

A possible advantage for immediate ADT in patients with lymph node metastases after radical prostatectomy was seen in a study, but the number of patients in the study was small [58].

In conclusion, the advantages and disadvantages of immediate and delayed ADT should be discussed with each patient individually, based on the present state of knowledge (Table 2).

5.3 Continuous Versus Intermittent Hormone Deprivation

The basis for intermittent hormone deprivation (IAD) is to simulate intermittent castration with normalization of the testosterone levels in the therapy-free intervals. IAD can only be performed with drugs that cause medical castration, essentially therefore LHRH agonists and antagonists. It was hoped that IAD, compared to continuous ADT, would reduce therapy-related adverse reactions with a subsequent improvement in quality of life in the therapy-free intervals and lower treatment costs. It was also thought that IAD might delay the occurrence of castration resistance, which almost always occurs under continuous ADT after a certain period [59]. A further advantage of IAD might also be an osteoprotective effect. With this approach it is also necessary to take into account that while the baseline testosterone level drops relatively quickly after treatment initiation, it usually takes some time to return to normal again in the therapy-free intervals [60]. Numerous studies investigated whether these hoped-for advantages would actually be realized with IAD while still achieving oncological results as good as with continuous treatment. The study protocols, types of androgen deprivation applied, and results were not consistent. Only a few studies enrolled only patients with metastatic carcinoma of the prostate, others also included locally advanced tumors or recurrent tumors after primary treatment with curative intent. One large-scale noninferiority study showed a difference in overall survival of 5.1 versus 5.8 years in favor of continuous ADT [59]. The results were not conclusive for methodological reasons and statistically significant inferiority was not able to be shown for either of the two treatments. Several recent meta-analyses and reviews of the current literature reach the conclusion that IAD is not inferior to continuous ADT in locally advanced or metastatic carcinoma of the prostate [60–63]. This appears to apply to overall survival, tumor-specific survival, and progression-free survival. Furthermore, advantages with regard to quality of life were shown, especially for sexual and physical activity [60]. Overall, however, the advantages do not seem to be as great as assumed. Hot flushes occur less frequently under IAD [62, 64]. Treatment costs can be reduced by using IAD [1]. Not all authors of the reviews and meta-analyses cited made recommendations regarding the value of IAD. Some recommend it as a thera-

Table 2 Immediate versus delayed castration

Population	Recommendation
M1 symptomatic	Offer immediate castration to palliate symptoms and reduce the risk for potentially catastrophic sequelae of advanced disease (spinal cord compression, pathological fractures, ureteral obstruction, extra-skeletal metastasis)
M1 asymptomatic	Offer immediate castration to defer progression to a symptomatic stage and prevent serious disease progression-related complications Discuss delayed castration with a well-informed patient since it lowers the treatment side-effects, provided the patient is closely monitored

Recommendations of EAU-guidelines for hormonal treatment of metastatic carcinoma of the prostate [1]

peutic alternative, and others see IAD as a valid standard therapy. The current EAU Guidelines state that IAD might be an option following a successful induction phase [1].

Not all patients qualify for IAD, as was shown by the SWOG 9346 Study [59]. An initial response to ADT is decisive. The following treatment schedule based on empiric data can be used for IAD [1]. If an adequate decrease in PSA to values <4 ng/ml occurs in patients with metastatic disease in the first 3–6 months after the start of ADT, the ADT can be temporarily interrupted to start the IAD. Frequent and regular laboratory investigations must be made in the therapy-free interval. If the PSA value increases to 10–20 ng/ml or clinical progression occurs during the break from ADT, the ADT should be restarted. The patient can undergo several therapy cycles until castration resistance occurs. Patients with a high metastatic burden at baseline and/or a high PSA value may not be ideal candidates for IAD.

IAD is no longer an experimental approach to treatment and, regardless of current recommendations in guidelines, is already a not infrequently used strategy in everyday clinical practice. The advantages and disadvantages of IAD as opposed to continuous ADT should be discussed with each patient individually in the light of the present state of knowledge (Table 3).

Table 3 Intermittent treatment

Intermittent treatment	Recommendation
M1 asymptomatic	Offer intermittent treatment to highly motivated, well-informed, and compliant men, with a major PSA response after the induction period
Threshold to start and stop ADT	Stop treatment when the PSA level is <4 ng/ml after 6–7 months of treatment (induction period) Resume treatment when the PSA level is >10–20 ng/ml (or to the initial level if <20 ng/ml) or disease progresses clinically
Follow up	Strict follow-up is mandatory, with clinical examination every 3–6 months The more advanced the disease, the closer the follow-up should be

Recommendations of EAU-guidelines for hormonal treatment of metastatic carcinoma of the prostate [1]

5.4 Monotherapy with Antiandrogens

The nonsteroidal pure antiandrogens act exclusively on the androgen receptor and have no direct gonadotropic effects [6]. With regard to the antiandrogen class, bicalutamide appears to have the most favorable adverse reaction profile [30]. Compared to orchiectomy and MAB, monotherapy with bicalutamide showed clinically relevant advantages with regard to maintaining quality of life, mainly in the areas of sexual interest and physical activity [6, 65]. Relatively frequent adverse reactions with bicalutamide are gynecomastia and breast tenderness. The frequency and extent can be reduced or alleviated by prophylactic irradiation of the breast [1]. Antiestrogen prophylaxis is also recommended. Surgical mastectomy can be considered as a last resort. Hot flushes occur much less frequently under treatment with nonsteroidal antiandrogens than after castration [65]. Libido and potency may be preserved.

The standard dosage of bicalutamide for monotherapy is 150 mg/day. A PSA response similar to that of castration was achieved with this dosage [36]. One study showed a slight but statistically significant survival advantage of castration over bicalutamide monotherapy in the treatment of metastatic carcinoma of the prostate [66]. In subgroup analyses, this result depended on the PSA value and tumor burden at study entry. With a PSA value <400 ng/ml, survival in both groups was similar, and in patients with a high tumor burden (defined by the number of bony metastases), survival after orchiectomy seemed to be better [30, 67]. According to a recent Cochrane analysis, the current literature indicates that antiandrogen monotherapy is inferior to medical or surgical castration for the treatment of metastatic carcinoma of the prostate with regard to overall survival, clinical progression,

Table 4 Antiandrogen monotherapy

Population	Recommendation
M1 patients	Do *not* offer antiandrogen monotherapy

Recommendations of EAU-guidelines for hormonal treatment of metastatic carcinoma of the prostate [1]

and number of discontinuations of treatment because of adverse reactions [68]. The effects on tumor-specific survival and biochemical progression remained unclear and the evidence with regard to GRADE is only moderate. Survival and the duration of progression-free survival were similar in both study arms in the treatment of locally advanced, nonmetastatic carcinoma (M0) of the prostate [65].

The current EAU Guidelines do not recommend antiandrogen monotherapy for the treatment of metastatic carcinoma of the prostate (M1) [1]. Under certain circumstances, however, bicalutamide monotherapy may be considered for selected patients with nonmetastatic disease after individual discussion of the advantages and disadvantages, for example, if medical or surgical castration is not an option and quality of life aspects are of primary importance. In this situation, the patient should be made aware of the potential risk of poorer overall survival (Table 4).

6 New Developments

6.1 First-Line Combination of Chemotherapy with Hormone Therapy

For many years, the standard therapy for metastatic hormone sensitive carcinoma of the prostate has been ADT in the form of medical or surgical castration. The early addition of cytotoxic chemotherapy with docetaxel to the ADT has been investigated in three large Phase III studies [7–9, 69–71].

The GETUG-AFU-15 Study was the first prospective, randomized comparison of ADT versus ADT plus docetaxel given for up to 9 cycles [7, 70, 71]. Overall survival in the overall study sample was about 14 months longer with chemohormonal therapy, but this difference was not statistically significant. With a median follow-up of 7 years, a statistically significant advantage of initial chemohormonal therapy was seen for progression-free survival. Subgroup analyses showed that this was observed in particular in patients with a high tumor burden.

The CHAARTED Study (Chemohormonal Therapy versus Androgen Ablation Randomized Trial for Extensive Disease in Prostate Cancer) also compared ADT and ADT combined with docetaxel (75 mg/m^2 KOF, every 3 weeks, maximum of 6 cycles) [9]. About twice as many patients were randomized to treatment as in the GETUG-AFU-15 Study. A recent publication states that after a median follow-up period of 28.9 months, median survival in the entire study sample was 13.6 months longer in the combination therapy group. This survival advantage amounted to as much as 17 months in the subgroup of patients with high volume disease. The survival advantage in patients with high volume disease was not only statistically significant but was also clinically relevant and is certainly impressive. At the time of publication, median survival had not yet been reached in either study arm in the subgroup of patients with low volume disease. A much longer follow-up period will therefore be necessary to show whether there was also a survival advantage in these patients. High volume disease was defined in the CHAARTED Study as the presence of visceral metastases and/or at least 4 boney metastases, with at least one of these outside the pelvis or on the spine.

Survival data from the largest randomized study, the STAMPEDE Study (Systemic Therapy in Advancing or Metastatic Prostate Cancer: Evaluation of Drug Efficacy) were published in 2015 [8, 69]. The STAMPEDE Study is a multi-arm study testing several different treatment options against ADT as standard therapy, with no differentiation between high and low volume diseases. Evaluation of the results for ADT plus docetaxel (maximum of 6 cycles) compared with ADT alone showed a 10-month overall survival advantage (81 versus 71 months) for the chemohormonal therapy in the whole group after a median follow-up of 43 months. Overall survival was as much as 15 months longer (60 versus 45 months) in the subgroup of patients with metastatic carcinoma of the prostate.

Not all of these studies are complete, and their results are not directly comparable because of differences between the patients recruited, and overall survival in the treatment arms with ADT alone shows considerable differences in some cases. A meta-analysis did, however, show that there was a statistically significant advantage for chemotherapy with docetaxel over ADT alone in the treatment of metastatic carcinoma of the prostate [72]. The authors conclude that combined chemohormonal therapy should be considered the new standard for the treatment of metastatic hormone-sensitive carcinoma of the prostate. Worthy of mention is that the meta-analysis reports on a total of 16 deaths in the context of treatment with docetaxel. In general, the toxic potential of additive chemotherapy is not inconsiderable and should be borne in mind when deciding on the therapeutic option chosen.

The current EAU Guidelines recommend that all patients with metastatic carcinoma of the prostate should be offered combined chemohormonal therapy at the time of diagnosis [1]. ADT alone should be offered to patients who are not suitable for chemotherapy or reject it. According to the present state of knowledge, particularly patients with high volume disease will benefit from this approach. It is a sensible approach to discuss all options in all patients with advanced metastatic hormone-sensitive carcinoma of the prostate at an interdisciplinary tumor board, and then to speak to the patients individually about the possibility of receiving combination chemohormonal therapy [73] (Tables 5 and 6).

Table 5 First-line combination of chemotherapy with hormone therapy

Treatment type	Recommendation
Castration combined with chemotherapy	Offer castration combined with chemotherapy (docetaxel) to all patients with newly diagnosed M1 disease and who are fit enough for chemotherapy
Castration alone	Offer castration alone to patients unfit for, or unwilling to consider, castration combined with chemotherapy

Recommendations of EAU guidelines for hormonal treatment of metastatic carcinoma of the prostate [1]

Table 6 Results of the CHAARTED, STAMPEDE, and GETUG-AFU-15 studies in the entire study populations [9, 69, 71]

	CHAARTED		STAMPEDE		GETUG-AFU-15	
Number of patients (n)	790		1776		385	
Number of cycles of docetaxel 75 mg/m^2	6		6		9	
Follow-up (months)	28.9		43		83.9	
	ADT	ADT & D	ADT	ADT & D	ADT	ADT & D
Number of patients (*n*)	393	397	1184	592	193	192
Overall survival (months)	44.0	57.6	71	81	48.6	62.1

ADT androgen deprivation treatment, *D* docetaxel

References

1. Heidenreich A, Bastian PJ, Bellmunt J, et al. EAU guidelines on prostate cancer. Part II: treatment of advanced, relapsing and castration-resistant prostate cancer. Eur Urol. 2014;65(2):467–79.
2. Huggins C, Hodges CV. Studies on prostate cancer. I. The effect of castration, of estrogen and of androgen injection on serum phosphatases in metastatic carcinoma of the prostate. Cancer Res. 1941;1:293–7.
3. Schally AV, Kastin AJ, Arimura A. Hypothalamic follicle-stimulating hormone (FSH) and luteinizing hormone (LH)-regulating hormone: structure, physiology, and clinical studies. Fertil Steril. 1971;22(11):703–21.
4. Schally AV, Arimura A, Baba Y, et al. Isolation and properties of the FSH and LH-releasing hormone. Biochem Biophys Res Commun. 1971;43(2):393–9.
5. Schally AV. Luteinizing hormone-releasing hormone analogues and hormone ablation for prostate cancer: state of the art. BJU Int. 2007;100:2–4.
6. Heidenreich A, Pfister D, Ohlmann CH, et al. Androgendeprivation in der Therapie des Prostatakarzinoms. Urologe A. 2008;47(3):270–83.
7. Gravis G, Fizazi K, Joly F, et al. Androgen-deprivation therapy alone or with docetaxel in non-castrate metastatic prostate cancer (GETUG-AFU 15): a randomised, open-label, phase 3 trial. Lancet Oncol. 2013;14(2):149–58.
8. James ND, Spears MR, Clarke NW, et al. Survival with newly diagnosed metastatic prostate cancer in the "docetaxel era": data from 917 patients in the control arm of the STAMPEDE Trial (MRC PR08, CRUK/06/019). Eur Urol. 2015;67(6):1028–38.
9. Sweeney CJ, Chen YH, Carducci M, et al. Chemohormonal therapy in metastatic hormone-sensitive prostate cancer. N Engl J Med. 2015;373(8):737–46.
10. Oefelein MG, Feng A, Scolieri MJ, et al. Reassessment of the definition of castrate levels of testosterone: implications for clinical decision making. Urology. 2000;56(6):1021–4.
11. Cassileth BR, Soloway MS, Vogelzang NJ, et al. Patients' choice of treatment in stage D prostate cancer. Urology. 1989;33(5):57–62.
12. Bonzani RA, Stricker HJ, Peabody JO. Quality of life comparison of lupron and orchiectomy. J Urol. 1996;155 Suppl 5:611A.
13. Vogelzang NJ, Chodak GW, Soloway MS, et al. Goserelin versus orchiectomy in the treatment of advanced prostate cancer: final results of a randomized trial. Urology. 1995;46(2):220–6.
14. Sun M, Choueiri TK, Hamnvik OR, et al. Comparison of gonadotropin-releasing hormone agonists and orchiectomy: effects of androgen-deprivation therapy. JAMA Oncol. 2016;2(4):500–7. doi:10.1001/jamaoncol.2015.4917.
15. Shahinian VB, Kuo YF, Freeman JL, et al. Risk of fracture after androgen deprivation for prostate cancer. N Engl J Med. 2005;352(2):154–64.
16. Schally AV. Luteinizing hormone-releasing hormone analogs: their impact on the control of tumorigenesis. Peptides. 1999;20(10):1247–62.
17. Redding TW, Schally AV. Inhibition of prostate tumor growth in two rat models by chronic administration of D-Trp6 analogue of luteinizing hormone-releasing hormone. Proc Natl Acad Sci U S A. 1981;78(10):6509–12.
18. Tolis G, Ackman D, Stellos A, et al. Tumor growth inhibition in patients with prostatic carcinoma treated with luteinizing hormone-releasing hormone agonists. Proc Natl Acad Sci U S A. 1982;79(5):1658–62.
19. Schlegel PN. Efficacy and safety of histrelin subdermal implant in patients with advanced prostate cancer. J Urol. 2006;175(4):1353–8.
20. Wilson HC, Shah SI, Abel PD, et al. Contemporary hormone therapy with LHRH agonists for prostate cancer: avoiding osteoporosis and fracture. Cent European J Urol. 2015;68(2):165–8.
21. Ross RW, Small EJ. Osteoporosis in men treated with androgen deprivation therapy for prostate cancer. J Urol. 2002;167(5):1952–6.
22. Van Poppel H, Klotz L. Gonadotropin-releasing hormone: an update review of the antagonists versus agonists. Int J Urol. 2012;19(7):594–601.
23. Van Poppel H, Nilsson S. Testosterone surge: rationale for gonadotropin-releasing hormone blockers? Urology. 2008;71(6):1001–6.
24. Klotz L, Boccon-Gibod L, Shore ND, et al. The efficacy and safety of degarelix: a 12-month, comparative, randomized, open-label, parallel-group phase III study in patients with prostate cancer. BJU Int. 2008;102(11):1531–8.
25. Van Poppel H, Tombal B, de la Rosette JJ, et al. Degarelix: a novel gonadotropin-releasing hormone (GnRH) receptor blocker-results from a 1-yr, multicentre, randomised, phase 2 dosage-finding study in the treatment of prostate cancer. Eur Urol. 2008;54(4):805–13.
26. Gittelman M, Pommerville PJ, Persson BE, et al. A 1-year, open label, randomized phase II dose finding study of degarelix for the treatment of prostate cancer in North America. J Urol. 2008;180(5):1986–92.
27. Debruyne F, Bhat G, Garnick MB. Abarelix for injectable suspension: first-in-class gonadotropin-releasing hormone antagonist for prostate cancer. Future Oncol. 2006;2(6):677–96.
28. Tombal B, Miller K, Boccon-Gibod L, et al. Additional analysis of the secondary end point of biochemical recurrence rate in a phase 3 trial (CS21) comparing degarelix 80 mg versus leuprolide in prostate cancer patients segmented by baseline characteristics. Eur Urol. 2010;57(5):836–42.

29. MacLean DB, Shi H, Faessel HM, et al. Medical Castration using the Investigational Oral GnRH antagonist TAK-385 (Relugolix): phase 1 Study in Healthy Males. J Clin Endocrinol Metab. 2015;100(12):4579–87.
30. Anderson J. The role of antiandrogen monotherapy in the treatment of prostate cancer. BJU Int. 2003;91(5):455–61.
31. Iversen P, Melezinek I, Schmidt A. Nonsteroidal antiandrogens: a therapeutic option for patients with advanced prostate cancer who wish to retain sexual interest and function. BJU Int. 2001;87(1):47–56.
32. Schröder FH, Whelan P, de Reijke TM, et al. Metastatic prostate cancer treated by flutamide versus cyproterone acetate. Final analysis of the "European Organization for Research and Treatment of Cancer" (EORTC) Protocol 30892. Eur Urol. 2004;45(4):457–64.
33. Moffat LE. Comparison of Zoladex, diethylstilbestrol and cyproterone acetate treatment in advanced prostate cancer. Eur Urol. 1990;18 Suppl 3:26–7.
34. Thorpe SC, Azmatullah S, Fellows GJ, et al. A prospective, randomised study to compare goserelin acetate (Zoladex) versus cyproterone acetate (Cyprostat) versus a combination of the two in the treatment of metastatic prostatic carcinoma. Eur Urol. 1996;29(1):47–54.
35. Boccon-Gibod L, Fournier G, Bottet P, et al. Flutamide versus orchiectomy in the treatment of metastatic prostate carcinoma. Eur Urol. 1997;32:391–6.
36. Tyrrell CJ, Denis L, Newling D, et al. Casodex 10–200 mg daily, used as monotherapy for the treatment of patients with advanced prostate cancer. An overview of the efficacy, tolerability and pharmacokinetics from three phase II dose-ranging studies. Casodex Study Group. Eur Urol. 1998;33(1):39–53.
37. Byar DP. The veterans administration cooperative urological research group's studies of cancer of the prostate. Cancer. 1973;32(5):1126–30.
38. Hedlund PO, Damber JE, Hagerman I, et al. Parenteral estrogen versus combined androgen deprivation in the treatment of metastatic prostatic cancer: part 2. Final evaluation of the Scandinavian Prostatic Cancer Group (SPCG) Study No. 5. Scand J Urol Nephrol. 2008;42(3):220–9.
39. Klotz L, McNeill I, Fleshner N. A phase 1–2 trial of diethylstilbestrol plus low dose warfarin in advanced prostate carcinoma. J Urol. 1999;161(1):169–72.
40. Labrie F, Dupont A, Belanger A, et al. New hormonal therapy in prostatic carcinoma: combined treatment with an LHRH agonist and an antiandrogen. Clin Invest Med. 1982;5(4):267–75.
41. Collette L, Studer UE, Schröder FH, et al. Why phase III trials of maximal androgen blockade versus castration in M1 prostate cancer rarely show statistically significant differences. Prostate. 2001;48(1):29–39.
42. Crawford ED, Blumenstein BA, Goodman PJ, et al. Leuprolide with and without flutamide in advanced prostate cancer. Cancer. 1990;66 Suppl 5:1039–44.
43. Crawford ED, Eisenberger MA, McLeod DG, et al. A controlled trial of leuprolide with and without flutamide in prostatic carcinoma. N Engl J Med. 1989;321(7):419–24.
44. Eisenberger MA, Blumenstein BA, Crawford ED, et al. Bilateral orchiectomy with or without flutamide for metastatic prostate cancer. N Engl J Med. 1998;339(15):1036–42.
45. Denis LJ, Carnelro de Moura JL, Bono A, et al. Goserelin acetate and flutamide versus bilateral orchiectomy: a phase III EORTC trial (30853). EORTC GU Group and EORTC Data Center. Urology. 1993;42(2):119–29.
46. Denis LJ, Keuppens F, Smith PH, et al. Maximal androgen blockade: final analysis of EORTC phase III trial 30853. EORTC Genito-Urinary Tract Cancer Cooperative Group and the EORTC Data Center. Eur Urol. 1998;33(2):144–51.
47. Denis L, Robinson M, Mahler C, et al. Orchidectomy versus Zoladex plus Eulexin in patients with metastatic prostate cancer (EORTC 30853). J Steroid Biochem Mol Biol. 1990;37(6):951–9.
48. Prostate Cancer Trialists Collaborative Group. Maximum androgen blockade in advanced prostate cancer: an overview of the randomised trials. Lancet. 2000;355(9214):1491–8.
49. Prostate Cancer Trialists' Collaborative Group. Maximum androgen blockade in advanced prostate cancer: an overview of 22 randomised trials with 3283 deaths in 5710 patients. Lancet. 1995;346(8970):265–9.
50. Moinpour CM, Savage MJ, Troxel A, et al. Quality of life in advanced prostate cancer: results of a randomized therapeutic trial. J Natl Cancer Inst. 1998;90(20):1537–44.
51. Loblaw DA, Virgo KS, Nam R, et al. Initial hormonal management of androgen-sensitive metastatic, recurrent, or progressive prostate cancer: 2006 update of an American Society of Clinical Oncology practice guideline. J Clin Oncol. 2007;25(12):1596–605.
52. Studer UE, Whelan P, Albrecht W, et al. Immediate or deferred androgen deprivation for patients with prostate cancer not suitable for local treatment with curative intent: European Organisation for Research and Treatment of Cancer (EORTC) Trial 30891. J Clin Oncol. 2006;24(12):1868–76.
53. Wilt T, Nair B, MacDonald R, et al. Early versus deferred androgen suppression in the treatment of advanced prostatic cancer. Cochrane Database Syst Rev. 2002(1):CD003506. doi:10.1002/14651858.CD003506.
54. Studer UE, Hauri D, Hanselmann S, et al. Immediate versus deferred hormonal treatment for patients with prostate cancer who are not suitable for curative local treatment: results of the randomized trial SAKK 08/88. J Clin Oncol. 2004;22(20):4109–18.
55. The Medical Research Council Prostate Cancer Working Party Investigators Group. Immediate versus deferred treatment for advanced prostatic cancer: initial

results of the medical research council trial. Br J Urol. 1997;79(2):235–46.
56. Studer UE, Whelan P, Wimpissinger F, et al. Differences in time to disease progression do not predict for cancer-specific survival in patients receiving immediate or deferred androgen-deprivation therapy for prostate cancer: final results of EORTC randomized trial 30891 with 12 years of follow-up. Eur Urol. 2014;66(5):829–38.
57. Studer UE, Collette L, Whelan P, et al. Using PSA to guide timing of androgen deprivation in patients with T0-4 N0-2 M0 prostate cancer not suitable for local curative treatment (EORTC 30891). Eur Urol. 2008;53(5):941–9.
58. Messing EM, Manola J, Sarosdy M, et al. Immediate hormonal therapy compared with observation after radical prostatectomy and pelvic lymphadenectomy in men with node-positive prostate cancer. N Eng J Med. 1999;341(24):1781–8.
59. Hussain M, Tangen CM, Berry DL, et al. Intermittent versus continuous androgen deprivation in prostate cancer. N Engl J Med. 2013;368(14):1314–25.
60. Magnan S, Zarychanski R, Pilote L, et al. Intermittent vs continuous androgen deprivation therapy for prostate cancer: a systematic review and meta-analysis. JAMA Oncol. 2015;1(9):1261–9.
61. Brungs D, Chen J, Masson P, et al. Intermittent androgen deprivation is a rational standard-of-care treatment for all stages of progressive prostate cancer: results from a systematic review and meta-analysis. Prostate Cancer Prostatic Dis. 2014;17(2):105–11.
62. Botrel TE, Clark O, dos Reis RB, et al. Intermittent versus continuous androgen deprivation for locally advanced, recurrent or metastatic prostate cancer: a systematic review and meta-analysis. BMC Urol. 2014;14:9.
63. Niraula S, Le LW, Tannock IF. Treatment of prostate cancer with intermittent versus continuous androgen deprivation: a systematic review of randomized trials. J Clin Oncol. 2013;31(16):2029–36.
64. Calais da Silva FE, Bono AV, Whelan P, et al. Intermittent androgen deprivation for locally advanced and metastatic prostate cancer: results from a randomised phase 3 study of the South European Uroncological Group. Eur Urol. 2009;55(6):1269–77.
65. Iversen P, Tyrrell CJ, Kaisary AV, et al. Bicalutamide monotherapy compared with castration in patients with nonmetastatic locally advanced prostate cancer: 6.3 years of followup. J Urol. 2000;164(5):1579–82.
66. Tyrrell CJ, Kaisary AV, Iversen P, et al. A randomised comparison of "Casodex" (bicalutamide) 150 mg monotherapy versus castration in the treatment of metastatic and locally advanced prostate cancer. Eur Urol. 1998;33(5):447–56.
67. Kaisary AV, Iversen P, Tyrrell CJ, et al. Is there a role for antiandrogen monotherapy in patients with metastatic prostate cancer? Prostate Cancer Prostatic Dis. 2001;4(4):196–203.
68. Kunath F, Grobe HR, Rücker G, et al. Non-steroidal antiandrogen monotherapy compared with luteinising hormone-releasing hormone agonists or surgical castration monotherapy for advanced prostate cancer. Cochrane Database Syst Rev. 2014(6):CD009266. doi:10.1002/14651858.CD009266.pub2.
69. James ND, Sydes MR, Clarke NW, et al. Addition of docetaxel, zoledronic acid, or both to first-line long-term hormone therapy in prostate cancer (STAMPEDE): survival results from an adaptive, multiarm, multistage, platform randomised controlled trial. Lancet. 2016;387:1163–77.
70. Gravis G, Boher JM, Joly F, et al. Androgen deprivation therapy (ADT) plus docetaxel (D) versus ADT alone for hormone-naïve metastatic prostate cancer (PCa): long-term analysis of the GETUG-AFU 15 phase III trial. Genitourinary Cancers Symposium. J Clin Oncol. 2015;33(7): 140.
71. Gravis G, Boher JM, Joly F, et al. Androgen Deprivation Therapy (ADT) plus docetaxel versus ADT alone in metastatic non castrate prostate cancer: impact of metastatic burden and long-term survival analysis of the randomized phase 3 GETUG-AFU15 trial. Eur Urol. 2016;70(2):256–62.
72. Vale CL, Burdett S, Rydzewska LH, et al. Addition of docetaxel or bisphosphonates to standard of care in men with localised or metastatic, hormone-sensitive prostate cancer: a systematic review and meta-analyses of aggregate data. Lancet Oncol. 2016;17(2):243–56.
73. Strebel RT, Sulser T, Schmid HP, et al. Multidisciplinary care in patients with prostate cancer: room for improvement. Support Care Cancer. 2013;21(8):2327–33.

Chemotherapy and Androgen Receptor-Directed Treatment of Castration Resistant Metastatic Prostate Cancer

S. Osanto and S.A.C. Luelmo

1 Introduction

Metastatic prostate cancer is sensitive to androgen deprivation in the majority of men. However, castration resistance inevitably occurs after a median of 18–24 months. Relatively few chemotherapeutic agents have been proven to be of benefit to patients. Single agent chemotherapeutic trials published in the late 1980s to early 1990s in men with castration-resistant disease found a response rate to various chemotherapeutic agents of less than 10 % in men with measurable disease with a median survival of 10–12 months [38].

2 Chemotherapy in Castration Resistant Prostate Cancer

2.1 Mitoxantone

In the early 1990s, PSA tests became available and have since been incorporated as response measurement in trials.

Two trials investigated the combination of mitoxantrone 12 mg/m^{2}on day 1 every 3 weeks plus daily prednisone 10 mg compared to prednisone alone. The first study investigated quality of life (clinical benefit consisting of a decrease in pain and use of analgesics) in 161 men with metastatic prostate cancer and found a significantly better pain control in the combination arm (Table 1, 29 % vs. 12 %, $p<0.0001$) [36]. There was no difference in PSA response and overall survival.

In the second randomized trial, 242 patients received hydrocortisone 40 mg/day or the combination of mitoxantrone 14 mg/m^2 on day 1 every 3 weeks plus hydrocortisone 40 mg daily (Table 1) [14]. The combination led to improved pain control, but there was no significant difference in overall survival between the combination of mitoxantrone and hydrocortisone and hydrocortisone alone.

In 1996, the American Food and Drug Administration (FDA) approved the use of the combination of mitoxantrone and prednisone for the treatment of symptomatic patients with hormone resistant prostate cancer. Mitoxantrone plus corticosteroids (prednisone or hydrocortisone) was considered the standard of care for palliation not for extending survival in metastatic castration-resistant prostate cancer (mCRPC) patients.

A multicenter randomized phase III trial in 121 men with asymptomatic, progressive, CRPC compared mitoxantrone intravenously once every 3 weeks plus 10 mg prednisone daily with prednisone alone and confirmed absence of survival

S. Osanto (✉) • S.A.C. Luelmo
Department of Oncology, Leiden University Medical Center (LUMC), Albinusdreef 2, 2333 ZA Leiden, The Netherlands
e-mail: S.Osanto@lumc.nl

M. Bolla, H. van Poppel (eds.), *Management of Prostate Cancer*,
DOI 10.1007/978-3-319-42769-0_22

Table 1 Randomized phase III chemotherapy trials: first-line treatment

Author/company	Trial	No. of patients	Treatment	Outcome
Tannock et al. [36]	NOV-22	161	Mitoxantrone + prednisone vs. prednisone	Palliative response: 29 % vs. 12 % Duration of palliation: 48 vs. 13 weeks OS: no difference
Kantoff et al. [14]	CALGB 9182	242	Mitoxantrone + hydrocortisone vs. hydrocortisone	OS: 12.3 vs. 12.6 months TTP or treatment failure (TTF) : 3.7 vs. 2.3 months ($P = .021$ and .025, resp) PSA response: 37.5 % vs. 21.5 % ORR: 7 % vs. 4 % QOL response: indication of better QOL with mitoxantrone
Berry et al. [8]		121	Mitoxantrone + prednisone vs. prednisone	OS: 23 vs. 19 months (not significant) TTP: 8.1 vs. 4.1 months ($p = 0.017$) ≥50 % PSA decrease: 48 % vs. 24 % ($p = 0.007$)
Tannock et al. [34]	TAX327	1,006	Docetaxel + prednisone vs. mitoxantrone + prednisone	OS: 18.9 vs. 16.5 months (HR, 0.76) (Δ *2.6 months*) PSA response: 45 % vs. 32 % ORR: 12 % vs. 7 % Pain response: 35 % vs. 22 % QOL response: 22 % vs. 13 %
Petrylak et al. [23]	SWOG 99-16	647	Docetaxel + estramustine vs. mitoxantrone + prednisone	OS: 17.5 vs. 15.6 months (HR, 0.80) (Δ *1.9 months*) PFS: 6.3 vs. 3.2 months PSA response: 50 % vs. 27 % ORR: 17 % vs. 11 %
Small et al. [32]	VITAL-2	408	GVAX + docetaxel + prednisone vs. docetaxel + prednisone	Terminated as there were more deaths in experimental (67) than in control (47) arm
Scher et al. [31]	ASCENT-2	953	DN-101 + docetaxel + dexamethasone vs. docetaxel + prednisone	OS: 16.6 vs. 19.9 months (HR, 1.33) More deaths in experimental arm
Kelly et al. [16]	CALGB 90401	1,050	Bevacizumab + docetaxel + prednisone vs. placebo + docetaxel + prednisone	OS: 22.6 vs. 21.5 months (HR, 0.91) PFS: 9.9 vs. 7.5 months (HR, 0.77) PSA response: 69.5 % vs. 57.9 % ORR: 53.2 % vs. 42.1 %
Nelson et al. [21]	ENTHUSE M1	594	Zibotentan (ZD4054) + standard therapy vs. placebo + standard therapy	OS: 24.5 vs. 22.5 months (HR, 0.87) PFS: 6.2 vs. 6.5 months (HR, 1.01)
Quin et al. [26]	SWOG S0421	930	Atrasentan + docetaxel + prednisone vs. placebo + docetaxel + prednisone	OS: 18 vs. 18 months (HR, 1.04) PFS: 9 vs. 9 months (HR, 1.02) PSA response: 50 % vs. 49 % ORR: 14 % vs. 14 %

Araujo et al. [2]	CA180-227	1,380	Dasatinib + docetaxel + prednisone vs. placebo + docetaxel + prednisone	OS: 21.5 vs. 21.2 months (HR, 0.99) PFS: 11.8 vs. 11.1 months (HR, 0.92) ORR: 30.5 % vs. 31.9 %
Tannock et al. [35]	VENICE	1,200	Aflibercept + docetaxel + prednisone vs. placebo + docetaxel + prednisone	OS: 22.1. vs. 21.2. months (HR, 0.94) PFS: 6.9 vs. 6.2 months (p 0.31) PSA response: 68.6 % vs. 63.5 %
Petrylak et al. [24]	MAINSAIL	1,059	Lenalidomide + docetaxel + prednisone vs. placebo + docetaxel prednisone	OS: 17.7 months. vs. not reached (HR, 1.53) PFS: 10.4 vs. 10.6 months (HR, 1.32) ORR: 22 % vs. 25 %
OncoGenex Pharmaceuticals	SYNERGY	1,022	Custirsen (OGX-011) + docetaxel + prednisone vs. docetaxel + prednisone	Primary endpoint: OS improvement not achieved OS: 23.4 vs. 22.2 months (HR. 0.93) (one-sided p value 0.207)

benefit for the combination of mitoxantrone and prednisone over prednisone alone (Table 1) [8].

2.2 Taxanes

2.2.1 Paclitaxel and Docetaxel

An early trial by the Eastern Cooperative Oncology Group in 23 patients administered a 24-h infusion of 135–150 mg/m² paclitaxel every 3 weeks [27]. Paclitaxel treatment induced considerable toxicity, including neutropenic sepsis in 26 % of patients and two toxic deaths, but no ≥50 % PSA declines and only a 4.3 % measurable response rate.

In a second study, in which 17 patients were treated with weekly paclitaxel, 150 mg/m² for 6 out of 8 weeks (6 weeks on, 2 weeks rest), a higher PSA decline rate of 39 %, a 50 % measurable response rate, and a median survival of 13.5 months was observed [37].

Docetaxel administered as a single agent administered either weekly or every 3 weeks, resulted in PSA decline rates in approximately 50 % of patients and measurable disease response rates ranging between 28 and 40 % [4, 7, 25].

2.2.2 Pivotal Phase III Trials Leading to Registration of Docetaxel in 2004

Two landmark phase III randomized trials, TAX327 and SWOG 99–16, were reported in 2004. They both demonstrated that docetaxel-based treatment administered every 3 weeks prolongs median OS by 2–3 months for men with mCRPC when compared with the palliative standard of care mitoxantrone and prednisone (Table 1) [23, 34]. The results of these two pivotal studies replaced mitoxantrone-based therapy as standard treatment.

TAX 327, a randomized phase III trial, was a three-arm trial with 1004 patients which included the standard arm (mitoxantrone combined with prednisone) and two experimental arms (docetaxel combined with prednisone at varying doses) (Table 1). Half of the men did not respond to docetaxel and did not benefit from chemotherapy and were only at risk for potential docetaxel-related toxicity.

The median survival was 16.5 months in the mitoxantrone group, 18.9 months in the group given docetaxel every 3 weeks, and 17.4 months in the group given weekly docetaxel. No significant difference in survival was observed of docetaxel once every 3 weeks compared with docetaxel once per week.

Among these three groups, 32 %, 45 %, and 48 % of men, respectively, had at least a 50 % decrease in the serum PSA level ($p<0.001$ for both comparisons with mitoxantrone). With regard to pain relief: 22 %, 35 % ($p=0.01$), and 31 % ($p=0.08$), respectively, had reductions in pain; and 13 %, 22 % ($p=0.009$), and 23 % ($p=0.005$), respectively, had improvements in the quality of life.

Adverse events were more common in the groups that received docetaxel. There were significantly more grade 3–4 adverse events with docetaxel administered every 3 weeks when compared with mitoxantrone and with once-per-week docetaxel. In the once-per-week docetaxel arm, clinical benefit was generally greater albeit not statistically significant, than that of mitoxantrone treatment and lower than that with docetaxel every 3 weeks. Using the Functional Assessment of Cancer Therapy–Prostate, functional status was significantly better with docetaxel administered every 3 weeks (22 %) or once per week (23 %) in comparison to mitoxantrone (13 %; $p=.009$ and .005, respectively).

The Southwest Oncology Group (SWOG) study 99–16 compared a 5-day course of estramustine 280 mg orally three times a day combined with docetaxel 60 mg/m² to continuous prednisone and mitoxantrone 12 mg/m² in 770 men (Table 1). Dose escalation was permitted to 70 mg/m² and 14 mg/m² for docetaxel and mitoxantrone, respectively.

In an intention-to-treat analysis, the median overall survival was longer in the group given docetaxel and estramustine than in the group given mitoxantrone and prednisone (17.5 months vs. 15.6 months, $p=0.02$ by the log-rank test), with a 20 % reduction in the risk of death (hazard ratio for death was 0.80; 95 % confidence interval, 0.67–0.97). Grade 3 or 4 neutropenic fevers ($p=0.01$), nausea and vomiting ($p<0.001$), and cardiovascular events ($p=0.001$) were more commonly observed in patients receiving docetaxel and estramustine than among those receiving mitoxantrone and prednisone. Pain relief was similar in both groups.

These two landmark studies TAX327 and SWOG 99–16 led to the registration of docetaxel for the treatment of castration-resistant prostate cancer.

2.2.3 Optimal Dose and Schedule of Docetaxel

Although the optimal dose and scheduling of docetaxel has not been assessed unequivocally and the administration dose and schedule of docetaxel may be associated with clinical outcome, the 75 mg/m^2 i.v. every 3 weeks TAX327 regimen is most widely used by clinicians. Interestingly, a Finnish study suggested that 50 mg/m^2 docetaxel administered i.v. on days 1 and 15 of a 4-week cycle was superior to 75 mg/m^2 docetaxel administered i.v. on day 1 of a 3-week cycle [15]. Overall survival was 19.5 months in the 2-weekly group (95 % CI, 15.9–23.1) versus 17 months in the 3-weekly group (95 % CI, 15.0–19.1), which was statistically significant (HR = 1.4; 95 % CI, 1.1–1.8; $p=.021$), and time to progression was 15.8 months (95 % CI, 13.6–18.1) and 14.6 months (95 % CI, 13.2–16.0), respectively (HR = 1.3; 95 % CI, 1.0–1.6; $P=.047$).

Another docetaxel trial reported that docetaxel administered every 2 versus every 3 weeks was associated with a longer time to treatment failure (5.6 vs. 4.9 months; $p=.016$) and fewer grade 3–4 toxicities. These findings suggest that more frequent docetaxel dosing might improve tolerability, efficacy, or both.

2.2.4 Prognostic and Predictive Factors

Four independent baseline factors (pain, visceral metastases, anemia, and bone scan progression) predicted PSA decline of ≥30 % within 3 months of treatment with chemotherapy could be identified after analysis of the TAX327 trial data [3]. Three risk groups were developed with a median OS of 25.7 months (zero to one risk factors), 18.7 months (two risk factors), and 12.8 months (three to four risk factors). These predictors of survival may be useful for prognostication as well as for stratification in and interpretation of clinical trials and sample size planning.

2.3 Estramustine

Estramustine phosphate, an ester of estradiol and microtubule-associated proteins binding mustard, leads to inhibition of cell mitosis and lowers plasma testosterone levels. Estramustine is an old drug which has been used many years in the clinic before the registration of docetaxel. Estramustine administered orally at a dose of 10 mg/kg/day has a response rate ranging from 19 to 69 % in metastatic CRPC [22]. Based on preclinical data showing synergy between estramustine and chemotherapeutic agents such as vinblastine, etoposide, paclitaxel, and docetaxel, estramustine has also been used in combination with cytotoxic agents. Combination of estramustine and vinblastine, vinorelbine, paclitaxel, and docetaxel were tested in various studies. Several phase II and III studies investigated whether addition of estramustine to chemotherapy leads to an improvement in clinical outcome. Data from randomized clinical trials that compared chemotherapy regimens with and without estramustine published between 1966 and 2004 were analyzed [12]. Hemoglobin ($p<0.0001$), use of chemotherapy plus estramustine ($p=0.008$), performance status ($p=0.002$), and serum PSA concentrations ($p=0.04$) were associated independently with overall survival. Overall survival was significantly better in patients who received chemotherapy plus estramustine (adjusted hazard ratio [HR] 0.77 [95 % CI 0.63–0.93], $p=0.008$) with an estimated absolute increase in overall survival of 9.5 % (SE 4.0) at 1 year after randomization. Patients who received chemotherapy plus estramustine had a better PSA response than those who received chemotherapy without estramustine (RR 0.53 [0.38–0.72], $p<0.0001$) but experienced more grade 3 or grade 4 thromboembolic events. It was concluded that the clinical benefits did not outweigh the additional risk of adverse events including thromboembolic events.

2.4 First-Line Chemotherapy: Phase III Randomized Clinical Trials of Docetaxel Combinations

Several new agents have been evaluated in combination with docetaxel plus prednisone in randomized phase III trials in chemo-naïve CRPC patients (Table 1).

2.4.1 GVAX

Prostate GVAX consists of two prostate cancer cell lines, LNCaP and PC3, transfected with a GM-CSF gene. A phase III trial comparing GVAX immunotherapy for prostate cancer in combination with docetaxel to docetaxel plus prednisone was initiated in 2005. The study was designed to enroll 600 patients with a primary endpoint of superiority in overall survival. CRPC patients with pain requiring opioid analgesics were treated with docetaxel (75 mg/m^2 q 3 weeks × 10 cycles) plus GVAX or docetaxel plus prednisone 10 mg daily in the control arm. CG1940/CG8711 (500 million cells prime/300 million cells boost doses q 3 weeks × 10 cycles) was administered 2 days following each docetaxel infusion in the experimental arm followed by maintenance immunotherapy alone (q 4 weeks). The study was prematurely terminated after accrual of 408 patients due to an imbalance in deaths, with 67 deaths in the docetaxel/GVAX arm and 47 deaths in the docetaxel plus prednisone arm [32]. Two phase III studies of single-agent prostate GVAX in patients with CRPC were also terminated early.

2.4.2 ASCENT-2

In preclinical experiments, DN-101 (high-dose calcitriol, the active form of vitamin D) was shown to upregulate apoptosis and inhibit cell proliferation in prostatic cancer cell lines treated with chemotherapy, including docetaxel. A large, randomized phase II study (ASCENT-1 [Androgen-Independent Prostate Cancer Study of Calcitriol Enhancing Taxotere 1], with 250 patients) of weekly docetaxel and prednisone with or without DN-101 did not meet its primary endpoint of a prespecified increase in PSA response, but there was better OS in the DN-101 arm with reduced toxicity. In the ASCENT-2 study, DN-101 given with weekly docetaxel was compared with standard 3-weekly docetaxel, the best arm of the TAX 327 study (Table 1) [31]. The study was terminated with 953 patients recruited after an interim analysis showed more deaths in the experimental arm (hazard ratio [HR], 1.33 for OS; $P = .019$). ASCENT treatment was associated with shorter survival than the control. This difference might be due to either weekly docetaxel dosing, which, in a prior study, showed a trend toward inferior survival compared with an every-3-weeks regimen, or DN-101 therapy.

2.4.3 Endothelin receptor antagonists

Endothelin-1 and the endothelin A (ET(A)) receptor have been implicated in prostate cancer progression in bone.

This study aimed to determine whether the specific ET(A) receptor antagonist, zibotentan, prolonged overall survival (OS) in patients with castration-resistant prostate cancer and bone metastases who were pain-free or mildly symptomatic for pain. Patients were randomized 1:1 to zibotentan 10 mg/day or placebo, plus standard prostate cancer treatment. The primary endpoint was OS. In this large, randomized, placebo-controlled phase III trial, treatment with zibotentan 10 mg/day did not lead to a statistically significant improvement in OS in this patient population. Zibotentan had an acceptable safety profile (Table 1) [21].

Atrasentan, another endothelin recetor antagonist in combination with docetaxel was compared to placebo in a phase III trial including 498 CRPC patients. No improvement in overall survival or progression free survival was seen when adding atrasentan to the standard docetaxel (Table 1).

2.4.4 Dasatinib

Src kinases regulate osteoclast functions and may play a role in the development of bone metastases. Preclinical observations suggested an association between src kinase activity and decreased sensitivity to androgen ablation. The addition of src-inhibitor dasatinib to docetaxel in a phase III placebo-controlled trial in 1,522 men with metastatic castration-resistant prostate cancer did not improve overall survival. Median time to PSA progression was also similar in the placebo and dasatinib groups. There was a small, nonsignificant difference in the time to first skeletal-related event in favor of the dasatinib arm (HR 0.81, 95 % CI 0.64–1.02) (Table 1) [2].

2.4.5 Antiangiogenic Drugs

The observation that increased microvessel density, increased expression of VEGF, high plasma and urine levels of VEGF are associated with poorer OS in men with CRPC, led to enthusiasm to study the addition of angiogenesis inhibitors to chemotherapy. Combinations of docetaxel and angiogenesis-inhibitors have been studied extensively in mCRPC patients.

2.4.6 Bevacizumab

Based on encouraging phase II data, the CALGB 90401 clinical trial compared docetaxel, prednisone, and bevacizumab with docetaxel and prednisone in 1,050 men with prognostically favorable mCRPC [17]. The primary endpoint was OS, which was not significantly different between the control and experimental arms (HR, 0.91; $p=0.18$). Bevacizumab led to significant improvements in secondary endpoints progression-free survival (PFS) and PSA response rate. Compared to docetaxel control, there were significantly more grade 3–4 adverse effects (75 % vs. 56 %; $P<0.001$) in the bevacizumab combination arm and a higher percentage deaths related to toxicity (3.8 % vs. 1.1 %).

2.4.7 VEGF Trap Aflibercept and Lenalomide

Two other large, randomized clinical trials evaluated antiangiogenic agents in combination with docetaxel and prednisone.

The VENICE trial (Aflibercept in Combination With Docetaxel in Metastatic Androgen Independent Prostate Cancer) evaluating aflibercept (VEGF trap) explored whether the combination of docetaxel and prednisone with aflibercept which targets a broader spectrum of angiogenic mediators than bevacizumab (VEGF-A, VEGF-B, and placental growth factor) was superior to docetaxel/prednisone alone (Table 1) [35].

Lenalidomide, a less toxic analog of thalidomide with immunomodulatory and antiangiogenic properties, has been evaluated in combination with docetaxel and prednisone in the Mainsail trial (Study to Evaluate Safety and Effectiveness of Lenalidomide in Combination With Docetaxel and Prednisone for Patients With Castrate-Resistant Prostate Cancer; Table 1). Overall survival with the combination of lenalidomide, docetaxel, and prednisone was significantly worse than with docetaxel and prednisone for chemotherapy-naive men with metastatic, castration-resistant prostate cancer (Table 1) [24].

Other antiangiogenic agents include monoclonal antibodies targeting $\alpha v\beta 3$ and $\alpha v\beta 5$ integrin receptors expressed on endothelial cells, i.e., CNTO 95 (intetumumab) and etaracizumab. These have been evaluated in phase II clinical trials for men with mCRPC. In a phase II trial for first-line CRPC, patients were treated with docetaxel plus prednisone and were randomized between placebo or intetumumab every 3 weeks. All the endpoints including OS, PFS, and PSA response favored placebo over intetumumab [13].

2.4.8 Custirsen

Clusterin is a chaperone protein associated with treatment resistance and upregulated by apoptotic stressors such as chemotherapy. Clusterin is upregulated in tumor cells after chemotherapy, hormonal therapy, and radiation therapy, and is overexpressed in prostate and other types of cancers. Clusterin production has been linked to treatment resistance and shorter survival.

Custirsen is a second-generation antisense that inhibits clusterin production, inhibits tumor growth, and reduces resistance to other treatments, e.g., chemotherapy. The SYNERGY trial evaluated docetaxel +/– custirsen as first-line therapy in men with mCRPC ($N=1022$). In 2014, OncoGenex announced that the phase III

SYNERGY trial showed that the addition of custirsen to standard first-line docetaxel/prednisone therapy did not meet the primary endpoint of improvement in overall survival in men with mCRPC compared to docetaxel/prednisone alone (median survival 23.4 months vs. 22.2 months, respectively; hazard ratio 0.93 and one-sided *p* value 0.207).

3 Second Line Treatment in Men with mCRPC Progressing After First-Line Chemotherapy

Since the two pivotal docetaxel/prednisone phase III randomized clinical trials demonstrating OS benefit in first-line treatment, the use of chemotherapy in the postdocetaxel setting has represented an unmet medical need. Various new cytotoxic drugs have been evaluated in second line in men with mCRPC progressing after first-line chemotherapy (e.g., satraplatin, cabazitaxel).

3.1 TROPIC Trial: Cabazitaxel with Prednisone

Cabazitaxel is a next-generation taxane, selected for clinical development based on its ability to overcome docetaxel resistance and its ability to cross the blood–brain barrier in preclinical animal models. For patients who experienced progression during or shortly after docetaxel treatment, a phase III trial comparing cabazitaxel plus prednisone versus mitoxantrone plus prednisone reported a significant OS benefit of 15.1 versus 12.7 months ($P<.001$) and median PFS of 2.8 versus 1.4 months with cabazitaxel (HR, 0.74; 95 % CI, 0.64–0.86; $P<.001$) [10]. This was the first time that a second-line chemotherapy had shown a survival benefit.

QOL benefit was not clearly demonstrated (small nonsignificant improvement in pain compared with mitoxantrone was seen, although rates of pain palliation in both arms were low; overall or prostate-specific QOL was not assessed). Grade 3–4 adverse events were more frequent with cabazitaxel compared to mitoxantrone: grade 3–4 neutropenia (82 % vs. 58 %; p not reported), with a concomitant increase in severe infections. Febrile neutropenia (8 % vs. 1 %; p not reported) and diarrhea (6 % vs. 1 %; p not reported) were greater in the cabazitaxel arm. More deaths were reported within 30 days of last drug administration in the cabazitaxel arm than in the mitoxantrone arm (18 patients (5 %) vs. 9 patients (2 %)).

Cabazitaxel with prednisone resulted in an OS benefit in men who have received prior docetaxel, without a substantial improvement in pain or QOL possibly due to increased toxicity from cabazitaxel.

Preliminary results of a large European compassionate use programme (CUP) and expanded access programme (EAP) showed that the adverse event (AE) profile is manageable in routine practice in both younger (<70 years) and elderly patients (70–74 years and ≥75 years) with mCRPC. Prophylactic G-CSF use was more common in older men, as recommended by international guidelines. In multivariate analysis, age ≥ 75 years, treatment cycle 1 and a neutrophil count <4000/mm^3 before cabazitaxel injection were associated with an increased risk of developing grade ≥3 neutropenia and/or neutropenic complications. In the presence of these factors, G-CSF significantly reduced this risk by 30 %.

Pooled phase I/II safety data suggested that doses of cabazitaxel <25 mg/m^2 showed a significantly decreased incidence of neutropenia. Postmarketing requirements asked for a comparative trial between 20 mg/m^2 and 25 mg/m^2 of cabazitaxel in mCRPC patients. A phase III randomized, open-label, noninferiority trial, PROSELICA, has been performed comparing the efficacy and toxicity of cabazitaxel 20 mg/m^2 plus prednisone versus cabazitaxel 25 mg/m^2 plus prednisone in the postdocetaxel space. The results reported at ASCO 2016 showed that the noninferiority endpoint in OS of 20 mg/m^2 of cabazitaxel versus 25 mg/m^2 was met, while 25 mg/m^2 resulted in more high grade toxicity than 20 mg/m^2.

3.2 Head-to-Head Comparison of Docetaxel Plus Prednisone with Cabazitaxel Plus Prednisone in First Line Chemotherapy Setting

The FIRSTANA trial comparing cabazitaxel plus prednisone at 20 and 25 mg/m^2 versus docetaxel (75 mg/m^2) plus prednisone in patients with chemotherapy-naïve mCRPC has recently completed enrollment. At ASCO 2016, the results of this randomized trial of "Cabazitaxel vs docetaxel in chemotherapy-naive (CN) patients with metastatic castration-resistant prostate cancer (mCRPC): A three-arm phase III study (FIRSTANA)" were presented (A. Oliver Sartor, Abstract Number: 5006). The RCT demonstrated no superiority of cabazitaxel 20 or 25 mg/m^2 plus prednisone over docetaxel 75 mg/m^2 plus prednisone in chemo-naïve patients with overall survival being identical in all three groups of patients.

3.3 Sunitinib Plus Prednisone

The clinical value of adding vascular endothelial growth factor receptor tyrosine kinase inhibitor (VEGFR-TKI) sunitinib was tested in a phase III trial. The SUN 1120 (Sunitinib Plus Prednisone in Patients With Metastatic Castration-Resistant Prostate Cancer After Failure of Docetaxel Chemotherapy) phase III clinical trial evaluated the antiangiogenic agent sunitinib in men with advanced mCRPC who progressed after treatment with docetaxel. Overall, 873 patients with progressive mCRPC after docetaxel-based chemotherapy were randomly assigned to receive sunitinib (n =584) or placebo ($n=289$). Patients also received oral prednisone 5 mg twice daily. The primary endpoint was overall survival (OS); secondary endpoints included progression-free survival (PFS). Two interim analyses were planned. The interim analysis by the data monitoring committee (DMC) found that the combination of sunitinib with prednisone was unlikely to improve OS when compared with prednisone alone and the trial was terminated after the second interim analysis for futility reasons.

After a median overall follow-up of 8.7 months, median OS was 13.1 months and 11.8 months for sunitinib and placebo, respectively (hazard ratio [HR], 0.914; 95 % CI, 0.762–1.097; stratified log-rank test, $p=.168$) [20]. PFS was significantly improved in the sunitinib arm (median 5.6 vs. 4.1 months; HR, 0.725; 95 % CI, 0.591–0.890; stratified log-rank test, $p<.001$). Toxicity and rates of discontinuations because of adverse events (AEs; 27 % vs. 7 %) were greater with sunitinib than placebo.

Based on this phase III trial, the role of antiangiogenic therapy in mCRPC is questionable.

3.4 Satraplatin Plus Prednisone

Satraplatin, an oral platinum analog was tested in a phase III trial in 950 mCRPC patients who progressed after one prior chemotherapy regimen [33]. Patients were randomized (2:1) to receive oral satraplatin 80 mg/m^2 on days 1–5 of a 35-day cycle and prednisone 5 mg twice daily or placebo and prednisone 5 mg twice daily. No difference was seen in the primary endpoint overall survival (HR = 0.98; 95 % CI, 0.84–1.15; $p=.80$). The secondary endpoint time to pain progression (TPP) was significantly better for satraplatin compared to placebo (HR = 0.64; 95 % CI, 0.51–0.79; $p<.001$). A 33 % reduction (hazard ratio [HR] = 0.67; 95 % CI, 0.57–0.77; $p<.001$) was observed in the risk of progression or death with satraplatin versus placebo irrespective of prior docetaxel treatment. Satraplatin was generally well tolerated, with myelosuppression and gastrointestinal disorders occurring more frequently with satraplatin than with placebo.

3.5 Novel Cytotoxic Agents and Overcoming Mechanisms of Resistance to Chemotherapy, e.g., by Inhibition of PARP

Epothilones are a class of chemotherapy that target microtubule disassembly, similar to taxanes. Results from phase II studies demonstrating a positive impact on serum prostate-specific antigen for patupilone and sagopilone, current epothilones in development, along with those of ixabepilone, are comparable with historical response rates to docetaxel. A phase II first-line study with sagopilone plus prednisone showed a PSA response rate of 37 % [5]. A phase II trial of weekly ixabepilone in CRPC patients who were either chemo naive, had received a prior taxane, or two previous chemotherapeutic lines showed PSA response rates of 34 %, 28 %, and 22 %, respectively [18]. Epothilones could be efficacious as an additional therapy in patients who respond to docetaxel chemotherapy.

Inhibiting the enzyme poly (ADP-ribose) polymerase (PARP) by small molecule inhibitors in tumors which have a defect in the homologous DNA recombination pathway, most characteristically due to BRCA mutations, may show efficacy in preselected patient cohorts. Olaparib, a highly potent PARP inhibitor, produced a response rate of 33 % in all patients and the response rate was 88 % among patients with tumors with defects in DNA repair genes.

In a phase II trial reported by Mateo et al. [19], 50 patients were treated with the PARP inhibitor olaparib at 400 mg twice daily. All patients had received prior treatment with docetaxel, 98 % with abiraterone (Zytiga) or enzalutamide (Xtandi), and 58 % with cabazitaxel. The primary endpoint was response rate, defined as objective response, reduction in prostate-specific antigen level of ≥50 %, or confirmed reduction in circulating tumor cell counts. Targeted next-generation sequencing, exome and transcriptome analysis, and digital polymerase chain reaction testing were performed on tumor biopsies from all patients.

Overall, response was observed in 16 of 49 evaluable patients (response rate = 33%, 95 % confidence interval = 20–48 %). Next-generation sequencing identified homozygous deletions, deleterious mutations, or both in DNA-repair genes, including BRCA1/2, ATM, Fanconi's anemia genes, and CHEK2, in 16 (335) of the 49. Of these, 14 (88 %, $p < .001$ vs. patients negative for biomarkers) had a response to olaparib, including each of seven patients with BRCA2 loss (four with biallelic somatic loss, three with germline mutations) and four of five with ATM aberrations.

Median radiologic PFS was 9.8 months in biomarker-positive patients versus 2.7 months in biomarker-negative patients ($p < .001$). Median OS was 13.8 versus 7.5 months ($p = .05$). The most common grade 3 or 4 adverse events were anemia (20 %) and fatigue (12 %).

In January 2016, the US Food and Drug Administration (FDA) granted Breakthrough Therapy designation (BTD) for the oral poly ADP-ribose polymerase (PARP) inhibitor Lynparza™ (olaparib), for the monotherapy treatment of BRCA1/2 or ATM gene mutated mCRPC patients who have received a prior taxane-based chemotherapy and at least one newer hormonal agent (abiraterone or enzalutamide).

4 Novel hormonal treatment

4.1 Abiraterone, an Androgen Biosynthesis Inhibitor

Biosynthesis of extragonadal androgen may contribute to the progression of castration-resistant prostate cancer.

Abiraterone acetate is converted in vivo to abiraterone, an androgen biosynthesis inhibitor, that inhibits 17 α-hydroxylase/C17,20-lyase (CYP17). This enzyme is expressed in testicular, adrenal, and prostatic tumor tissues and is required for androgen biosynthesis. CYP17 catalyzes two sequential reactions: 1) the conversion of pregnenolone and progesterone to their 17α-hydroxy derivatives by 17α-hydroxylase activity and 2) the subsequent formation of dehydroepiandrosterone (DHEA) and androstenedione, respectively, by C17, 20 lyase activity. DHEA and androstenedione are androgens and are precursors of testosterone. Inhibition of CYP17 by abiraterone can also result in increased mineralocorticoid production by the adrenals.

Androgen sensitive prostatic carcinoma responds to treatment that decreases androgen levels. Androgen deprivation therapies, such as treatment with GnRH agonists or orchidectomy, decrease androgen production in the testes but do not affect androgen production by the adrenals or in the tumor.

A phase III double-blind multicenter trial testing the efficacy of abiraterone was performed in 1,195 patients whose metastatic prostate cancer had previously been treated with one of two chemotherapy regimens that included docetaxel. Among the 797 patients randomly assigned to receive abiraterone acetate plus the corticosteroid prednisone, median overall survival was 14.8 months. Among the 398 who received prednisone plus placebo, median survival was 10.9 months [9].

After an interim analysis, the Independent Data Monitoring Committee recommended unblinding the trial and offering abiraterone acetate to patients in the placebo arm. Based on this trial the Food and Drug Administration (FDA) approved abiraterone in April 2011 for men with metastatic castration-resistant prostate cancer that had previously been treated with a chemotherapy regimen containing docetaxel.

In another phase III double-blind multicenter trial, 1,088 patients were randomized to receive abiraterone acetate (1000 mg) plus prednisone (5 mg twice daily) or placebo plus prednisone [28]. The COU-AA-302 study was unblinded after a planned interim analysis showing 43 % of the expected deaths had occurred. The median radiographic progression-free survival was 16.5 months with abiraterone–prednisone and 8.3 months with prednisone alone (hazard ratio for abiraterone–prednisone vs. prednisone alone, 0.53; 95 % confidence interval [CI], 0.45–0.62; $P<0.001$). Over a median follow-up period of 22.2 months, overall survival was improved with abiraterone–prednisone (median not reached, vs. 27.2 months for prednisone alone; hazard ratio, 0.75; 95 % CI, 0.61 to 0.93; $P=0.01$) but did not cross the efficacy boundary. Abiraterone–prednisone showed superiority over prednisone alone with respect to time to initiation of cytotoxic chemotherapy, opiate use for cancer-related pain, prostate-specific antigen progression, and decline in performance status. Grade 3 or 4 mineralocorticoid-related adverse events and abnormalities on liver-function testing were more common with abiraterone–prednisone.

In December 2012, the FDA expanded the approval of abiraterone (ZYTIGA®) (in combination with prednisone) to treat men with metastatic castration-resistant prostate cancer who have not previously undergone chemotherapy.

In the final analysis of the pivotal Phase III trial abiraterone acetate + prednisone achieved a median overall survival (OS) of almost 3 years (34.7 months median overall survival) for abiraterone acetate + prednisone versus 30.3 months with placebo plus prednisone, achieving a 4.4 months improvement in median overall survival compared with placebo plus prednisone [29]. Coprimary endpoint—overall survival: hazard ratio (HR) = 0.81; 95 % CI: 0.70, 0.93; $P=0.0033$. Coprimary endpoint—rPFS: at the prespecified rPFS analysis, median not reached for ZYTIGA® + prednisone versus a median of 8.28 months for placebo + prednisone; HR = 0.425; 95 % CI: 0.347, 0.522; $P=0.0001$.

4.2 Enzalutamide and Other AR-Inhibitors

Enzalutamide (formerly called MDV3100) targets multiple steps in the androgen receptor signaling pathway, the major driver of prostate cancer growth. Enzalutamide, a synthetic, nonsteroidal pure oral, once-daily androgen receptor inhibitor, has been investigated in various early and phase III trials. In the AFFIRM study 1,199 postdocetaxel mCRPC patients were randomized in a 2:1 ratio to receive enzalutamide 160 mg or placebo once daily. Patients were stratified according to performance-status score and pain intensity [30]. Enzalutamide was shown to be superior over placebo in the primary endpoint of overall survival; 18.4 months (95 % confidence interval [CI], 17.3 not yet reached) versus 13.6 months (95 % CI, 11.3–15.8) with a hazard ratio for death in the enzalutamide group of 0.63 (95 % CI, 0.53 to 0.75; $p<0.001$) as well as the secondary endpoints of PSA level response rate (54 % vs. 2 %, $p<0.001$), the soft-tissue response rate (29 % vs. 4 %, $p<0.001$), the quality-of-life response rate (43 % vs. 18 %, $p<0.001$), the time to PSA progression (8.3 vs. 3.0 months; hazard ratio, 0.25; $p<0.001$), radiographic progression-free survival (8.3 vs. 2.9 months; hazard ratio, 0.40; $p<0.001$), and time to the first skeletal-related event (16.7 vs. 13.3 months; hazard ratio, 0.69; $p<0.001$). A higher incidence of all grade fatigue (34 vs. 29 %), diarrhea (21 vs. 18 %), hot flashes (20 vs. 10 %), musculoskeletal pain (14 vs. 10 %), and headache (12 vs. 6 %) was seen in the enzalutamide group than in the placebo group with a lower incidence of grade 3 or higher adverse events (45 vs. 53 %). In the enzalutamide group five of the 800 patients (0.6 %) were reported to have seizures; no seizures were reported in the placebo group. In August 2012, the FDA initially approved enzalutamide (XTANDI), for use in patients with metastatic CRPC who previously received docetaxel (chemotherapy).

Subsequently, enzalutamide was also tested in 1,717 mCRPC patients before chemotherapy [6]. In the PREVAIL trial, enzalutamide 160 mg daily was compared with placebo (not with chemotherapy as the study population consisted of men with asymptomatic or minimally symptomatic advanced prostate cancer who usually do not have chemotherapy at this stage). This in contrast to the comparator arm prednisone, which has activity in mCRPC patients, in the pre-docetaxel phase III COU-AA-302 study testing abiraterone.

Coprimary endpoints for the PREVAIL study were radiographic progression-free survival and overall survival. Treatment with enzalutamide resulted in a significant improvement in radiographic PFS at 12 months of 65 % compared with 14 % in the placebo group (81 % risk reduction; hazard ratio in the enzalutamide group, 0.19; 95 % confidence interval [CI], 0.15–0.23; $p<0.001$). At the planned interim analysis conducted after 540 deaths, the median follow-up for survival was approximately 22 months. At that time 72 % in the enzalutamide group and 63 % in the placebo group were still alive resulting in a 29 % decrease in risk of death (hazard ratio, 0.71; 95 % CI, 0.60–0.84; $p<0.001$). The estimated median overall survival was 32.4 months in the enzalutamide group compared with 30.2 months in the placebo group. Enzalutamide was superior with respect to all secondary endpoints, including time until the initiation of cytotoxic chemotherapy (hazard ratio, 0.35), time until the first skeletal-related event (hazard ratio, 0.72), a complete or partial soft-tissue response (59 % vs. 5 %), time until prostate-specific antigen (PSA) progression (hazard ratio, 0.17), and a rate of decline of at least 50 % in PSA (78 % vs. 3 %) ($p<0.001$ for all comparisons). Enzalutamide significantly decreased the risk of radiographic progression and death and delayed the initiation of chemotherapy in men with metastatic prostate cancer.

Updated results show that enzalutamide delayed the radiographically detected progression of the disease by 81 % (rPFS: hazard ratio [HR], 0.19; $p<.0001$) with a disease control rate in soft tissue of 59 % (20 % complete responses and 39 % partial responses) compared with 5 % in patients on placebo. On average, patients treated with enzalutamide received chemotherapy about 17 months later than those in the placebo arm (28 months vs. 10.8 months; HR, 0.35; $p<.0001$).

In 2014, the FDA approved enzalutamide for use in men with metastatic CRPC who have not received chemotherapy. Enzalutamide is generally well tolerated and results in relatively few side effects.

Next-generation AR inhibitors, such as ARN- 509 and ODM-201 with more potent AR-inhibitory capacity than enzalutamide, are currently being tested in various clinical trials.

4.3 Acquired Resistance Mechanisms

Prostate cancer cells demonstrate “addiction” to androgen receptor (AR) signaling in all stages of disease progression, but it has now been shown that various molecular alterations indicating treatment resistance may arise in patients treated with AR-directed therapies. Second-generation androgen receptor antagonist enzalutamide and abiraterone are major breakthroughs in the treatment of mCRPC, but primary resistance occurs in approximately 20–40 % of patients typified by failure to exhibit a PSA response or clinical or radiological improvements. Moreover, in all patients who respond initially in time resistance will develop. Various mechanisms may account for resistance under selection pressure by abiraterone and enzalutamide. Examples are gene amplification of androgen receptor and/or CYP17 upregulation, emergence of AR splice variants and AR point mutations.

4.3.1 AR and CYP17 Upregulation

AR gene amplification and protein overexpression have been observed in a high proportion of tumors during treatment with androgen deprivation therapy (ADT) and this may account for resistance to novel antiandrogens such as abiraterone and enzalutamide. AR amplification and AR gene aberrations were also noted in circulating cell-free DNA and this was associated with resistance to enzalutamide and abiraterone in mCRPC. Upregulation of CYP17 or other androgen-synthetic enzymes also seems to play a role in resistance to novel antiandrogens. Intratumoral CYP17A1 upregulation was associated with tumor relapse in preclinical studies.

4.3.2 AR Splice Variants

Alternative splicing of AR mRNA resulting in AR splice variants has been put forward as a mechanism for the resistance to both enzalutamide and abiraterone. Multiple AR splice variants have now been reported. Such AR splice variants encode for a truncated AR protein that lacks the C-terminal ligand binding domain (LBD) while retaining the trans-activating N-terminal domain. Thus, the truncated AR protein is no longer able to bind the ligand but is still constitutively active as transcription factors and able to promote the activation of target genes (as it would do after ligand binding).

Following inhibition of the AR pathway with abiraterone and enzalutamide, such selection pressure results in expression of ARV7 and other splice variants.

Antonarakis and coworkers [1] elegantly demonstrated the prognostic value of AR-V7. In mCRPC patients about to start abiraterone or enzalutamide treatment, AR-V7 mRNA expression could be detected in their circulating tumor cells (CTCs).

PSA responses (PSA decline ≥50 %), progression-free survival (PFS), and OS were compared between patients positive for AR-V7 and patients without AR-V7 expression. Eighteen of the 62 patients (29 %) tested positive for AR-V7 at baseline (12 of 31 enzalutamide-treated patients and 6 of 31 abiraterone-treated patients). None of these 18 AR-V7-positive patients had a PSA response with enzalutamide or abiraterone, compared with AR-V7-negative patients who had a 53 and 68 % PSA response rate to enzalutamide and abiraterone, respectively. PFS and OS were also decreased for the AR-V7-positive patients. The study results indicated that AR-V7 detection in CTCs might be associated with primary resistance to novel antiandrogen therapies and suggested that expression of alternative AR splice variants is increased as a consequence of continued androgen-directed therapies. AR-V7 testing had been performed in CTCs which means that only a proportion of circulating tumor cells are tested whereas at the site of the metastases tumor cells displaying other types of resistance may exist in vivo.

Efstathiou et al. [11] evaluated 60 men with mCRPC for AR-V7 expression at the protein level from bone marrow biopsies prior to treatment with enzalutamide and after 8 weeks of therapy. Given the high incidence of the splice variant expression noted in this study, AR-V7 appears to be a frequent cause of drug resistance to enzalutamide in this setting. AR-V7 can thus be reliably measured in both tissue and circulating tumor cells derived from mCRPC patients, and detection of AR-V7 in mCRPC has potential clinical utility as a treatment selection marker.

4.3.3 AR Point Mutations and Other Mechanisms of Resistance, Including Escape via Other Tumor Histologies

AR point mutations have also been found in CRPC patients undergoing hormonal therapy and novel antiandrogens during progression. Another mechanism of resistance by which tumors escape to AR inhibition may be the upregulation or induction of the glucocorticoid receptor (GR), which could subsequently form the driver pathway in mCRPC patients exposed to AR blockade. Other mechanisms of resistance may lead to changes in the histological type of the tumor cells, e.g., emergence of small cell carcinoma whether this results from transformation to another type of cell or results from selection of preexisting tumor cell clones. Another cell type may be the recently reported intermediate atypical carcinoma (IAC). The prognosis for patients harboring the IAC histology approximates that of small cell cancer and is more unfavorable than that of the classical adenocarcinoma histology. Other mechanisms of tumor cell scape may be induction of expression of programmed death-ligand 1 (PD-L1) on tumor cells as has been observed in enzalutamide-resistant prostate cancer cell lines and increased amounts of circulating PD-L1/2-positive dendritic cells. Clinical trials with checkpoint inhibitors in enzalutamide-refractory mCRPC and in AR-V7-positive mCRPC are currently ongoing.

4.3.4 Novel Drugs That May Overcome Resistance to Second Generation Androgen-Receptor Inhibitors

Galeterone (Gal) is a small molecule that disrupts androgen receptor (AR) signaling via inhibition of CYP17, AR antagonism, and AR degradation. Galeterone may overcome resistance to current therapy resulting from upregulation of full-length AR, splice variants AR and AR mutations, and is now tested in clinical trials.

5 Overall Conclusion

Since 2004, there have been rapid advancements in the treatment of CRPC with two chemotherapeutic agents and several other novel agents which demonstrated OS improvement being approved for CRPC. Various combinations of docetaxel with targeted agents have been extremely disappointing and docetaxel had proven to be a poor partner with regard to combinations with other classes of agents.

Interestingly, molecular targeting of previously treated mCRPC patients with a defect in DNA repair genes with the PARP inhibitor olaparib led to a high response rate has been shown to be an effective approach.

Novel therapies such as abiraterone and enzalutamide that maximally decrease androgen receptor (AR) signaling activity in metastatic castration-resistant prostate cancer (mCRPC) meant a major step forward in prostate cancer therapeutics and have been added to our armamentarium in recent years. Even though abiraterone and enzalutamide have demonstrated significant survival benefits in mCRPC patients, a significant proportion of patients have primary resistance to these agents and virtually all patients develop secondary resistance. AR-dependent and AR-independent mechanisms, including upregulation of AR and cytochrome P450 17α-hydroxylase/17,20-lyase (CYP17), induction of AR splice variants, AR point mutations, upregulation of glucocorticoid receptor, activation of alternative oncogenic signaling pathways, neuroendocrine transformation, and immune evasion via programmed death-ligand 1 upregulation, may be drivers of therapeutic resistance.

There is an unmet need to develop biomarkers to select patients who may benefit from a particular therapy. Ongoing trials using agents with novel mechanisms of action may further revolutionize the therapeutic landscape. In the coming years we will hopefully be able to add new agents to the current armamentarium.

References

1. Antonarakis ES, Lu C, Wang H, et al. AR-V7 and resistance to enzalutamide and abiraterone in prostate cancer. N Engl J Med. 2014;371:1028–38.
2. Araujo JC, Trudel GC, Saad F, et al. Docetaxel and dasatinib or placebo in men with metastatic castration-resistant prostate cancer (READY): a randomised, double-blind phase 3 trial. Lancet Oncol. 2013;14(13):1307–16. doi:10.1016/S1470-2045(13)70479-0. Epub 2013 Nov 8.
3. Armstrong AJ, Tannock IF, de Wit R, et al. The development of risk groups in men with metastatic castration-resistant prostate cancer based on risk factors for PSA decline and survival. Eur J Cancer. 2010;46:517–25.

4. Beer TM, Pierce WC, Lowe BA, Henner WD. Phase II study of weekly docetaxel in symptomatic androgen-independent prostate cancer. Ann Oncol. 2001;12:1273–9.
5. Beer TM, Smith DC, Hussain A, et al. Phase II study of first-line sagopilone plus prednisone in patients with castration-resistant prostate cancer: a phase II study of the Department of Defense Prostate Cancer Clinical Trials Consortium. Br J Cancer. 2012;107(5):808–13. doi:10.1038/bjc.2012.339. Epub 2012 Jul 31.
6. Beer TM, Armstrong AJ, Rathkopf DE, et al. Enzalutamide in metastatic prostate cancer before chemotherapy. N Engl J Med. 2014;371:424–33.
7. Berry W, Dakhil S, Gregurich MA, Asmar L. Phase II trial of single-agent weekly docetaxel in hormone-refractory, symptomatic, metastatic carcinoma of the prostate. Semin Oncol. 2001;4 suppl 15:8–15.
8. Berry W, Dakhil S, Modiano M, et al. Phase III study of mitoxantrone plus low dose prednisone versus low dose prednisone alone in patients with asymptomatic hormone refractory prostate cancer. J Urol. 2002;168:2439–43.
9. de Bono JS, Logothetis CJ, Molina A, et al. COU-AA-301 Investigators Abiraterone and increased survival in metastatic prostate cancer. N Engl J Med. 2011;364(21):1995–2005.
10. de Bono JS, Oudard S, Ozguroglu M, et al. Prednisone plus cabazitaxel or mitoxantrone for metastatic castration-resistant prostate cancer progressing after docetaxel treatment: a randomised open-label trial. Lancet. 2010;376:1147–54.
11. Efstathiou E, Titus M, Wen S, et al. Molecular characterization of enzalutamide-treated bone metastatic castration-resistant prostate cancer. Eur Urol. 2015;67(1):53–60.
12. Fizazi K, Le Maitre A, Hudes G, Berry WR, Kelly WK, Eymard JC, Logothetis CJ, Pignon JP, Michiels S. Addition of estramustine to chemotherapy and survival of patients with castration-refractory prostate cancer: a meta-analysis of individual patient data. Lancet Oncol. 2007;8:994–1000.
13. Heidenreich A, Real SK, Szkarlat K, Bogdanova N, et al. A randomized, double-blind, multicenter, phase 2 study of a human monoclonal antibody to human αν integrins (intetumumab) in combination with docetaxel and prednisone for the first-line treatment of patients with metastatic castration-resistant prostate cancer. Ann Oncol. 2013;24(2):329–36. doi:10.1093/annonc/mds505. Epub 2012 Oct 26.
14. Kantoff PW, Halabi S, Conaway M, et al. Hydrocortisone with or without mitoxantrone in men with hormone-refractory prostate cancer: results of the cancer and leukemia group B 9182 study. J Clin Oncol. 1999;17:2506–13.
15. Kellokumpu-Lehtinen P-L, Harmenberg U, Joensuu T, et al. 2-weekly versus 3-weekly docetaxel to treat castration resistant advanced prostate cancer: a randomised, phase 3 trial. Lancet Oncol. 2013;14(2):117–24.
16. Kelly WK, Halabi S, Carducci MA, et al. A randomized, double-blind, placebo-controlled phase III trial comparing docetaxel, prednisone, and placebo with docetaxel, prednisone, and bevacizumab in men with metastatic castration-resistant prostate cancer (mCRPC): survival results of CALGB 90401. J Clin Oncol. 2010;28(suppl):344s, abstr LBA4511.
17. Kelly WK, et al. Randomized, double-blind, placebo-controlled Phase III trial comparing docetaxel and prednisone with or without bevacizumab in men with metastastic castration-resistant prostate cancer: CALGB 90401. J Clin Oncol. 2012;30(13):1534–40.
18. Liu G, Chen YH, Dipaola R, et al. Phase II trial of weekly ixabepilone in men with metastatic castrate-resistant prostate cancer (E3803): a trial of the Eastern Cooperative Oncology Group. Clin Genitourin Cancer. 2012;10(2):99–105. doi:10.1016/j.clgc.2012.01.009. Epub 2012 Mar 3.
19. Mateo J, Carreira S, Sandhu S, et al. DNA-repair defects and olaparib in metastatic prostate cancer. N Engl J Med. 2015;373(18):1697–708. doi:10.1056/NEJMoa1506859.
20. Michaelson MD, Oudard S, Ou YC, et al. Randomized, placebo-controlled, phase III trial of sunitinib plus prednisone versus prednisone alone in progressive, metastatic, castration-resistant prostate cancer. J Clin Oncol. 2014;32(2):76–82. doi:10.1200/JCO.2012.48.5268. Epub2013Dec9.
21. Nelson JB, Fizazi K, Miller K, Higano C, Moul JW, Akaza H, Morris T, McIntosh S, Pemberton K, Gleave M. Phase 3, randomized, placebo-controlled study of zibotentan (ZD4054) in patients with castration-resistant prostate cancer metastatic to bone. Cancer. 2012;118:5709–18. doi:10.1002/cncr.27674. Epub 2012 Jul 11.
22. Perry CM, McTavish D. Estramustine phosphate sodium. A review of its pharmacodynamic and pharmacokinetic properties, and therapeutic efficacy in prostate cancer. Drugs Aging. 1995;7:49–74.
23. Petrylak DP, Tangen CM, Hussain MH, et al. Docetaxel and estramustine compared with mitoxantrone and prednisone for advanced refractory prostate cancer. N Engl Med. 2004;351:1513–20.
24. Petrylak DP, Vogelzang NJ, Budnik N, Wiechno PJ, Sternberg CN, Doner K, Bellmunt J, Burke JM, de Olza MO, Choudhury A, Gschwend JE, Kopyltsov E, Flechon A, Van As N, Houede N, Barton D, Fandi A, Jungnelius U, Li S, de Wit R, Fizazi K. Docetaxel and prednisone with or without lenalidomide in chemotherapy-naïve patients with metastatic castration-resistant prostate cancer (MAINSAIL): a randomised, double-blind, placebo-controlled phase 3 trial. Lancet Oncol. 2015;16(4):417–25. doi:10.1016/S1470-2045(15)70025-2. Epub 2015 Mar 3.
25. Picus J, Schultz M. Docetaxel (Taxotere) as monotherapy in the treatment of hormone refractory prostate cancer: preliminary results. Semin Oncol. 1999;26((5) Suppl 17):14–8.
26. Quin et al. Docetaxel and atrasentan versus docetaxel and placebo for men with advanced castration-resistant prostate cancer (SWOG S0421): a randomised phase 3

trial. Lancet Oncol. 2013;14(9):893–900. doi: 10.1016/S1470-2045(13)70294-8. Epub 2013 Jul 17.
27. Roth BJ, Yeap BY, Wilding G, et al. Taxol in advanced, hormone-refractory carcinoma of the prostate. Cancer. 1993;72:2457–60.
28. Ryan CJ, Smith MR, de Bono JS, et al. Abiraterone in metastatic prostate cancer without previous chemotherapy. N Engl J Med. 2013;368(2):138–48. doi:10.1056/NEJMoa1209096. Epub 2012 Dec 10.
29. Ryan CJ, Smith MR, Fizazi K. et al; for the COU-AA-302 Investigators. Abiraterone acetate plus prednisone versus placebo plus prednisone in chemotherapy-naive men with metastatic castration-resistant prostate cancer (COU-AA-302): final overall survival analysis of a randomised, double-blind, placebo-controlled Phase 3 study. Lancet Oncol. 2015;16(2):152–60.
30. Scher HI, Fizazi K, Fred Saad F, et al. for the AFFIRM Investigators*. Increased survival with enzalutamide in prostate cancer after chemotherapy. N Engl J Med. 2012;367:1187–97. 27 Sept 2012. doi:10.1056/NEJMoa1207506.
31. Scher HI, Jia X, Chi K, et al. Randomized, open-label phase III trial of docetaxel plus high-dose calcitriol versus docetaxel plus prednisone for patients with castration-resistant prostate cancer. J Clin Oncol. 2011;29(16):2191–8. doi:10.1200/JCO.2010.32.8815. Epub 2011 Apr 11.
32. Small E, Demkow T, Gerritsen WR, et al. Proceedings genitourinary cancer symposium (February 26–28, 2009, Orlando, FL), A phase III trial of GVAX immunotherapy for prostate cancer in combination with docetaxel versus docetaxel plus prednisone in symptomatic, castration-resistant prostate cancer, suppl, abstr 7.
33. Sternberg CN, Petrylak DP, Sartor O, et al. Multinational, double-blind, phase III study of prednisone and either satraplatin or placebo in patients with castrate-refractory prostate cancer progressing afterprior chemotherapy: the SPARC trial. J Clin Oncol. 2009;27(32):5431–8. doi:10.1200/JCO.2008.20.1228. Epub 2009 Oct 5.
34. Tannock IF, de Wit R, Berry WR, et al. Docetaxel plus prednisone or mitoxantrone plus prednisone for advanced prostate cancer. N Engl J Med. 2004;351:1502–12.
35. Tannock IF, Fizazi K, Ivanov S, et al. VENICE investigators. Aflibercept versus placebo in combination with docetaxel and prednisone for treatment of men with metastatic castration-resistant prostate cancer (VENICE): a phase 3, double-blind randomised trial. Lancet Oncol. 2013;14(8):760–8. doi:10.1016/S1470-2045(13)70184-0. Epub 2013 Jun 4.
36. Tannock IF, Osoba D, Stockler MR, et al. Chemotherapy with mitoxantrone plus prednisone or prednisone alone for symptomatic hormone-resistant prostate cancer: a Canadian randomized trial with palliative end points. J Clin Oncol. 1996;14:1756–64.
37. Trivedi C, Redman B, Flaherty LE, et al. Weekly 1-hour infusion of paclitaxel. Clinical feasibility and efficacy in patients with hormonerefractory prostate carcinoma. Cancer. 2000;89:431–43.
38. Yagoda A, Petrylak D. Cytotoxic chemotherapy for advanced hormone-resistant prostate cancer. Cancer. 1993;71:1098–109.

Bone-Targeted Therapies in Prostate Cancer

Abdulazeez T. Salawu, Catherine Handforth, and Janet E. Brown

1 Introduction

The bone is by far the most common site for metastasis in prostate cancer (PCa) with around 70–80 % patients with advanced disease having bone involvement on imaging and an even greater proportion displaying micro-metastases on autopsy [1]. Bone involvement in PCa leads to profound local consequences in terms of bone integrity, and can be associated with significant morbidity. Improvements in survival have been seen as newer, systemic treatments emerge for metastatic PCa, but all these currently remain non-curative and do not specifically address the local consequence of metastatic bone disease. This means that patients with bone metastatic PCa carry the risk of skeletal morbidity for longer, the reduction of which is of paramount importance in order to maintain a good quality of life [2]. The use of bone-targeted agents are central to modalities used to achieve this aim because, not only do they address the local consequences of bone metastases, but the newer agents have direct effects on the tumour itself at this site.

Even outside the bone metastatic setting, key PCa treatments including androgen-deprivation therapy (ADT) and corticosteroids contribute to significant decreases in bone mineral density (BMD) collectively termed cancer treatment-induced bone loss (CTIBL), which is associated with an increased risk of fractures and other skeletal morbidity. The use of bone-targeted agents has emerged as an important tool in the preservation of bone health among these patients, as they have been shown to increase BMD and reduce fracture risk [3].

This chapter describes the current understanding of the cellular and molecular pathophysiology of bone disease, its consequences and the current and emerging evidence for the use of bone-targeted agents in clinical practice.

2 Pathophysiology of Bone Metastases from Prostate Cancer

Initially proposed by Paget in 1889, the 'seed and soil' theory describes the preferential interaction between metastatic cancer cells (seeds) with the environment (soil) at specific organs to facilitate their growth and forms the basis of our current understanding of cancer metastasis to bone. The bone microenvironment comprises a mineralised extracellular matrix (ECM) and a range of specific cells that are regulated by various systemic and paracrine factors that provide a perfect milieu that PCa cells are able to co-opt and utilise for their growth and survival [4]. Using a molecular mechanism similar to that utilised by haemotopoietic stem cells (HSCs) for homing to their bone marrow

A.T. Salawu (✉) • C. Handforth • J.E. Brown
Academic Unit of Clinical Oncology, University of Sheffield, Weston Park Hospital,
Whitham Road, Sheffield S10 2SJ, UK
e-mail: a.salawu@sheffield.ac.uk

M. Bolla, H. van Poppel (eds.), *Management of Prostate Cancer*,
DOI 10.1007/978-3-319-42769-0_23

niche, PCa tumour cells disseminated in the circulation express the chemokine receptor CXRCR4, which interacts with the chemoattractant protein CXCL12 expressed by endothelial cells and osteoblasts present in the bone microenvironment. On arrival in the HSC niche, evidence suggests that the PCa cells act as molecular parasites that out-bind HSCs for receptors such as ANXA2 with which they remain anchored within their niche and release factors that drive HSCs differentiation to progenitor cell pools or into the peripheral circulation [5]. Additional interactions between PCa tumour cell surface proteins such as αvβ3 integrins with bone marrow extracellular matrix (ECM) proteins have been shown to promote colonisation and survival. Local influences of the bone microenvironment including physical factors such as hypoxia and low pH trigger molecular signalling via the HIF-1a, NF-kB and AP-1 pathways, which have been shown to promote PCa cell growth [4].

Normal bone metabolism involves continuous, tightly regulated remodelling that balances bone matrix resorption by osteoclasts with matrix formation by osteoblasts. The key molecular signalling mechanism that promotes osteoclast activation involves an interaction between the receptor activator of nuclear factor-kB (RANK) that is expressed on the surface of osteoclast precursors with its ligand (RANKL), a soluble factor that is produced by mainly by osteoblasts [4]. Negative regulation exists in the form of osteoprotegerin, a soluble decoy receptor to RANKL that is also produced by osteoblasts in response to factors (such as oestrogens and androgens) and inhibits osteoclast activation and bone resorption by preventing RANKL-RANK interaction [4].

PCa cells present in bone secrete several factors such as parathyroid hormone-related protein (PTHrP), which stimulates osteoblastic release of soluble RANKL. The resultant RANKL-RANK signalling causes increased osteoclastogenesis and resorption of the mineralised bone ECM, with breakdown of type 1 collagen fibres and the release of stores of calcium and growth factors such as TGFβ. The release of TGFβ in turn causes increased proliferation of tumour cells and further PTHrP secretion, thus setting up a self-propagating 'vicious cycle' that promotes growth of bone metastasis with attendant osteolysis. Further, evidence suggests that tumour cells can exhibit 'osteomimicry', whereby they acquire osteoclastic properties themselves or promote formation of giant, multinucleated cells from osteoclast precursors with increased bone resorptive function [4].

PCa cells also release factors that directly or indirectly influence an increase in osteoblast activity. Tumour cells secrete Endothelin-1 (ET1), a soluble factor that directly stimulates osteoblast activity via the ETA receptor pathway. Interestingly N-terminal fragments of PTHrP bear strong sequence homology with ET1, suggesting that they may also play a role in osteoblast activation, while TGFβ has also been shown to promote osteoblast growth [6]. The result is that PCa bone metastases have a predominantly sclerotic appearance on radiologic imaging in spite of clear evidence of increased bone resorption [6]. Further, PCa bone metastases are associated with an increase in markers of both bone formation and resorption reflecting elevated both osteoclast and osteoblast activity (discussed later in this chapter).

3 Consequences of Metastatic Bone Disease in Prostate Cancer

3.1 Clinical and Socioeconomic Implications

The clinical sequelae of PCa bone metastases arise predominantly as a result of increased bone resorption. They include severe bone pain; pathological fractures necessitating surgery or radiotherapy; spinal cord and nerve root compression, bone marrow infiltration and hypercalcaemia. These can also have significant health implications for patients in terms of their physical, emotional and functional well-being in the form of fatigue, pain, depression, anxiety, impaired mobility and reduced independence, as well as an increased risk of mortality. With increased survival rates of metastatic PCa patients, the cumulative effect is that of increased stress on health and social care systems.

Objective measures of skeletal morbidity from bone metastases include the frequency or time to development of skeletal-related events (SREs) and symptomatic skeletal events (SSEs). SREs by definition include pathological fractures, (symptomatic or incidental finding), spinal cord compression, necessity for radiation to bone (for pain or impending fracture) or surgery to bone. SSEs are very similar to SRE by definition, but exclude asymptomatic pathologic fractures [7]. SREs and SSEs have been defined for use as composite endpoints for clinical trials of bone-targeted agents. SRE/SSEs occur with a very high frequency in patients with bone metastases from PCa with one study report showing that up to half of patients experience at least one SRE within 2 years in the absence of treatment with bone-targeted agents and that an increased risk of further SREs exists following an initial event [8]. In addition, the degree of skeletal involvement, an increase in bone turnover markers and progression of disease are all factors that increase the risk of SRE [8].

3.2 Biochemical Consequences

The cellular and metabolic processes involved in bone matrix resorption and formation result in the release of proteins, peptide fragments and mineral components of the bone ECM into the circulation, which can be measured in blood and urine. These bone turnover markers may be broadly divided into markers of bone resorption and bone formation. Examples of bone resorption markers include the N- and C- terminal cross-linked telopeptide breakdown products of type I collagen, termed NTX and CTX respectively and measurable in both serum and urine. Bone formation markers measureable in serum include bone-derived alkaline phosphatase (BALP) which is released by osteoblasts during matrix formation, and the N- and C-terminal propeptides formed by cleavage of type I procollagen to native collagen (P1NP and P1CP, respectively).

Several studies have demonstrated correlation between bone turnover marker levels and the extent of bone disease in PCa both before and during treatment and suggested that they may be used to identify either a need for treatment with bone-targeted agents, or treatment failure [9]. Bone turnover markers have also been found to be predictive of the risk of SREs and overall survival and have potential to be used as surrogate end points in clinical trials. However, these require further evaluation in large prospective studies before they can be validated for this purpose. Routine clinical use of bone turnover markers to monitor response to bone-targeted agent treatment is also currently limited, as a result of diurnal and interlaboratory variations in measured levels that require further research and optimisation so they can be standardised.

4 Bone-Targeted Agents in Prostate Cancer: Bisphosphonates

4.1 Mechanisms of Action, Mode of Administration and Side Effects

Bisphosphonates are a group of compounds that contain two phosphonate groups and have a molecular structure similar to pyrophosphate. This molecular similarity confers on them a high affinity for mineralised bone matrix where they bind to hydroxyapatite and accumulate. Bisphosphonates are subsequently released during bone resorption and ingested by osteoclasts, with resultant inhibition of osteoclast bone resorptive function. The molecular mechanism by which they achieve this inhibition depends on whether or not they contain nitrogenous groups. Non-nitrogen-containing bisphosphonates (such as clodronate) disrupt cellular energy metabolism leading to osteoclast apoptosis. The more potent nitrogen-containing bisphosphonates (such as ibandronate, pamidronate, zoledronate) inhibit the HMG CoA reductase pathway and prevent the formation of metabolites required for lipid modification of G-proteins required for normal cytoskeletal function that is key to osteoclastogenesis, survival and bone resorptive ability [10]. Bisphosphonates that have been evaluated in phase 3 trials of PCa include alendronate, etidronate, pamidronate, clodronate and zoledronate. Some bisphosphonates (such as clodronate) are administered orally and others by the intravenous route such as zoledronate, which is given as a 30-min intravenous infusion. Zoledronate is not metabolised and around 40 % of the drug is excreted unchanged by the kidneys in the first 24 h with the rest bound to bone tissue and slowly released into circulation.

Bisphosphonates in clinical use and in trials are generally well tolerated with few and infrequent adverse effects. Orally administered bisphosphonates such as clodronate may incur gastrointestinal side effects and, for zoledronate, dose modifications may be required in mild to moderate renal impairment (creatinine clearance 30–60 L/min) and it is contraindicated in patients with creatinine clearance <30 L/min. Other reported side effects of intravenous bisphosphonates include flu-like symptoms and hypocalcaemia.

A rare, but potentially serious side effect of potent bisphosphonates, for example, zoledronate, is osteonecrosis of the jaw (ONJ). This is defined as an area of exposed jaw bone that persists for more than 8 weeks in patients without previous craniofacial radiation [11]. Its severity can range from mild pain, swelling or infection that can be treated conservatively with mouthwashes and antibiotics, to severe symptoms that require surgical debridement and bone resection. Risk factors identified for ONJ development include higher frequency and longer duration of BP use, poor baseline dental hygiene, invasive dental procedures such as extractions, systemic comorbidities and concomitant use of corticosteroids [11]. Precautionary dental health measures are now recommended for patients receiving potent bisphosphonates such as zoledronic acid.

4.2 Bisphosphonates in Prevention of SREs in Patients with Metastatic Castrate-Resistant Prostate Cancer (mCRPC)

In the Zoledronic acid 039 trial, 643 patients with mCRPC were randomised to receive 4-weekly IV zoledronate at a dose of 4 mg or 8 mg or placebo (Table 1). The primary endpoint of SRE incidence was 38 % in the zoledronate arms after 24 months compared with 49 % in the placebo arm ($p = 0.028$) [8]. Time to first SRE and the rate of development of SREs per year in both groups also showed favourable results in the zoledronate arms ($p = 0.009$ and $p = 0.005$, respectively) and continued administration of zoledronate following one SRE was shown to reduce the risk of further SREs by approximately 36 % (risk ratio [RR] 0.64, 95 % confidence interval [CI] 0.485–0.845; $p = 0.002$). This efficacy response was accompanied by a sharp reduction in bone resorption markers, with urinary NTX to creatinine (uNTX:Cr) ratios falling by approximately 70 % within the first month of zoledronate treatment, independent of dose, and remaining suppressed. This demonstration of efficacy led to its approval for reduction of SRE risk in mCRPC by the European Medicines Agency (EMA) and United States Food and Drug Administration (US FDA). No significant benefit with zoledronate was however seen in imaging or biomarker parameters of progression free survival (PFS) or in overall survival (OS) [8]. In their combined analysis of three phase 3 trials involving around 5700 patients, Saad and colleagues reported 1.3 % frequency of ONJ in patients receiving zoledronic acid, the majority of which was treated conservatively [11].

Less potent bisphosphonates are not widely used routinely for SRE prevention in PCa.

4.3 Zoledronate in Castration-Sensitive Patients

CALGB 90202 was a phase 3 randomised placebo controlled trial that evaluated zoledronate in the castration-sensitive, PCa bone metastasis setting [12]. Patients in the experimental arm were given IV zoledronate every 4 weeks and all patients were switched to this arm on development of castration resistance. It recruited 645 out of a planned 680 patients and recorded 299 of an expected 470 SREs before it was terminated prematurely due to withdrawal of sponsor support. The median time to first SRE was 31.9 *vs.*

Table 1 Notable phase 3 trials of bone-targeted agents in prostate cancer

Agent/trial	Accrual	Eligibility criteria	Arms	Primary outcome measure	Results of primary outcome	Comments
Non-metastatic PCa						
Clodronate						
MRC PR04 [14]	508	Non-metastatic PCa	Clodronate 2080 mg *vs.* placebo daily for 5 years	Symptomatic BPFS or OS	107 vs 131 mo HR 1.22; $p = 0.23$	Clodronate does not alter the natural history of non-metastatic PCa
Zoledronate						
704 [16]	398 (991 planned)	Non-metastatic CRPC rising PSA	Zoledronate 4 mg *vs.* placebo every 4 weeks	NA	NA	Trial terminated early due to low event rate
ZEUS [17]	1433	High-risk localised PCa Gleason Score 8–10 PSA > 20 node positive	Zoledronate 4 mg *vs.* Observation every 3 months	Proportion with bone metastases	17.1 % *vs.* 17.0 % $p = 0.95$	No role for zoledronate in patients with high-risk localised PCa
Denosumab						
147 [18]	1432	Non-metastatic Castrate-resistant PCa PSA ≥8 ng/ml or PSA DT ≤10 months	Denosumab 120 mg *vs.* placebo every 4 weeks	BMFS	29.5 *vs.* 25.2 months HR: 0.85; $p = 0.028$	– No difference in PFS or OS – ONJ in 4.6 % with denosumab
Metastatic castration-sensitive PCa						
Clodronate						
MRC PR05 [15]	311	Castration-sensitive PCa with bone metastases	Clodronate 2080 mg vs placebo daily for 3 years	Symptomatic BPFS	26.3 vs 19.6 months HR: 0.79; $p = 0.066$	No significant benefit on either bone or non-bone metastatic disease progression
Zoledronate						
CALGB 90202 [12]	645	Castration-sensitive PCa with bone metastases	Zoledronate 4 mg *vs.* placebo every 4 weeks	Time to first SRE	31.9 *vs.* 29.8 months HR: 0.97; $p = 0.39$	Terminated prior to full accrual

(continued)

Table 1 (continued)

Agent/trial	Accrual	Eligibility criteria	Arms	Primary outcome measure	Results of primary outcome	Comments
[a]STAMPEDE [13]	2962	Castration-sensitive PCa (high risk, locally advanced or metastatic) on first-line hormone therapy	+no other agents vs +zoledronate 4 mg vs + docetaxel vs + docetaxel + zoledronate 4 mg	Overall survival	No OS benefit when zoledronate added to SOC alone ($p=0.416$) or to docetaxel + SOC ($p = 0.592$)	No survival role for zoledronate in castration-sensitive PCa patients
Metastatic castrate-resistant PCa (mCRPC)						
Zoledronate						
039 [8]	643	mCRPC with bone metastases	Zoledronate 4 mg *vs.* placebo every 3 weeks	Proportion with SRE	38 % *vs.* 49 % $p=0.028$	Time to SRE: 488 *vs.* 321 days $p=0.009$
TRAPEZE [19]	757	mCRPC with bone metastases on Docetaxel + Prednisolone	Zoledronate *vs.* Sr-89 *vs.* Zoledronate + Sr-89 *vs.* No BTA	CPFS	no CPFS benefit with Zoledronate $p=0.46$	SRE-free interval HR = 0.76, $p=0.008$
Denosumab						
103 [20]	1904	mCRPC with bone metastases	Denosumab 120 mg *vs.* Zoledronate 4 mg every 4 weeks	Time to first SRE	20.7 *vs.* 17.1 month HR: 0.82; $p=0.0002$	No difference in PFS or OS
Radium-223						
ALSYMPCA [21]	921	mCRPC with symptomatic bone metastases and no visceral metastases	Radium-223 50KBq/kg *vs.* Placebo every 4 weeks x 6	OS	14.9 *vs.* 11.3 months HR: 0.70; $p<0.001$	Time to first SSE 15.6 *vs.* 9.8 months HR: 0.66; $p<0.001$

[a]Trial also involved non-metastatic prostate cancer patients

PCa prostate cancer, *PSA* prostate-specific antigen, *SOC* standard of care, *BPFS* bone progression-free survival, *DT* Doubling Time, *CPFS* clinical progression-free survival, *BMFS* bone metastasis-free survival, *SRE* skeletal-related event, *SSE* symptomatic skeletal event, *HR* Hazard Ratio, *BTA* bone-targeted agent

29.8 months in the zoledronate and placebo arms, respectively (hazard ratio [HR]: 0.97; $p = 0.39$) and therefore did not support the use of BP prior to castration resistance in PCa patients with bone metastases (Table 1).

The STAMPEDE trial is a large, multiarm, multistage trial in castrate-sensitive PCa patients in which all patients receive ADT. The trial is ongoing, but has recently reported data from the zoledronate arms (Table 1). The results show that addition of zoledronate to first-line hormonal therapy did not improve failure-free or OS in PCa patients with high risk, locally advanced or metastatic disease (HR 0.93, 95 % CI 0.77–1.11; $p = 0.416$) [13]. While the study reported a significant OS advantage with the addition of six cycles of docetaxel (75 mg/kg every 3 weeks) in this patient population (HR 0.76, 95 % CI 0.62–0.92; $p = 0.005$), concurrent administration of zoledronate did not show additional benefit (HR 1.06, 95 % CI 0.86–1.30; $p = 0.593$) and is therefore not recommended [13].

4.4 Attempts to Use Bisphosphonates to Prevent Bone Metastases

Oral clodronate at a daily dose of 2080 mg failed to show significant benefit in the time to development of bone metastases or symptomatic bone progression-free survival in non-metastatic PCa patients (MRC PC04 trial) [14] or castration-sensitive PCa patients with bone metastases (MRC PC05 trial) [15], respectively (Table 1). While long term overall survival analysis suggested some benefit in the bone metastatic setting (HR 0·77, 95 % CI 0·60–0·98; $p = 0{\cdot}032$), significantly more frequent gastrointestinal side effects were reported in the clodronate groups of both trials and attention was focused on other more potent BPs such as zoledronate (zoledronic acid or ZA).

To evaluate its efficacy in prevention of bone metastases, non-metastatic CRPC patients with rising PSA levels (at least 3 consecutive rises) enrolled in the zoledronate 704 trial (Table 1) were randomised to receive either IV zoledronate 4 mg every 4 weeks or placebo [16]. While this study had to be terminated prematurely after recruitment of only 398 out of a planned 991 patients due to a low event rate, it contributed important insights into the design of future trials of bone-targeted agents. The reported rate of development of bone metastases was only 33 % after 2 years (median bone metastasis-free survival of 30 months). It was noted however that a high baseline PSA (>10 ng/ml) or rapidly rising PSA were independent predictors of shorter bone metastasis-free survival and even OS [16]. A subsequent phase 3 trial (ZEUS) was conducted in high-risk localised PCa (Gleason Score 8–10, node-positive disease or PSA >20) that involved 1433 men randomised to receive either IV zoledronate 4 mg every 3 months for 4 years or observation only [17] (Table 1). Zoledronate did not show a significant reduction in the primary outcome measure, which was the proportion of patients that developed bone metastases [17].

5 Bone-Targeted Agents in Prostate Cancer: RANKL-RANK Inhibition

5.1 Denosumab

Denosumab is a fully humanised monoclonal IgG2 antibody that targets RANKL. It binds competitively to RANKL, preventing its interaction with RANK on osteoclast precursors thereby inhibiting their differentiation and activation in a molecular mechanism identical to the physiological regulation of osteoclast function by OPG [10]. It is administered as a subcutaneous bolus injection and at doses of 60 mg or higher every 4 weeks. Its clearance is independent of renal and hepatic function and following discontinuation, and it has a mean half-life of approximately 28 days.

5.2 Denosumab and Prevention of SREs

Denosumab was compared with zoledronate in a phase 3 randomised trial (Protocol 103) that aimed to evaluate its efficacy in the reduction of skeletal morbidity in bone metastatic CRPC (Table 1). A total of 1904 patients were assigned randomly to receive either IV zoledronate 4 mg or SC denosumab 120 mg every 4 weeks, with the time to first on-study SRE as the primary endpoint [20]. A statistically significant reduction in the time to first on-study SRE was seen with denosumab compared to zoledronate (20.7 *vs.* 17.1 months; HR 0.82, 95 % CI 0.71–0.95; $p=0.0002$ for non-inferiority and 0.008 for superiority). Patients in the denosumab arm also had a delayed time to first and subsequent SRE in a multievent analysis (HR 0.82, 95 % CI 0.71–0.94; $p=0.008$). There were fewer SSEs with denosumab (25.4 % *vs.* 30.4 %; HR 0.78; $p<0.01$) and greater decrease in the uNTX: Cr ratio (−40.3 % *vs.* −28 %; $p<0.0001$) and BALP (−7.9 % *vs.* −4.8 %; $p<0.0001$) after 13 weeks of treatment. There was however no significant difference in PFS or OS between the groups [20].

Denosumab and zoledronate share common side effects, the most important of which are ONJ and hypocalcaemia. In the Protocol 103 trial, hypocalcaemia was more frequent (13 % *vs.* 6 %; $p<0.0001$) among patients on denosumab although many of these were asymptomatic and only observed biochemically [20]. However, biochemical monitoring is recommended and, in clinical practice, calcium and vitamin D supplementation is given routinely while on treatment to ameliorate this side effect. Denosumab caused ONJ with a similar frequency as zoledronate (1.1 % *vs.* 0.7 % per 100 patient years) in the blinded phase of the 103 trial, but subsequent analysis of the open-label extension phase reported that the incidence rate rises with continued denosumab treatment to around 4.1 % per 100 patient years [22].

While the evidence suggests that denosumab is superior to zoledronate for the prevention of SREs and SSEs in metastatic CRPC, is more conveniently administered and has become part of the standard of care, data about the sequencing of these agents are currently limited [7]. A phase 2 trial that involved 111 patients with bone metastases from various cancers (including 50 with PCa) who had persistently elevated uNTX levels despite BP treatment showed that those whose were switched to SC denosumab 180 mg every 4 or 12 weeks achieved uNTX suppression more frequently than those who remained on bisphosphonate treatment (69 % *vs.* 19 % at 13 weeks) [23]. No additional toxicity was reported, suggesting that a transition from zoledronate to denosumab, particularly in cases of suspected treatment failure is a practicable strategy that has potential SRE benefits that will need to be proven by larger prospective trials [7].

5.3 Denosumab and Prevention of Bone Metastases

The Denosumab 147 trial evaluated a possible role for denosumab in the prevention of bone metastases in 1432 men with localised castrate-resistant PCa with PSA>8 ng/ml and/or PSA doubling time <10 months (Table 1). They were randomised to receive either SC denosumab 120 mg or placebo every 4 weeks. Denosumab showed a favourable effect on the primary end point of bone metastasis-free survival (29.5 *vs.* 25.2 months; HR 0.85; 95 % CI 0.73–0.98; $p=0.028$) and drastic reduction in BTMs (uNTX:Cr ratio decreased by 68 % and BALP by 49 %), but no significant improvement was seen in PFS or OS [18]. An ONJ frequency of 4.6 % was reported in the denosumab arm and it failed to get US FDA approval for this indication on the basis of an unfavourable risk-benefit ratio [18]. It was however noted in a subset analysis that patients with aggressive PSA kinetics such as a doubling time of <6 months had a shorter time to development of bone metastasis and appeared to benefit significantly more from denosumab treatment (18.3 *vs.* 25.9 months; HR 0.77; $p=0.006$) [18].

6 Bone-Targeted Agents in Prostate Cancer: Radiopharmaceuticals

Although external beam radiation is still very important in symptomatic treatment of bone metastases, a range of alpha- and beta-emitting bone-seeking systemic radiopharmaceuticals are available. They emit high energy alpha and/or beta particles that cause DNA double-strand breaks that lead to apoptosis. Although they are administered systemically (IV route), their selective toxicity derives from their affinity for areas of the bone with high turnover. Alpha emitters in particular have a short range of penetration of their ionising radiation, which limits damage to normal bone marrow and is therefore a major advantage [7].

6.1 Strontium-89 (Sr-89) and Samarium-153 (Sm-153)

Sr-89 is a divalent ion similar to calcium that is incorporated into bone ECM, preferentially at sites of metastatic disease and emits beta particles that deliver an energy of 1.5 MeV with a penetration range of around 3 mm in bone. It is excreted via the renal route and has a long half-life of 50.5 days. Sr-89 chloride was the first radiopharmaceutical approved for use in bone metastatic CRPC after early studies demonstrated a quick, sustained pain response in about a third of these patients [24].

Sm-153 conjugated to ethylenediaminetetramethylenephosphonic acid (Sm-153-EDTMP) forms a complex with hydroxyapatite that accumulates in areas of high bone turnover. Bone metastases retain around 5 times more Sm-153-EDTMP than normal bone, and it emits mostly beta particles with maximum energy of 0.81 MeV and average penetration of approximately 0.8 mm. Its beta decay is associated with around 28 % gamma emission that can be detected by nuclear imaging cameras. It is renally excreted but has a much shorter half-life than Sr-89 of 1.9 days. It showed rapid and sustained pain response in bone metastatic CRPC and is licensed for this indication [24].

Neither agent however showed significant improvement in survival and their use is limited by myelosuppression, which is somewhat milder with Sm153. They have therefore been largely confined to use in pain palliation in metastatic PCa bone disease and are only suitable for use in patients in whom baseline myelosuppression, exposure to recent radiation (in the preceding 2 months), impending spinal cord compression and significant renal impairment have been excluded [24].

6.2 Radium-223 (Ra-223 or Alpharadin)

A major practice-changing development has recently emerged using Ra-223, which is a calcium-mimetic that forms complexes with ECM hydroxyapatite in areas of high bone turnover. It decays with a half-life of 11.4 days with 95 % of its energy released as alpha particles. These deliver high energy radiation (5.78 MeV) but have a very short range of penetration (<100 μm) in bone that translates to only mild, reversible myelosuppression as observed in Phase 1 studies. A phase 2 study recruited men with mCRPC, rising PSA and multiple or at least one painful bone metastasis. Treatment with Ra-223 (at 50 kBq/kg) was found to have an acceptable haematological toxicity profile, longer time to PSA progression, greater reduction in BALP levels and a better pain response than external beam radiotherapy [24].

This led to the phase 3 trial (ALSYMPCA) in which 921 patients with symptomatic bone metastases from CRPC and no visceral disease were randomised 2:1 to receive either 4-weekly IV Ra-223 for 24 weeks or placebo (Table 1). OS was chosen as the primary endpoint based on encouraging results from the phase 2 study [21]. The results showed that there was a significant improvement in OS seen with Ra-223 (14.9 *vs.* 11.3 months; HR 0.70; $p<0.001$), the first of its kind with a bone-targeted agent that led to early trial termination for efficacy [21] as well as fast track approval by the US FDA [24]. Ra-223 also showed favourable results with the secondary end points of this trial, including an increased time to first SSE (15.6 *vs.* 9.8 months; HR 0.66; $p<0.001$) and time to PSA rise (HR 0.64, 95 % CI 0.54–0.77: $p < 0.001$). The overall rates of myelosuppression were comparable in both trial arms. Grade ≥3 thrombocytopaenia was slightly more frequent in the Ra-223 arm, but on subgroup analysis, this was found to be predominantly among patients who had prior treatment with docetaxel [21]. While its role in PCa patients with asymptomatic bone metastases is yet to be determined, phase 3 trials in this patient population are ongoing (discussed below).

Of patients in the treatment arm of the ALSYMPCA trial, around 41 % (250 patients) were already on BP therapy prior to recruitment and this was continued as best standard of care. Concurrent administration of the two bone-targeted agents was presumed to be safe given the different mechanisms of action and adverse effect profiles of the two agents. Subgroup analysis showed that the survival benefit of Ra-223 was independent of BP use [21]. However, a greater delay in SSE was noted in those patients who received concurrent BP (19.6 *vs.* 10.2 months; HR 0.49; $p=0.00048$) compared with those who did not (11.8 *vs.* 8.4 months: HR 0.77; $p=0.07$), suggesting a synergistic effect of the two bone-targeted agents on skeletal morbidity. Very little data are currently available on the combination of Ra-223 with denosumab (it was yet to be approved at the start of the ALSYMPCA trial) but for the same reasons as with BPs, there does not appear to be any evidence for discontinuation of denosumab on initiation of Ra-223 treatment [7].

7 Combination of Bone-Targeted Agents with Other Systemic Therapeutic Agents

7.1 Combination with Cytotoxic Agents

In current clinical practice, concomitant administration of direct osteoclast-targeted (zoledronate) and cytotoxic agents such as docetaxel is common and appears to be well tolerated. Additional benefits of the combination over docetaxel alone were evaluated in a phase 3 trial (TRAPEZE) in which 757 CRPC patients with bone metastases treated with docetaxel and prednisolone were randomised to receive zoledronate, SR-89, both bone-targeted agents, or no additional bone-targeted agents (Table 1). The primary endpoint of PFS was not achieved and there was no OS benefit with addition of either agent, but the zoledronate group did have a significantly increased SRE-free interval (HR 0.76, 95 % CI 0.63–0.93; $p=0.008$) and there were no additional toxicities reported [19]. There is no clear evidence addressing the combination of denosumab and docetaxel, but as with zoledronate they appear to be well tolerated in clinical practice.

Both docetaxel and Ra-223 independently show OS benefit in CRPC with painful bone metastases. Combining both agents would therefore suggest potential additive or even synergistic benefit, but tolerability in view of their overlapping side effect of myelosuppression is a source of concern. This is being investigated in a Phase 1/2a clinical trial, early results from which suggest however that the combination is well tolerated and may cause a greater reduction in BALP compared with single agent treatment [25]. In terms of sequencing these treatments, subgroup analysis in the ALSYMPCA trial showed that prior docetaxel exposure (57 % of patients) added no OS advantage over being docetaxel-naïve [21]. The time to first SSE was however significantly delayed in these patients (HR 0.62; $p=0.0009$) compared to the docetaxel-naïve subgroup in whom it did not reach significance (HR 0.77; $p=0.12$). Grade ≥3 thrombocytopaenia and neutropaenia were reported slightly more frequently among patients who had previously received docetaxel (9 % and 3 %, respectively) compared with the docetaxel naive patients (3 % and 1 %, respectively), but this was considered to be within acceptable limits [7].

7.2 Combination with Novel Hormone-Targeted Agents

The introduction of androgen-axis-targeted agents (AATAs) including enzalutamide and abiraterone have been practice-changing developments in the systemic management of metastatic CRPC. While bone-targeted agents have been shown to improve pain from bone disease in metastatic CRPC, they may also have benefit in delaying the onset of pain. This is supported by an unplanned analysis following the COU-AA-302 trial (Table 1) that evaluated abiraterone with prednisolone *vs.* prednisolone alone in asymptomatic docetaxel-naïve metastatic CRPC patients, which showed that the patients who were on concomitant bone-targeted agents had a delayed time to opioid use (HR 0.80; $p=0.036$) and improved survival (HR 0.75; $p=0.012$) [26]. Importantly, the currently available bone-targeted agents have no overlapping side effects with AATAs. Combinations of enzalutamide and abiraterone with Ra-223 in similar patient populations will therefore be evaluated in the phase 3 PEACE trial (NCT02194842) and ERA 223 trial (NCT02043678), respectively [7].

8 Bone Health in Prostate Cancer

Maintaining bone health is an important consideration for men with both localised and metastatic PCa in view of CTIBL that results primarily as a result of androgen deprivation therapy (ADT), the cornerstone of treatment prior to development of castration resistance. Androgens and oestrogens are vital in the physiological maintenance of bone mass and ADT reduces their serum levels to less than 5 % and 20 % of normal, respectively, with accelerated bone loss as a consequence [27]. Further, CTIBL in PCa is often superimposed upon normal age-related loss of BMD as the highest incidence is in the seventh decade [28]. Fracture risk is doubled with a 10–15 % reduction in BMD [29]. ADT results in a 5–10 % decrease in BMD during the first year, with subsequent gradual decline over years of continued treatment. Men receiving ADT have been shown to be five times as likely to develop a fracture than healthy age-matched controls. Long-term ADT also results in sarcopenia, further increasing the risk of fracture as it often occurs along with reduced mobility and falls. Development of one fracture predisposes to future fractures, has a profound impact on quality of life and is associated with significant increase in risk of mortality [30].

Assessment of BMD should therefore be undertaken in all men prior to the initiation of ADT with subsequent monitoring in line with current ESMO guidelines. Dual emission X-ray absorptiometry (DXA) scans are suitable for this as they are widely available, use low dose radiation and identify men with osteopenia (T score < -1) and osteoporosis (T score < -2.5) who are at risk of fracture. The WHO FRAX tool can be used to estimate baseline 10-year risk of fracture and may be a more sensitive measure of those likely to benefit from initiation of bone-targeted agents [31]. Several important lifestyle modifications are recommended in order to minimise CTIBL in PCa. These include smoking cessation, avoidance of excessive alcohol consumption and regular exercise. In addition to improving BMD, exercise may also reduce the incidence of sarcopenia and improve both fatigue and quality of life. Calcium and vitamin D supplementation is also advisable as PCa patients are frequently deficient.

Bone-targeted agents may also be used to ameliorate CTIBL in PCa. BPs are licensed for the treatment of osteoporosis and evidence suggests that BPs are superior to placebo in the prevention CTIBL [32] and may also reduce the vertebral fracture risk. The strength of available studies in PCa is however limited by small size, heterogeneous populations, variations in the type and frequency of BP administration and different follow-up schedules. Large prospective studies are required to determine the extent of the benefits associated with BP use in this setting, and to compare the efficacy of different BPs, particularly with regard to fracture rates. Denosumab has been shown to increase BMD and reduce the incidence of vertebral fractures when compared to placebo [33] and is currently specifically licensed for the prevention of ADT-associated bone loss. Selective oestrogen receptor modulators such as raloxifene and toremifene may also increase BMD and reduce the risk of fracture while on ADT. They however confer a significant risk of thromboembolic events in older patients and are not used in routine clinical practice.

Box 1: Summary and Guidelines for Use of BTAs in Prostate Cancer

Non-Metastatic PCa

- Clinical trials do not support a role for BTAs in delaying metastasis, PFS or OS
- In non-metastatic CRPC with aggressive PSA kinetics, there is limited evidence that Denosumab may delay the development of bone metastases
- Routine BTAs are therefore not recommended as standard of care outside of the clinical trial setting

Metastatic Castration -Sensitive PCa

- Clinical trials do not support a role in improving PFS or OS
- BTAs are not recommended as standard of care outside the clinical trial setting

Metastatic Castrate-resistant PCa

- Clinical trials of Zoledronate, Denosumab and Radium 223 all show reduction in the risk of SRE/SSEs
- Available evidence suggests that it is safe to switch from zoledronate to denosumab with potential benefit
- Sr-89 and Sm-153 have symptomatic benefit but are limited by myelotoxicity and have been largely superseded by Ra-223
- Ra-223 was shown to improve overall survival in patients with symptomatic, predominantly bone metastases
- Zoledronate and Denosumab are recommended for patients with bone metastases and should be started at diagnosis of bone metastases and continued while they remain fit for treatment
- Ra-223 is recommended for patients with symptomatic bone disease without visceral metastases

Bone health while on ADT

- BMD monitoring is recommended in patients on ADT
- Lifestyle modifications including regular exercise, smoking cessation and alcohol reduction can ameliorate CTIBL and improve quality of life
- BP can be used to treat osteoporosis
- Denosumab is licensed for prevention of ADT-associated bone loss

9 Conclusions and Future Directions

Elucidation of the molecular interactions within the bone microenvironment and the mechanisms responsible for bone metastasis have resulted in the development of several targeted agents that are effective in reducing skeletal morbidity in metastatic PCa. Some of these agents have also shown additional benefits such as improvement in overall survival and even delay in the development of bone metastasis when used in the selected patient populations. While the current roles of these agents promises less morbidity for patients, optimisation of combination and sequencing strategies for bone-targeted agents and other systemic antitumour agents has the potential to further improve management options. A number of clinical trials are planned or already in progress to address these questions.

Application of recent technological advances in genomic analysis methods, for example, next-generation sequencing for candidate identification and genome editing techniques such as the CRISPR/Cas9 system for translational animal model development promises newer insights into the molecular mechanisms that drive PCa bone disease in the near future. This will facilitate the development of novel therapeutic-targeted agents as well as predictive biomarkers, which will guide precision treatment of PCa in the bone as well as other metastatic sites.

References

1. Bubendorf L, Schöpfer A, Wagner U, et al. Metastatic patterns of prostate cancer: an autopsy study of 1,589 patients. Hum Pathol. 2000;31(5):578–83.
2. Vasudev NS, Brown JE. Medical management of metastatic bone disease. Curr Opin Support Palliat Care. 2010;4(3):189–94.
3. Coleman RE, Rathbone E, Brown JE. Management of cancer treatment-induced bone loss. Nat Rev Rheumatol. 2013;9(6):365–74.
4. Weilbaecher KN, Guise TA, McCauley LK. Cancer to bone: a fatal attraction. Nat Rev Cancer. 2011;11(6):411–25.
5. Shiozawa Y, Pedersen EA, Havens AM, et al. Human prostate cancer metastases target the hematopoietic stem cell niche to establish footholds in mouse bone marrow. J Clin Invest. 2011;121(4):1298–312.
6. David Roodman G, Silbermann R. Mechanisms of osteolytic and osteoblastic skeletal lesions. Bonekey Rep. 2015;4:753.
7. Gartrell BA, Coleman R, Efstathiou E, et al. Metastatic prostate cancer and the bone: significance and therapeutic options. Eur Urol. 2015;68(5):850–8.
8. Saad F, Gleason DM, Murray R, et al. A randomized, placebo-controlled trial of zoledronic acid in patients with hormone-refractory metastatic prostate carcinoma. J Natl Cancer Inst. 2002;94(19):1458–68.
9. Brown JE, Sim S. Evolving role of bone biomarkers in castration-resistant prostate cancer. Neoplasia. 2010;12(9):685–96.
10. Kardamakis D, Vassiliou V, Chow E. Bone metastases : a translational and clinical approach. 2014. http://search.ebscohost.com/login.aspx?direct=true&scope=site&db=nlebk&db=nlabk&AN=664555.
11. Saad F, Brown JE, Van Poznak C, et al. Incidence, risk factors, and outcomes of osteonecrosis of the jaw: integrated analysis from three blinded active-controlled phase III trials in cancer patients with bone metastases. Ann Oncol: Off J Eur Soc Med Oncol/ESMO. 2012;23(5):1341–7.
12. Smith MR, Halabi S, Ryan CJ, et al. Randomized controlled trial of early zoledronic acid in men with castration-sensitive prostate cancer and bone metastases: results of CALGB 90202 (alliance). J Clin Oncol: Off J Am Soc Clin Oncol. 2014;32(11):1143–50.
13. James ND, Sydes MR, Clarke NW, et al. Addition of docetaxel, zoledronic acid, or both to first-line long-term hormone therapy in prostate cancer (STAMPEDE): survival results from an adaptive, multiarm, multistage, platform randomised controlled trial. Lancet. 2016;387(10024):1163–77.
14. Mason MD, Sydes MR, Glaholm J, et al. Oral sodium clodronate for nonmetastatic prostate cancer–results of a randomized double-blind placebo-controlled trial: Medical Research Council PR04 (ISRCTN61384873). J Natl Cancer Inst. 2007;99(10):765–76.
15. Dearnaley DP, Sydes MR, Mason MD, et al. A double-blind, placebo-controlled, randomized trial of oral sodium clodronate for metastatic prostate cancer (MRC PR05 Trial). J Natl Cancer Inst. 2003;95(17):1300–11.
16. Smith MR, Kabbinavar F, Saad F, et al. Natural history of rising serum prostate-specific antigen in men with castrate nonmetastatic prostate cancer. J Clin Oncol: Off J Am Soc Clin Oncol. 2005;23(13):2918–25.
17. Wirth M, Tammela T, Cicalese V, et al. Prevention of bone metastases in patients with high-risk nonmetastatic prostate cancer treated with zoledronic acid: efficacy and safety results of the Zometa European Study (ZEUS). Eur Urol. 2015;67(3):482–91.
18. Smith MR, Saad F, Coleman R, et al. Denosumab and bone-metastasis-free survival in men with castration-resistant prostate cancer: results of a phase 3, randomised, placebo-controlled trial. Lancet. 2012;379(9810):39–46.
19. James ND, Pirrie S, Barton D, et al. Clinical outcomes in patients with castrate-refractory prostate cancer (CRPC) metastatic to bone randomized in the factorial TRAPEZE trial to docetaxel (D) with strontium-89 (Sr89), zoledronic acid (ZA), neither, or both (ISRCTN 12808747). J Clin Oncol. 2013;31(18_suppl):LBA5000.
20. Fizazi K, Carducci M, Smith M, et al. Denosumab versus zoledronic acid for treatment of bone metastases in men with castration-resistant prostate cancer: a randomised, double-blind study. Lancet. 2011;377(9768):813–22.
21. Parker C, Nilsson S, Heinrich D, et al. Alpha emitter radium-223 and survival in metastatic prostate cancer. N Engl J Med. 2013;369(3):213–23.
22. Stopeck AT, Fizazi K, Body JJ, et al. Safety of long-term denosumab therapy: results from the open label extension phase of two phase 3 studies in patients with metastatic breast and prostate cancer. Support Care Cancer. 2016;24(1):447–55.
23. Fizazi K, Bosserman L, Gao G, Skacel T, Markus R. Denosumab treatment of prostate cancer with bone metastases and increased urine N-telopeptide levels after therapy with intravenous bisphosphonates: results of a randomized phase II trial. J Urol. 2009;182(2):509–15; discussion 515–506.
24. El-Amm J, Aragon-Ching JB. Targeting bone metastases in metastatic castration-resistant prostate cancer. Clin Med Insights Oncol. 2016;10 Suppl 1:11–9.
25. Morris MJ, Hammers HJ, Sweeney C, et al. Safety of radium-223 dichloride (Ra-223) with docetaxel (D) in patients with bone metastases from castration-resistant prostate cancer (CRPC): A phase I Prostate Cancer Clinical Trials Consortium Study. J Clin Oncol. 2013;31(15_suppl):5021.
26. Rathkopf DE, Smith MR, de Bono JS, et al. Updated interim efficacy analysis and long-term safety of abiraterone acetate in metastatic castration-resistant prostate cancer patients without prior chemotherapy (COU-AA-302). Eur Urol. 2014;66(5):815–25.
27. LeBlanc ES, Nielson CM, Marshall LM, et al. The effects of serum testosterone, estradiol, and sex hormone

binding globulin levels on fracture risk in older men. J Clin Endocrinol Metab. 2009;94(9):3337–46.
28. Brown JE, Sherriff JM, James ND. Osteoporosis in patients with prostate cancer on long-term androgen deprivation therapy: an increasing, but under-recognized problem. BJU Int. 2010;105(8):1042–3.
29. Faulkner KG. Bone matters: are density increases necessary to reduce fracture risk? J Bone Miner Res. 2000;15(2):183–7.
30. Oefelein MG, Ricchiuti V, Conrad W, Resnick MI. Skeletal fractures negatively correlate with overall survival in men with prostate cancer. J Urol. 2002;168(3):1005–7.
31. Kanis JA, McCloskey E, Johansson H, Oden A, Leslie WD. FRAX(®) with and without bone mineral density. Calcif Tissue Int. 2012;90(1):1–13.
32. Serpa Neto A, Tobias-Machado M, Esteves MA, et al. Bisphosphonate therapy in patients under androgen deprivation therapy for prostate cancer: a systematic review and meta-analysis. Prostate Cancer Prostatic Dis. 2012;15(1):36–44.
33. Smith MR, Egerdie B, Hernández Toriz N, et al. Denosumab in men receiving androgen-deprivation therapy for prostate cancer. N Engl J Med. 2009;361(8):745–55.

Immunotherapy and Targeted Therapies in Advanced Castration Resistant Prostate Cancer

Joaquim Bellmunt and Irene Moreno

1 Introduction

Over the last decade, the management of PC has become increasingly complex and controversial for both early and advanced disease. Androgen deprivation therapy (ADT) remains a mainstay of treatment in a noncurative setting but progression to castration-resistant PC (CRPC), where the ADT is not anymore useful, eventually occurs. Exploring other therapeutics is key to further improving the quality and quantity of life of our patients.

In the last few years, cancer immunotherapy has changed the natural history and treatment strategies of a number of solid tumors, including melanoma, lung cancer, renal cell carcinoma, and bladder cancer. Immunotherapy is now becoming a mainstay in the management strategy for this type of patients. PC was historically not considered immunogenic in its nature, and first attempts to stimulate an immune response in the prostate cancer were unsuccessful [1, 2]. However, PC generates a variety of tumor-associated antigens, as PSA, prostatic acid phosphatase, and prostatic-specific membrane antigen, which are potentially capable of producing a clinical response through inducing immunogenicity [3]. In fact, PC was the first solid tumor to demonstrate improved survival with a cancer-specific vaccine [4], encouraging researchers to further explore immunotherapy in prostate cancer and other solid tumors.

In this chapter, we will start discussing the basic biology of PC, focusing on issues that relates to immune environment and immune response in PC to then outline some of the immunotherapy approaches that have been approved and the investigational ones that are currently being studied. We will emphasis on the immunologic biomarkers that can help us on the selection of patients. Finally, we will explore some others targeted therapies that are currently available for PC treatment.

2 Rationale

The concept that the immune system acts as a tumor suppressor was introduced in the early twentieth century by Ehrlich [5]. Since then, several studies have provided evidence supporting the role of immunity in cancer development, progression and suppression, conceptually under the term "immune surveillance" [6].

J. Bellmunt (✉)
Dana-Farber/Brigham and Women's Cancer Center, Harvard Medical School,
450 Brookline Ave, Boston, MA
02215 (DANA 1230), USA
e-mail: Joaquim_Bellmunt@DFCI.HARVARD.EDU

I. Moreno
Fundación Jiménez Díaz Hospital, Autonomous University of Madrid, Avenida Reyes Católicos 2, Madrid, 28040, Spain

M. Bolla, H. van Poppel (eds.), *Management of Prostate Cancer*,
DOI 10.1007/978-3-319-42769-0_24

In order to better understand immunotherapy, we will first briefly discuss the normal response of the human immune system. This system can be classified into subsystems, such as the innate immune system [7] versus the adaptive immune system [8], or humoral immunity versus cell-mediated immunity. Both divisions have been shown to be involved in tumor immune surveillance.

2.1 Innate Immune System

The innate response is usually triggered when foreign organisms or particles are identified by pattern recognition receptors [9] or when damaged or stressed cells send out alarm signals. Thus, innate immune cells are responsible for the initial response [10]. The main components of this type of immune response include macrophages, natural killer cells, and antigen-presenting cells. The macrophages are initially recruited and can be classified as pro-inflammatory M1 (CD68+) cells and anti-inflammatory M2 (CD163+) cells [11]. Inducers or inhibitors of these different types of macrophages are now targets of the new immunthera-peutic agents. In the cancer context the relationship between M1 and M2 cells can become unbalanced [12], resulting in a gain of M2 cells. A recent study reported that in localized PC, the prevalent macrophage phenotype was M1, whereas in PC with extracapsular extension, M2 macrophages were more frequently seen [13]. These findings, together with another observation of reduced infiltration of CD68+ macrophages, associated with higher clinical stage and lymph node positivity, indicate that reduced numbers of macrophages with cytotoxic capabilities parallel more aggressive disease [14].

Natural killer cells (NK) are the responsible of targeting tumor cells without prior sensitization. They recognize altered cells by detecting the loss of human leukocyte antigen (HLA) class I molecules (a change that is associated with injured cells) or by recognition of specific ligands (tumor associated antigens or TAAs) that are expressed by these altered cells [15]. In PC these include the serine protease prostate-specific antigen (PSA), prostate-specific membrane antigen (PSMA), prostatic acid phosphatase (PAP), mucin-1 (MUC-1), prostate stem cell antigen (PSCA), and NY-ESO-1 [16]. Preclinical data show that PC cells induce the expression of inhibitory receptor (ILT2/LILRB1) and down-regulate the expression of activating receptors NKp46 (NCR1), CD16 (FCGR3) and NKG2D (KLRK1) by NK cells, thus preventing their recognition of tumor cells. Notably, blood levels of NKp46 also decrease in PC patients and are inversely correlated with levels of PSA, PC [17].

Antigen-presenting cells (macrophages and dendritic cells)(APC) are the link between the innate and adaptive immunity. The role of these professional antigen-presenting cells is to get ready the naïve T cells for being activated when contacting with foreign antigens.

Cancer employs numerous immune escape strategies such as down regulation of HLA class I antigens and beta-2 microglobulin to escape killing by cytotoxic T cells.

2.2 Adaptive Immune System

This division of the immune system is composed of T and B lymphocytes which develop highly specialized functions via cell surface or secreted effector molecules. The main effector cells in cancer immune response are the CD8+ cytotoxic T-lymphocytes. The TAAs (peptide fragments from the initial tumor cell destruction by innate effectors) can activate this type of lymphocytes, undergoing clonal expansion after that. CD4+ T cells (helper T cells) induce antibody production in B cells and activate macrophages [18]. CD4+ T cells can be divided in: Th1 (involved in intra-cellular immunity), Th2 (involved in extracellular-humoral immunity), Th17, and regulatory T cells. The last ones are able to suppress effector T cells in order to maintain immune tolerance [19]. CD8+ T cells constitutively express cytotoxic T-lymphocyte-associated protein 4-CTLA-4 (a well-known immunotherapy target [20, 21]).

T cells recognize antigens presented by the MHC on the surface of cancer cells through their T-cell receptor. Activation of T cells requires two signals: first antigens need to be presented on the setting of HLA receptor and second a signal delivered by the B7 stimulatory molecules in APC is required interacting with CD28 receptor on T cells. In order to maintain self-tolerance and prevent hyperactivation, there is a co-inhibitory signal that binds B7 with greater affinity, inactivating T cells-like CTAL-4. The interaction between CTLA-4 and the costimulatory molecules happens primarily in the priming phase of a T-cell response within lymph nodes. Activated T cells can also upregulate programmed cell death protein 1 (PD1), a cell surface receptor that is expressed on T cells and pro-B cells. The PD1 inhibitory receptor is expressed by T cells during long-term antigen exposure and results in negative regulation of T cells. Inflammatory signals in the tissues induce the expression of PD1 ligands, downregulate the activity of T cells binding PD1 in lymphocytes, and thus limit collateral tissue damage in the light effect her face of a T-cell response in peripheral tissues.

Regulatory T cells can be found in large proportions of tumor infiltrating lymphocytes (which has been associated with poor prognosis of certain cancers [22], including prostate cancer). Early studies reported that greater tumor infiltration of CD4+ T-reg cells can predict poorer prognosis [23] in PC, and a high tumor infiltration of forkhead box P3- (foxp3-) expressing cells (T-regs) was also found to correlate with higher baseline PSA levels [24]. This data suggest that therapeutic blockade of these cells may induce beneficial clinical responses.

2.3 Androgen Deprivation and Immune System Response

Early results in this field show that neoadjuvant androgen deprivation (before PC surgery) results in a CD4+ T cell infiltration into the gland [25]. Contrarily, the analysis of a postcastration PC tissue reveals a CD8+ T cell infiltration [26]. These findings are also observed in mice models, where it was found that androgen ablation decreases CD4+ T cell tolerance to a PC-associated antigen, showing that clonotypic CD4+ T cells could respond to specific vaccination after androgen deprivation but not in intact, tumor-bearing mice [27]. Moreover, androgen deprivation is related to an increase in the number of cells expressing the co stimulatory molecules B7.1 and B7.2, which are necessary for effective T cell activation [28]. According to these data hormone ablation may have an additive effect with immunotherapy, taking in consideration the timing of treatments (obtaining better results if the immunotherapy is given prior to castration) [29].

2.4 Tumor Immune Scape (Immunoediting)

As described in the beginning of the chapter, functional cancer immunosurveillance process indeed exists that acts as an extrinsic tumor suppressor. However, it has also become clear that the immune system can facilitate tumor progression, at least in part, by sculpting the immunogenic phenotype of tumors as they develop. The recognition that immunity plays a dual role in the complex interactions between tumors and the host prompted a refinement of the cancer immunosurveillance hypothesis into one termed "cancer immunoediting." Tumor cells are normally suppressed by the immune system, however, as part of tumor immunoediting, they sometimes gain properties to escape detection and present themselves as disease [5]. This modern hypothesis, first put forth by Schreiber, describes the three phases (elimination, equilibrium, and escape) where the balance between the tumor and the immune system is discussed. In the first stage, the immune system recognizes and eliminates the high immunogenic tumor cells by effectors such as NK cells or CD8+ T-lymphocytes. This can result in the selection of tumor cells with reduced immunogenicity and thus become resistant to immune effectors, leading the process to the equilibrium phase (where the elimination of tumor cells is balanced by the selection of less immunogenic variants, known as functional dormancy) [30]. As tumor size increases, tumor-derived soluble factors help to modify the microenvironment causing several mechanisms of immune escape. Some of them are the increasing extracellular matrix that binds tumor antigens (reducing the amount of TAAs) or the attraction of immature DCs which inhibit T cell activation [31]. New immunological therapies try to force the tumor backs towards either the equilibrium phase or, in the best scenario, to the elimination stage (meaning a complete response of the disease).

Sipuleucel T is one potential example that immunoediting plays a role in the immunotherapy of prostate cancer. Despite a benefit seen in terms of overall survival, it has been quite worrisome as patient's tumors very rarely shrink on this treatment with few objective responses described.

If we think about the cancer immunoediting hypothesis, maybe what is happening is not elimination, but maybe the vaccine is just pushing patients back toward an equilibrium phase, where both tumor and an antitumor response are present, but neither one is really winning.

In conclusion, all these data show that PC remains an attractive target for immunotherapy. This type of treatment can also be potentially useful in the biochemical recurrence setting, where the immunosuppressive mechanisms (such as TReg cells, myeloid-derived suppressor cells) and transforming growth factor-β (TGFβ) [32], usually seen associated with an advanced tumor stage-, are expected to be at a minimum at this stage.

Another characteristic of PC which can predict a good response to immunotherapy is that it is a slowly progressing disease, allowing sufficient time for the immunologic response to be build [33]. In terms of a potential risk of adverse events with a prostate cancer-specific immunotherapy, we can take into account that the prostate is a nonessential organ for life, meaning that even if immunotherapy destroys normal prostatic tissue, it would not be life-threatening.

3 Approved Agents

3.1 Immunomodulating Properties of Standard ("Nonimmunotherapy-Based") Agents

It is now believed that many conventional treatments for prostate and others cancers have beneficial immunological effects, making combinatorial trials an attractive strategy. ADT, radiation therapy and chemotherapy (which was broadly viewed as immunosuppressive in the past), might to some extent boost an antitumor response, modulating immune cells and their milieu. For example, ADT may produce changes in the patient immune system and an additive effect with immunotherapy might be expected.

In the setting of chemotherapy and targeted therapies, multiple studies (both in murine and in human models) have shown that various agents (such as the VEGF TKI sunitinib, specific inhibitors of $BRAF^{V600E}$, gemcitabine, 5-fluorouracil or doxorrubicin-cyclophosphamide) can promote a more active anticancer immune environment by enhancing dendritic cell function and decreasing inhibitory T cell populations such as regulatory T cells (Tregs) and myeloid-derived suppressor cells (MDSCs) [34–39].

There are also some early studies with taxanes (widely used in advanced PC) that report their capability of modulation the immune system in tumor-bearing mice [40] and in human samples of nonsquamous cell carcinoma [41], breast cancer [42], or melanoma [43]. For example, in a phase II clinical trial [44] published in 2012, the levels of circulating MDSC were assessed in 41 women diagnosed with HER-2 neu-negative breast cancer in stages II-IIIa. They received three chemotherapeutic drugs: doxorubicin-cyclophosphamide followed by docetaxel every 3 weeks followed by NOV-002, a disodium glutathione disulfide. In this study, 15 out of 39 patients achieved a pCR. It was found that patients who achieved pathologic complete response (pCR) had lower levels of circulating MDSC ($Lin^{-}HLA\text{-}DR^{-}CD11b^{+}CD33^{+}$) in the blood compared to patients who did not achieve pCR. The authors contended that MDSC suppression may increase the efficacy of chemotherapy regimens currently used in the clinic.

There is increasing evidence that radiation therapy may induce or help synergize immunotherapeutic effects on PC [45]. Evidence for an immunological effect of radiotherapy is provided by data showing that the tumoricidal effects of radiation require CD8+ T cells. It seems that the uptake of dying tumor cells by APCs plays an important role [46] where new antibody specificities appear following radiotherapy treatment [47], as well as the induction of a proinflammatory microenvironment by this type of treatment [48]. Radiation may modulate host immunity by increasing CD8+ effector T cells and dendritic cells at the radiation site; increasing antigen availability; inducing immune stimulating cytokines such as Type 1 interferon and chemokines and reducing immunosuppressive cell populations such as MDSCs [49–51]. Some recent work has also shown that HMGB1 (high mobility group box 1) released from dying tumor cells can function as a TLR4 agonist, activating APCs in either the tumor parenchyma or in the lymph nodes [33, 45].

It has been also described in case reports from several cancers [52] that radiation therapy may induce tumor cell death through a rare indirect out-of-field phenomenon described as the abscopal effect [53], in which distant metastatic lesions regress following radiation to an unrelated primary treatment field. The etiology of this scenario is not well known but evidence suggests that is immune mediated [54].

Identification of the optimal dose, fractionation regimens, and timing are an important issue to be planned in future clinical trials.

A study of TRAMP (Transgenic Adenocarcinoma of the Mouse Prostate) mice demonstrated optimal mitigation of tolerance with a tumor vaccine at 3–5 weeks following radiotherapy, when tumor burden is at its lowest [56].

Following these observations, there is a remarkable potential for synergistic combinations of radiation therapy with such immune-based agents. Several preclinical studies support this notion in terms of the antitumor response. This concept has been evaluated clinically in a randomized trial of men undergoing primary radiotherapy for PC [57], that will be described in Sect. 4.2.

3.2 Sipuleucel-T (Provenge)

Sipuleucel-T is an autologous cellular immunotherapy, approved in 2010 by the US Food and Drug Administration (FDA) for the treatment of asymptomatic or minimally symptomatic metastatic castrate-resistant PC [58]. It has been shown to increase overall survival [59] and generate antigen-specific immune responses that correlate with increased overall survival [60]. Similar to traditional vaccines, cellular immunotherapy tries to engage the immune system by activating effector T cells and dampening immunosuppressive factors, facilitating the infiltration of lymphocytes into the tumor microenvironment. The concept of this type of treatment approach was originated in lymphoma, where antigen-loaded, autologous APCs showed clinical promise [61].

Sipuleucel-T is a personalized product that is individually manufactured for each patient with PC. First, leukopheresis is carried out, and monocytes are enriched in the leukopheresis product through density–gradient centrifugation. Autologous cells are cultured in vitro with a proprietary protein cassette (PA2024) that couples the vaccine target (prostatic acid phosphatase, PAP; chosen based on preclinical studies in a murine model [62]) to the granulocyte–macrophage colony-stimulating factor (GM-CSF), before intravenous administration. The infusion contains at least 50 million autologous activated CD54+ dendritic cells, and a variable number of T cells, B cells, natural killer cells, and others [63]. Treatment is repeated three times over 4–6 weeks [33, 64]. Once infused, it is thought that these autologous monocytes present the PAP antigen to host T cells (PAP-specific CD4+ and CD8+ T cells), resulting in the T-cell activation and proliferation [65] (Fig. 1).

An analysis of culture during the manufacture process showed an increase in APC activation

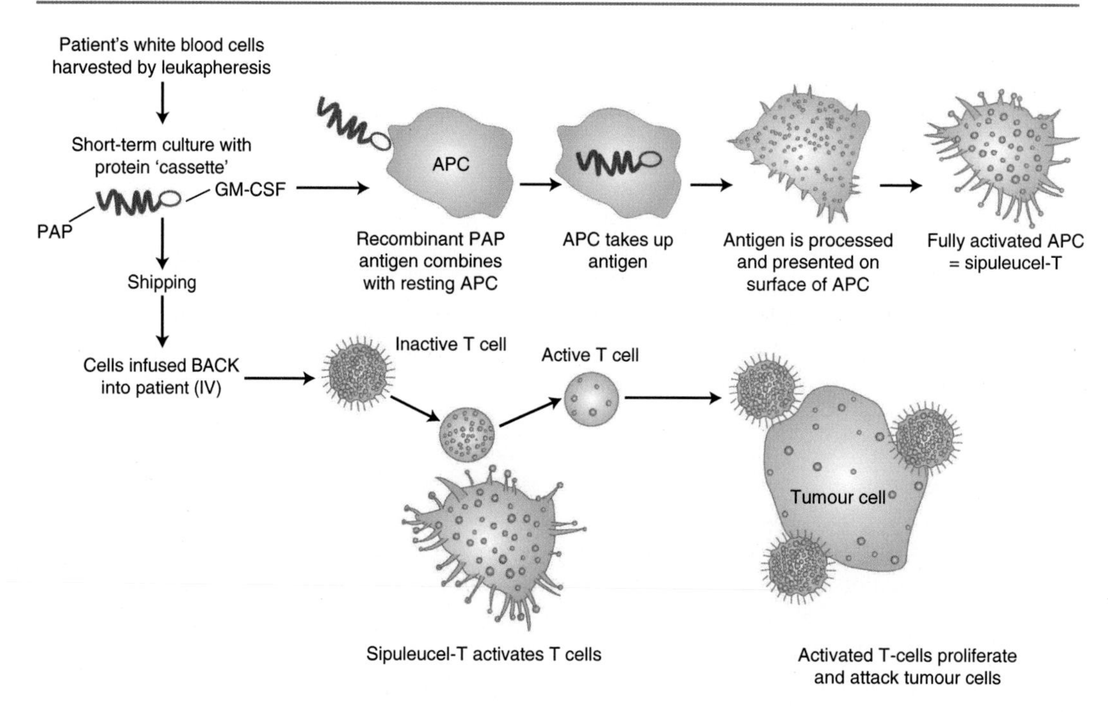

Fig. 1 The predicted mechanism of action and stages of Sipuleucel-T treatment for patients with castration-resistant prostate cancer (CRPC)

cytokines (macrophage inflammatory protein (MIP)-1a and -1b; interleukin (IL)-1a, IL-23), T cell activation markers (IL-2, IL-3, IL-4, IL-5, IL-10, and IL-17) and APC/T cell activation-associated cytokines (IL-12, tumor necrosis factor-TNF) [60]. The GM-CSF component of the fusion protein is an immune modulatory cytokine that stimulates the development and maturation of APCs, including type 1 dendritic cells (DC1), the subset responsible for initiation of cytotoxic immune responses [65, 66].

Sipuleucel-T is the first antigen-specific immunotherapy approved for cancer treatment. Three Phase III studies have been completed.

The first sipuleucel-T phase-3 trials (D9901 and D9902A) used the traditional measure of response, time to disease progression (TTP) as the primary endpoint. The improvement in the primary end point TTP did not achieve statistical significance [67]. There was, however, a significant benefit in the prespecified endpoint of 3-year survival with sipuleucel-T versus placebo in D9901 (median survival benefit 4.5 months; $p=0.01$; hazard ratio [HR] 0.586; 95 % confidence interval [CI] 0.39–0.88), suggesting that sipuleucel-T may provide a survival advantage to asymptomatic HRPC patients. The subsequent IMPACT (IMmunotherapy Prostate AdenoCarcinoma Treatment) trial met its primary end-point of significantly improved overall survival (OS) with sipuleucel-T versus placebo (median survival benefit 4.1 months: 25.8 months versus 21.7 months; $p=0.03$; HR 0.78; 95 % CI 0.61–0.98) [4]. This trial, where 512 patients with asymptomatic or minimally symptomatic metastatic castration-resistant PC were studied, served as the basis for the licensing approval of sipuleucel-T. Overall, in an integrated analysis of survival across the three trials (D9901, D9902A, and IMPACT; $n=737$), sipuleucel-T provided a survival benefit compared with placebo ($p<0.001$; HR 0.735 [95 % CI 0.613–0.882]) [68]. The greatest magnitude of benefit was observed among patients with better baseline prognostic factors, particularly among patients with lower baseline PSA values [69].

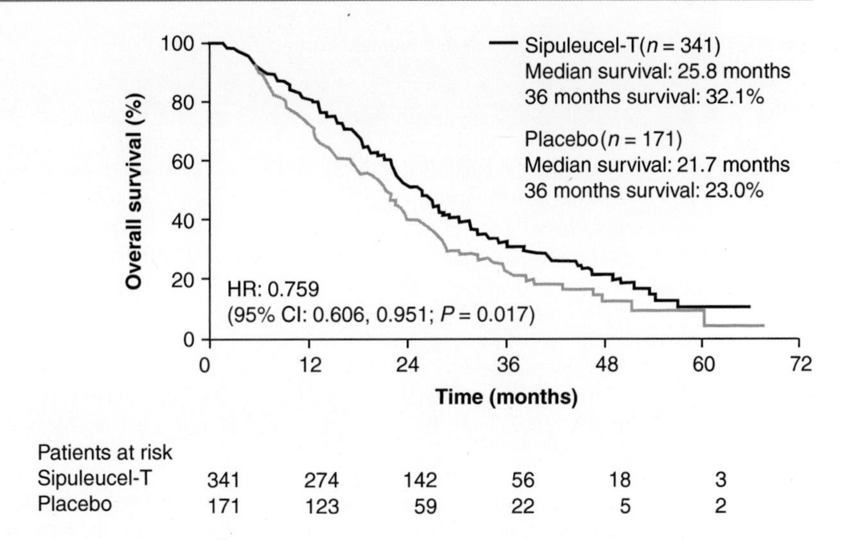

Fig. 2 Kaplan-Meier estimates of overall survival from the phase III (IMPACT) trial of sipuleucel-T in patients with metastatic CRPC

Although the median survival time was greater for sipuleucel-T-treated patients over placebo in all the trials, no difference in progression-free survival was observed between the two groups. Possible explanations relate to how progression is defined (in which a responding scenario can be interpreted as progression) or the idea that the treatment gradually slows down progression, being reflected in prolongation of overall survival, but short-term improvements are not apparent [14].

In the study, sipuleucel-T was generally well tolerated. Adverse events were reported more commonly by patients in the treatment group than in the placebo. These included chills, fever, myalgia, headache, influenza-like illness, hyperhidrosis, hypertension, and groin pain, most of which occurred within 1 day after infusion and resolved in a few days. Grade 3/4 adverse events were uncommon, being reported in 23 of 338 patients (6.8 %) in the sipuleucel-T group and 3 of 168 patients (1.8 %) in the placebo group (Fig. 2).

Sipuleucel-T has also been studied in the neoadjuvant setting with the single-arm phase 2 NeoACT (NEOadjuvant Active Cellular immunotherapy) trial. It was undergone in 42 patients with localized and treatment-naive PC prior to radical prostatectomy to characterize the immune infiltrate in this type or tumor before and after treatment with sipuleucel-T, and not to look at patient-specific outcomes [70]. The NeoACT trial was the first to demonstrate that sipuleucel-T induced a local immune effect, with an increased T and B cell infiltration (such as CD3+ cells, CD4+ cells, CD8+ cells, CD4+/FOXP3+-T helper, and CD20+ cells) at tumor interface after treatment with Sipuleucel-T. In addition, an examination of peripheral blood mononuclear cells revealed a significant change in antigen-specific T-cell circulation at 12 weeks postradical prostatectomy relative to baseline. This fact was also shown in a subsequent study where it was examined whether sipuleucel-T altered adaptive T cell responses by expanding preexisting T cells or by recruiting new T cells to prostate tissue [71]. Next-generation sequencing of the T cell receptor (TCR) genes from blood or prostate tissue was used to quantitate and track T cell clonotypes in these treated subjects with PC. A significantly greater diversity of circulating TCR sequences in subjects with PC compared with healthy donors was seen, supporting the hypothesis that sipuleucel-T treatment facilitates the recruitment of T cells into the prostate.

Despite all the controversy, sipuleucel-T is the first anticancer therapeutic vaccine that has demonstrated an overall survival improvement in solid cancer patients. It is also interesting the way that this approach can be adaptable to other tumor types by changing the nature of the immunogen–the antigen coupled to GM-CSF in the fusion protein.

Key clinical trials based on the four selected immunotherapies for prostate cancer.

Drug	Trial design	Number of patients	Phase	Key finding	Reference
Sipuleucel-T	Randomized, double-blind, placebo-controlled trial for asymptomatic metastatic CRPC	127	III	Improved OS by sipulcucel-T compared to placebo (25.9 versus 21.4 months)	Pasero et al. [17]
	Randomized, double-blind, placebo-controlled trial for asymptomatic metastatic CRPC	98	III	Improved OS by sipuleucel-T compared to placebo (19 versus 15.7 months)	Zhu and Paul [18]
	Randomized, double-blind, placebo-controlled trial for asymptomatic metastatic CRPC	512	III	Improved OS by sipuleucel-T compared to placebo (25.8 versus 21.7 months)	Wing and Sakaguchi [19]
Ipilimumab	Randomized, double-blind, placebo-controlled trial for metastatic CRPC after docetaxel	799	III	No difference in OS between the two groups, but trend of improved PFS rate by ipilimumab at 6 months (30.7 % versus 18.1 %)	Wei et al. [20]
Prostvac-VF	Randomized placebo-controlled trial of Prostvac-VF for metastatic CRPC	125	II	Improved OS by Prostvac-VF compared to control vector placebo (25.1 versus 16.6 months)	Hodi et al. [21]
	Nonrandomized trial for chemotherapy-naive CRPC	32	II	Improved OS by Prostvac-VF compared to historical controls (Halabi nomogram): (26.6 versus 17.4 months)	Nishikawa and Sakaguchi [22]
GVAX	Randomized trial of GVAX with docetaxel versus docetaxel with prednisone in taxane-naïve patients with symptomatic CRPC	408	III	Trial terminated early due to excess deaths in GVAX plus docetaxel group compared to control (docetaxel plus prednisone) (67 versus 47), and shorter median OS (12.2 versus 14.1 months).	Dalgleish et al. [23]
	Randomized trial of GVAX with docetaxel versus docetaxel with prednisone in taxane-naïve patients with asymptomatic CRPC	626	III	Trial terminated early based on futility analysis showing <30 % chance of meeting primary endpoint (improved OS)	Dunn et al. [24]

Tse et al. [14]

4 Investigational Agents

Multiple immune approaches beyond sipuleucel-T are under development, including monoclonal antibodies against immune checkpoints as well as antigen-directed therapies. Moreover, combinations of these immunotherapies and conventional therapies are also under investigation. In addition, finding the ideal setting and timing for these therapies is also a priority. It is at early stages of the disease when the immune system of patients may be more intact. That might be the best setting where to apply this approach.

4.1 PROSTVAC-VF Tricom

The use of viral vectors is a promising area in treating cancer. Using this approach, with proven efficacy in infectious disease, might have several advantages as they can mimic natural infection and lead to the induction of potent immune responses against the tumor antigens they encode. An increased number of tumor antigens are available for intersection into these vectors. The poxvirus-based vaccines are the most established and well studied. One example of these vaccines is PROSTVAC®-VF, which employs a recombinant poxvirus-based vector encoded with PSA and TRICOM (three immune co stimulatory molecules: B7.1, ICAM-1, and LFA-3). Vaccination is often enhanced by the subcutaneous co administration of GM-CSF, which acts to further boost immune function [72]. The rationale behind this treatment is that the virus will directly infect the APCs (resulting in expression of the costimulatory molecules), or somatic cells (epithelial and/or fibroblasts) at the site of injection, leading to cell death and subsequent uptake of cellular debris containing PSA by the APCs [14]. APCs will lead to the promotion of a T cell-mediated immune response that destroys PSA-expressing cancer cells. The vaccine virus-based vector is followed by fowl pox virus-based vector boots, helping to overcome the host antivector antibody responses to the original vector and maintaining the level of immunity (Fig. 3).

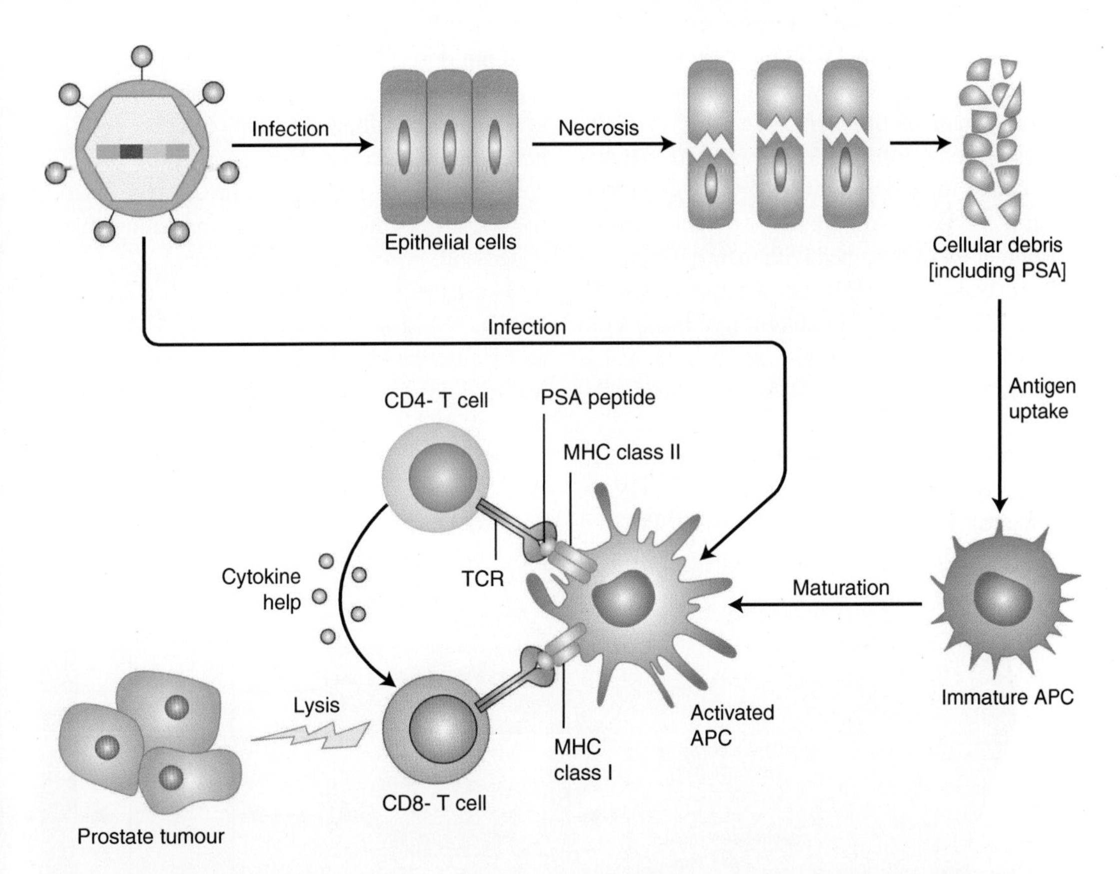

Fig. 3 The ProstVac VF 'vaccine' consists of a DNA plasmid encoding the target antigen (PSA) and a series of co-stimulatory molecules. Then viral vectors are injected intradermally, where they probably infect the patient's epithelial cells. This in turn leads to epithelial cell death, following which the cellular debris (including the target antigen PSA) is taken up by host antigen´presenting cells (APCs) and presented to host CD4+ and CD8+ T cells. The incorporation of CD80 into viral vector facilitates the activation of T cells, through the provision of a co-stimulatory signal for T cell activation

The therapy has been studied in two phases II trials. The first one enrolled 32 patients and evaluated PSA-specific T-cell responses as the primary endpoint, finding a trend towards increased overall survival and a decreased in regulatory T-cell (Treg) suppression in patients with longer survival [18]. These data suggest that PSA-specific T-cell responses and Treg functionality can be used as prognostic markers of efficacy in future trials. The largest phase II randomized 125 patients with minimally symptomatic, metastatic castration resistant PC to treatment or control vectors. The primary end point of progression-free survival was similar between 82 patients treated with PROSTVAC®-VF and 40 patients who received placebo. However, with 3 years of follow-up, patients receiving the vaccine had an 8.5 month improvement in median OS [73]. The therapy was well-tolerated. Most adverse effects were injection site reactions, with only a few patients experiencing associated systemic symptoms such as fatigue, nausea, or fever.

Based on this information, a phase III trial was designed, with and without GM-CSF, in asymptomatic or minimally symptomatic, chemotherapy-naïve, men with metastatic castration resistant PC with or without GM-CSF (NCT01322490). This three-arm trial has overall survival as primary endpoint, and the accrual is already completed ($n=1200$) with results maturing (Fig. 4).

Another type of vaccine that has been studied is the whole-cell-based vaccine or GVAX (BioSante). It is an allogenic cell-based PC vaccine that is composed of both homono-sensitive (LNCaP) and naive (PC3) PC cell lines and that have been genetically modified to constitutively secrete GM-CSF and irradiated to prevent cell replication [74]. The whole tumor cell is used as the antigen, facilitating both humoral and cellular immune responses, with GM-CSF enhancing this process by functioning as chemo attractant for dendritic cells [75]. The use of allogeneic tumor cells as the main component also has advantages in being faster and less expensive to manufacture as compared to autologous cells. Initial phase I/II studies confirmed clinical activity [74]. One phase II trial involving 55 men with chemotherapy-naive metastatic CRPC showed a trend of increased survival time by GVAX in a dose-dependent fashion. Another phase II clinical trial comprised of 80 men with the same clinical characteristics, treatment with high dose was associated with longer median survival time (35 months) as compared with those given medium dose (20 months) and low dose therapy (23.1 months). The proportion of patients that generated an antibody response to either cell line had a median survival of 34 months ($n=30$), compared to 16 months for those who did not ($n=6$), suggesting that immune reaction is associated with better clinical outcomes.

These results lead to two phase III clinical trials (VITAL-2 and VITAL-1). VITAL-2 was a multicenter, randomized, controlled phase 3 clinical trial designed to evaluate the safety and efficacy of GVAX immunotherapy for prostate cancer used in combination with docetaxel chemotherapy compared to the use of docetaxel chemotherapy and prednisone in hormone-refractory prostate cancer (HRPC) patients with metastatic

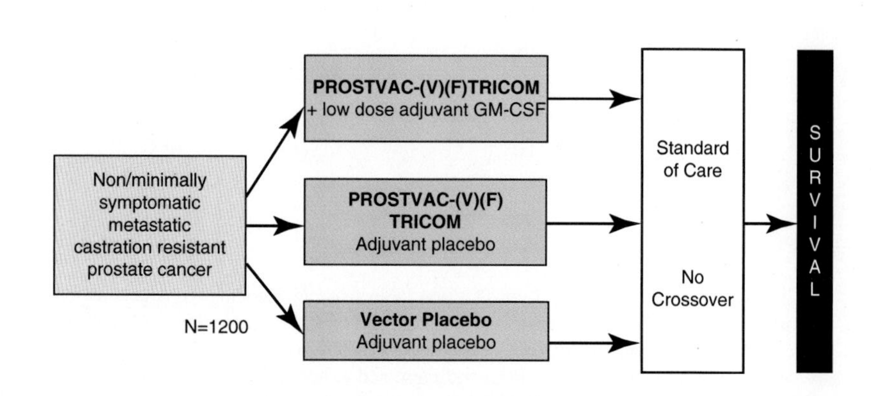

Fig. 4 Phase III ProstVac VF +/- GM-CSF trial study design

disease who were symptomatic with cancer-related pain. The primary endpoint of the trial was an improvement in survival. The trial ended after the Independent Data Monitoring Committee (IDMC) observed an imbalance in deaths between the two treatment arms of the study. VITAL-2 enrolled 408 patients. The IDMC based its recommendation on 114 deaths of which 67 occurred in the GVAX plus docetaxel combination treatment arm and 47 deaths occurred in the docetaxel control arm [76]. VITAL-1, the other Phase 3 clinical trial of GVAX immunotherapy for prostate cancer, was designed to compare GVAX cancer immunotherapy as a monotherapy to docetaxel chemotherapy plus prednisone in earlier stage HRPC patients with metastatic disease who were asymptomatic with respect to cancer-related pain. The primary endpoint of the trial was an improvement in survival. The trial was fully enrolled in 2007 with 626. The study was terminated trial based on the results of a previously unplanned futility analysis conducted by the study's IDMC which indicated that the trial had less than a 30 % chance of meeting its predefined primary endpoint of an improvement in survival.

Despite these disappointing results, GVAX is currently being trialed in combination with other immunotherapies, for example, Ipilimumab [77] or mitoxantrone [78] for PC.

4.2 Immune Checkpoint Blockade

As previously mentioned, immune responses are kept in balance by immune checkpoints that oppose co-stimulatory pathways. Alteration of these pathways in tumor cells can provoke sending negative signal into the binding T cells, thus leading to its exhaustion (Fig. 5).

4.1 Anti-CTLA-4 Therapies

Several phase II trials have investigated the role of ipilimumab in PC. A phase I/II study evaluated ipilimumab at up to 10 mg/kg dose with or without radiotherapy in patients with metastatic CRPC who received no more than one prior chemotherapy. PSA decline and radiographic responses were observed in all dose cohorts [79]. A subsequent phase II study randomized 43 chemotherapy naive CRPC patients to ipilimumab at 3 mg/kg versus ipilimumab and docetaxel [80]. These trials lead to plan two phase III trials, which have been completed accrual. The first study evaluated the impact of ipilimumab and radiation (in an effort to prime an initial antitumor immune response) versus radiation alone in the postdocetaxel setting looking for an overall survival (OS) advantage. The study's primary endpoint of OS did not reach statistical significance with median OS at 11.2 months with ipilimumab and 10 months with the placebo (HR = 0.85; 95 % CI = 0.72–1.00; $p = 0.053$). Median progression-free survival favored ipilimumab over placebo (HR = 0.70; 95 % CI = 0.61–0.82) as did prostate-specific antigen (PSA) response rates. A post hoc analysis was done showing that patients with favorable prognosis (three baseline factors defined by: alkaline phosphatase level, hemoglobin level and no visceral metastases) may derive clinical benefit from ipilimumab [81]. The results of the second study that evaluates ipilimumab versus placebo in metastatic CRPC patients who have not received chemotherapy are still pending (NCT01057810) (Fig. 6).

Tremelimumab, another monoclonal antibody, has been studied in a phase I trial in PSA-recurrent setting. It does show dose-limiting toxicities (diarrhea and skin rash) and PSA doubling time prolongation was observed in 3/11 patients [82].

4.2 Anti-PD1 Therapies

PD1 has been less well studied in PC, although it was found that the CD8+ T cells that infiltrate the prostate gland in men with cancer seem to express PD1 [83].

An earlier phase I study of nivolumab in multiple cancer types enrolled 17 patients with castration-resistant PC, but no objective responses were seen in these patients [84]. Also, there is a phase II trial in the metastatic PC setting, currently ongoing, studying the efficacy of pembrolizumab after androgen-deprivation therapy

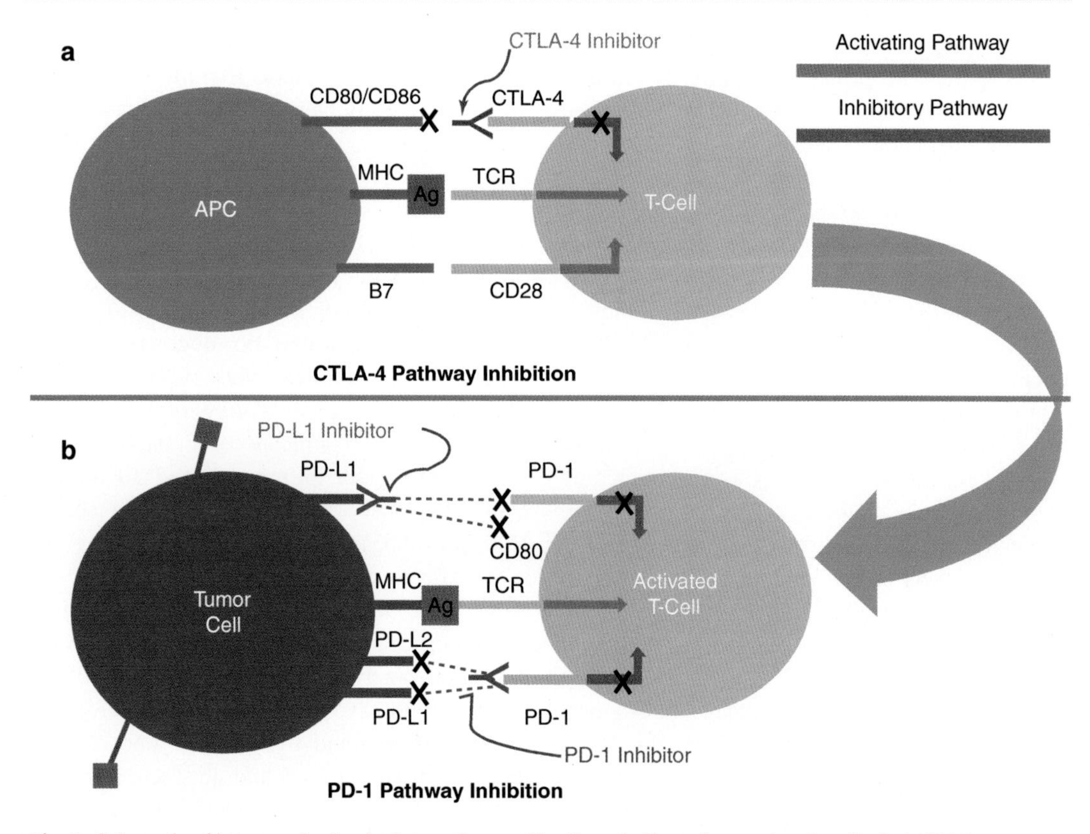

Fig. 5 Schematic of immune checkpoint interactions on T cells and effect of monoclonal antibody inhibition

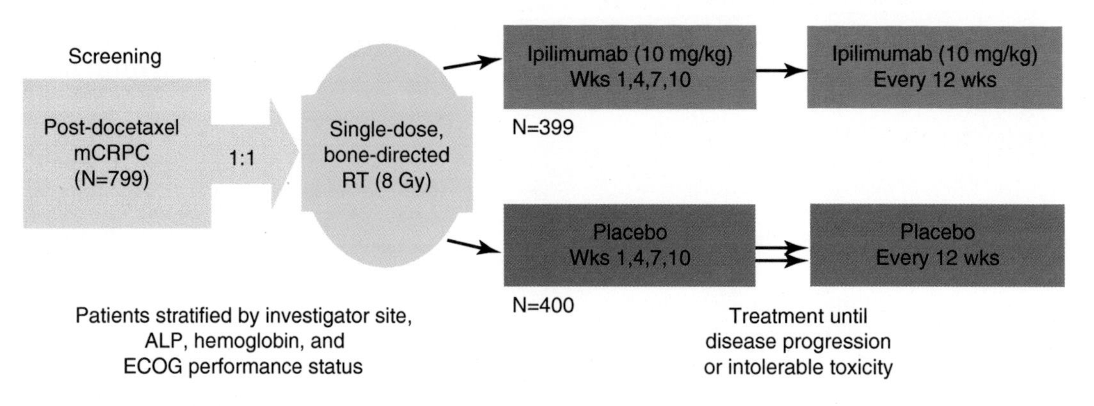

Fig. 6 Phase III trial which evaluates radiation +/- ipilimumab in the post-docetaxel setting. Study design

(NCT02312557). Besides, there are some studies that are focused on the combination of immunotherapy (pembrolizumab) with other types of treatment, such as radium-223, in castration-resistant PC with bone metastases (Investigator initiated trail at Dana Farber)

Pidilizumab, another PD-1 antibody, is being evaluated in a phase II trial for the treatment of androgen-independent PC in combination with sipuleucel-T and cyclophosphamide (NCT01420965).

A promising field of PC treatment is the combination of radiation and immunotherapy. This concept has been evaluated in the previously mentioned phase III clinical trials that combines ipilimumab and radiotherapy and also, in a small randomized trial of men undergoing primary radiotherapy [57];

13 out of 17 patients in the radiotherapy and immunotherapy combination treatment group had a greater than threefold increase in the number of PSA-specific T cells, whereas no increase in the number of PSA-specific T cells was noted in the group that received radiotherapy alone.

New emerging immune checkpoint targets have been identified and include LAG-3, TIM-3, VISTA, and co-stimulatory molecules OX40, ICOS, and 4-1BB [85]. In addition, new next generation sequencing techniques sequencing could help to identify a spectrum of mutation frequencies that can respond to immunotherapy. Some select patients with advanced heavily pretreated PC might harbor microsatellite instability making them more suitable for PD1/PDL1 blockade (P.Nelson, *ASCO* 2016).

4.3 Biomarkers in PC

Due to the emerging development of new therapies, including immune agents, predictive and surrogate biomarkers will be needed. Such biomarkers could identify responders in the earlier phases of treatments, in which the full effects are often not apparent before weeks to months after initiation. Because OS is a more reliable endpoint than PFS with immunotherapy, such biomarkers could provide intermediate surrogate endpoints for trials (while final end points would otherwise take years to complete). Multiple categories of immune biomarkers have already been investigated in PC, in the following table there is a selection of these [86].

Biomarker	Description/examples	Applications	Sampling specimen	Routine clinical availability	Prognostic	Predictive	Pharmacodynamic	Surrogate
Inflammatory biomarkers								
Individual cytokines	IL-6, IL-8, TGF-β1	Diagnostic and prognostic utility in various stages of disease Prediction of responses with chemotherapy, vaccines and Sipuleucel-T	Serum	No	Yes	Yes	FSN	FSN
C-reactive protein (CRP)	Acute-phase protein involved in inflammation, necrosis, and carcinogenesis	Prognostic utility in various stages of disease	Serum	Yes	Yes	FSN	FSN	FSN
Toll-like receptors (TLRs)	Family of transmembrane proteins that can recognize highly conserved molecules in invading pathogens	Postdiagnostic prognostic utility	Serum	No	Yes	FSN	FSN	FSN
Neutrophil-to-lymphocyte ratio	Ratio of peripheral neutrophil to lymphocite count	Postdiagnostic prognostic utility Possible predictive value in enzalutamide-treated-patients	Serum	Yes	Yes	Yes	FSN	FSN
Cellular response to PC								
Increase in Th1 T cell response	Subtype of T-helper cell response	Possible favorable prognostic utility	Serum	No	Yes	FSN	FSN	FSN
Increase in Th2 T cell response	Subtype of T-helper cell response	Possible negative prognostic utility	Serum	No	Yes	FSN	FSN	FSN
Cellular response to immunotherapeutic agents								
Increase in various T cell responses	Cytotoxic and T-helper lymphocytes	Possible prognostic and pharmacodynamic utility in patients treated with vaccines	Serum	No	Yes	FSN	Yes	FSN
Decrease in Treg response	Regulatory T cells	Role to be defined in patients treated with ipilimumab, Sipuleucel-T, and other vaccines	Serum	No	FSN	FSN	FSN	FSN
Increase in eosinophil response	Peripheral eosinophil count	Possible prognostic and predictive utility in Sipuleucel-treated patients	Serum	No	Yes	FSN	FSN	FSN

Humoral response to PC								
Tumor-associated antigens (TAAs) other than PSA	p90, p62	Possible diagnostic and prognostic utility	Serum	No	Yes	FSN	FSN	FSN
Auto-antibody signatures	Combination of various serum auto-antibodies	Possible diagnostic and prognostic utility	Serum	No	Yes	FSN	FSN	FSN
Humoral response to immunotherapeutic agents								
Antigen spreading	Vaccine-associated response to ubiquitously expressed self-antigens	Possible pharmacodynamic, prognostic and predictive Serum utilities in patients treated with vaccines including Sipuleucel-T	Serum	No	FSN	FSN	FSN	FSN
Immune checkpoints								
PD-1/PD-L1 (B7- H1)	PD-1: Immunoglobulin superfamily member PD-L1: Ligand of PD-1, member of the B7 super-family of costimulatory molecules	Predictive role in patients treated with anti-PD-L1 and tissue anti-PD-1 monoclonal antibodies Possible predictive role in enzalutamide-resistant patients Possible prognostic role in ipilimumab- and Sipuleucel-T-treated patients	Tissue	Yes	Yes	Yes	FSN	FSN
CD276 (B7-H3)	Member of the B7 super-family of costimulatory molecules	Possible postdiagnostic, prognostic and predictive tissue roles New immunotherapy target	Tissue	No	Yes	Yes	FSN	FSN
CD73	Ectonucleotidase catabolizing the hydrolysis of extracellular adenosine monophosphate (AMP) to adenosine	Possible postdiagnostic, prognostic and predictive tissue roles New immunotherapy target	Tissue	No	Yes	Yes	FSN	FSN
Immunologic biomarkers of tumor microenvironment								
Tumor-associated macrophages (TAMs)		Possible adverse prognostic role tissue	Tissue	No	Yes	FSN	FSN	FSN
Cytotoxic CD8 tumor-infiltrating lymphocytes (TILs)		Possible adverse prognostic role tissue	Tissue	No	Yes	FSN	FSN	FSN
Treg tumor- infiltrating lymphocytes (TILs)		Possible adverse prognostic role tissue	Tissue	No	FSN	FSN	FSN	FSN
Mast cells		Role remains to be defined tissue	Tissue	No	FSN	FSN	FSN	FSN

Immunotherapy with check point inhibitors is now a newly rediscovered therapeutic strategy in PC that was initially dismissed. Like in colorectal cancer, in selected patients these agents might be of benefit.

5 Targeted Therapies

In the field of PC, bevies of novel therapeutics with distinct mechanisms of action have been recently tested. Unfortunately although preliminary data were promising, in unselected patients, no one of these new agents has been able to provide clinically meaningful benefit. Here, we briefly report some new therapies that can potentially be useful in PC treatment if the adequate target patient population is identified. An example has been the potential benefit seen with PARP inhibitors is select patient harboring DNA repair genomic alterations (see Sect. 5.8)

5.1 Angiogenesis Inhibitors

Angiogenesis mechanisms play an important role in cancer. It is also well known that a high microvascular density in prostate gland is a poor prognostic factor in PC [87]. There are several angiogenesis-related agents which have been studied, such as thalidomide [88], bevazicumab [89], lenalidomide [90], sorafenib (NCT00619996) [91], most of them with no success in phase III trials.

5.2 Next-Generation Androgen Synthesis Inhibitors and Androgen Receptor Signaling Inhibitors

PC progression usually occurs despite continued castration in patients receiving standard androgen deprivation therapy. There are several mechanisms that have been implicated in castration resistance; such as, overexpression of AR, androgen synthesis by PC cells; alterations in expression of coactivators and corepressors of AR signaling; and constitutively active, ligand-independent AR splice variants [92]. There are currently several androgen synthesis inhibitors in development beyond the ones already approved abiraterone and enzalutamide [93]. AR antagonist in development like ARN-509, competitively inhibits AR signaling in the setting of AR overexpression, with potentially improved efficacy compared with enzalutamide in xenograft models. Phase III studies with ARN-509 are ongoing (NCT01946204).

5.3 HSP90 Inhibitors (Olanespib)

The transcriptional activity of steroid receptors, including AR, is dependent on interactions with the HSP90 chaperone machinery, this is way some early studies are checking the utility of HSP90 inhibitors, specially on PC with androgen receptor variant 7 [94].

5.4 mTOR (Mammalian Target of Rapamycin) Inhibitors (Everolimus, RAD 001)

MTOR inhibition appears to reverse dysregulation of Akt system, thus avoiding the effect of PTEN mutation, which is a common characteristic in 50 % of advanced PC [95].

5.5 EGFR (Epidermal Growth Factor Receptor)-Tyrosine-kinase Inhibitors (Gefitinib, Erlotinib, Pertuzumab)

There are several studies published with poor results, although in vitro test results were promising [96, 97].

5.6 mRNA-Based Therapies

Such as oblimersen, a Bcl-2 antisense oligonucleotide, with negative results in a phase II trial performed in patients with castration-resistant PC [98].

5.7 Histone Deacetylase Inhibitors (HDACs)

HDACs are part of a transcriptional corepressor complex that influences various tumor suppressor genes, included in PC scenario [99]. There are some examples of HDACs that have been studied in this disease with controversial results, such as vorinostat (with a phase II trial where it showed significant toxicities that limited efficacy assessment in the patient population) [100].

5.8 PARP (poly(ADP-ribose) Polymerase) Inhibitors

Previous PC genomic sequencing efforts have identified genetic aberrations, including mutations in DNA repair genes. The researchers hypothesized that olaparib, which targets those tumor cells that are particularly vulnerable to DNA repair defects, may work in this subset of PC patients. A phase II trial [TOPARP, NCT01682772], which is currently recruiting patients will try to determine if this approach can be useful in PC.

Conclusions

PC is a target for immunotherapy approaches. It has a unique natural history characterized by a relatively indolent course, which allows immunotherapies, time to achieve an effect via stimulation of the immune machinery. It was the first type of solid cancer where an immunotherapy drug was the standard of care (sipuleucel-T) upon improving survival. Since that achievement, there are multiple novel therapeutics under investigation (off the shelf vaccines such as PROSTVAC-VF, GVAX; checkpoint inhibitors; or novel homegrown vaccines). However, still some questions remain according to the immune approach: timing and combination with other modalities of treatment need to be explored. Establishing the optimal combination and sequencing of treatment will prove crucial. Also, it is important to keep on finding predictive immune biomarkers as the response is often gradual, and the usual monitored clinical markers are not always affected immediately after treatment initiation. Identifying the best method to measure and quantify such immune responses remains a challenge because of the difficulty in obtaining an adequate quantity of samples and the limitations of current functional assays.

New technologies or platforms, such as T cells receptor (TCR) clonotyping, chimeric antigen receptor T-cell therapies (CARTs), computational analysis approach, or home grown vaccines, are welcomed in this fight against PC.

Achieving long-term remission in most treated patients is an ambitious goal for the scientific community and requires the integration of several modalities in a rational combination therapeutic approach.

Bibliography

1. Saad F, Miller K. Current and emerging immunotherapies for castration-resistant prostate cancer. Urology. 2015;85:976–86.
2. Harris DT, Matyas GR, Gomella LG, et al. Immunologic approaches to the treatment of prostate cancer. Semin Oncol. 1999;26(4):439–47.
3. Fernandez-Garcia EM, Vera-Badillo FE, Perez-Valderrama B, Matos-Pita AS, Duran I. Immunotherapy in prostate cancer: review of the current evidence. Clin Transl Oncol. 2015;17(5):339–57.
4. Kantoff PW, Higano CS, Shore ND, et al. Sipuleucel-T immunotherapy for castration-resistant prostate cancer. N Engl J Med. 2010;363(5):411–22.
5. Schreiber RD, Old LJ, Smyth MJ. Cancer immunoediting: integrating immunity's roles in cancer suppression and promotion. Science. 2011;331:1565–70.
6. Swann JB, Smyth MJ. Immune surveillance of tumors. J Clin Invest. 2007;117(5):1137–46.
7. Hagerling C, Casbon AJ, Werb Z. Balancing the innate immune system in tumor development. Trends Cell Biol. 2014;25:214–20.
8. Coffelt SB, Visser KE. Immune-mediated mechanisms influencing the efficacy of anticancer therapies. Trends Immunol. 2015;36:198–216.
9. Medzhitov R. Recognition of microorganisms and activation of the immune response. Nature. 2007;449(7164):819–26.
10. Alberts B, Johnson A, Lewis J, Raff M, Roberts K, Walters P. Molecular biology of the cell. 4th ed. New York/London: Garland Science; 2002.

11. Noy R, Pollard JW. Tumor-associated macrophages: from mechanisms to therapy. Immunity. 2015;41:49–61.
12. Wang N, Liang H, Zen K. Molecular mechanisms that influence the macrophage m1-m2 polarization balance. Front Immunol. 2014;5:614.
13. Lanciotti M, Masieri L, Raspollini MR, et al. The role of M1 and M2 macrophages in prostate cancer in relation to extracapsular tumor extension and biochemical recurrence after radical prostatectomy. Biomed Res Int. 2014;2014:486798. 6 pages.
14. Tse BW, Jovanovic L, Nelson CC, et al. Review article from bench to bedside: immunotherapy for prostate cancer. Biomed Res Int. 2014:981434, 11 pages.
15. Huntington ND. NK cell recognition of unconventional ligands. Immunol Cell Biol. 2014;92:208–9.
16. Westdorp H, Skold AE, Snijer BA, et al. Immunotherapy for prostate cancer : lessons from responses to tumor-associated antigens. Front Immunol. 2014;5:191.
17. Pasero C, Gravis G, Guerin M, et al. Inherent and tumor-driven immune tolerance in the prostate microenvironment impairs natural killer cell antitumor activity. Cancer Res. 2016;76(8):2153–65.
18. Zhu J, Paul WE. CD4 T cells: fates, functions, and faults. Blood. 2015;112:1557–70.
19. Wing K, Sakaguchi S. Regulatory T cells exert checks and balances on self-tolerance and autoimmunity. Nat Immunol. 2010;11:7–13.
20. Wei XX, Fong L, Small EJ. Prospects for the use of ipilimumab in treating advanced prostate cancer. Expert Opin Biol Ther. 2016;16(3):421–32.
21. Hodi FS, O'Day SJ, McDermott DF, et al. Improved survival with ipilimumab in patients with metastatic melanoma. N Engl J Med. 2010;363(8):711–23.
22. Nishikawa H, Sakaguchi S. Regulatory T cells in tumor immunity. Int J Cancer. 2010;127:759–67.
23. Dalgleish A, Featherstone P, Vlassov V, et al. Rituximab for treating CD20+ prostate cancer with generalized lymphadenopathy: a case report and review of the literature. Invest New Drugs. 2014;32:1048–5.
24. Dunn GP, Bruce AT, Ikeda H, et al. Cancer immunoediting: from immunosurveillance to tumor escape. Nat Immunol. 2002;3:991–8.
25. Mercader M, et al. T cell infiltration of the prostate induced by androgen withdrawal in patients with prostate cancer. Proc Natl Acad Sci U S A. 2001;98:14565–70.
26. Gannon PO, et al. Characterization of the intraprostatic immune cell infiltration in androgendeprived prostate cancer patients. J Immunol Methods. 2009;348:9–17.
27. Drake CG, et al. Androgen ablation mitigates tolerance to a prostate/prostate cancer -restricted antigen. Cancer Cell. 2005;7:239–49.
28. Mercader M, Bodner BK, Moser MT, et al. T cell infiltration of the prostate induced by androgen withdrawal in patients with prostate cancer. Proc Natl Acad Sci U S A. 2001;98(25):14565–70.
29. Koh YT, Gray A, Higgins SA, Hubby B, Kast WM. Androgen ablation augments prostate cancer vaccine immunogenicity only when applied after immunization. Prostate. 2009;69:571–84.
30. Greaves M. Evolutionary determinants of cancer. Cancer Discov. 2015;5:806–20.
31. Mahnke K, Schmitt E, Bonifaz L, et al. Immature, but not inactive: the tolerogenic function of immature dendritic cells. Immunol Cell Biol. 2002;80:477–83.
32. Drake CG, Jaffee E, Pardoll DM. Mechanisms of immune evasion by tumors. Adv Immunol. 2006;90:51–81.
33. Drake CG. Prostate cancer as a model for tumor immunotherapy. Nat Rev Immunol. 2010;10(8):580–93.
34. Ozao-Choy J, et al. The novel role of tyrosine kinase inhibitor in the reversal of immune suppression and modulation of tumor microenvironment for immune-based cancer therapies. Cancer Res. 2009;69(6):2514–22.
35. Xin H, et al. Sunitinib inhibition of Stat3 induces renal cell carcinoma tumor cell apoptosis and reduces immunosuppressive cells. Cancer Res. 2009;69(6):2506–13.
36. Schilling B, Sucker A, Griewank K, Zhao F, et al. Vemurafenib reverses immunosuppression by myeloid derived suppressor cells. Int J Cancer. 2013;133(7):1653–63.
37. Suzuki E, Kapoor V, Jassar AS, Kaiser LR, Albelda SM. Gemcitabine selectively eliminates splenic Gr-1+/CD11b+myeloid suppressor cells in tumor-bearing animals and enhances antitumor immune activity. Clin Cancer Res. 2005;11(18): 6713–21.
38. Vincent J, et al. 5-Fluorouracil selectively kills tumor-associated myeloid-derived suppressor cells resulting in enhanced T cell-dependent antitumor immunity. Cancer Res. 2010;70(8):3052–61.
39. Diaz-Montero CM, Salem ML, Nishimura MI, et al. Increased circulating myeloid-derived suppressor cells correlate with clinical cancer stage, metastatic tumor burden, and doxorubicin-cyclophosphamide chemotherapy. Cancer Immunol Immunother. 2009;58(1):49–59.
40. Young MR, Lathers DM. Combination docetaxel plus vitamin D(3) as an immune therapy in animals bearing squamous cell carcinomas. Otolaryngol Head Neck Surg. 2005;133(4):611–8.
41. Walker DD, et al. Immunological modulation by 1alpha,25-dihydroxyvitamin D3 in patients with squamous cell carcinoma of the head and neck. Cytokine. 2012;58(3):448–54.
42. Kodumudi KN, et al. A novel chemoimmunomodulating property of docetaxel: suppression of myeloid-derived suppressor cells in tumor bearers. Clin Cancer Res. 2010;16(18):4583–94.

43. Sevko A, et al. Application of paclitaxel in low non-cytotoxic doses supports vaccination with melanoma antigens in normal mice. J Immunotoxicol. 2012;9(3):275–81.
44. Montero AJ, et al. Phase 2 study of neoadjuvant treatment with NOV-002 in combination with doxorubicin and cyclophosphamide followed by docetaxel in patients with HER-2 negative clinical stage II-IIIc breast cancer. Breast Cancer Res Treat. 2012;132(1):215–23.
45. Apetoh L, et al. Toll-like receptor 4-dependent contribution of the immune system to anticancer chemotherapy and radiotherapy. Nat Med. 2007;13:1050–9.
46. Lugade AA, et al. Local radiation therapy of B16 melanoma tumors increases the generation of tumor antigen-specific effector cells that traffic to the tumor. J Immunol. 2005;174:7516–23.
47. Nesslinger NJ, et al. Standard treatments induce antigen-specific immune responses in prostate cancer. Clin Cancer Res. 2007;13:1493–502.
48. Chakraborty M, et al. Irradiation of tumor cells up-regulates Fas and enhances CTL lytic activity and CTL adoptive immunotherapy. J Immunol. 2003;170:6338–47.
49. Deng L, Liang H, Burnette B, et al. Irradiation and anti-PD-L1 treatment synergistically promote antitumor immunity in mice. J Clin Invest. 2014;124:687–95.
50. Lee Y, Auh SL, Wang Y, et al. Therapeutic effects of ablative radiation on local tumor require CD8+ T cells: changing strategies for cancer treatment. Blood. 2009;114:589–95.
51. Takeshima T, Chamoto K, Wakita D, et al. Local radiation therapy inhibits tumor growth through the generation of tumor-specific CTL: its potentiation by combination with Th1 cell therapy. Cancer Res. 2010;70:2697–706.
52. Postow MA, Callahan MK, Barker CA, et al. Immunologic correlates of the abscopal effect in a patient with melanoma. N Engl J Med. 2012;366:925–31.
53. Levy A, Chargari C, Marabelle A, Perfettini JL, Magné N, Deutsch E. Can immunostimulatory agents enhance the abscopal effect of radiotherapy? Eur J Cancer. 2016;62:36–45.
54. Demaria S, Ng B, Devitt ML, et al. Ionizing radiation inhibition of distant untreated tumors (abscopal effect) is immune mediated. Int J Radiat Oncol Biol Phys. 2004;58:862–70.
55. Dewhirst MW, Burnette B, Weichselbaum RR. Radiation as an immune modulator. Semin Radiat Oncol. 2013;23:273–80.
56. Harris TJ, Hipkiss EL, Borzillary S, et al. Radiotherapy augments the immune response to prostate cancer in a time-dependent manner. Prostate. 2008;68:1319–29.
57. Gulley JL, et al. Combining a recombinant cancer vaccine with standard definitive radiotherapy in patients with localized prostate cancer. Clin Cancer Res. 2005;11:3353–62.
58. PROVENGE® (sipuleucel-T) prescribing information. Dendreon Corporation, Seattle, Washington, USA. Last revision Oct 2014. Available at: http://www.provenge.com/pdf/prescribing-information.pdf. Accessed 8 June 2015.
59. Kantoff PW, Higano CS, Shore ND, Berger ER, Small EJ, Penson DF, et al. Sipuleucel-T immunotherapy for castration-resistant prostate cancer. N Engl J Med. 2010;363:411–22.
60. Sheikh NA, Petrylak D, Kantoff PW, Dela Rosa C, Stewart FP, Kuan LY, et al. Sipuleucel-T immune parameters correlate with survival: an analysis of the randomized phase 3 clinical trials in men with castration-resistant prostate cancer. Cancer Immunol Immunother. 2013;62:137–47.
61. Hsu FJ, Benike C, Fagnoni F, Liles TM, Czerwinski D, Taidi B, Engleman EG, Levy R. Vaccination of patients with B-cell lymphoma using autologous antigen-pulsed dendritic cells. Nat Med. 1996;2:52–8.
62. Fong L, Ruegg CL, Brockstedt D, Engleman EG, Laus R. Induction of tissue-specific autoimmune prostatitis with prostatic acid phosphatase immunization: implications for immunotherapy of prostate cancer. J Immunol. 1997;159:3113–7.
63. Paller CJ, Antonarakis ES. Sipuleucel-T for the treatment of metastatic prostate cancer: promise and challenges. Hum Vaccin Immunother. 2012;8(4):509–19.
64. Gulley JL, Drake CG. Immunotherapy for prostate cancer: recent advances, lessons learned, and areas for further research. Clin Cancer Res. 2011;17:3884–91.
65. Fang LC, Dattoli M, Taira A, True L, Sorace R, Wallner K. Prostatic acid phosphatase adversely affects cause specific survival in patients with intermediate to high-risk prostate cancer treated with brachytherapy. Urology. 2008;71(1):146–50.
66. Arellano M, Lonial S. Clinical uses of GM-CSF, a critical appraisal and update. Biologics Targets Ther. 2008;2(1):13–27.
67. Small EJ, Schellhammer PF, Higano CS, et al. Placebo-controlled phase III trial of immunologic therapy with sipuleucel-T (APC8015) in patients with metastatic, asymptomatic hormone refractory prostate cancer. J Clin Oncol. 2006;24:3089–94.
68. Petrylak DP, Dawson NA, Gardner T, Klotz L, Curti BD, Flanigan RC, Fishman MN, Xu Y, Whitmore JB, Frohlich MW. Persistence of immunotherapy survival effects of sipuleucel-T and relationship to postrandomization docetaxel use in phase III studies. J Clin Oncol. 2010;28 Suppl 15:4551.
69. Schellhammer PF, Chodak G, Whitmore JB, Sims R, Frohlich MW, Kantoff PW. Lower baseline prostate-specific antigen is associated with a greater overall survival benefit from sipuleucel-T in the Immunotherapy for Prostate Adenocarcinoma

Treatment (IMPACT) trial. Urology. 2013;81: 1297–302.
70. Fong L, Carroll P, Weinberg V, Chan S, et al. Activated lymphocyte recruitment into the tumor microenvironment following preoperative sipuleucel-T for localized prostate cancer. J Natl Cancer Inst. 2014;106(11):1–9.
71. Sheikh N, Cham J, Zhang L, DeVries T, Letarte S, Pufnock J, Hamm D, Trager J, Fong L. Clonotypic diversification of intratumoral T cells following sipuleucel-T treatment in prostate cancer subjects. 2016. doi:10.1158/0008-5472.CAN-15-3173.
72. May Jr KF, Gulley JL, Drake CG, et al. Prostate cancer immunotherapy. Clin Cancer Res. 2011;17:5233–8.
73. Kantoff PW, Schuetz TJ, Blumenstein BA, et al. Overall survival analysis of a phase II randomized controlled trial of a Poxviral-based PSA-targeted immunotherapy in metastatic castration-resistant prostate cancer. J Clin Oncol. 2010;28:1099–105.
74. Small EJ, Sacks N, Nemunaitis J, et al. Granulocyte macrophage colony-stimulating factor-secreting allogeneic cellular immunotherapy for hormone-refractory prostate cancer. Clin Cancer Res. 2007;13:3883–91.
75. Ward JE, McNeel DG. GVAX: an allogeneic, whole-cell, GM-CSF-secreting cellular immunotherapy for the treatment of prostate cancer. Expert Opinion on BiologicalTherapy. 2007;7(12):1893–902.
76. Higano CS, Schellhammer PF, Small EJ, et al. Integrated data from 2 randomized, double-blind, placebo-controlled, phase III trials of active cellular immunotherapy with sipuleucel-T in advanced prostate cancer. Cancer. 2009;115:3670–9.
77. Schweizer MT, Drake CG. Immunotherapy for prostate cancer: recent developments and future challenges. Cancer Metastasis Rev. 2014;33(2–3):641–55.
78. Van Dodewaard-de Jong JM, Santegoets SJ, van de Ven PM, et al. Improved efficacy of mitoxantrone in patients with castration-resistant prostate cancer after vaccination with GM-CSF-transduced allogeneic prostate cancer cells. Oncoimmunology. 2015;5(4):e1105431.
79. Slovin SF, Higano CS, Hamid O, et al. Ipilimumab alone or in combination with radiotherapy in metastatic castration-resistant prostate cancer: results from an open-label, multicenter phase I/II study. Ann Oncol. 2013;24:1813–21.
80. Small E, Higano C, Tchekmedyian N, et al. Randomized phase II study comparing 4 monthly doses of ipilimumab (MDX-010) as a single agent or in combination with a single dose of docetaxel in patients with hormone-refractory prostate cancer. JClinOncol(MeetingAbstracts).2006;24(Suppl):4609.
81. Kwon ED, Drake CG, Scher HI, Fizazi K, Bossi A, van den Eertwegh AJ, Krainer M, Houede N, Santos R, Mahammedi H, Ng S, Maio M, Franke FA, Sundar S, Agarwal N, Bergman AM, Ciuleanu TE, Korbenfeld E, Sengeløv L, Hansen S, Logothetis C, Beer TM, McHenry MB, Gagnier P, Liu D, Gerritsen WR, CA184-043 Investigators. Ipilimumab versus placebo after radiotherapy in patients with metastatic castration-resistant prostate cancer that had progressed after docetaxel chemotherapy (CA184-043): a multicentre, randomised, double-blind, phase 3 trial. Lancet Oncol. 2014;15(7):700–12.
82. McNeel DG, Smith HA, Eickhoff JC, et al. Phase I trial of tremelimumab in combination with short-term androgen deprivation in patients with PSA-recurrent prostate cancer. Cancer Immunol Immunother. 2012;61:1137–47.
83. Sfanos KS, et al. Human prostate-infiltrating CD8$^+$ T lymphocytes are oligoclonal and PD-1 $^+$. Prostate. 2009;69:1694–703.
84. Topalian SL, Hodi FS, Brahmer JR, et al. Safety, activity, and immune correlates of anti-PD-1 antibody in cancer. N Engl J Med. 2012;366:2443–54.
85. Sharma P, Allison JP. Immune checkpoint targeting in cancer therapy: toward combination strategies with curative potential. Cell. 2015;161:205–14.
86. Gaudreau P-O, Stagg J, Soulières D, Saad F. The present and future of biomarkers in prostate cancer: proteomics, genomics, and immunology advancements. Biomark Cancer. 2016;8 Suppl 2:15–33.
87. Buhmeida A, Pyrhönen S, Laato M. Prognostic factors in prostate cancer. Diagn Pathol. 2006;1:4.
88. Figg WD, Aragon-Ching JB, Steinberg SM, Gulley JL, Arlen PM, Sartor O, Petrylak DP, Higano CS, Hussain MH, Dahut WL. Randomized phase III trial of thalidomide (Th) or placebo (P) for non-metastatic PSA recurrent prostate cancer (PCa) treated with intermittent therapy. J Clin Oncol. 2008;26(May 20 suppl; abstr 5016).
89. Kelly WK, Halabi S, Carducci M. Randomized, double-blind, placebo-controlled phase III trial comparing docetaxel and prednisone with or without bevacizumab in men with metastatic castration-resistant prostate cancer: CALGB 90401. J Clin Oncol. 2012;30(13):1534–40.
90. Moss R, Mohile S, Shelton G, et al. A phase I open-label study using lenalidomide and docetaxel in and rogen-independent prostate cancer (AI). Paper presented at: American Society for Clinical Oncology Prostate cancer Symposium; February 22–24. Orlando; 2007.
91. Beardsley EK, Ellard SL, Holte SJ, North SA, Winquist E, Chi KN. A phase II study of sorafenib in combination with bicalutamide in patients with chemo-naive hormone refractory prostate cancer (HRPC). J Clin Oncol. 2008;26(May 20 suppl; abstr 16098).
92. Mostaghel EA, Page ST, Lin DW, et al. Intraprostatic androgens and androgen-regulated gene expression persist after testosterone suppression: therapeutic implications for castration-resistant prostate cancer. Cancer Res. 2007;67:5033–41.
93. Dreicer R, Agus DB, MacVicar GR, et al. Safety, pharmacokinetics, and efficacy of TAK-700 in meta-

static castration-resistant prostate cancer: a Phase I/II, open-label study. J Clin Oncol. 2010;28(Suppl): 15S. Abstract 3084

94. Ferraldeschi R, Welti J, Powers MV. Second-generation HSP90 inhibitor onalespib blocks mRNA splicing of androgen receptor variant 7 in prostate cancer cells. Cancer Res. 2016;76(9):2731–42.
95. Cao C, Subhawong T, Albert JM, et al. Inhibition of mammalian target of rapamycin or apoptotic pathway induces autophagy and radiosensitizes PTEN null prostate cancer cells. Cancer Res. 2006;66:10040–7.
96. Boccardo F, Rubagotti A, Tacchini L, et al. Conti. Gefitinib plus prednisone versus placebo plus prednisone in the treatment of hormonerefractory prostate cancer (HRPC): a randomized phase II trial. J Clin Oncol. 2007;25(18 Suppl):5070.
97. Schlomm T, Erbersdobler A, Simon R, et al. Epidermal growth factor receptor family memebers (EGFR and Her2) are prognostic markers and potential therapeutic targets in prostate cancer. Paper presented at: 2006 Prostate cancer Symposium; February 24–26, 2006; San Francisco.
98. Sternberg CN, Dumez H, Van Poppel H. Docetaxel plus oblimersen sodium (Bcl-2 antisense oligonucleotide): an EORTC multicenter, randomized phase II study in patients with castration-resistant prostate cancer. Ann Oncol. 2009;20(7):1264–9.
99. Conley BA, Wright JJ, Kummar S. Targeting epigenetic abnormalities with histone deacetylase inhibit ors. Cancer. 2006;107:832.
100. Bradley D, Rathkopf D, Dunn R. Vorinostat in advanced prostate cancer patients progressing on prior chemotherapy (National Cancer Institute Trial 6862): trial results and interleukin-6 analysis: a study by the Department of Defense Prostate cancer Clinical Trial Consortium and University of Chicago Phase 2 Consortium. Cancer. 2009;115(23):5541–9.

How to Interpret Numeric Results in Publications?

Laurence Collette

1 Introduction

The number of specialist medical journals and the number of scientific publications relating to the medical interventions against cancer increase constantly. Just for 2015, PubMed search for the year 2015 with Medical Subject Heading term "prostatic neoplasm/therapy" in the human species revealed 1657 citations of which 158 were clinical trials (including 112 controlled ones) and 123 other comparative studies. Interestingly 74 systematic reviews were published that year that included 22 formal meta-analyses.

Obviously a practising clinician will hardly find the time to appraise such amount of information, and this does not include the more recent findings reported in abstract format at international and national congresses! And importantly, even if one would have the ability to take in all that new information, this would still not be sufficient, because of the presence of intentional or unintentional bias in the way the data are reported and interpreted.

However, every clinician needs to make up his mind about the value of emerging treatments and therapeutic interventions. Most clinicians today are familiar with the hierarchy of clinical evidence ([30], http://www.cebm.net/wp-content/uploads/2014/06/CEBM-Levels-of-Evidence-2.1.pdf) and will rightly give more weight to reports from more controlled and preferably randomized studies than to those of non-randomized or ill-controlled observational studies. The medical reader may however be less aware of the other various biases that may be introduced at every step of a clinical experiment, all of which have the potential to undermine the validity of the results. Bias may be inherent to the trial design itself, or may result from systematic differences in the way the endpoints are assessed, in the process of data collection and in the methods used for data analysis that together or separately result in observed differences in outcome being erroneously attributed to an impact of the experimental treatment. Bias may also take the form of systematic favouritism in the way results are reported or in the way they are interpreted in the discussion and conclusion of the report. We will illustrate with examples from the prostate cancer research field, a number of misuses of statistics and various types of bias that exist with the aim to help you identify them when appraising a clinical trial report at congresses or in journal.

To ensure the clarity of these examples, we will however start by demystifying a few basic statistical concepts that are commonly found in clinical study reports.

L. Collette
European Organisation for Research and Treatment of Cancer, Headquarters, Statistics Department, Avenue Emmanuel Mounier 83/11, B-1200 Brussels, Belgium
e-mail: Laurence.collette@eortc.be

M. Bolla, H. van Poppel (eds.), *Management of Prostate Cancer*,
DOI 10.1007/978-3-319-42769-0_25

2 Statistical Concepts Demystified

To illustrate the concepts, we will use the hypothetical example of a randomized phase III trial in advanced prostate cancer. Phase III randomized trials are designed to compare two or more forms of therapies by quantification of their respective effect on one or several pre-specified evaluation criteria, the primary endpoint(s). In this example, we take overall survival as single primary endpoint. We consider a superiority study: the trial is built to test if the overall survival with a new oral compound "WonderPill" is superior to that achieved with the current standard (intravenous) treatment "MarvelDrug".

2.1 Do the Trial Results Apply to My Practice?

Patients who enter a clinical trial are regarded as forming a (pseudo-random) sample from the target patient population of interest, thought to be susceptible of benefit from the new treatment. The clinician is not as interested in the treatment effect observed in the study sample as he is to extrapolate the results to the broader population of patients from whom the study sample is (hopefully) representative (Fig. 1) and to know whether the study results are broadly applicable to the patients he/she is seeing in his/her practice.

The clinical trial is a controlled experiment that is carried out according to a protocol that defines all circumstances of the patient management (eligibility criteria to the study, examinations, frequency of visits, treatments, diagnostic of disease progression) but also the methodological circumstances of the trial (treatment allocation method, data collection, data cleaning processes, endpoint adjudication, statistical analysis methods, etc.,) as well as legal or ethical aspects. From the methodological perspective, the WonderPill vs. MarvelDrug study protocol should ensure that the two studied groups will differ only by the treatment they were given, only this (which is achieved through randomization and "control", i.e., compliance to the detailed protocol) will allow to causally attribute observed differences between the two survival curves to the treatment difference.

However, one should keep in mind that protocol eligibility criteria (that often require that patients be free of severe comorbidity, be in good performance status, etc.) define the target population of interest in a rather restrictive way and that the protocol also specifies a very specific clinical practice (diagnostic methods, imaging and other examinations, frequency of follow-up). This per se may be detrimental to generalization of the trial results to clinical practice.

In reading a study report, it is also essential to carefully consider the description of the "Patient Characteristics" (in a table and in Results) to assess if the patient population actually recruited to the study covered the whole range of the population eligible according to the study protocol.

If a subset of the target population is underrepresented (e.g., only low burden disease entered the trial and high burden disease were rarely recruited), the results may not apply to the entire target population (evidence in this case would mostly apply to low burden disease). In addition, one should read all other aspects of the report with that same question of applicability of results in the clinic in mind. Results may not be directly applicable if for instance the diagnostic and follow-up work-up in routine practice is not as intensive as the ones in the trial, or if different imaging or diagnostic devices were used that bare very different predictive values than the ones in use in your practice.

We illustrate this with the report by Briganti et al. [9] that shows that among patients with node-positive disease, those with up to two positive nodes experienced excellent cancer-specific survival, which was significantly higher compared to that of patients with more than two positive nodes. The authors suggest that this should be considered in the next revision of the TNM classification. However, they clearly state that their results were obtained in a series of patients in whom pathological nodal staging was based on an extensive lymph node dissection. The mean number of nodes removed in their series was 13.9, which is significantly higher compared to limited

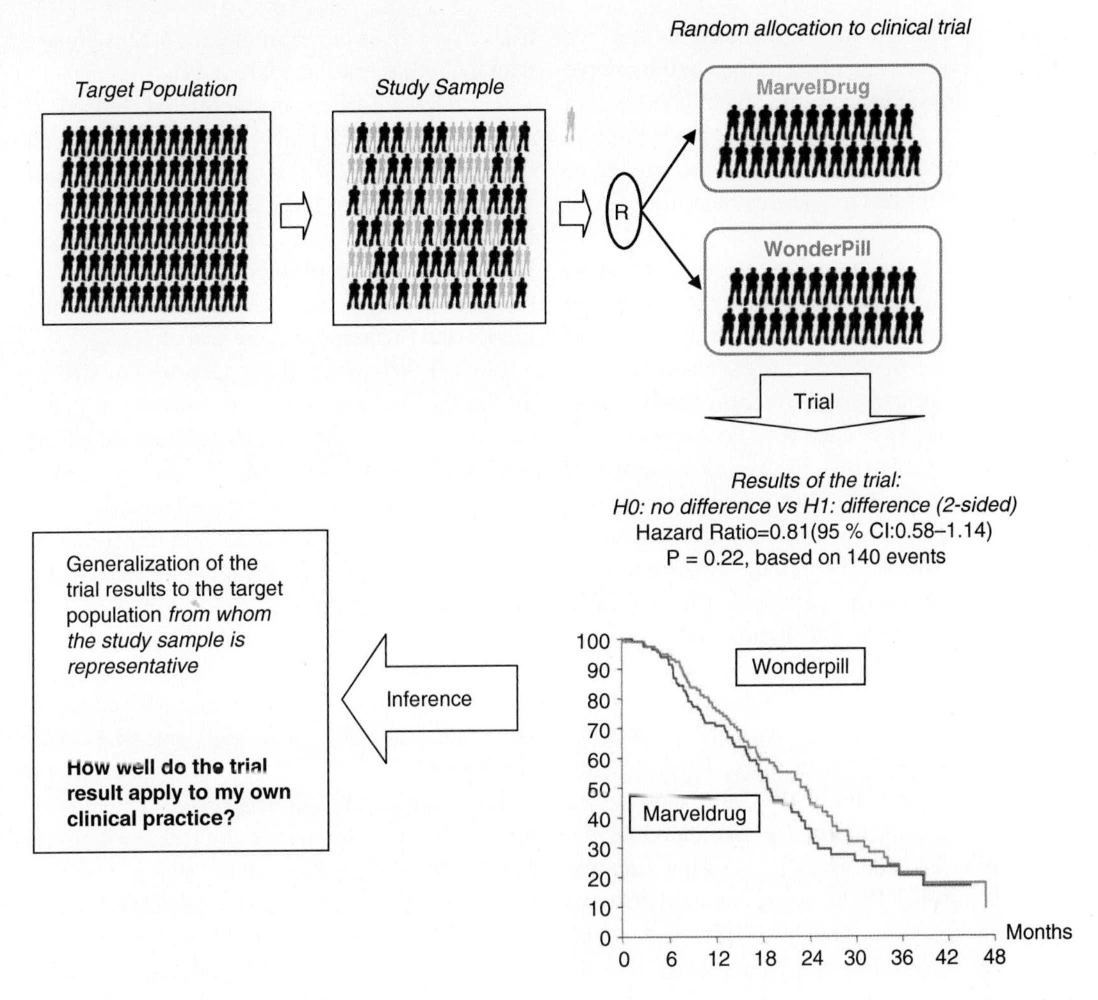

Fig. 1 A hypothetical phase III clinical trial testing the superiority of WonderPill over MarvelDrug for overall survival in advanced prostate cancer

nodal dissection series, with mean number of nodes removed as low as 5.8. Because the number of positive nodes that can be found during pathological assessment is directly related to the number of nodes available for examinations; it would be incorrect to blindly apply the threshold of two positive lymph nodes when less extended lymph node dissection is performed.

2.2 The Truth About *P*-Values and Significance Level

The cornerstone of phase III clinical trials is the eventual statistical test that is used to assess the effect of the treatment on the outcome of interest. In our next example (Fig. 1), a statistical test is performed to determine if the impact of WonderPill on overall survival differs from that of MarvelDrug. The value of the statistical test itself (a test statistic) is then converted into a *P* value.

The null hypothesis (denoted as "H_0") states that overall survival in the two treatment groups is equal and that any observed difference in would be solely due to random fluctuations due to sampling ("chance"). The *P* value measures the likelihood that the difference observed in the study is due to such chance fluctuations alone, in absence of any effective difference, when there is no systematic bias between the groups being compared. The alternative (denoted by "H_1" or "H_a") hypotheses that observations in the sample at hand are influenced by some non-random cause, which, thanks to the control made through the study protocol and adherence to it, can legitimately be identified as the treatment the patient received.

When there are compelling reasons to a priori believe that the difference will only occur in one direction (generally favouring the experimental treatment), one-sided tests and *P*-values are used. When it is expected that differences may occur in both directions, two-sided tests are then used.

In our example (Fig. 1), we use a two-sided test. Comparison of the survival curves yielded a *P*-value of 0.22 for an observed hazard ratio of 0.81. This indicates that if the two treatments were truly equivalent, we would still have 22 % chance of observing a difference of similar or larger magnitude than the one observed, due to random fluctuations only. *P*-values can take any value between 0 and 1, as any probability measure.

When this probability P is low enough, we make the judgement that the likelihood of the observations at hand under H_0 is so low (i.e., the evidence against H_0 is strong enough) that we conclude that some non-zero difference in the effects of WonderPill and MarvelDrug is truly present.

Because we need to make a dichotomous decision: either there is a difference or there is not, we will select a threshold (α, the statistical significance level, usually taken to be 0.05 for two-sided tests and 0.025 for one-sided tests) and we require $P<\alpha$ to decide that *P* is "low enough" to declare that a non-null treatment effect is present. The choice of the significance level alpha, usually 0.05, is an entirely arbitrary cut-off. It means that we are willing to accept a 5 % chance of incorrectly concluding that a difference is present (Table 1) where none is. Thus by definition using the 5 % significance level, on average 5 % of perfectly conducted trials with new treatments that have no added benefit over standard treatment will lead to false positive findings. In practice, however, when $P<\alpha$, one will never know if it is a true or a false-positive finding. Only repeated trials may tell. In our example, $P=0.22$ is greater than 0.05; thus, we cannot reject H_0.

P-values are often misinterpreted. Indeed, *P* does not measure the probability that the observed difference is true (in our example $P=0.22$ does not mean that there is 22 % chance that the true HR = 0.81)! The *P*-value only quantifies the likelihood that such a difference arises by chance alone, in absence of systematic bias between the groups and in absence of any real effect.

Next, *P*-values are influenced by the size of the sample and amount of information at hand: the larger the sample size, the greater the precision, and thus the lower the *P*-value associated with a given observed treatment effect size. Thus, theoretically, any size of treatment effect can be made statistically significant by sufficiently increasing the sample size!

Furthermore, *P*-values directly refer to the summary and test statistic used. Two alternative rank-tests (Logrank or Wilcoxon), applied to the same survival data, may not give the same conclusion!

Last, statistical significance is no guarantee for the clinical relevance of the treatment effect. Indeed, *P*-values only indicate that a *non-zero* treatment effect is present. The medical relevance of the results must be assessed from the estimated magnitude of treatment effect, through its point estimate and its associated 95 % confidence interval.

The confidence interval, calculated from the observed data, gives a range of plausible values for the unknown true treatment effect with which the data are compatible. Its width gives an impression of the precision of the results

Table 1 Hypothesis testing for a difference

	Reality (unknown)	
Our conclusion	H_0 is true (there is no difference)	H_0 is not true (there is a difference)
$P \geq \alpha$: Accept H_0 (conclude there is no difference)	Correct decision	False negative (β)
$P<\alpha$: Reject H_0 (conclude there is a difference)	False positive (α)	Correct decision *(power 1-β)*

(with narrower intervals obtained in studies having larger event numbers). If the trial was to be repeated independently under same conditions and a 95 % confidence interval calculated each time, then on average 95 % of these intervals would contain the true HR. We will see below that a significant *P*-value may also be obtained when the true treatment effect is smaller than the minimum clinically relevant treatment effect specified in the trial sample size calculation.

2.3 The Statistical Power Is Not a Number!

Table 1 above shows that a second type of erroneous conclusion may occur during statistical inference, namely, the false-negative conclusion that H_0 is true when it is not (type-II error β). This error is directly related to the statistical power of the test, or probability to correctly conclude to a non-null treatment effect when a non-trivial effect is present.

A common misbelief is that the statistical power is a *number* (80 % or 90 %). However, the statistical power is a *function* of the true (and unknown!) treatment effect. The size of a trial is indeed calculated to ensure a sufficiently high (≥80 %) power of rejecting the null hypothesis under a specific alternative that a (preferably minimum) clinically meaningful difference of interest is effectively present.

In our example randomized trial comparing WonderPill versus MarvelDrug, the study would need to be sized to produce 640 deaths, in order to have 80 % power to detect a treatment effect hazard ratio of 0.80 (which corresponds to a median increase from 18.5 months with MarvelDrug to 23.1 months survival with WonderPill). In this example using a time to event endpoint, the information contained in a study is measured in terms of the number of events, not the number of patients. Therefore two studies that differ in number of patients and total duration may provide the same power, as long as the data in both are analysed when the 640 events are observed.

Figure 2a shows how the statistical power decreases as the size of the true (unknown) treatment effect decreases. For a trial of given size (number of events) the risk of erroneously concluding to no treatment effect thus increases as the size of the true treatment effect decreases. For the trial results given in Fig. 1, Fig. 2b shows that with 140 events, the trial has no more than 25 % chance to declare statistically significant a treatment effect of size HR = 0.80 when present. Thus, the non-significant *P*-value obtained in the results does not prove that the two treatments are equivalent. The trial was merely inconclusive due to inadequate statistical power, a common feature in the urological literature [8] as well as in the oncological literature [3].

Figure 2a also shows that the likelihood of detecting a non-null treatment effect (i.e., getting a significant *P*-value $P < \alpha$) with a study that was sized to detect a target HR of 0.80, is still 50 % when the true treatment effect is 0.85 and 25 % when the true treatment effect is 0.90! Thus, statistical significance may also be attained for *true* treatment effects that are smaller than the minimum clinically important difference pre-specified as the target effect size of interest. I indeed, statistically significant superiority tests only reject the hypothesis that the effect size is null. One should not mistake the estimated treatment effect with the true treatment effect.

2.4 Meaningless *P*-Values

Statistical significance based on *P*-value is often reported in the medical literature to support claims of association between two measurements, such as a continuous biomarker and a surrogate measure of activity such as a measure of tumour size or another expression of another biomarker such as Ki-67. In that case, the association is measured by a correlation coefficient (ρ). Most often, only the *p*-value is reported and the researcher overlooks the actual hypothesis that this claim supports. Indeed, most often, the quoted *P*-value relates to a test that the correlation is *not null* (i.e., H_1:

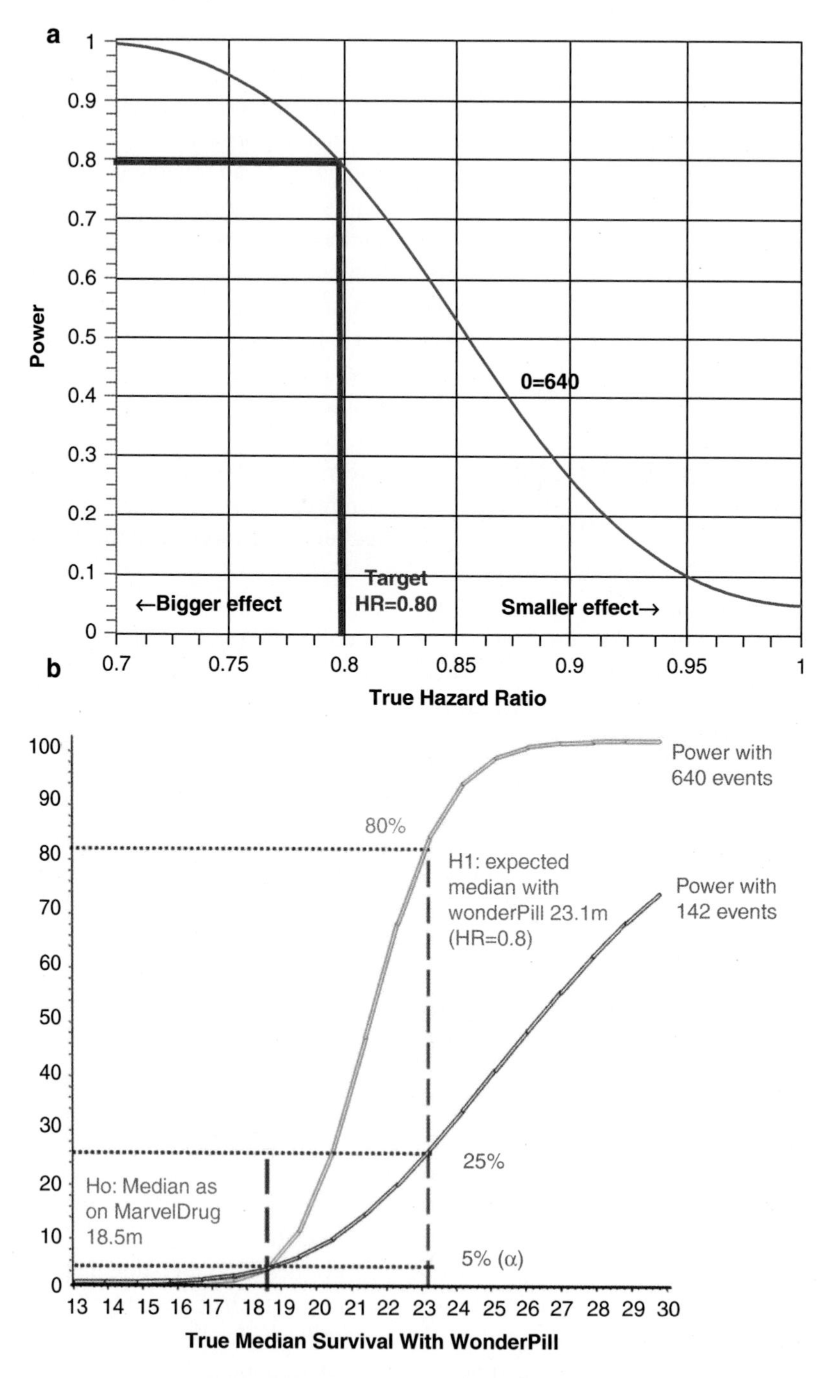

Fig. 2 Statistical power for a trial comparing overall survival with WonderPill versus MarvelDrug, with 640 events, i.e., sized for 80 % power to reject the null hypothesis if the a target hazard ratio (HR) of 0.80 is real. (**a**) Shows the statistical power versus the true hazard ratio: the statistical power is 50 % if the true HR is 0.85 and it equals α when there the two treatments are equal. (**b**) Shows the power in relation to the median survival in the experimental arm

$\rho > 0$ against H_0: $\rho = 0$). Figure 3 illustrates the patterns of association between two biomarkers that correspond to various values of the correlation coefficient. Importantly, few observations are needed to guarantee statistical power for this kind of hypothesis test, so that

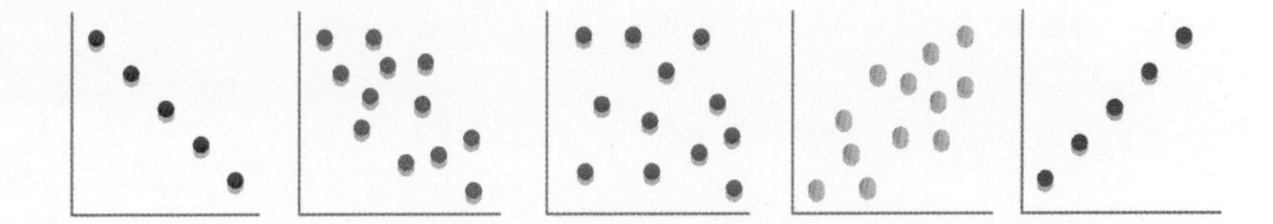

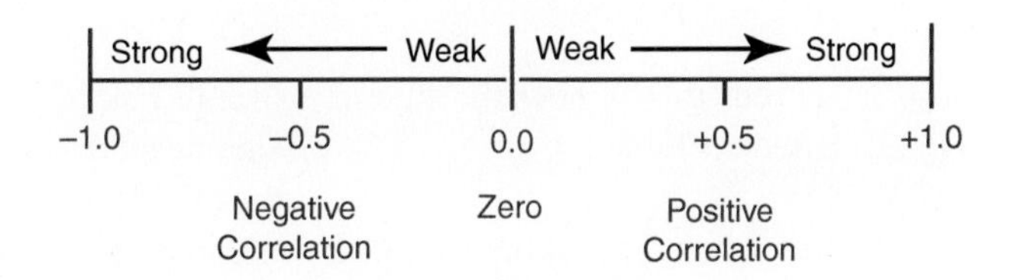

Fig. 3 The correlation coefficient and the corresponding patterns observed in the data

with 200 observations, statistical significance may be reached for $\rho = 0.15$ and with just 50 observations, as is common in early biomarker studies, statistical significance may be reached at $\rho = 0.30$, a value that effectively does not suggest a very meaningful degree of association between the two studied measurements. It would be more meaningful to test the hypothesis that the correlation is greater than some relevant threshold $\rho 0$, selected in the range above 0.5, depending on the research objectives.

3 Reading the Literature with a Critical Eye

The reasoning involved when reading a publication is, from the statistical point of view, very similar to that of designing and conducting a clinical trial to its end. When reading a scientific paper, the reader should first identify the primary and planned secondary objectives of the research, then read the methods and the results, and then make his own judgement about their value. This should be done *before* reading/writing the discussion and conclusion! Indeed, biased reporting is not uncommon and arguments in a discussion may seem very persuasive although the evidence supporting them is lacking in the results.

We will now illustrate some of the most commonly encountered biases.

3.1 Impressing with Numbers

When reading research reports, the reader will naturally be more impressed by numerically larger numbers. There exists a variety of ways of numerically reporting the difference between the treatments in a randomized comparative trial, some of which may impress more than others. Table 2 below summarizes the survival results with 10-year median follow-up in the EORTC 22863 phase III trial of external irradiation with or without long-term androgen suppression for prostate cancer with high metastatic risk by Bolla et al. [7].

If all of the following statements are correct statements, some certainly suggest a stronger magnitude of treatment difference than others:

(a) Median survival of the combined treatment group is 158 % of the median with irradiation alone.
(b) A 58 % improvement in median survival with androgen suppression.
(c) A 40 % reduction in risk of death with androgen suppression.
(d) A 18.3 % absolute improvement in 10-year overall survival rate.
(e) A 46 % relative improvement in 10-year survival rate.
(f) Irradiation alone had a 67 % higher risk of death.
(g) The number needed to treat for 10-year overall survival is 5.5 patients.

Table 2 Survival results in the EORTC phase III trial 22863

Irradiation alone		Irradiation plus long term androgen suppression	
Median	95 % CI	Median	95 % CI
6.9 years	6.0–8.3 years	10.9 years	10.0–14.5 years
		Hazard ratio	95 % CI
		0.60*	0.45–0.80
10-year survival	95 % CI	10-year survival	95 % CI
39.8%	31.9–47.5 %	58.1 %	49.2–66.0 %

P=0.0004

For those interested, this is how the figures were computed, based on Table 2.

(a) The ratio of the medians is 10.9/6.9 = 1.58, so 158 %.
(b) Is the same as (a), but concentrating on the increase of 58 %.
(c) The hazard ratio is 0.60, thus a 40 % reduction of the risk of death.
(d) 58.1–39.8 % at 10 years makes + 18.3 % *absolute* improvement.
(e) 58.1/39.8 = 1.46 thus a 46 % *relative* improvement.
(f) The hazard ratio was 0.60, which is the ratio of the risk of death with irradiation and androgen suppression compared to irradiation alone; thus, the hazard ratio for irradiation versus the combined modality treatment is 1/0.60 = 1.67, or a 67 % higher risk of death.
(g) As in (d) the absolute improvement at 10 years is 18.3 % = 0.183, the number of patients to treat to spare one death at 10 years is 1/0.183 = 5.46, rounded to 5.5.

3.2 The Temptation of Subgroup Analyses

In today's world of personalized medicine, subgroup analyses of clinical trial data aiming at segmenting the disease population seem a logical step in data analysis. However, especially when the overall trial results are statistically or medically not significant, subgroup analyses carry serious concerns and the associated risks of over-interpretation. Indeed, the probability of at least one false-positive finding rapidly increases with the number of subgroups analysed. If K tests are conducted at the 0.05 significance level, the overall risk of one or more of them turning out significant due to chance alone equals $(1\text{-}[1\text{-}\alpha]^K)$, thus for 10 tests with significance level $\alpha = 0.05$ that risk is 40.1 %! Thus, reporting $p < 0.05$ has little meaning for any single test among a large number. If all attempted subgroup analyses were reported, the reader could in theory adjust for multiplicity by adopting for his interpretation a more stringent significance level for each test. The use of α/K would conservatively protect against type I errors. However, comparisons are often not reported [35] so that the number K is unknown to the reader, making such adjustment impossible. When subgroups are extremely numerous, as in the case of search for association between genomic alterations and prognosis, more advanced methods such as control of the false discovery rate should be used. The reader may refer to the work of Goeman and Solari [26] for further details regarding these methods.

By the law of averages, the whole being the sum of the parts, it is always possible to define a grouping of the patients such that the treatment effect in one group is more extreme than the overall effect in the trial and is less extreme in another. Furthermore, breaking down the study sample into numerous subgroups (for instance, age at baseline into four categories, or attempting several cut-points dichotomizing a biomarker) induces multiplicity if tests are conducted in all subgroups. To protect against false-positive results conducting formal statistical tests of heterogeneity (also known as interaction tests) is recommended. Demonstration of significant heterogeneity, possibly at a relaxed statistical significance level, owing to the lack of power of such tests, should be a prerequisite to making strong interpretation of within-subgroup findings.

To illustrate the multiplicity problem, we used the data of the historical EORTC trial

30892 comparing cyproterone acetate (CPA) to flutamide in metastatic prostate cancer [38]. The choice of the example does not however matter to our argument. This study of 310 patients of which 250 died showed no statistically significant differences with respect to overall mortality (HR for CPA/flutamide = 1.22, 95 % CI: 0.95–1.57, $P=0.1252$). We created 20 completely random splits of the data into two subgroups of equal probability. Each time we then tested for treatment effect in both subgroups. In two instances, the treatment effect turned out significant in one subgroup and not in the other. Figure 4 shows the survival curves in two subgroups for the 18th split, for which the test for heterogeneity of the treatment effect is even statistically significant ($P=0.032$)! In the first half of the patients, those on CPA fare significantly worse (HR = 1.59, 95 % CI: 1.10–2.30, $P=0.013$) with 3-year survival rate of 45 % compared to 55 % for those on flutamide. In the second half of the patient, there is absolutely no difference between the two groups (HR = 0.92, 95 % CI: 0.65–1.31, $P=0.657$) and the 3-year overall survival is 54 % in both groups.

Another kind of misleading subgroup analyses is that of subgroups defined on the basis of postbaseline assessments. Such problems will be

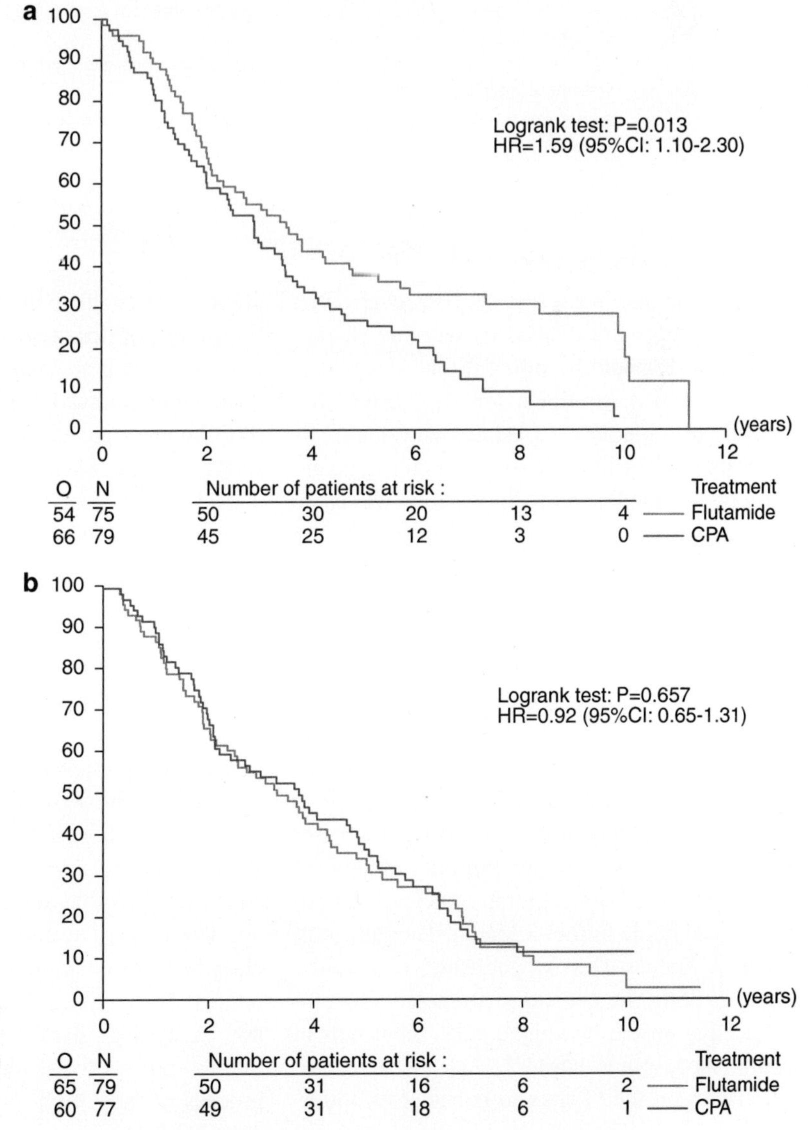

Fig. 4 Survival outcomes in two randomly created subgroups of patients from EORTC trial 30892. (**a**) shows the first subgroup and figure (**b**) shows the complementary subgroup

Table 3 Guidelines for subgroup analyses

In the protocol	Planned subgroup analyses must be specified in the protocol, with the methods intended for the analyses, and the multiplicity adjustment that will be applied to control type I errors
	Subgroup analyses should be conducted only if there is a sound biological rationale for conducting them!
In the abstract	If any, only preplanned subgroup analyses for the primary endpoint should be reported in the abstract. Post hoc findings are only hypothesis generating and should not take prominence in the abstract
In the methods	The number of pre-specified subgroup analyses performed and reported should be indicated. For each, the endpoint and the method used to assess heterogeneity should be indicated The number of post hoc subgroup analyses performed and reported should be indicated. These should be clearly identified, as well as the rationale for conducting them. For each, the endpoint and the method used to assess heterogeneity should be indicated Indicate the potential effect on type I errors (false positives) due to multiplicity and how this effect is addressed. Describe the adjustments that were used
In the results	First assess heterogeneity of treatment effects across subgroups. Report effect estimates and confidence intervals in all subgroups. Interpret statistical tests of significance only if there is evidence of heterogeneity across subgroups Clearly distinguish the subgroup analyses that were pre-specified from those that were generated by the data themselves
In the discussion	Avoid overinterpretation of subgroup differences. Be properly cautious in appraising their credibility, acknowledge the limitations. Confront the findings with those from other studies

Adapted from Rui Wang et al. [35]

illustrated in the next section. However, even when subgroups are defined by baseline characteristics, one should be mindful that unless randomization was stratified for the factor that defined the subgroups imbalances between treatments may exist within the subgroup. If a dynamic allocation method such as minimization was used, further covariates used for the stratification may also be imbalanced between treatments within the sub-groups Indeed, these methods do not balance combination of stratification factors between treatments, only each factor taken separately. Furthermore, false-negative results are also more likely within subgroups, because of lack of power due to reduced numbers, which may lead to apparently inconsistent conclusions.

Subgroup analyses are not wrong in themselves, as long as they are carefully conducted and interpreted. Data exploration is important to inform and guide further research. The European Medical Agency (EMA) published two guidelines covering the questions discussed above: a "Guideline on the investigation of subgroups in confirmatory clinical trials" [21] and a recommendation on the "Points to consider on multiplicity issues in clinical trials" [22] in the framework of drug registration studies, the principles of which are more broadly relevant. Both documents are available from the EMA website (http://www.ema.europa.eu)

We summarize in Table 3 some key points to consider when conducting or interpreting subgroup analyses (adapted from [35]).

3.3 Comparing the Apples and Pears and Claiming All Are Oranges

The most common problem encountered when reviewing published research is that of "length time" or selection bias, i.e., attempts to compare groups that are not defined at baseline, but by characteristics that are observed during follow-up. These carry serious risks of bias when the classification is influenced by the outcome of interest itself. Such biases are pernicious and not easily identified by the untrained reader. Such reports do get through the peer-review process of very high-quality journals. Because

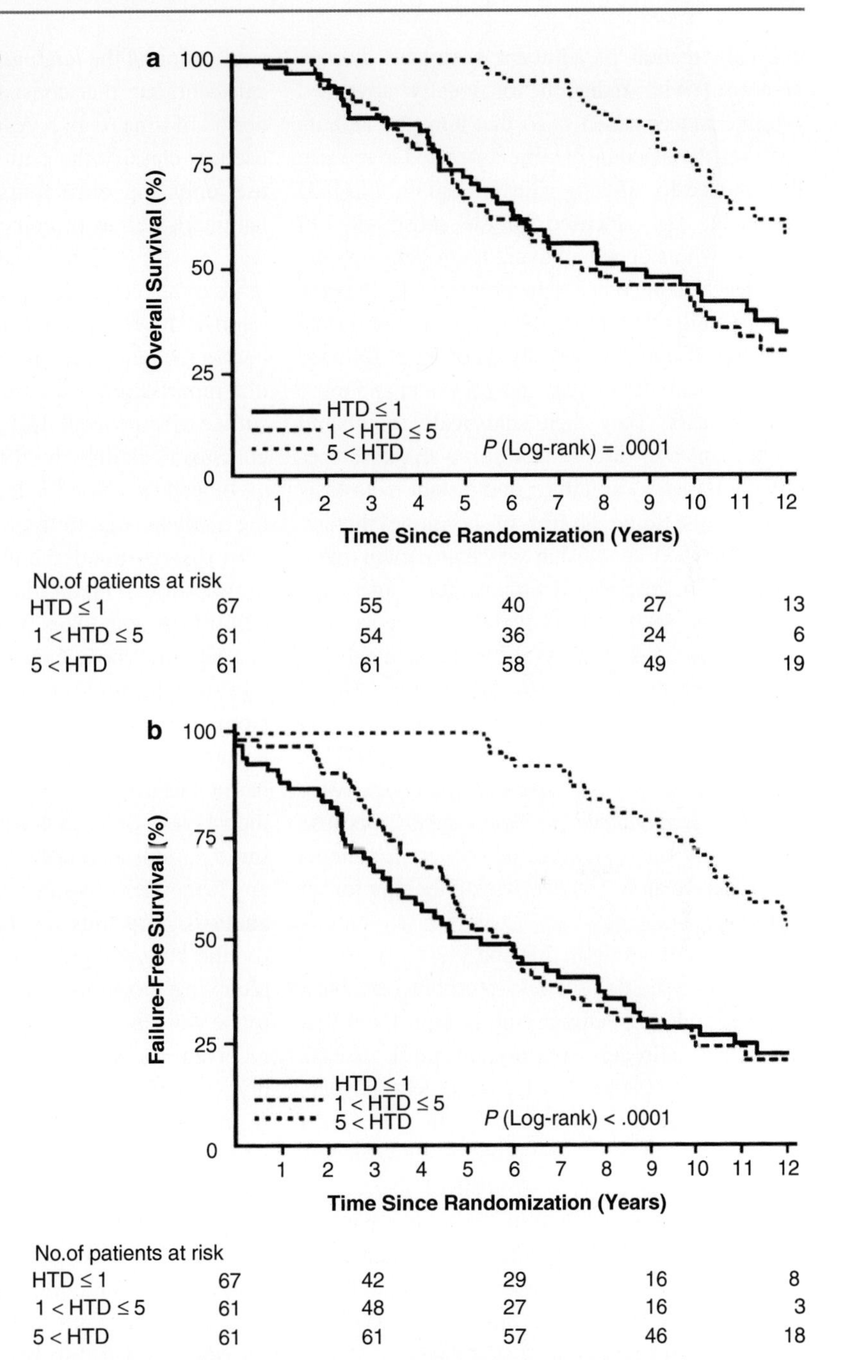

Fig. 5 Overall survival (**a**) and disease-free survival (**b**) by hormone therapy duration (HTD) in RTOG trail 85-31 (Reproduced with permission Souhami et al. [41])

they often produce largely overestimated effect sizes, they also tend to receive much greater attention than is legitimate. In the best instance, they will be criticized in letters to the editors, but these are less likely to be read than the original report.

A number of examples are discussed below that illustrate the problem.

3.4 Length Time Bias: Post hoc Analysis of Duration of Androgen Deprivation Therapy in RTOG 85-31 (JCO)

In 2009, Souhami et al. reported a secondary analysis of the RTOG 85-31 in the *Journal of Clinical Oncology* [41, 42] that attempted to identify the optimal duration of adjuvant hormonal therapy combined with radiation for locally advanced prostate cancer patients. To that aim, the authors analysed the outcome of patients treated in the arm that intened for lifelong adjuvant monthly LHRH treatment. They focused on the subset of 189 patients who stopped adjuvant androgen suppression for reasons other than progression. Patients were then divided into three groups based on the quantiles of hormone therapy duration as follows: ≤1 year, more than 1 year and ≤5 years, and more than 5 years. They then statistically compared overall survival, disease-free survival, cause-specific mortality, local failure, and distant metastasis between the three groups of hormone therapy duration. Their conclusion was that patients with androgen deprivation treatment for more than 5 years had an improved overall disease-specific and progression-free survival compared to patients with shorter duration of hormonal therapy. Based on these findings, the authors concluded that "*decreasing hormonal therapy duration (HTD) to ≤5 years may have a detrimental effect on patients with locally advanced prostate cancer*" because overall survival is significantly better in patients who received androgen deprivation therapy for >5 years (Fig. 5).

What went wrong in this analysis?

First, one should note that in order to receive x years of androgen suppression in a protocol that mandated androgen suppression until disease progression, a patient has to live at least x years and be disease-free for x years! Thus all patients in group 3 (HTD>5 years, group 3) *by definition of the grouping* enjoy a survival of 5 years or more. If a patient died within less than 5 years of radiation therapy for any other reason than prostate cancer, then, obviously, he had to be included in the group with HTD<1 (group 1) or HTD of 1–5 (group 2) years.

The presence of bias is easily identified from the overall survival curves in Fig. 1a that show no event in group 2 (HTD of 1–5 years) for the first year on study and no event (no drop of the survival curves) in group 3 (HTD >5 years) until year 5. This is a very good example of *length-time bias,* a specific form of selection bias. This kind of bias may sometimes be removed by application of the *landmark* method [1], a statistical technique that consists in defining an initial period of time (e.g., 5 years, the *landmark*) that is used to classify the patients into groups and to use only the observations obtained after that landmark period to compare the groups. In this way, a new baseline is defined (the end of the landmark, here 5 years) and the selection bias is removed by exclusion of all observations obtained before the new baseline. However, for the particular report discussed here, that method would not suffice to remove all the bias and to support to the conclusion claimed by the authors.

Indeed, a second selection bias is present in the analysis, due to the exclusion of all patients who discontinued therapy because of disease progression. This is discussed in a letter to the editor [29] who takes two examples. Example 1 is a patient whose cancer is simply not responsive to hormonal modulation. If the patient stops the hormonal therapy for any reason before the recurrence is detected, that patient has a failure and is classed in either the less than 1-year or 1- to 4-year HTD group. But the same patient who continued the hormonal therapy long-term would be excluded from the analysis (and thus not be counted as a failure for the >5 year group) as long as he was still receiving hormonal therapy when the recurrence was detected. Example 2 is a patient who received therapy for 4 years, then develops myocardial infarction and dies 2 years later from cardiovascular complications. If upon myocardial infarction at year 4, hormonal therapy is stopped, the patient is counted as a death in the 1- to 4-year hormone therapy group but if that same patient believes in the benefits of >5-year HTD and continues his hormonal therapy, he would *not* count as a death in the >5-year HTD group because patients who die on hormone therapy are excluded from the analysis. This shows how this second selection of patients for the study that excludes 41 % of patients allocated to the combined treatment group in the RTOG study induces further bias in favour of the longer duration group (group 3) by selecting out the non-hormone-responsive patients. It also leads to underestimation of the detrimental effects of hormones because patients who die while on treatment are excluded from the analysis, even if the longer duration of hormonal treatment contributed to that death [29].

This paper raised a number of reactions through letter to the editors. The authors diligently replied to these, but did not recognise fully the limitations of their analyses, which only report an artificial correlation built-in the analysis methods used. They however recognized that their "secondary analysis was a hypothesis-generating exercise; only a properly designed phase III randomized trial can conclusively and unequivocally clarify this issue" [41, 42]. One may wonder however if such explorations are worth a publication.

3.5 Selection Bias in Assessing the Value of Radical Prostatectomy for Node-Positive Patients

Selection bias is present whenever selection of patients for the studied intervention is confounded by patient factors that are also related to clinical endpoint of interest. To illustrate the reasoning involved in identifying possible selection bias in a publication, we will use a report by Engel et al. [20] discussing the value of continuing versus abandoning radical prostatectomy when positive lymph nodes are found during the surgery. The authors used a series of 938 lymph node-positive patients from the Munich Cancer Registry: in 688 the radical prostatectomy (RP) was conducted

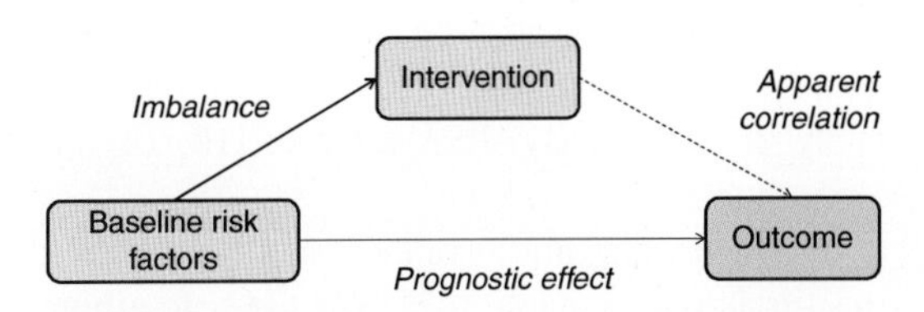

Fig. 6 Mechanisms of selection bias in a study assessing the effect of a non-randomized intervention on an outcome. Both *solid arrows* are necessary for an apparent correlation to be induced between the intervention and the outcome. In randomized trials, randomization ensures that the *top left solid arrow* is absent

and in 250 the RP was abandoned. Data about age, grade, and PSA were available. The authors used multivariate Cox regression analysis to compare overall survival between the two groups. Here, the reader must pay a particular attention to the following question: are the two groups comparable in terms of risk factors? Was the decision to stop the surgery independent of baseline risk factors? Were appropriate and sufficiently effective statistical adjustments made to attempt to correct for selection bias? If the answer to any of these questions is negative, there is a risk to erroneously attribute the effect of patient selection to that of the studied intervention itself. When this mechanism is present (as illustrated in Fig. 6), the correlation between the tested intervention (here radical prostatectomy) and the outcome (here survival) is induced in whole or in part by a third factor (here baseline risk of both pN+ disease and shorter overall survival) that is correlated to both the intervention and the outcome. It is important to note that imbalances in strong prognostic factors between the intervention groups need not to be statistically significant for the above mechanism to be present!

To address the first question above, a careful inspection of the tables showing the distribution of the available risk factors in the study is needed. Such an inspection shows that the two patient groups differ in many ways: PSA was >20 ng/ml in only 42 % of the patients who underwent RP compared to 66 % in the patients whose surgery was aborted; stage T4 was also five times less frequent in the operated group (4 % vs 20.9 %), reflecting the fact that these parameters may have played a role in the decision to abort the surgery. Thus, in this study, the two groups are not balanced for risk factors and there is suggestion that these factors that are known risk factors for outcome, may have been used in treatment decision [43].

The fact that a single positive node was found in 50.7 % of the patients who underwent prostatectomy but only in 27.9 % of the patients in whom RP was aborted speaks in the same direction, as well as the figure showing that node negative patients who underwent radical prostatectomy in the study have a better life expectancy – despite their prostate cancer – than the survival estimate for the general population [20, 43].

Were appropriate statistical measure taken to adjust for these imbalances? The authors made due diligence in attempting to correct for these, by means of multivariate modelling. However, this is made very difficult by the large amount of missing data for the very same prognostic factors (that are also not balanced in the two groups): the clinical T stage was unknown in 16.1 % of the analysed node-positive patients who underwent prostatectomy and in 6.0 % of those with aborted prostatectomy, and the number of positive lymph nodes retrieved was unknown in 40 % and 62.8 % of the patients, respectively. Despite multivariate analysis, the selection bias in baseline factors cannot be properly accounted for due to the large amount of missing data. More efficient methods of statistical adjustment for confounding such as propensity score adjustment or matching exist [15] but could not have been used in this report, because of the missing data. Furthermore, as it is impossible to adjust for unknown or unmeasured factors, the best method to date to ensure group comparability remains randomization, when sufficiently large numbers are included. For further discussion about adjustment methods for confounding, the reader may refer to Wunsch et al. [50] for a review of the statistical techniques that are available (matching, stratification, multivariable adjustment, propensity scores, and instrumental variables) to adjust for confounders and the issues that need to be addressed when interpreting the results.

To illustrate the diverging conclusions that may be obtained through properly randomized study and an adjusted non-randomized comparison of two treatments one may contrast the results of two reports comparing short-term and long-term androgen suppression plus external beam radiation therapy and survival in men with node negative high risk prostate cancer. In a the pooled analysis, D'Amico et al. [16] concluded that after adjusting for known prognostic factors, the treatment of node-negative, high-risk prostate cancer using 3 years as compared with 6 months of AST with RT was not associated with prolonged survival in men of advanced age. In the randomized trial EORTC 22961, Bolla et al. [5], the authors concluded that the combination of radiotherapy plus 6 months of androgen suppression provides inferior survival as compared with radiotherapy plus 3 years of androgen suppression in the treatment of locally advanced prostate cancer.

3.6 Biases in Nonrandomized Reports Comparing Immediate and Deferred Therapeutic Interventions

In a number of clinical circumstances, the decision to initiate the treatment of prostate cancer immediately or to defer treatment until further signs of disease evolution present (symptoms, or more commonly PSA increases) is made: it may be a the decision to treat locally for small asymptomatic localized disease, the decision to initiate systemic hormonal therapy in patients who cannot receive local treatment with curative intent, or it may concern the timing of adjuvant treatment after radical local treatment. If several randomized clinical trials were conducted to address each of those three questions, all those studies took a long time to complete due to the naturally long history of the disease. These results are being criticized for not reflecting the current practice of initial treatment or of follow-up and decision to initiate therapy. For example, the three major trials assessing immediate postoperative irradiation versus observation for patients with pathologically high-risk disease after radical prostatectomy [6, 45, 49] were criticized for not using PSA criterion by current assay sensitivity or PSA doubling time to decide on treatment initiation. This lead to a number attempts to address the question using retrospective non-randomized patient series that were treated either immediately or upon (early) PSA relapse ([10, 12, 44, 46] among others).

However, the validity of these non-randomized results is questionable [32]. We list below how several of the biases discussed earlier in this chapter influence these analyses:

(a) All retrospective analyses attempt to compare disease-free or survival rates in men who have received adjuvant radiotherapy with patients who had established biochemical relapse and therefore received salvage radiotherapy. As noted by Patel and Stephenson [32], if the second group has *effective* biochemical relapse, patients in the comparator group who all had adjuvant radiotherapy only have a *theoretical* risk of biochemical relapse and this group includes a proportion of patients who, had they not been given adjuvant radiotherapy, would never have experienced biochemical relapse. There is selection bias in the analysis, since the patients with similar features who never recurred are de facto excluded from the salvage irradiation group. None of these retrospective studies could account for the true denominator in the salvage irradiation group.

(b) By the same mechanism, there is also length time bias in the comparison, since patients who would die of a cause unrelated to prostate cancer before experiencing biochemical failure are excluded from the salvage group but are included in the adjuvant irradiation group. Length time bias is also evident in the studies that counted the survival time *from the date of (end of) irradiation*, such as the report by Budiharto et al. [10]. Indeed, as illustrated in Fig. 7, the time to event is *by definition* shorter in the group with salvage irradiation as compared to the group with immediate irradiation.

(c) Finally, confounding is likely to be present in such comparisons as the intention for treatment was not randomized but was chosen for each patient individually. Therefore, risk factors for final outcome likely influenced the decision to treat immediately or later so that the mechanism illustrated in Fig. 7 are all in place for bias to be present.

Given these limitations, we can safely conclude that randomized evidence is needed to provide the definitive proof regarding the timing of an intervention, when the decision to treat is triggered by signs of disease evolution.

3.7 Issues with the Endpoint "Progression-Free Survival"

Due to the long protracted natural history of prostate cancer and a new effective treatments emerge to control the later stages of the disease, the use of overall survival as the primary endpoint of phase III randomized trials in earlier stages of the disease becomes extremely difficult and costly. As a result, many trials have progression-free survival as primary or co-primary endpoint.

Depending on the setting, this composite endpoint may encompass different types of events such as skeletal-related events or symptomatic bone progression in studies assessing bisphosphonates or more commonly a combination of biochemical failure, clinical disease progression (loco-regional and/or distant) and death. Common to all such endpoints is that they require repeated diagnostic tests (markers such as PSA or imaging such as CT-scans, MRI, bone scans) at regularly scheduled follow-up intervals. Because of this and unlike overall survival, a progression-free endpoint is subject to measurement errors and imprecision, and to a risk of interpretation bias whenever their assessment require diagnostics such as bone imaging that involve a degree of subjective interpretation.

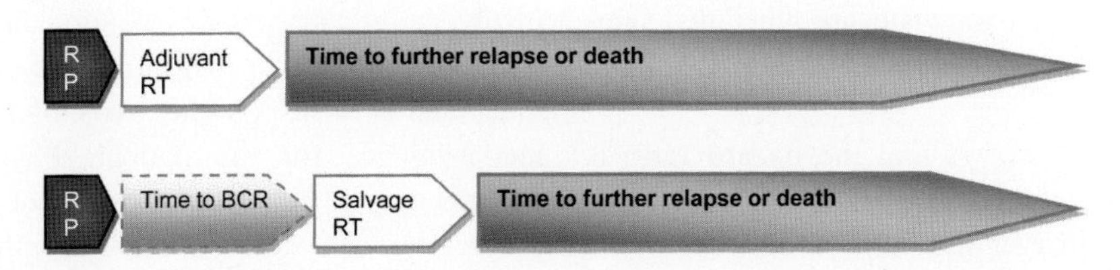

Fig. 7 Hypothetical timeline after radical prostatectomy (*RP*) for two patients receiving either adjuvant or salvage radiotherapy (*RT*) delivered upon biochemical relapse (*BCR*)

3.7.1 Inflation of the Median Time to Event due to the Discreteness of the Assessments

Even for more objectively measurable events such as biochemical failure, a failure that is identified at a given follow-up visit would in fact have occurred in the time interval from the preceding assessment to the present visit. This leads to over estimation of the time to failure [11, 31]. Gignac et al. [25] showed that when the true median progression-free survival was 12 weeks, the information lag inherent in lengthening the interval between assessment inflated the estimated median progression-free survival times to 15.6, 16.6, and 18.7 weeks for every 6, 8, and 12 week schedules, respectively. Further simulation studies by Panageas et al. [31] show that the bias in estimation does however not necessarily increase with an increase in the length of the assessment interval. Instead, it depends on the timing of the interval relative to the true median. The bias will be smallest when the true median progression-free survival time is a multiple of the interval between visits (thus if the true median is 12 weeks, the bias will be larger if visits are scheduled every 5 weeks than if they are scheduled every 3 or 4 weeks).

Importantly because the visit schedule directly influences the reported median progression-free survival times, results from studies that used varying assessment schedules are not directly comparable!

3.7.2 Loss of Power and Biased Estimation of the Treatment Hazard Ratio in Relation to Infrequent Assessments

The frequency of assessments also directly impacts the estimated treatment differences [11, 25, 31], even when the visits are scheduled symmetrically in the two randomized treatment groups.

Caroll 2007 shows that the hazard ratio is increasingly biased toward the null hypothesis of no difference as the interval between visits lengthens and the frequency of visits decreases. Consequently, the statistical power is reduced and more events are needed to achieve the desired power. He suggests that to maintain statistical power to detect hazard ratios between 0.80 and 0.667, the interval between visits can afford to be no more than about one half of the median progression-free survival in the control arm.

3.7.3 Biased Treatment Effect Estimation due to Imbalances in the Assessment Schedules Between Arms

From the remarks above, it becomes apparent that artificial treatment effect differences may result from asymmetric visit schedules between the two groups. This may occur by design, or if for some reason, systematically longer or more frequent visit delays occur in one arm compared to the other. If for instance visits in arm A take place every 4 weeks and visits in arm B every 5 weeks, the median time to event for arm B take place will be inflated, since the events will systematically be attributed to a later time in the arm where visits are less frequent. This type of bias is referred to as *evaluation-time bias* by Dancey in her review of the possible sources of bias and variability in studies that use a progression-free survival endpoint [17]. Simulation studies showed that differences in the timing of disease evaluations can significantly bias PFS analyses to the point of causing an apparent improvement in outcome when none existed [4, 24, 31].

3.7.4 Evaluation Bias

In that same review, Dancey et al. [17] recommend blinding in trials that use a progression-free survival endpoint. This is to prevent that knowledge of the treatment group influences the investigator in his assessment of the endpoint that involve a greater degree of subjectivity (e.g., review of images), or his decision to delay treatment and/or visits on the basis of toxicity or inconvenience for the patient. Physicians or patients may be biased towards earlier claim that progression has occurred in the arm that is considered to be the less intensive treatment option. Since then the FDA revised its view regarding the need for systematic central review and opened the door to less costly approaches such as audit central review [19]

3.7.5 Bias-Induced by the Statistical Methods

In the FDA Guidance for Industry Clinical Trial Endpoints for the Approval of Cancer Drugs and Biologics [47], a whole section is devoted to the statistical analysis of progression-free survival endpoints. The guidance is often interpreted as recommending that patients who stop taking randomized therapy prior to documented progression should be censored at the time when the treatment is stopped [11]. However, this causes obvious problems in the analysis as censoring inevitably becomes informative in this case. Indeed, patients who stop treatment in absence of progression generally do so because of either toxicity or general deterioration of the patient status that may be indicative of treatment failure. In such circumstances, if the prevalence of censoring differs between arms, naive censoring could lead to extremely biased results: taken to the extreme, a treatment that would be so toxic that all patients would stop treatment due to toxicity would have an estimated progression-free survival rate of 100 % when using the method described above.

The impact of varying analysis methods and other sensitivity analyses are discussed in detail by Bhattacharya [4] in a study of bevacizumab in late stage breast cancer.

3.7.6 Further Challenges When Using a PSA or Other Biomarker-Based Endpoint

The definition of what constitutes biochemical failure differs according to disease setting and treatments. The updated Prostate Cancer Clinical Trials Working Group 3 suggest that PSA outcomes should be interpreted within the context of a drug's mechanism of action, and the anticipated timing of a potential favourable/unfavourable effect on PSA should be considered when designing studies [37]. For the assessment of biochemical relapse after primary local treatment with curative intent distinct definitions are adopted depending on the local therapy (AUA guidelines after radical prostatectomy [14] and ASTRO-Phoenix definition after primary irradiation with or without neoadjuvant hormone therapy [34]).

Because biochemical failure is defined differently depending on the treatment given, the use of this endpoint for randomized comparisons of treatment with varying modalities of action and specifically actions on PSA are at greater risk of bias. Differences between treatment groups in terms of PSA-based endpoints do not necessarily translate into differences in more clinically relevant endpoints (clinical progression-free survival or overall survival). For example, further analyses of RTOG trial 92-02 in which patients received differing durations of androgen suppression in combination with irradiation showed that observed differences in terms of time to biochemical progression or in terms of PSA-doubling time did not translate into differences in overall survival [36, 48]. There is in fact no definitive statistical proof that time to biochemical-relapse or biochemical progression-free survival is surrogate for overall survival in prostate cancer [2, 13, 18, 33].

PSA-based endpoints are indeed subject to a number of confounding factors such as recovery of testosterone after adjuvant ADT and institution of ADT for rising PSA after the local therapy or institution of salvage curative therapy (e.g., radiation post-prostatectomy) [28]. As such, it is subject to many confounders from treatment. Furthermore, in the adjuvant trials, the long lead time to metastases and death from prostate cancer results in patients dying of other diseases, which makes PSA-based endpoints unlikely surrogates for overall survival.

3.7.7 Surrogate Endpoints

Because of the long history of prostate cancer, the use of intermediate endpoints that would be surrogate for the longer term outcome would greatly facilitate the therapeutic progress by speeding up the clinical trials. However, surrogacy of an endpoint for another (usually survival) is dependent on the disease state and mechanism of action of the drug in question, so that a surrogate for one state or one therapy cannot necessarily be extrapolated to other disease states or drugs [2]. Efforts were made to try to demonstrate surrogacy of intermediate endpoints in the advanced stages of the disease such as the work of Sonpavde et al. [40] who attempted to show surrogacy of radiographic progression by Prostate Cancer Working Group (PCWG)-2 criteria in metastatic castration-resistant prostate cancer. However, evidence of formal validation remains limited. The Intermediate Clinical Endpoints in Cancer of the Prostate Working Group [28] is now collating several thousands of individual patient data from all available clinical trials of radiation or prostatectomy for localized disease and conduct the requisite analyses to determine whether an intermediate clinical endpoint that is surrogate for survival can be identified in this setting.

3.8 Conclusions and Recommendations

The discussion in this chapter should hopefully provide hints to the reader of clinical reports for assessing the quality and medical relevance of published reports. A level of familiarity with statistics and methodology in the broader sense as well as a good dose of critical thinkng are indeed essential to reduce the vulnerability of the reader to misinterpretation.

Readers of medical reports must always keep the presence of publication bias in mind. Publication bias is the decision to publish or not publish a study based on its results [27]. This bias is inherent to the process whereby editorial and journalistic criteria emphasize the newest and most striking research findings. These findings are often exaggerated in magnitude and may not be confirmed by later research that for the same reasons is less likely to get published.

The requirement for complete and transparent reporting of results through the adoption by most scientific journals of reporting guidelines such as CONSORT (http://www.consort-statement.org) and the further requirement to submit the study protocol with the manuscript should help the reader scrutinize the quality of the evidence presented in journals. Further requirements are the honest and full declaration of conflicts of interest and the correct assignment of authorship [39]. We suggest that readers of medical reports should get familiar with the reporting guidelines and their accompanying checklists. Such guidelines have been developed for a large number of types of studies. All existing guidelines are accessible through the website of the EQUATOR-Network (http://www.equator-network.org). The EQUATOR Network is an international initiative that seeks to enhance reliability and value of medical research literature by promoting transparent and accurate reporting of research studies.

More recently, the European Union (EU) adopted a new version of the clinical trial regulation [23] that aims to increase transparency and availability of information on clinical trials and their results. According to this regulation that was implemented in 2016, all trials that use investigational new agents must be registered with the EU and their results must be disclosed on the portal provided by the European Medical Agency within one year of the end of the trial. With this new regulation in place, one is hopeful that publication bias will be drastically reduced in the future.

The Center for Evidence Based Medicine of the University of Oxford (http://www.cebm.net) offers further tools and downloads for the critical appraisal of medical evidence, including appraisal sheets for the assessment of randomized clinical trials. Completing these checklists or appraisal sheets when reading reports of studies is certainly an efficient method for gradually gaining the methodological expertise needed for a correct interpretation of research reports.

References

1. Anderson JR, Cain KC, Gelber RD. Analysis of survival by tumor response. J Clin Oncol. 1983;1(11):710–9.
2. Armstrong AJ, Febbo FG. Using surrogate endpoints to predict clinical benefit in men with castration-resistant prostate cancer: an update and review of the literature. Oncologist. 2009;14(8):816–27.

3. Bedard PL, Kryzanowska MK, Pintilie M, et al. Statistical power of negative randomized controlled trials presented at American Society for Clinical Oncology Annual Meetings. J Clin Oncol. 2007;25(23):3482–7.
4. Bhattacharya S, Fyfe G, Gray RJ, et al. Role of sensitivity analyses in assessing progression-free survival in late-stage oncology trials. J Clin Oncol. 2009;27(35):5958–64.
5. Bolla M, de Reijke THM, Van Tienhoven G, et al. Duration of androgen suppression in the treatment of prostate cancer. N Engl J Med. 2009;364(24): 2516–27.
6. Bolla M, van Poppel H, Collette L, et al. Postoperative radiotherapy after radical prostatectomy: a randomized controlled trial (EORTC trial 22911). Lancet. 2005;366(9485):572–8.
7. Bolla M, Van Tienhoven G, Warde P, et al. External irradiation with or without long-term androgen suppression for prostate cancer with high metastatic risk:10-year results of an EORTC randomised study. Lancet Oncol. 2010;11(11):1066–73.
8. Breau RH, Carnat TA, Gaboury I. Inadequate statistical power of negative clinical trials in the urological literature. J Urol. 2006;176(1):263–6.
9. Briganti A, Karnes JR, Da Pozzo LF, et al. Two positive nodes represent a significant cut-off value for cancer specific survival in patients with node positive prostate cancer. A new proposal based on a two-institution experience on 703 consecutive N+ patients treated with radical prostatectomy, extended pelvic lymph node dissection and adjuvant therapy. Eur Urol. 2009;55(2):261–70.
10. Budiharto T, Perneel C, Haustermans K, et al. A multi-institutional analysis comparing adjuvant and salvage radiation therapy for high-risk prostate cancer patients with undetectable PSA after prostatectomy. Radiother Oncol. 2010;97(3):474–9.
11. Carroll KJ. Analysis of progression-free survival in oncology trials: some common statistical issues. Pharm Stat. 2007;6(2):99–113.
12. Catton C, Gospodarowicz M, Warde P, et al. Adjuvant and salvage radiation therapy after radical prostatectomy for adenocarcinoma of the prostate. Radiother Oncol. 2001;59(1):51–60.
13. Collette L. Prostate-specific antigen (PSA) as a surrogate endpoint for survival in prostate cancer clinical trials. Eur Urol. 2008;53(1):6–9.
14. Cookson MS, Aus G, Burnett AL, et al. Variation in the definition of biochemical recurrence in patients treated for localized prostate cancer: the American Urological Association prostate guidelines for localized prostate cancer update panel report and recommendations for a standard in the reporting of surgical outcomes. J Urol. 2007;177(2):540–5.
15. D'Agostino Jr RB. Propensity score methods for bias reduction in the comparison of a treatment to a non-randomized control group. Stat Med. 1998;17(19):2265–81.
16. D'Amico AV, Denham JW, Bolla M, et al. Short- vs long-term androgen suppression plus external beam radiation therapy and survival in men of advanced age with node negative high risk adenocarcinoma of the prostate. Cancer. 2007;109(10):2004–10.
17. Dancey JE, Dodd LE, Ford R, et al. Recommendations for the assessment of progression in randomized cancer treatment trials. Eur J Cancer. 2009;45(2):281–9.
18. Denham JW, Steigler A, Wilcox C, et al. Time to biochemical failure and prostate-specific antigen doubling time as surrogates for prostate cancer-specific mortality: evidence from the TROG 96.01 randomised controlled trial. Lancet Oncol. 2008;9(11):1058–68.
19. Dodd LE, Korn EL, Freidlin B, Gray R, Bhattacharya S. An audit strategy for progression-free survival. Biometrics. 2011;67(3):1092–9.
20. Engel J, Bastian PJ, Baur H, et al. Survival benefit of radical prostatectomy in lymph node positive patients with prostate cancer. Eur Urol. 2010;57(5):754–61.
21. European Medicines Agency. Guideline on the investigation of subgroups in confirmatory clinical trials. EMA/CHMP/539146/2013. 2014. Available at: http://www.ema.europa.eu/docs/en_GB/document_library/Scientific_guideline/2014/02/WC500160523.pdf. Accessed 19 Apr 2016.
22. European Medicines Agency. Points to consider on multiplicity issues in clinical trials. CPMP/EWP/908/99. 2002. Available at: http://www.ema.europa.eu/docs/en_GB/document_library/Scientific_guideline/2009/09/WC500003640.pdf. Accessed 19 Apr 2016.
23. European Union. Regulation (EU) 536/2014 of the European Parliament and of the Council of 16 April 2014 on clinical trials on medicinal products for human use, and repealing Directive 2001/20/EC. Available at: http://ec.europa.eu/health/files/eudralex/vol-1/reg_2014_536/reg_2014_536_en.pdf. Accessed 19 Apr 2016.
24. Freidlin B, Korn EL, Hunsberger S, et al. Proposal for the use of progression-free survival in unblinded randomized trials. J Clin Oncol. 2007;25(15):2122–6.
25. Gignac GA, Morris MJ, Heller G, et al. Assessing outcomes in prostate cancer clinical trials: a twenty-tirst century tower of babel. Cancer. 2008;113(5):966–74.
26. Goeman JJ, Solari A. Multiple hypothesis testing in genomics. Stat Med. 2014;33(11):1946–78.
27. Howland RH. What you see depends on where you're looking and how you look at it: publication bias and outcome reporting bias. J Psychosoc Nurs Ment Health Serv. 2011;49(8):13–5. J Psychosoc Nurs Ment Health Serv. 15:1–3.
28. ICECaP working group. The development of intermediate clinical endpoints in cancer of the prostate (ICECaP). J Natl Cancer Inst. 2015;107(12):1–8.
29. Lin K, Lee SP, Steinberg ML. Selection bias clouds apparent benefit of longer hormone duration. J Clin Oncol. 2010;28(5):e79.
30. OCEBM Levels of Evidence Working Group*. "The oxford 2011 levels of evidence". Oxford centre for evidence-based medicine. http://www.cebm.net/index.aspx?o=5653. Last Accessed 19 Apr 2016.* OCEBM Table of Evidence Working Group = Jeremy

Howick, Iain Chalmers (James Lind Library), Paul Glasziou, Trish Greenhalgh, Carl Heneghan, Alessandro Liberati, Ivan Moschetti, Bob Phillips, Hazel Thornton, Olive Goddard and Mary Hodgkinson.
31. Panageas KS, Ben-Porat L, Dickler MN, et al. When you look matters: the effect of assessment schedule on progression-free survival. J Natl Cancer Inst. 2007; 99(6):428–32.
32. Patel AR, Stephenson AJ. Radiation therapy for prostate cancer after prostatectomy: adjuvant or salvage? Nat Rev Urol. 2011;8(7):385–92.
33. Ray ME, Bae K, Hussain MH, Hanks GE, et al. Potential surrogate endpoints for prostate cancer survival: analysis of a phase III randomized trial. J Natl Cancer Inst. 2009;101(4):228–36.
34. Roach MI, Hanks G, Thames HJ, et al. Defining biochemical failure following radiotherapy with or without hormonal therapy in men with clinically localized prostate cancer: recommendations of the RTOG–ASTRO Phoenix Consensus Conference. Int J Radiat Oncol Biol Phys. 2006;65(4):965–74.
35. Rui Wang MS, Lagakos SW, Ware JH, et al. Statistics in medicine – reporting of subgroup analyses in clinical trials. N Engl J Med. 2007;357(21):2189–94.
36. Sandler HM, Pajak TF, Hanks GE, et al. Can biochemical failure (ASTRO definition) be used as a surrogate endpoint for prostate cancer survival in phase III localized prostate cancer clinical trials? Analysis of RTOG protocol 92–02. J Clin Oncol. 2003;22:381 (abstract 1529).
37. Scher HI, Morris MJU, Stadler WM, et al. Trial design and objectives for castration-resistant prostate cancer: updated recommendations from the Prostate Cancer Clinical Trials Working Group 3. J Clin Oncol. 2016;34(12):1402–18.
38. Schroeder FH, Whelan P, de Reijke TM, et al. Metastatic prostate cancer treated by flutamide versus cyproterone acetate: final analysis of the European Organisation for Research and Treatment of Cancer (EORTC) protocol 30892. Eur Urol. 2004;45(4):457–64.
39. Sharrock G, Graf C, Fitzpatrick JM. The role of ethical publishing in promoting the evidence-based practice of urology. World J Urol. 2011;29(3):319–24.
40. Sonpavde G, Pond GR, Armstrong AJ, et al. Radiographic progression by Prostate Cancer Working Group (PCWG)-2 criteria as an intermediate endpoint for drug development in metastatic castration-resistant prostate cancer. BJU Int. 2014;114(6b):E25–31.
41. Souhami L, Bae K, Pilepich M, et al. Impact of the duration of adjuvant hormonal therapy in patients with locally advanced prostate cancer treated with radiotherapy: a secondary analysis of RTOG 85-31. J Clin Oncol. 2009;27(13):2137–43.
42. Souhami L, Bae K, Sandler H. Reply to Collette et al. and Tangen et al. J Clin Oncol. 2009;27(33):e204.
43. Studer UE, Collette L, Sylvester R. Can radical prostatectomy benefit patients despite the presence of regional metastases? Eur Urol. 2010;57(5):762–3.
44. Taylor N, Kelly JF, Kuban DA. Adjuvant and salvage radiotherapy after radical prostatectomy for prostate cancer. Int J Radiat Oncol Biol Phys. 2003;56(3): 755–63.
45. Thompson IM, Tangen CM, Paradelo J, et al. Adjuvant radiotherapy for pathologically advanced prostate cancer: a randomized trial. JAMA. 2006;296(19):2329–35.
46. Trabulsi EJ, Valicenti RK, Hanlon AL, et al. A multi-institutional matched-control analysis of adjuvant and salvage postoperative radiation therapy for pT3–4N0 prostate cancer. Urology. 2008;72(6):1298–304.
47. U.S. Department of Health and Human Services Food and Drug Administration. Guidance for industry clinical trial endpoints for the approval of cancer drugs and biologics. 2007. Available at: http://www.fda.gov/downloads/Drugs/Guidances/ucm071590.pdf. Accessed 19 Apr 2016.
48. Valicenti R, Deslivio M, Hanks G, et al. Posttreatment prostatic-specific antigen doubling time as a surrogate endpoint for prostate cancer-specific survival: an analysis of Radiation Therapy Oncology Group Protocol 92–02. Int J Radiat Oncol Biol Phys. 2006;66(4): 1064–71.
49. Wiegel T, Bottke D, Steiner U, et al. Phase III postoperative adjuvant radiotherapy after radical prostatectomy compared with radical prostatectomy alone in pT3 prostate cancer with postoperative undetectable prostate- specific antigen: ARO 96-02/AUO AP 09/95. J Clin Oncol. 2009;27(18):2924–30.
50. Wunsch H, Linde-Zwirble W, Angus DC. Methods to adjust for bias and confounding in critical care health services research involving observational data. J Crit Care. 2006;21(1):1–7.

Management of Prostate Cancer: EAU Guidelines on Screening, Diagnosis and Local Primary Treatment

Hocine Habchi and Nicolas Mottet

1 Introduction

The latest version of European Association of Urology (EAU) guidelines on prostate cancer (PCa) was published and posted on the EAU website Uroweb: https://uroweb.org/guideline/prostate-cancer/ in 2016 [24]. In this most recent summary, the radiotherapy section has been developed jointly with the European Society for Radiotherapy & Oncology (ESTRO) as well as with the Society for Oncogeriatrics (SIOG). Therefore, they should now be considered as the EAU-ESTRO-SIOG guidelines on prostate cancer.

2 Epidemiology

Prostate cancer is the most common non-skin cancer in elderly males in Europe. It is a major health concern, especially in developed countries with a greater proportion of elderly men in the general population. The incidence is highest in Northern and Western Europe (>200 per 100,000 men), while rates in Eastern and Southern Europe have showed a continuous increase. With the expected increase in the life expectancy of men and the subsequent rise in the incidence of PCa, the disease's economic burden in Europe is also expected to increase. It is estimated that the total economic costs of PCa in Europe exceed € 8.43 billion [24].

3 Risk Factors

Epidemiological studies have shown strong evidence for a genetic predisposition to PCa, based on two of the most important factors, ethnical origin and family history. The third well-established risk factor is the increasing age. Genome-wide association studies have identified 100 common susceptibility loci who contribute to the risk for PCa [3]. As for breast cancer, a genetic abnormality (BRCA2) likely to be associated with an increased risk has been shown prospectively. About 9 % of individuals with prostate PCa have true hereditary PCa, defined as three or more affected relatives (both paternal and maternal families), or at least two relatives who have developed early-onset disease, i.e., before the age of 55. Patients with hereditary PCa usually have a disease onset 6–7 years earlier than spontaneous cases, but do not differ in other ways.

H. Habchi • N. Mottet (✉)
Department of Urology, CHU Saint-Etienne,
42055 St Etienne, France
e-mail: nicolas.mottet@chu-st-etienne.fr

M. Bolla, H. van Poppel (eds.), *Management of Prostate Cancer*,
DOI 10.1007/978-3-319-42769-0_26

The incidence of clinical PCa varies widely between different geographical areas, being high in the USA and Northern Europe and low in South-East Asia. These findings indicate that exogenous factors affect the risk of progression from so-called latent PCa to clinical PCa. Factors such as diet, sexual behaviour, alcohol consumption, exposure to ultraviolet radiation, chronic inflammation and occupational exposure have all been discussed as being aetiologically important. However, there is currently no strong evidence to suggest that dietary interventions can reduce the risk of PCa.

4 Classification

The UICC 2010 Tumour Node Metastasis (TNM) classification for staging of PCa and the EAU risk group classification essentially based on D'Amico's classification system for PCa should be used.

The 2005 International Society of Urological Pathology (ISUP)-modified Gleason score of biopsy-detected PCa consists of the Gleason grade of the most extensive pattern (primary pattern) *plus* the second most common pattern (secondary pattern). For three grades, the Gleason score comprises the most common grade plus the highest grade, irrespective of its extent. The key change in pathology is the 2014 ISUP Gleason grading conference of prostatic carcinoma [12] has introduced the concept of the grade groups of PCa, to further codify the clinically highly significant distinction between Gleason score 7 (3+4) and 7 (4+3) PCa. It is summarised in the Table 1.

5 Prostate Cancer Screening and Early Detection

An updated Cochrane review [17] presents the main overview. It highlights that screening is associated with an increased diagnosis of PCa (RR: 1.3; 95 % CI: 1.02–1.65) as well as with detection of more localised disease (RR: 1.79; 95 % CI: 1.19–2.70) and less advanced PCa (T3-4, N1, M1) (RR: 0.80; 95 % CI: 0.73–0.87). Neither the PCa-specific survival (RR: 1.00; 95 % CI: 0.86–1.17) nor the OS (RR: 1.00; 95 % CI: 0.96–1.03) was observed from 5 to 4 randomised controlled trials (RCTs) respectively.

Table 1 The 2014 ISUP grading system for PCa

Gleason score	Grade group
2–6	1
7 (3+4)	2
7 (4+3)	3
8 (4+4) or (3+ 5) or (5+3)	4
9–10	5

The ERSPC (European Randomized Study of Screening for Prostate Cancer) data have now 13 years of follow up [28]. Even if the mortality reduction remains unchanged (21 and 29 % after non-compliance adjustment), the number needed to screen and to treat, 781 and 27, respectively, is decreasing, and is now below the number needed to screen observed in breast cancer trials.

An individualised risk-adapted strategy for early detection might be offered to a well-informed man with at least 10–15 years of life expectancy. However, this approach may still be associated with a substantial risk of overdiagnosis. Men at elevated risk of having PCa are those > 50 years, or with a family history of PCa and age > 45 years, or African-Americans. Informed men requesting an early diagnosis should be given a PSA test and undergo a digital rectal examination (DRE). The optimal intervals for PSA testing and DRE follow-up are unknown. A risk-adapted strategy might be considered based on the initial PSA level [15]. Men at 40 years of age with a PSA < 1 ng/ml, or better at 60 years with a PSA < 2 ng/ml, have such a minimal risk of further metastatic PCa during their lifetime that any further testing is questionable. Men who have less than a 15-year life expectancy are unlikely to benefit from screening. Furthermore, although there is no simple tool to evaluate individual life expectancy, co-morbidity is at least as important as age.

Mass screening of PCa is not indicated anywhere. Early diagnosis on an individual basis is possible. This requires an informed consent from the patient following a full discussion on the pros and cons of the complete procedure, taking into account the patient's risk factors, age and life expectancy. Furthermore, breaking the link between diagnosis and active treatment is the only way to decrease the overtreatment risk, while still maintaining the potential benefit of individual early diagnosis for men requesting it.

6 Clinical Diagnosis

Prostate cancer is usually suspected on the basis of DRE and/or PSA levels. Definitive diagnosis depends on histopathology on prostate biopsy cores or specimens from transurethral resection of the prostate (TURP) or prostatectomy for benign prostatic hyperplasia (BPH).

In about 18 % of cases, PCa is detected by suspect DRE alone, irrespective of PSA level. Suspect DRE in patients with PSA level ≤ 2 ng/ml has a positive predictive value up to 30 %. Abnormal DRE is associated with an increased risk of higher Gleason score [25].

As an independent variable, PSA is a better predictor of cancer than either DRE or transrectal ultrasound (TRUS). PSA is a continuous parameter, with higher levels indicating greater likelihood of PCa. Many men may harbour PCa despite having low serum PSA and there is no absolute PSA value to rule out any PCa. The use of nomograms may help in predicting indolent PCa.

To improve the PSA specificity for PCa detection, several modifications of serum PSA have been described such as the PSA density, free/total (f/t) PSA ratio and age-specific reference ranges.

The f/t PSA ratio stratifies the risk of PCa in men with 4–10 ng/ml total PSA and negative DRE: 56 % of PCa positive biopsy with f/t PSA < 0.10, compared to only 8 % with f/t PSA > 0.25. However, f/t PSA must be used cautiously because it may be adversely affected by several pre-analytical and clinical factors.

Based on the background noise (prostate volume and BPH), different intervals between PSA determinations and acceleration/deceleration of PSAV and PSA-DT over time, PSA velocity, and PSA-DT do not provide additional information compared with PSA alone.

Prostate Health Index (PHI) test (a combination of total PSA, free PSA and [−2] pro-PSA) and the four kallikrein (4 K) score test (measuring free, intact and total PSA and kallikrein-like peptidase 2 [hK2]) have been developed. Both tests outperformed f/t PSA for the prediction of clinically significant PCa, in men with a PSA between 2 and 10 ng/ml and are intended to reduce the number of unnecessary prostate biopsies [7]

The Prostate Cancer Antigen 3 (PCA3) is a prostate-specific, non-coding mRNA biomarker that is detectable in urine after prostatic massage. The PROGENSA urine test for PCA3 is superior to total and percent-free PSA for detection of PCa in men with elevated PSA. PCA3 score increases with PCa volume, but there are conflicting data about whether it independently predicts Gleason score. Currently, its main indication is to determine whether repeat biopsy is needed after an initially negative biopsy. Its clinical effectiveness is uncertain.

The role of imaging in the early diagnosis of prostate cancer is based on mpMRI. Grey-scale TRUS is not reliable at detecting PCa, and there is a need for improvement such as sonoelastography and contrast-enhanced US which have still an unclear position.

Multiparametric MRI (mpMRI) associates T2-weighted with diffusion-weighted imaging, dynamic contrast-enhanced imaging has excellent sensitivity for the detection and localisation of Gleason score ≥ 7 cancers. Furthermore, the higher the tumour volume, the better the detection rate. For example, if the tumour volume is greater than 2 ml, the detection rate by mpMRI for Gleason score 7 is about 97 %. Many single-centre studies suggest that mpMRI can reliably detect significant PCa in candidates for prostate biopsy with a negative (NPV) and positive predictive value (PPV) ranging from 63 to 98 % and from 34 to 68 %, respectively [14]. MRI-ultrasound fusion biopsy may also better predict the final pathological grade found at prostatectomy with greater accuracy than conventional methods (81 % vs. 40–65 %).

This is in line with a recent meta-analysis included 16 studies used both MRI-targeted biopsies (TBx) and TRUS-TBx. The overall prostate cancer detection did not significantly differ but MRI-TBx had a higher rate of detection of significant prostate cancer (sensitivity 0.91, 95 % CI 0.87–0.94 vs. 0.76, 95 % CI 0.64–0.84) and a lower rate of detection of insignificant prostate cancer (sensitivity 0.44, 95 % CI 0.26–0.64 vs. 0.83, 95 % confidence interval 0.77–0.87). However, subgroup analysis revealed an improvement in significant prostate cancer detection by MRI-TBx in men with previous negative biopsy, rather than in men with initial biopsy (relative sensitivity 1.54, 95 % CI 1.05–2.57 vs. 1.10, 95 % CI 1.00–1.22) [27]. Therefore, the need for a systematic mpMRI before a first round of biopsy remains unclear.

And it remains uncertain whether a negative mpMRI can justify omitting biopsy. Another limitation to the widespread use of mpMRI is the inter-reader variability and the heterogeneity in definitions of positive and negative examinations [33]. The EAU-ESTRO-SIOG guidelines recommend mpMRI should be systematically considered before repeated biopsy. It is mandatory to include systematic biopsies and targeting of any mpMRI lesion seen.

The first elevated PSA level should not prompt an immediate biopsy. PSA level should be verified after a few weeks using the same assay under standardised conditions in the same laboratory. Empiric use of antibiotics in an asymptomatic patient in order to lower the PSA should not be undertaken.

Before performing biopsy, the coagulation must be checked. Biopsy is possible in patients receiving aspirin 75 mg/day. Other regimen or oral anticoagulant or anti-aggregant must be stopped and replaced if needed before biopsying. Oral or intravenous quinolones are the drugs of choice, with ciprofloxacin being superior to ofloxacin. Nevertheless, increased quinolone resistance is associated with a rise in severe post-biopsy infection.

Ultrasound (US)-guided 18 G core prostate biopsy is the standard way to obtain materiel. A transrectal approach is used for most prostate biopsies, although a perineal approach might also be used. Cancer detection rates are comparable with both approaches. Ultrasound-guided periprostatic block is recommended.

On baseline biopsies, the sample sites should be as far posterior and lateral as possible in the peripheral gland. Additional cores should be obtained from suspect areas by DRE/TRUS. For a prostate volume of 30–40 ml, ≥ 8 cores should be sampled. Ten to 12 core biopsies are recommended, with more than 12 cores not being significantly more conclusive. The incidence of PCa detected by saturation repeat biopsy (>20 cores) is 30–43 % and depends on the number of cores sampled during earlier biopsies. Saturation biopsy may be performed with the transperineal technique, which detects an additional 38 % of PCa. The high rate of urinary retention (10 %) is a shortcoming. Indications for seminal vesicle biopsies are poorly defined. Its added value compared with mpMRI is questionable.

The indications for repeat biopsy are rising and/or persistently elevated PSA, suspicious DRE, atypical small acinar proliferation, multifocal high grade prostatic intraepithelial neoplasia (HGPIN), atypical glands immediately adjacent to HGPIN, intraductal carcinoma which is associated in 90 % of cases with a high-grade prostate carcinoma and a positive mpMRI findings. However, the optimal timing is still uncertain. The later the repeat biopsy is done, the higher the detection rate.

Prostate core biopsies from different sites are processed separately. Each biopsy site should be reported individually, including its location and histopathological findings, which include the histological type, the Gleason score using the modified system adopted in 2005, the length (mm) or proportion (%) of tumour involvement per biopsy. A global Gleason score comprising all biopsies is also reported as well as the ISUP 2014 grade group. Intraductal carcinoma, lymphovascular invasion and extraprostatic extension must each be reported, if identified [12].

7 Clinical Staging

The extent of PCa is evaluated by DRE and PSA, and may be supplemented with bone scanning (BS) and computerised tomography (CT) or mpMRI. The decision to proceed to a tumour staging is only recommended if it directly affects treatment decisions.

Local staging (T-staging) is based on finding from DRE, PSA level, biopsy finding and possibly mpMRI. DRE is positively correlated with tumour stage in less than 50 % of cases, although it often underestimates tumour extension. Serum PSA levels increase with tumour stage, but it is inaccurate for predicting the pathological stage. The percentage of cancer per biopsy is a strong predictor of positive surgical margins, seminal vesicle invasion (SVI) and extra-prostatic extension. An increase in tumour-positive biopsies is an independent predictor of extraprostatic extension, margin involvement and lymph node invasion. Serum PSA, Gleason score and clinical T stage are more useful together than alone in predicting final pathological stage [10].

Transrectal ultrasound even with the advent of colour Doppler and contrast agents is inaccurate for local staging. Multiparametric MRI has good specificity but low sensitivity for detecting pT3 stages, and cannot detect microscopic (<1 mm) extracapsular extension (ECE). Pooled data for ECE, SVI and overall pT3 detection showed sensitivity and specificity of 0.57 (95 % CI: 0.49–0.64) and 0.91 (95 % CI: 0.88–0.93), 0.58 (95 % CI: 0.47–0.68) and 0.96 (95 % CI: 0.95–0.97), and 0.61 (95 % CI: 0.54–0.67) and 0.88 (95 % CI: 0.85–0.91), respectively [9]. The use of functional imaging in addition to T2-weighted imaging improves sensitivity for ECE or SVI detection. But the experience of the reader remains of paramount importance.

N-staging is only important when curative treatment is planned. Patients with low- and intermediate-risk PCa may be spared N-staging before potentially curative treatment. Nomograms can define patients at low risk (<5 %) of nodal metastasis, although they may be more accurate in establishing the extent of nodal involvement [10]. Sensitivity of imaging by either abdominal CT or mpMRI is low to detect lymph nodes invasion. For CT or mpMRI, detection of microscopic lymph node invasion is less than 1 % in patients with a Gleason score < 8, PSA < 20 ng/ml, or localised disease. This justifies to limit the use of CT or mpMRI for high-risk cancer. The imaging by 11C- or 18F-choline positron emission tomography (PET)/CT have good specificity for lymph node metastases, but a sensitivity of between 10 and 73 %, therefore, it has no place for up-front staging in nodal metastasis. Lymphadenectomy remains the reliable staging method in clinically localised PCa. Primary removal of sentinel lymph nodes (SN) might be an option. But the lack of data from large multicentre cohorts is a major limitation of this technique which should still be considered as experimental.

For skeletal metastasis, BS has been the most widely used method. However, it suffers from relatively low specificity. This may not be indicated in asymptomatic patients if PSA < 20 ng/ml in the presence of well or moderately differentiated tumours. It remains unclear whether choline PET/CT is more sensitive than conventional bone scanning, but it has higher specificity, with fewer indeterminate bone lesions. Diffusion-weighted whole-body and axial MRI are more sensitive than bone scanning and targeted radiography in detecting bone metastases in high-risk PCa. A recent meta-analysis found that mpMRI is more sensitive than choline PET/CT and BS for detecting bone metastases on a per-patient basis, although choline PET/CT had the highest specificity [29].

8 Primary Local Treatment of Prostate Cancer

8.1 Active Surveillance

Up to 45 % of men with PSA-detected PCa would be candidates for deferred management. In men with comorbidity and limited life expectancy, treatment of localised PCa may be deferred to avoid bothersome symptoms and loss of quality of life (QoL).

Active surveillance (AS) must be differentiated from watchful waiting (WW). The former aims to achieve correct timing for curative treatment and patients remain under close surveillance with a predefined schedule. The latter is a conservative management for frail patients until the development of local or systemic progression, leading to symptomatic treatment. AS was conceived with the aim to reduce over-treatment without compromising cure rates. AS is only proposed for highly selected low-risk patients.

A systematic review including more than 3,900 patients [32] is the best available evidence so far. There is considerable variation between studies regarding patient selection, follow-up policies and when active treatment should be instigated. According to these data, AS is a curative treatment options that must be systematically discussed with patients suitable for it, as well as surgery and radiotherapy. It should only be offered to patients with the lowest risk of cancer progression (i.e. cT1/2, PSA ≤ 10 ng/ml, biopsy Gleason score ≤ 6, ≤ 2 positive biopsies, minimal biopsy core involvement (≤50 % cancer per biopsy)), and at least 10 years life expectancy. mpMRI is of particular interest due to its high NPV value for lesion upgrading and for staging anterior prostate lesions. Its important place in AS programmes has been highlighted [27], but it cannot replace follow-up biopsies and should not be used alone as an assessment tool to prompt active treatment.

The follow-up strategy is based on repeated DRE, PSA and repeated biopsy and patients must be aware about the possibility of needing further treatment in the future. The decision to suggest active treatment should be based on a change in the biopsy results or clinical stage. A PSA change is a less powerful indication for changed management based on its weak link with grade progression. Active treatment may also be instigated upon a patient's request.

8.2 Watchful Waiting

PCa often progresses slowly, and is predominantly diagnosed in older men with a high incidence of comorbidity and other causes of mortality. Patients with well-, moderately- and poorly differentiated tumours had 10-year cancer-specific survival (CSS) rates of 91 %, 90 % and 74 %, respectively, without any active upfront treatment [22]. Recently 731 men with clinically organ-confined PCa were randomised to RP or WW [35]. After a mean follow-up of 10 years, there was no significant difference between the treatments for overall mortality (47 % for RP vs. 49.9 % for the WW group) and PCa-specific death (5.8 % for the RP group vs. 8.4 % for the WW group). There were no significant differences in OS when considering patient age, Gleason score, performance status and Charlson comorbidity index (CCI) score. Only patients with intermediate- or high-risk PCa had a significant OS benefit from RP.

The major impact of comorbidity has been confirmed in a recent analysis at 5 and 10 years follow up in 19,639 patients aged more than 65 years who were not given curative treatment [2]. If the CCI score was greater than two, tumour aggressiveness had little impact on OS, suggesting that patients could have been spared biopsy and diagnosis of cancer. Thus, evaluation of initial comorbidity and survival probability before proposing biopsy or treatment is important.

For locally advanced PCa, the final analysis of the largest RCT focusing on the question of deferred or immediate treatment was published in 2013 [30]. A total of 985 M0 PCa patients, who are not eligible for local treatment with curative intent, were randomly assigned to immediate androgen-deprivation therapy (ADT) or only on disease progression or occurrence of serious complications. After a median follow-up of 12.8 years, the OS hazard ratio (HR) was 1.21 (95 % CI: 1.05–1.39), favouring immediate treatment. The time from randomisation to progression to castrate resistant status did not differ significantly, nor did CSS. The median time to start of deferred treatment was 7 years. In this group, 126 patients died without requiring treatment (44 % of deaths in this arm). A baseline PSA > 50 ng/ml was associated with a 3.5-fold higher mortality compared to those with ≤ 8 ng/ml. If baseline PSA was

8–50 ng/ml, the mortality risk was about 7.5-fold higher in patients with a PSADT of <12 months compared with >12 months.

8.3 Radical Prostatectomy

Histopathological examination of radical prostatectomy (RP) specimens describes the pathological stage, histopathological type, grade, cancer location and surgical margins of PCa. Grading of prostatic adenocarcinoma using the Gleason system is the strongest prognostic factor for clinical behaviour and treatment response. On the other hand, the independent prognostic value of PCa volume in RP specimens has not been established. Compared to the biopsy Gleason score, the same ISUP rules must be used, with two major differences. A grade comprising ≤5 % of the cancer volume is not incorporated in the Gleason score (5 % rule). The tertiary grade 4 or 5, and its approximate proportion of the cancer volume should also be reported, as it is an unfavourable prognostic indicator for BCR.

Radical prostatectomy (RP) is the only treatment for localised PCa to show a benefit for OS and CSS, compared with WW, based on at least 1 RCT. [4]. The SPCG-4 trial showed that RP was associated with a reduction of all-cause mortality, with a relative risk (RR) of death at 18 years of 0.71 (95 % CI: 0.59–0.86). RP was also associated with a reduction in PCa-specific mortality (PCSM) at 18 years (RR: 0.56; 95 % CI: 0.41–0.77). The overall benefits in OS and CSS were not reproduced in PIVOT trial [35]. However, according to a pre-planned subgroup analysis among men with intermediate-risk tumours, RP significantly reduced all-cause mortality (HR: 0.69 [95 % CI: 0.49–0.98]), but not specific mortality (0.50; 95 % CI: 0.21–1.21). It must be highlighted that the populations included in these 2 RCTs are different; the SPCG trial includes a larger proportion of intermediate or high-risk patients while mainly low-intermediate risk patients were included in the PIVOT trial. Nowadays there is still no clear evidence that any surgical approach is better than another (open, laparoscopic or robotic).

In case of low-risk PCa, the decision to offer RP opposed to AS should be based upon the probabilities of clinical progression, side effects and potential benefit to survival, based on the tumour characteristics and the patients expectations and comorbidities. In intermediate risk group, RP is one of the standard treatment options. In patients with high-risk PCa, there is an increased risk of metastatic progression and death from PCa. The optimal treatment of this group is still unknown. Proposing a RP in a multimodality setting to selected patients with a low tumour volume and a life expectancy greater than 10 years may be reasonable. For patients with a biopsy Gleason score ≥ 8, up to 39 % biochemical progression-free survival at 10-years might be obtained through a multimodal treatment. This might be associated with a CSS at 5, 10 and 15 years of 96 %, 84–88 % and 66 %, respectively.

The high risk of positive margins and/or lymph node involvement associated with a high-risk locally advanced T3 situation deserves a multimodality approach. Several retrospective series have been published, showing a CSS at 5, 10 and 15 years ranging between 90–99 %, 85–92 % and 62–84 %, respectively, and an OS at 5 and 10 years ranging between 90–96 % and 76–77 %, respectively [24]. The key question remains the patient selection that has neither nodal involvement nor seminal vesicle invasion. Nomograms, including PSA level and Gleason score, may be useful in predicting the pathological stage of disease [6]. A cohort of 1360 high risk patients has clarified the heterogeneity of this group of patients. With a multimodal treatment if needed, based on postoperative characteristics, the 10-year-specific survival was 95.4 % when 1 risk factor was present (i.e. PSA > 20 ng/ml or cT3-4, or biopsy Gleason > 7), 88.3 % when PSA > 20 ng/ml and Gleason > 7 were present, and 79.7 % when the 3 risk factors were present [18].

Pelvic nodal dissection has no place in low-risk situations. In intermediate situations, it is mandatory for those patients with a greater than 5 % risk of pN+, based on the validated Briganti nomogram [6]. It is mandatory in all high risk situations. When performed, it must be systematically extended, meaning removing the nodes overlying the external iliac artery and vein, the nodes within the obturator fossa located cranially and caudally to the obturator nerve and the nodes medial and lateral to the internal iliac artery. An absolute minimal number of nodes is almost impossible to suggest, as this depends on other factors than just the template, especially the pathological processing.

Neoadjuvant androgen-deprivation therapy (ADT) has no place as it is not associated with an improved PFS or OS. Adjuvant ADT has no place in pN0 patients.

In case of pN+ situations, adjuvant androgen-deprivation therapy following RP has been shown to achieve a 10-year CSS rate of 80% [24]. Furthermore, two retrospective observational studies have shown a significant improvement in CSS and OS in favour of completed RP vs. abandoned RP in patients who were found to be N+ at the time of surgery [11]. Therefore, frozen sections on nodes are no longer recommended. Adjuvant radiotherapy is part of this multimodal approach in pN1 disease. Its beneficial impact on survival in these patients with pN1 PCa is highly influenced by tumour characteristics. Men with low-volume nodal disease (<3 lymph nodes) and GS 7–10 and pT3-4 or R1 as well as men with 3–4 positive nodes were more likely to benefit from RT after surgery [1]. No recommendations can be made on the RT fields, although whole pelvis RT was given in more than 70% of men in a large retrospective series that found a benefit for adding RT to androgen ablation in pN1 patients (Table 2). Finally, a close follow-up without any adjuvant treatment might be an option for those patients with an undetectable PSA and a minimal nodal involvement (i.e. 1 or 2 nodes without a capsular penetration) after and extended nodal dissection.

Table 2 EAU Guidelines for radical prostatectomy

Recommendation	Grade of recommendation
Discuss AS and radiotherapy with suitable patients	A
Offer RP to patients with low- and intermediate-risk PCa and a life expectancy >10 years	A
Nerve-sparing surgery may be attempted in pre-operatively potent patients with low risk of extracapsular disease (T1c, GS<7 and PSA<10 ng/ml, or refer to Partin tables/nomograms)	B
In intermediate- and high-risk disease, use multiparametric MRI as a decision tool to select patients for nerve-sparing procedures	B
Offer RP in a multimodality setting to patients with high-risk localised PCa and a life expectancy of >10 years	A
Offer RP in a multimodality setting to selected patients with locally advanced (cT3a) PCa, and a life expectancy >10 years	B
Offer RP in a multimodality setting to highly selected patients with locally advanced PCa (cT3b-T4 N0 or any T N1)	C
Do not offer neoadjuvant hormonal therapy before RP	A
Do not offer adjuvant hormonal therapy for pN0	A
Offer any surgical approach (i.e. open, laparoscopic or robotic) to patients who are surgical candidates for radical prostatectomy	A

8.4 Radiation Therapy

There are no published RCTs comparing RT with WW or AS. The only randomised trial in the modern era is the ProtecT study which has not yet reported its first results. The development of technology has been associated with improvement of radiotherapy dose results, and a decrease of side effects. These technology improvements allow an increased dose, as well as hypofractionation. Table 3 summarizes the EAU guidelines for definitive radiotherapy.

Intensity-modulated radiotherapy (IMRT), with or without image-guided radiotherapy (IGRT), is the gold standard for external beam radiotherapy (EBRT). Real-time verification of the irradiation field using portal imaging allows comparison of the treated and simulated fields,

Table 3 Summary of evidence and EAU guidelines for definitive radiotherapy

Recommendation	Grade of recommendation
Discuss AS and surgery with all patients who would be suitable for these treatment options	A
Offer EBRT to all risk groups of non-metastatic PCa	A
In low-risk PCa, use a total dose of 74–78 Gy	A
In patients with low-risk PCa, without a previous TURP and with a good IPSS and a prostate volume <50 ml, offer LDR brachytherapy	A
In intermediate- risk PCa use a total dose of 76–78 Gy, in combination with short-term ADT (4–6 months)	A
In patients with high-risk localised PCa, use a total dose of 76–78 Gy in combination with long-term ADT (2–3 years)	A
In patients with locally advanced cN0 PCa, offer radiotherapy in combination with long-term ADT (2–3 years)	A
Offer IMRT for definitive treatment of PCa by EBRT	A
In patients with cN+ PCa offer pelvic external irradiation in combination with immediate long-term ADT	B
In patients with pT3N0M0 PCa and an undetectable PSA following RP, discuss adjuvant EBRT because it improves at least biochemical-free survival	A
Inform patients with pT3N0M0 PCa and an undetectable PSA following RP about salvage irradiation as an alternative to adjuvant irradiation when PSA increases	A

and correction for prostate movements if needed. With dose escalation using IMRT, organ movement becomes a critical issue. Several randomised studies have shown that dose escalation (range 74–80 Gy) has a significant impact on 5-year relapse-free survival. An OS has been clearly suggested for intermediate- or high-risk PCa but not with low-risk PCa [19].

Fractionated RT utilises differences in the DNA repair capacity of normal and tumour tissue. In fast growing tissue, cells have little time to repair photon-induced DNA damage, leading to an α/β ratio around 10 Gy. In contrast, tissue with a low cell renewal has a good opportunity for repair between fractions, with an α/β ratio of 3 Gy or lower. These latter cells are very sensitive to an increased dose per fraction. PCa, has an α/β ratio of approximately 1.5 Gy, suggesting a strong interest for hypofractionation (HFX). Studies on moderate HFX (2.5–4 Gy/fx) delivered with conventional 3D-CRT/IMRT have sufficient follow-up to support the safety of this therapy, but long-term efficacy data are still lacking. Extreme HFX (5–10 Gy/fx) typically requires IGRT and stereotactic body radiotherapy (SBRT). Short-term biochemical control is comparable to conventional fractionation. However, there are concerns about high-grade genito-urinary and rectal toxicity, long-term side effects may not all be known yet and therefore this modality should still be considered as experimental. Whatever the techniques and their degree of sophistication, quality assurance plays a major role in the management of RT, requiring the involvement of physicians, physicists, dosimetrists, radiologists and computer scientists.

In cases of low-risk PCa, the decision to offer radiotherapy opposed to AS should be based upon the probabilities of clinical progression, side effects and potential benefit to survival, based on the tumour characteristics and the patients' expectations and comorbidities. In patients with low-risk PCa, IMRT with escalated dose without ADT may be an alternative to brachytherapy.

For intermediate-risk PCa, IMRT can be combined with a short-term ADT (4–6 months). For patients unsuitable or unwilling to accept ADT, the recommended treatment is IMRT at an escalated dose ranging from 76 to 80 Gy or a combination of IMRT and brachytherapy.

In patients with localised high-risk PCa, the use of a combined modality approach is mandatory, consisting of dose-escalated IMRT, possibly including the pelvic lymph nodes and a long-term ADT (at least 2–3 years). It is important to know that short-term ADT did not improve OS in these patients, as has been demonstrated by the Boston and RTOG trials [24]. However, the patient health profile must be considered to adapt the duration of ADT based on comorbidities such as metabolic or cardiac.

In locally advanced disease, RCTs have clearly established that the additional use of long-term ADT combined with RT produces better OS. While RT is effective in this patient group, combined RT + ADT is clearly superior to ADT alone as observed in RCT such as the NCIC PR3 trial where 1205 patients with locally advanced PCa were randomly assigned to lifelong ADT with or without RT. At a median follow-up of 8 years, OS was significantly improved in the combined group (HR: 0.70; 95 % CI: 0.57 to 0.85; $p<0.001$). Specific survival was also reduced in the combined group (HR: 0.46; 95 % CI: 0.34 to 0.61; $p<0.001$) [23].

The impact of neoadjuvant chemotherapy was evaluated by the GETUG 12 trial that randomised 413 patients with localised high-risk PCa to ADT plus chemotherapy (four cycles of docetaxel and estramustine) or to ADT alone [13]. Most patients (87 %) received RT. With a median follow-up of 4.6 years, the 4-year progression free survival was 85 % vs. 81 % in arm 2 ($p=0.26$), but the data need to mature.

8.4.1 Lymph Node Irradiation

There is no level 1 evidence for whole-pelvic irradiation in clinically N0 PCa, since randomised trials, including the RTOG 77–06 study, the Stanford study and the GETUG 01 trial [24], have failed to show any benefit from prophylactic irradiation (46–50 Gy) of the pelvic lymph nodes in high-risk cases. However, all the trials conducted in high risk situations combined with ADT used a whole pelvis template. With regard to clinical node positive (N1M0), the RTOG 85–31 trial, with a median follow-up of 6.5 years, suggested that 95 of the 173 pN1 patients who received pelvic RT with immediate long-term ADT had a better 5-year and 9-year PFS rates (54 % and 10 % respectively) compared to EBRT alone (33 % and 4 %, respectively), with a significant impact on the OS (multivariate analysis) [21]. Recent data from the STAMPEDE trial suggest that pelvic RT could be beneficial for N1 disease, but not based on an RCT.

8.5 Innovative Techniques

8.5.1 Proton Beam Therapy

Proton beams are a potentially attractive alternative to photon-beam RT as they deposit almost all their radiation dose at the end of the particle's path in tissue (the Bragg peak), in contrast to photons, which deposit radiation along their path. There is also a very sharp fall-off beyond their deposition depth, leading to normal tissue sparing beyond this depth. In contrast, photon beams continue to deposit energy until they leave the body, including an exit dose. Only one randomised trial on dose escalation (70.2 vs. 79.2 Gy) has incorporated protons for the boost doses of either 19.8 or 28.8 Gy. This trial shows improved outcome with the higher dose, but cannot be used as evidence for the superiority of proton therapy [36]. Thus, the real place of proton therapy remains unclear. It must be considered as a costly potentially promising, but experimental, alternative to photon-beam therapy.

8.5.2 Low-Dose Rate and High-Dose Rate Brachytherapy

LDR Brachytherapy

Transperineal low-dose rate brachytherapy (LDR) is a safe and effective technique for low-risk PCa. It is only indicated in patients with a cT1b-T2a N0M0, Gleason score 6 with no more than 50 % of biopsy cores involved with cancer or Gleason 7 (3 + 4) score with no more than 33 % of biopsy cores involved with cancer, an initial PSA < 10 ng/ml, a prostate <50 cc and good International Prostatic Symptom Score (IPSS). As for RP or EBRT, there is no RCT comparing LDR to anything. Outcome data are available from a number of large population cohorts with mature follow-up. 1 relapse free survival at 10 years between 65 and 85 % can be expected [16]. Neoadjuvant or adjuvant ADT has almost no place combined with LDR. In a retrospective analysis of 5,621 men who had undergone LDR brachytherapy [8], the urinary, bowel and erectile morbidity rates were 33.8 %, 21 % and 16.7 %, respectively. Previous TURP for benign prostatic hyperplasia increases the risk of post-implantation incontinence and urinary morbidity.

HDR Brachytherapy

High-dose-rate brachytherapy uses a radioactive source temporarily introduced into the prostate to deliver radiation. It can be delivered in single or multiple fractions and is often combined with EBRT. Data suggest an equivalent outcome in terms of recurrence-free survival in comparison with high-dose EBRT (HD-EBRT). Quality-of-life changes were similar, but the frequency of erectile dysfunction was significantly increased with HDR (86 vs. 34 %). A single randomised trial of EBRT vs. EBRT plus HDR boost showed a significant improvement in the biochemical relapse-free in the combined group (p=0.04) [20].

8.5.3 Adjuvant Post-operative EBRT After RP (cN0 or pN0)

After three RCT, the real place of adjuvant EBRT after RP remains controversial. The EORTC 22911, with a cohort of 1005 patients, compared immediate post-operative RT with RT delayed until local recurrence in pT2-3 pN0 with risk factors (such as positive margins) after RP. For patients younger than 70 years, the immediate post-operative RT significantly improved the 10-year biological PFS (60.6 % vs. 41.1 %) [5]. This was not linked to any survival benefit. The conclusions of ARO trial 96–02 (n = 385) appear to support those of the EORTC study. After a median follow-up period of 112 months, the RT group demonstrated a significant improvement in biochemical disease-free survival of 56 % vs. 35 %, respectively (p=0.0001) in patients with a post operative undetectable PSA [34]. However, no survival benefit was observed. The updated results of the SWOG 8794 trial, with a median follow-up of more than 12 years of 425 pT3 patients, showed a significant improvement in the metastasis-free survival, with a 10-year metastasis-free survival of 71 % vs. 61 % and a 10-year OS of 74 % vs. 66 % [31]. However, all these trial suffer from major limitations, such as the number of patients of post-operative detectable PSA or the lack of prespecified PSA threshold for salvage EBRT.

Thus, for patients classified as pT3 pN0 with a high risk of local failure after RP due to positive margins (highest impact), capsule rupture and/or invasion of the seminal vesicles and undetectable PSA level, two options can be offered within the frame of an informed consent: either an immediate EBRT to the surgical bed after recovery of urinary function during the 6 post-operative months, or a clinical and biological monitoring followed by salvage radiotherapy before the PSA exceeds 0.5 ng/ml.

8.6 Options Other Than Surgery and Radiotherapy for the Primary Treatment of Localised Prostate Cancer

Besides RP, EBRT and brachytherapy, cryosurgery (CSAP) and high-intensity-focused US (HIFU) have emerged as therapeutic options in patients with clinically localised PCa. Both HIFU and CSAP have been developed as minimally invasive procedures with the aim of providing equivalent oncological safety, reduced toxicity and improved functional outcomes.

Patients who are potential candidates for CSAP are those with low- or intermediate-risk PCa, prostate size should be <40 ml at the time of therapy. A recent systematic review [26] and meta-analysis compared CSAP vs. RP and EBRT. Because of the high risk of bias across studies, the findings in relation to cancer-specific outcomes were considered inconclusive. There was evidence that the rate of urinary incontinence at 1 year was lower for CSAP than for RP, but the size of the difference decreased with longer follow-up. There was no significant difference between CSAP vs. EBRT for urinary incontinence at 1 year and no significant difference for erectile dysfunction compared with RP. The only difference that reached statistical significance was for urethral stricture, which was less frequent after CSAP than after RP.

For HIFU, the same systematic review [26] compared HIFU vs. RP and EBRT as primary treatment for localised PCa. There was some evidence that biochemical failure rates were significantly higher at 1 year with HIFU than with EBRT. However, the difference was no longer statistically significant at 5 years. In terms of toxicity, there were insufficient data on urinary incontinence or erectile dysfunction to draw any conclusions. The quality of the evidence was poor, due to high risks of bias across studies and heterogeneity of outcome definition, measurement and reporting. No controlled trial was available for analysis, and no survival data were presented. No validated biochemical surrogate end-point was available for HIFU therapy. The review found HIFU to be associated with a progression-free survival of 63–87 % (projected 3- to 5-year data), but median follow-up in the studies ranged from 12 to 24 months only.

Conclusion

Based mainly on systematic revue and formal methodology, these 2016 EAU-ESTRO-SIOG guidelines should be helpful in the patient management. They will evolve based on systematic updated literature searches. However, they cannot cover all the individual situations. They have to be considered as guidance for the multidisciplinary team but will never replace the face-to-face discussion with the patient, based on its individual expectations and fears.

References

1. Abdollah F, Karnes J, Suardi N, et al. Impact of adjuvant radiotherapy on survival of patients with node-positive prostate cancer. J Clin Oncol. 2014;32:3939–47.
2. Albertsen PC, Moore DF, Shih W, et al. Impact of comorbidity on survival among men with localized prostate cancer. J Clin Oncol. 2011;29:1335–41.
3. Al Olama AA, Kote-Jarai Z, Berndt SI, et al. A meta-analysis of 87,040 individuals identifies 23 new susceptibility loci for prostate cancer. Nat Genet. 2014;46:1103–9.
4. Bill-Axelson A, Holmberg L, Garmo H, et al. Radical prostatectomy or watchful waiting in early prostate cancer. N Engl J Med. 2014;370:932–42.
5. Bolla M, van Poppel H, Tombal B, et al. Postoperative radiotherapy after radical prostatectomy for high-risk prostate cancer: long-term results of a randomised controlled trial (EORTC trial 22911). Lancet. 2012;380:2018–27.
6. Briganti A, Larcher A, Abdollah F, et al. Updated nomogram predicting lymph node invasion in patients with prostate cancer undergoing extended pelvic lymph node dissection: the essential importance of percentage of positive cores. Eur Urol. 2012;61:480–7.
7. Bryant RJ, Sjoberg DD, Vickers AJ, et al. Predicting high-grade cancer at ten-core prostate biopsy using four kallikrein markers measured in blood in the ProtecT study. J Natl Cancer Inst. 2015. doi: 10.1093/jnci/djv095.
8. Chen AB, D'Amico AV, Neville BA, Earle CC. Patient and treatment factors associated with complications after prostate brachytherapy. J Clin Oncol Off J Am Soc Clin Oncol. 2006;24:5298–304.
9. de Rooij M, Hamoen EHJ, Witjes JA, et al. Accuracy of magnetic resonance imaging for local staging of prostate cancer: a diagnostic meta-analysis. Eur Urol. 2015. doi: 10.1016/j.eururo.2015.07.029.
10. Eifler JB, Feng Z, Lin BM, et al. An updated prostate cancer staging nomogram (Partin tables) based on cases from 2006 to 2011. BJU Int. 2013;111:22–9.
11. Engel J, Bastian PJ, Baur H, et al. Survival benefit of radical prostatectomy in lymph node-positive patients with prostate cancer. Eur Urol. 2010;57:754–61.
12. Epstein JI, Egevad L, Amin MB, et al. The 2014 International Society of Urological Pathology (ISUP) consensus conference on Gleason grading of prostatic carcinoma: definition of grading patterns and proposal for a new grading system. Am J Surg Pathol. 2016;40:244–52.
13. Fizazi K, Faivre L, Lesaunier F, et al. Androgen deprivation therapy plus docetaxel and estramustine versus androgen deprivation therapy alone for high-risk localised prostate cancer (GETUG 12): a phase 3 randomised controlled trial. Lancet Oncol. 2015;16:787–94.
14. Fütterer JJ, Briganti A, De Visschere P, et al. Can clinically significant prostate cancer be detected with multiparametric magnetic resonance imaging? A systematic review of the literature. Eur Urol. 2015;68:1045–53.
15. Gelfond J, Choate K, Ankerst DP, et al. Intermediate-term risk of prostate cancer is directly related to baseline prostate specific antigen: implications for reducing the burden of prostate specific antigen screening. J Urol. 2015;194:46–51.

16. Grimm PD, Blasko JC, Sylvester JE, et al. 10-year biochemical (prostate-specific antigen) control of prostate cancer with (125)I brachytherapy. Int J Radiat Oncol Biol Phys. 2001;51:31–40.
17. Hayes JH, Barry MJ. Screening for prostate cancer with the prostate-specific antigen test: a review of current evidence. JAMA. 2014;311:1143–9.
18. Joniau S, Briganti A, Gontero P, et al. Stratification of high-risk prostate cancer into prognostic categories: a European multi-institutional study. Eur Urol. 2015;67:157–64.
19. Kalbasi A, Li J, Berman A, et al. Dose-escalated irradiation and overall survival in men with nonmetastatic prostate cancer. JAMA Oncol. 2015;1:897–906.
20. Kupelian PA, Potters L, Khuntia D, et al. Radical prostatectomy, external beam radiotherapy <72 Gy, external beam radiotherapy>or =72 Gy, permanent seed implantation, or combined seeds/external beam radiotherapy for stage T1-T2 prostate cancer. Int J Radiat Oncol Biol Phys. 2004;58:25–33.
21. Lawton CA, DeSilvio M, Roach M, et al. An update of the phase III trial comparing whole pelvic to prostate only radiotherapy and neoadjuvant to adjuvant total androgen suppression: updated analysis of RTOG 94–13, with emphasis on unexpected hormone/radiation interactions. Int J Radiat Oncol Biol Phys. 2007;69:646–55.
22. Lu-Yao GL, Albertsen PC, Moore DF, et al. Outcomes of localized prostate cancer following conservative management. JAMA. 2009;302:1202–9.
23. Mason MD, Parulekar WR, Sydes MR, et al. Final report of the intergroup randomized study of combined androgen-deprivation therapy plus radiotherapy versus androgen-deprivation therapy alone in locally advanced prostate cancer. J Clin Oncol. 2015;33:2143–50.
24. Mottet N, Bellmunt J, Bolla M, et al. EAU-ESTRO-SIOG guidelines on prostate cancer. 2016. http://uroweb.org/wp-content/uploads/EAU-Guidelines-Prostate-Cancer-2016.pdf.
25. Okotie OT, Roehl KA, Han M, et al. Characteristics of prostate cancer detected by digital rectal examination only. Urology. 2007;70:1117–20.
26. Ramsay CR, Adewuyi TE, Gray J, et al. Ablative therapy for people with localised prostate cancer: a systematic review and economic evaluation. Health Technol Assess Winch Engl. 2015;19:1–490.
27. Schoots IG, Roobol MJ, Nieboer D, et al. Magnetic resonance imaging-targeted biopsy may enhance the diagnostic accuracy of significant prostate cancer detection compared to standard transrectal ultrasound-guided biopsy: a systematic review and meta-analysis. Eur Urol. 2015;68:438–50.
28. Schröder FH, Hugosson J, Roobol MJ, et al. Prostate-cancer mortality at 11 years of follow-up. N Engl J Med. 2012;366:981–90.
29. Shen G, Deng H, Hu S, Jia Z. Comparison of choline-PET/CT, MRI, SPECT, and bone scintigraphy in the diagnosis of bone metastases in patients with prostate cancer: a meta-analysis. Skeletal Radiol. 2014;43:1503–13.
30. Studer UE, Collette L, Whelan P, et al. Using PSA to guide timing of androgen deprivation in patients with T0-4 N0-2 M0 prostate cancer not suitable for local curative treatment (EORTC 30891). Eur Urol. 2008;53:941–9.
31. Thompson IM, Tangen CM, Paradelo J, et al. Adjuvant radiotherapy for pathological T3N0M0 prostate cancer significantly reduces risk of metastases and improves survival: long-term followup of a randomized clinical trial. J Urol. 2009;181:956–62.
32. Thomsen FB, Brasso K, Klotz LH, et al. Active surveillance for clinically localized prostate cancer–a systematic review. J Surg Oncol. 2014;109:830–5.
33. Vaché T, Bratan F, Mège-Lechevallier F, et al. Characterization of prostate lesions as benign or malignant at multiparametric MR imaging: comparison of three scoring systems in patients treated with radical prostatectomy. Radiology. 2014;272:446–55.
34. Wiegel T, Bartkowiak D, Bottke D, et al. Adjuvant radiotherapy versus wait-and-see after radical prostatectomy: 10-year follow-up of the ARO 96-02/AUO AP 09/95 trial. Eur Urol. 2014;66:243–50.
35. Wilt TJ, Brawer MK, Jones KM, et al. Radical prostatectomy versus observation for localized prostate cancer. N Engl J Med. 2012;367:203–13.
36. Zietman AL, Bae K, Slater JD, et al. Randomized trial comparing conventional-dose with high-dose conformal radiation therapy in early-stage adenocarcinoma of the prostate: long-term results from proton radiation oncology group/american college of radiology 95–09. J Clin Oncol. 2010;28:1106–11.

The Millenium Patients' Perspective

Louis J. Denis

1 Introduction

In the estimated rates of European cancer incidence and mortality rates in 2012, prostate cancer ranks third in incidence (359,900) but drops to the fifth place in mortality (71.0) in the European Union (EU-27) [1].

This high incidence can be explained by the now-functioning cancer registries in many European countries, the ageing of its populations but primarily by the use of the prostate specific antigen (PSA) test used in population screening programmes. This explains the variation in incidence rates by more than sevenfold (25–193 per 100,000) in contrast to the mortality rates (13–36 per 100,000).

Recent public health policies on population screening of prostate cancer by decreasing the use of the PSA test may lower the incidence but slow an ongoing decrease in overall mortality. Also it is clear that a number of improved treatments, not only in surgery or radiotherapy but also in newly developed drugs, have shown survival benefit for localised, advanced and metastatic disease [2]. This extended survivorship and the ageing of our male citizens will increase rather than decrease the high prevalence (hovering around three million men) in the next decades.

One is ready to believe that modern urology turned prostate cancer from a lethal into a chronic disease. This conviction leads us patients to our ultimate expectation to receive up to date, optimal treatment for all European citizens coupled to an increased quality of life (QoL) and decreased health cost to society.

This philosophy is expressed in the vision and mission of Europa Uomo, the European Prostate Cancer Coalition (Table 1).

This ambitious goal depends mainly on the continuous clinical and basic research results from the professional organisations and the increasing interest in holistic care and advocacy.

Failure to reduce the still substantial mortality of prostate cancer may be due to increased incidence, failure to meet the goals of primary prevention, failure to early diagnosis in a curable stage and failure to improve treatment.

2 Increased Incidence

It is our belief that a better understanding of the natural history and biology of cancer in general and prostate cancer in particular has changed our management of the disease in a dramatic way. Despite the acceptance that prostate cancer has become a high profile disease in the affluent nations of the world and that it presented, before

L.J. Denis
Oncology Centre Antwerp (OCA),
Lange Gasthuisstraat 35-37, 2000 Antwerp, Belgium
e-mail: louis.denis@skynet.be

M. Bolla, H. van Poppel (eds.), *Management of Prostate Cancer*,
DOI 10.1007/978-3-319-42769-0_27

Table 1 Europa Uomo

Vision:	*A future where no man suffers with or dies from prostate cancer*
Mission:	*To achieve better treatment, care and quality of life for all prostate cancer patients across Europe*
	To provide an effective EU-wide voice representing the needs and priorities of National Organisations

the PSA era, mostly in the advanced, metastatic stage where it is incurable we face huge controversies on the value of population screening where we hope to catch the disease when it is curable by surgery or radiotherapy.

Let us start with simple arithmetic. Prostate cancer presents clinically as a common disease after the age of 55 years to reach its zenith around 70 years of age. With the ever-increasing life expectancy of our populations, it is obvious that we are going to find more cancer. But there is more. The clinically asymptomatic early stages of prostate cancer called 'latent carcinoma' of the prostate are found at autopsy in 30 % of the cases in men over 50 to rise to 80 % in the eight decade. This observation was already published by Rich about 80 years ago [3].

These latent tumours were called incidental when discovered at the occasion of prostate surgery and listed as T1 disease in the UICC TNM & US AJCC classification. Historically, no treatment was given to T1a tumours (histologic finding in 5 % or less prostatic tissue removed), while treatment was initiated in T1b tumours where more than 5 % of tumour tissue was identified. See Table 2 [4].

This relaxed attitude changes dramatically with the introduction of the PSA test as a complementary screening test for prostatic cancer next to the classical digital rectal examination (DRE) to detect early prostate cancer.

2.1 The PSA Era

The PSA test heralded correctly as the best cancer marker in solid tumours coupled to the introduction of the painless biopsy gun opened a tsunami of T1c prostate tumours waiting to be cured. The frustrated urologists having faced incurable, metastatic disease as the prime diagnosis for a century followed this simple, clinical axioma with enthusiastic curative treatments including laparoscopic and robot-assisted surgery, improved techniques of radiation from IMF to cyberknife, brachytherapy as well as cryosurgery and high-frequency ultrasound.

This initial enthusiasm slowly decreased and finally met resistance from public health authorities ending sometimes in legislative rules limiting the use of the PSA test. The main downstream effects were seen as massive overtreatment of localised disease and the complications caused by prostatic biopsies and curative treatments.

Is the PSA test saving the lives of thousands of cancer patients or is it the Patient Scaring Antigen leading to impotence and incontinence in the hands of urologists and oncologists. One recent publication stands out as the meanest blow to the use of the PSA test in clinical practice [5].

The PSA story started around 1960. A number of investigators studied prostate proteins, their enzymatic activities and its metabolism. Using electrophoresis to separate proteins in an electric field a number of proteins were described in semen and prostate fluid.

Forensic specialists thought to use the presence of these antigens to confirm cases of rape but the characterised bands later identified as acid phosphatase, prostate-specific antigen and much later prostate-specific membranous antigen (PSA and PSMA) were studied as markers in clinical prostate diseases including prostatitis, benign hyperplasia and cancer.

Table 2 TNM classification, T1 clinically inapparent tumour not palpable or visible by imaging

T1a	Tumour incidental histological finding in 5 % or less of tissue resected
T1b	Tumour incidental histological finding in more than 5 % of tissue resected
T1c	Tumour identified by needle biopsy (e.g. because of elevated prostate-specific antigen (PSA) level)

Indeed, the PSA test based on the immunologic properties of the protein took off, after this first decade of confusion, as the rising star in cancer of the prostate evaluation and diagnosis. In the first decade, we could identify 58 papers in English, in the second decade from 1990 to 2000 some 2262 articles and from 2000 till now more than 20,000 articles.

Equimolarity, measuring both free and complexed PSA in the serum with the identified 83 PSA antibodies finally resulted in a more or less exact measurement for clinical use. This is the reason that any follow-up or clinical use should be measured with the same methodology.

PSA test results depend on the measuring methodology and biological variations in relation to our daily activities.

The most important weakness is that PSA is not specific for cancer but specific for prostate diseases. This lack of specificity for cancer has the advantage that the PSA test is useful in prostatitis and benign hyperplasia where elevated levels correlate with the infectious process or the volume of the functional gland. There is no question in our clinical work that a diagnosis of prostate disease should be examined by a DRE and a PSA test.

Unfortunately, an elevated PSA test is frequently wrongly believed to be cancer, causing anxiety in the patient and the general practitioner, leading to unnecessary biopsies and overtreatment.

To remember all trauma to the prostate (digital examination, biopsy, bicycling and even sex) may result in elevated levels. This is NO diagnosis of cancer and any PSA test needs the interpretation as a possible risk of having prostate cancer. We advise to control an elevated PSA test after 6 weeks and compare the controls after an antibiotic treatment for infection or the congestion of the prostate when lower urinary tract symptoms are present or after a few days without bicycle racing or sex. The human prostate is not made out of plastic and can be congested just as any other organ.

The actual status of the PSA test as a tumour marker is evident after removing the prostate (radical prostatectomy). Here one expects 0 or <0.2 ng/ml. A decline is also noted after successful radiotherapy and PSA testing is useful in the follow-up of cancer treatment and/or relapse after treatment.

The cut-off value used to define sensitivity and specificity is set empirically (the common cut-off level of 4 ng/ml was casted in a huge retrospective study). This screening test will result in false positive (75 % for PSA) or false negative (15 % for PSA).

The problem in the use of the PSA test is not the test result itself but the interpretation in a clinical situation where it is used as an excuse for repeated, excessive blind biopsies and subsequent overtreatment.

To summarise the clinical usefulness of the PSA test:

1. PSA is a good tumour marker but not ideal due to limitations in sensitivity and specificity.
2. The clinical value is clear in treating prostatic diseases but controversial in population screening for prostate cancer.
3. Improvements are possible by combining free and complexed PSA (PSA is a protease destroying proteins and neutralised by antichymotrypsine in the serum).
4. The laboratory results are variable as well as the biological variation (the latter up to 20 %).
5. Part of the PSA is occult in the serum gobbled up by macroglobulines.
6. All derivations or measurements carry some lack of sensitivity for cancer.

We can conclude that the PSA test is useful in our clinical work if correctly interpreted in particular situations.

The message of this contribution is that the PSA test, of use in prostate diseases and not only for prostate cancer, is an excellent biomarker of these diseases but its interpretation requires knowledge of the natural (treated) history of the same diseases.

We are confident that the PSA test will regain its status as a useful biomarker in prostatic diseases if we are patient and adhere to evidence-based medicine and continue dedicated clinical and basic research to this diagnostic problem where individualised management and personalised care will determine future policies.

There is a place for great expectations in new, molecular biomarkers, improved imaging in ultrasound and multiparametric magnetic resonance imaging (MRI) to complement the DRE/PSA combination as the first step to suspect a possible localised prostate cancer.

A most important multidisciplinary success has been the ISUP 2014 grade groups of prostate cancer merging the Gleason scores and the WHO grading in five distinct WHO 2016 grade groups. Here Gleason score 3 + 3 = 6 becomes grade I recognised as a quiet, resting cancer that could be observed rather than treated [6].

The PSA test is vital to follow-up and treatment as it remains the top marker for successful curative surgery and it fills the niche in the definition of low, intermediate- and high-risk disease described in other chapters of this book.

2.2 Conclusion

Increased incidence caused by the ageing of our populations will bring more cancer deaths limited by the competitive mortality of co-morbidity. Increased incidence by the correct use of the PSA test can save lives by improved methodology of mass and/or personalised screening for prostate cancer.

3 Failure to Meet the Goals of Primary Prevention

Epidemiology studies of these latent (incidental, indolent occult), small T1 tumours revealed that they were found in all races from both Eastern and Western countries and should be considered as an early clinical stage, following premalignant lesions as prostate epithelial neoplasia (PIN), possibly leading to a full blown cancer phenotype in about 1 % of the cases.

It is believed that this process may take years before it is detectable by our actual technology and that it will take another 15–20 years for the clinical cancers to die specifically from metastatic dissemination or complications of the cancer.

Furthermore, the available data indicate that this cancer progression is observed much less in the Oriental males than in his Western counterpart. This difference disappears in the second generation of Oriental males after immigration to the West [8]. This observation possible suggest a promoting factor in the Western countries or a restraining influence in the East drawing our attention to the influence of environmental or dietary factors leading to the opportunity of proactive primary prevention.

Massive programmes to contain the burden of cancer have been launched in Europe and the USA even including a US National Prostate Cancer Program during the last decades of the previous century. These efforts led to major changes in diagnosis (the PSA test) and treatment (the cult of the randomised clinical trials, active surveillance, minimal endocrine treatment and chemotherapy) and a number of initiatives in lifestyle and nutrition [7]. Despite the explosive impact of the development of the genomics in this millennium, it is still felt that at least 50 % of all cancer is avoidable through lifestyle changes focusing on tobacco and alcohol, vaccinations or treatment of chronic infections. Cancer is a multicausal disease. This long list contains hereditary (5 %), hormonal (30 %), infection (10 %), physical Rx/UV (5 %), tobacco (30 %) and nutrition (20 %) [9].

Unfortunately, the outcomes in prostate cancer are restricted to circumstantial evidence in most, if not all, nutritional research. It is clear that in the myriad of recommendations there is no magic bullet to prevent prostate or any other cancer. There is no scientific proof that any single product prevents cancer although these over the counter (OTC) or complementary (CAM) products represent a multibillion market in Europe.

The soundest advice is found in the European Cancer Code. The advice is to eat more vegetables and fruits and eat moderate amounts of red meat. It is more practical to follow a Mediterranean (tomatoes) or Oriental diet (tofu) according to personal taste. Recent nutritional advises are published (British Eatwell Guide and the Dutch Schijf van Vijf). Less meat and more vegetables/fruits remain on the list. No surprise that the patients always remember the 'true' benefit of red wine in moderate amounts.

The emphasis has shifted towards the obesity of our citizens in affluent countries and the absolute need for physical exercise that is consensually accepted as a keystone to extended life expectancy and increased QoL. Our Feel+ programme devised by Prof. Tombal became a European favourite among prostate cancer patients [10].

4 Failure to Detect Prostate Cancer in a Curable Stage

If we cannot prevent prostate cancer let us at least try to find it when the cancer is still localised to the prostate which up till now remains the only curable stage of the disease. Screening for prostate cancer based on a DRE, a PSA test and a transrectal ultrasound (TRUS) examination looks easy but there is nothing easy about screening for cancer [11].

Prostate cancer screening remains controversial despite evidence from the European Randomised Study of Screening for Prostate Cancer (ERSPC) showing at least a 20% reduction in prostate cancer mortality after 9 years of follow-up [12]. We started this project with enthusiasm in 1991 looking for early cancer in patients between 55 and 74 years by checking the DRE (hard zones), the PSA test (10 ng/ml) and TRUS. In the following years, we dropped first TRUS (early technology), DRE (poor results), decreased the PSA value from 10 ng/ml to 4 and then 3 ng/ml to detect most cancers by transrectal TRUS-guided biopsy with the lowest number of biopsies and false positive diagnosis as well as lowering the age to 69 years. This randomised study reached 13 years of follow-up on 162,388 men in eight European countries. We were the first to report on the overdetection and subsequent overtreatment in screened prostate cancer, the limitations of the PSA test and harms done by unnecessary biopsy and treatment. However, the obtained, objective results are too promising to stop looking for early diagnosis, but we do advise to limit population screening until the overtreatment is stopped and streamlined needs of methodology introduced. The optimal balance is still unclear but improvement will come by regulated, multivariate risk-based programmes focused on high risk cancer.

5 Failure to Improve Treatment to Cure All

Major progress has been reached in the primary local treatment of prostate cancer by high-tech improvements in surgery and radiation treatment.

However the complications following prostatectomy or curative irradiation remain important enough, mainly incontinence and impotence, to reserve even the most minimal treatment to life-saving indications where QoL and cost-efficiency are accounted in a joint patient doctor decision.

Three major trends are noted in the new millennium. First the needed respect for the co-morbidity of the patient and the biologic low-risk tumours, the restrictions in endocrine treatment and last but not least the treatment of castrate (mostly metastatic)-resistant disease (mCRPC).

Our mantra remains treat the patient and then his cancer.

5.1 First the Patient Before His Cancer

The ERSPC study showed a decrease of mortality in the screened patients concomitant to a clear shift in the diagnosis to localised disease. Unfortunately, it became clear that overtreatment in these small early cancers with low-risk characteristics overtreatment was observed in about 40 % of treated cases. The famous one liner of pussycats and tigers! The confusion on the best choice of treatment was best quoted by Whitmore (a world class urologists who died of prostate cancer) in 1994: 'Appropriate treatment implies that therapy be applied neither to those patients for whom it is unnecessary nor to those for whom it will prove ineffective. Furthermore, the therapy should be that which will most assuredly permit the individual a qualitatively and quantitatively normal life. It need not necessarily involve an effort at cancer cure!'

In response to this dilemma two types of conservative 'non'-treatment were introduced in the clinic. The first one, Watchful Waiting (WW), is widely accepted since decades. It advises to withhold treatment from patients with a limited life expectancy of <10 years by biological age or by important co-morbidity. Here treatment is based on symptoms. Of course it follows the logic that you don't look for the diagnosis of prostate cancer in these patients.

This approach is completely different from withholding invasive treatment in fit individuals of any age when a low-risk, low-volume prostate cancer is diagnosed. This 'non-'treatment is called Active Surveillance (AS). After two decades of debate, the rationale of AS is now widely accepted and listed in most or all guidelines on treatment involving about half of the patients diagnosed with prostate cancer driven by the PSA test or lower urinary tract symptoms (LUTS) caused by the common benign hyperplasia (BPH). A problem remains the rationale and discipline of the evaluation of these patients or clinical controls to suggest a switch to active treatment [13].

There is sometimes a confusion between these two options although AS patients can move to WW within the years of the follow-up controls.

The two forms are compared in Table 3.

Table 3 Active surveillance vs. watchful waiting

Active surveillance	Watchful waiting
Fit patient	Co-morbidity/age
Low-risk cancer	Any cancer
PSA evolution define treatment (+ biopsies)	Symptoms define treatment
Option: cure	Option: palliation

Active Surveillance (AS) and Watchful Waiting (WW) are treatments based on the knowledge of the natural history of prostate cancer

5.2 Endocrine (Hormonal) Treatment

Not less than two Nobel prizes were awarded in the last half of the previous century for research in the endocrine management of prostate cancer (C. Huggins and A. Schally). Still from the very start of endocrine treatment after World War II it was clear that endocrine treatment (the new term is androgen deprivation treatment (ADT)) does not cure prostate cancer, is the cause of a number of serious side-effects and finally contributes to enhanced cardio-vascular complications and death. Already Nesbit and Plumb [14] published a follow-up on 795 patients prior to the endocrine era followed for up to 54 months. In comparing later series among patients with metastatic disease it shows that endocrine treatment has a beneficial influence on survival in advanced metastatic cases. This publication compares to the EORTC-study, published 50 years later, that patients with a baseline PSA >50 ng/ml and/or a PSDT (<12 months) where at increased risk to die from prostate cancer and might have benefited from immediate ADT [15].

Next to lifestyle changes heart healthy supplements intended to lessen the side-effects of ADT require extra attention from their treating physician [16].

Intermittent androgen deprivation has been widely tested to diminish the toxicity of ADT and has gained acceptance in the urological practice [17].

So far there is a trend to delay or avoid ADT (especially surgical or medical castration) in the long-term treatment of prostate cancer.

Two indications remain clear:

1. Any prostate cancer with symptomatic disease be it locally advanced or metastatic.
2. In patients selected for curative radiotherapy, a combination with a short or long-term ADT is advisable.

5.3 Conclusion

Deciding on an ADT is a serious decision that merits prospective patient information and has to be seen in the context of individual holistic treatment and care.

6 The Treatment of mCRPC

ADT was originally limited to castration or oestrogen treatment later replaced by the reversible medical castration by luteotrope hormone releasing hormone agonists (LRHR A) or antagonist supplement treatment with anti-androgens, occupying the androgen receptor, is called CAB or MAB (complete or maximal androgen blockade).

Most cancers show some effect on progression although sometimes the effect is limited to a partial decrease in serum PSA levels. This effect can be short-lived or impressive for long periods of time, but ultimately the effect wears off and then we are faced with so-called castration-resistant disease.

Serum testosterone (T) at castrate levels has to be confirmed for a correct diagnosis.

Here we deal with a patient with locally advanced and/or metastatic disease following the final, lethal pathway of the cancer. Recent interest and new technology aims for radical, local therapy for oligo-metastatic disease by metastasis-directed therapy (MDT).

On further progression after this localised effort or in a patient with multiple metastatic disease, resistant to hormonal treatment, we enter a phase of personalised management to the patient and his tumour. Here the endpoint of treatment is not mere overall or prostate cancer-specific survival but progression-free survival and QoL are the attainable targets of treatment. Classic management aims to palliate pain, prevent clinically significant skeletal related events and palliative care. New management aims to study the efficiency of new drugs as abiraterone and enzalutamide, radium-223 as well as chemotherapy with docetaxel/cabazitaxel already known to boost survival in hormone sensitive metastatic prostate cancer together with hormonal treatment.

All these forms of treatment have their own specific indications making outcomes comparisons difficult to impossible.

Several randomised trials are ongoing involving active surveillance, radiation and surgery in the hope to clarify some choices for the doctor and patient. At this moment in time the outcomes for the patient not only in terms of specific cancer survival but especially in measuring health-related quality of life (HRQOL) as well as cost-efficacy are unknown as the many subclassifications on cancer stage, grade and biological aggression leave room for debate.

We expect the treating physician to inform the patient on all treatments currently available and the expected side effects. Unfortunately, physicians quote the best outcomes published in the literature while the patients have unrealistic expectations based on statistical counselling that does not reflect on the individual. Consulting the Internet without guidance is a prescription for misled confusion but even professional journals print questionable P-results and omit relative risk and odds ratios on treatment results. Worse the perception of the patients especially on psychosocial and wellness problems are not fully evaluated in our culture of cancer-centered treatment rather than patient-centered care. It must be clear that a 50-year-old prostate cancer patient has different care needs as compared to the elderly cancer patients. As Harry Belafonte sings on the birds and the bees, 'now that I am ninety three I don't care a damn you see'.

The complexity of the treatment introduces the concept of prostate cancer units (PCU) of excellence as centres with a critical patient load and multifunctional collaboration and having the expertise of innovative health technology available to improve outcomes [18]. We do agree on these advantages while we plead for keeping track of the emotional and social patient needs by interactive communication and continuous information between the intra- (hospital) and extramural (community medicine) to assist all patients in all needs.

We believe that this development will provide better outcomes for scientific evaluation, quality of care control, and general, holistic patient care.

We will not discuss the merits for better outcomes by evidence-based research as it is clear from the recent publications that chemo, endocrine and immunological treatments showed life extending and QOL results in a number of trials. We live in hope to see not only the mortality of PCa reduced but as important the life of the patients enhanced with quality and hope for long-term survival in acceptable, functional health.

7 Europa Uomo: The European Prostate Coalition

We have witnessed a continuation of improvement in all aspects of optimal medical management centring on the disease. Most of these improvements were steps in a chronic interaction between clinical research and best practice. It remains evident that the prime stakeholders of clinical progress remain the patients aspiring for cure, control of the disease, and enhanced quality of life.

There is little that patient groups can do in this progress except to plead for research support, access and service of best quality practice, tailored treatment for the individual patient, and overcome the inequalities in treatment and care in Europe.

However, we feel strongly that our advocacy role is focused on holistic patient care involving a treatment policy on the patient first and then on his disease involving quality of life and wellness in psycho-social and financial domains. We enjoy a number of rights in some European nations which we would like to balance with patient obligations. The latter directed towards a fair distribution of scarce health funds, facilitation of translational research, and support of existing, functional partnerships with many professional and patient societies.

Europa Uomo, established in 2004, advocates patient-centred management that we expressed in a manifesto presented in Table 4.

7.1 Europa Uomo Management

The management of Europa Uomo is assigned to a seven man Board, aided by a number of ex-officio officers whose knowledge and expertise are of great help in the activities of the Board, which must report back to the annual assembly where every project or initiative is duly approved and later reported on its successful conclusion.

The Board is composed by a chairman, two vice-chairmen, a treasurer, a secretary and two members. The office and secretariat is located in

Table 4 Manifesto Europa Uomo

1.	To find ways and means to promote quality of life for prostate cancer patients and their families
2.	To promote the dissemination and exchange of evidence-based as well as factual and up-to-date information on prostate cancer
3.	To promote prostate awareness and appropriate diagnosis and prognosis
4.	To emphasise the need for appropriate early detection
5.	To campaign for provision of and access to optimum treatment
6.	To ensure quality, supportive care throughout and after treatment
7.	To promote multiprofessional quality care and appropriate medical infrastructure
8.	To acknowledge good clinical practice and promote its development
9.	To ensure that all men fully understand any proposed treatment options, including entry into clinical trials and their right to a second opinion
10.	To promote the advancement of prostate cancer research

Antwerp, Belgium where there is a permanent coordination with the Board of a Newsletter, a Website and social media to follow.

Membership is restricted to patient organisations who are responsible in their respective countries (23 in 2015) to organize events to sensitize the general public on prostate cancer and raise, if needed, the standards in quality treatment and care to the European standard.

Europa Uomo aspires for representation and collaboration with the most important professional bodies as EAU and ESO, and patient organisations as ECPC and EAPM. It is also represented in European Institutes as EMA and Cancer organisations as ECCO, ESMO, ESTRO, ESSO, etc.

The annual activities are focused on a General Assembly, Masterclass sessions and a traditional European Prostate Awareness Day in the European Parliament.

The Coalition is an independent, international, non-profit association of patient-led prostate cancer support groups. It was founded by the European School of Oncology (ESO) and the Oncologic Centre Antwerp (OCA) as well as sponsored by the EAU and international Companies [19].

After our first years we launched a proactive prostate cancer call out to the European Parliament (Table 5).

We are far from reaching our mission in healthcare but we are convinced that transparency of our healthcare system and policies will improve patient-related outcomes as well as professional satisfaction as well-being. A close collaboration with our general practitioners and specialists in a multidisciplinary setting will open frontiers and better perspective in a new paradigm of prostate cancer treatment and care.

Table 5 Prostate cancer proactive call out

Governments to be aware of prostate diseases
Governments to support coordinated research on biomarkers, genomics
Tailored individualised treatment and personalised care to patients
Standards of management and patient outcomes following good clinical practice
Creation of centers of excellence (prostate cancer units) to deliver optimal treatment and care
Partnership building to receive updated, objective guidelines and share social needs to identify common action and overcome inequality in medical treatment and holistic care

We would like to conclude with the Prostate Cancer Patients' Etiquette:

- Every patient is not just a non-identity object for treatments, trials or tests.
- Every patient should be considered as a valuable human being to be reintegrated in society.
- When a patient does not recognize his needs for understanding his disease, professionals have to give guiding council.
- Any question by a patient is not irrelevant to him even if not related to his disease.
- Patients should respect professionals' expertise and follow given orders.

Suaviter in modo, fortiter in re.

References

1. Ferlay J, Steliarov-Foucher E, et al. Cancer incidence and mortality patterns in Europe: estimates for 40 countries in 2012. Eur J Cancer. 2013;49:1374–403.
2. Bolla M, Van Poppel H. Management of prostate cancer. Berlin: Springer; 2016: in press.
3. Rich AR. On frequency of occurrence of occult carcinoma of the prostate. J Urol. 1935;33:215–23.
4. UICC. TNM classification of malignant tumours. 7th ed. New York: Wiley-Blackwell; 2016. ISBN 978-1-4443-3241-4.
5. Richard J. Ablin with professional writer Roland Rana. The great prostate hoax. New York: Palgrave McMillan; 2014. ISBN 9781137278746.
6. Epstein JI, Zelefsky MJ, et al. A contemporary prostate cancer grading system: a validated alternative to the Gleason score. Eur Urol. 2016;69:428–35.
7. Renehan AG, Soerjomataram I, et al. Implementing cancer prevention in Europe. Eur J Cancer. 2010;46(14):2523–4.
8. Griffiths K, Adlerkrenz H, et al. Nutrition and cancer. Oxford: Printek Bilbao; 1996. ISBN: 1-899-066-349.
9. Khayat D. Prévenir le cancer, ça depend aussi de vous. Paris: Odile Jacon; 2014. ISBN 978-2-7381-2924-6.
10. Bourke L, Smith D, et al. Exercise for men with prostate cancer: a systematic review and meta-analysis. Eur Urol. 2016;69(4):693–703.
11. Welch HG. Should I be tested for cancer? Maybe not and here's why. Berkeley: Regents of the University of California. 2004. ISBN 0-520-23976-8.

12. Schröder FH, Hugosson J, et al. Screening and prostate-cancer mortality in a randomized European study. N Engl J Med. 2009;360(3):1320–8.
13. Newcomb LF, Thompson IM, et al. Outcomes of active surveillance for clinically localized prostate cancer in the prospective, multi-institutional Canary PASS cohort. J Urol. 2016;195:313–20.
14. Nesbit RM, Plumb RT. Prostatic carcinoma. A follow-up on 795 patients treated prior to the endocrine era and a comparison of survival rates between these and patients treated by endocrine therapy. Presented at the 3rd annual meeting of the Central Surgical Association, Chicago, 1946.
15. Studer UE, Colette L, et al. Using PSA to guide timing of androgen deprivation in patients with T0-4 N0-2 M0 prostate cancer not suitable for local curative treatment (EORTC 30891). Eur Urol. 2008;53:941–9.
16. Moyad MA, Roack M. Promoting wellness for patients on androgen deprivation therapy: why using numerous drugs for drug side effects should not be first-line treatment. Urol Clin North Am. 2011;38:303–12.
17. Hussain M, Tangen C, et al. Evaluating intermittent androgen-deprivation therapy phase III clinical trials: the devil is in the details. J Clin Oncol. 2016;34(3):280–5.
18. Valdagni R, Albers P, et al. The requirements of a specialist Prostate Cancer Unit: a discussion paper from the European School of Oncology. Eur J Cancer. 2011;47(1):1–7.
19. Hudson T, Denis L. Europa Uomo, the European Prostate Cancer Coalition. In: Ramon J, Denis L, editors. Recent results in cancer research. Berlin: Springer; 2006.

Printed by Printforce, the Netherlands